# Macleod's
## Clinical Examination

## John Macleod (1915–2006)

John Macleod was appointed consultant physician at the Western General Hospital, Edinburgh, in 1950. He had major interests in rheumatology and medical education. Medical students who attended his clinical teaching sessions remember him as an inspirational teacher with the ability to present complex problems with great clarity. He was invariably courteous to his patients and students alike. He had an uncanny knack of involving all students equally in clinical discussions and used praise rather than criticism. He paid great attention to the value of history taking and, from this, expected students to identify what particular aspects of the physical examination should help to narrow the diagnostic options.

His consultant colleagues at the Western welcomed the opportunity of contributing when he suggested writing a textbook on clinical examination. The book was first published in 1964, and John Macleod edited seven editions. With characteristic modesty he was very embarrassed when the eighth edition was renamed *Macleod's Clinical Examination*. This, however, was a small way of recognising his enormous contribution to medical education.

He possessed the essential quality of a successful editor – the skill of changing disparate contributions from individual contributors into a uniform style and format without causing offence; everybody accepted his authority. He avoided being dogmatic or condescending. He was generous in teaching others his editorial skills, and these attributes were recognised when he was invited to edit *Davidson's Principles and Practice of Medicine*.

# Macleod's

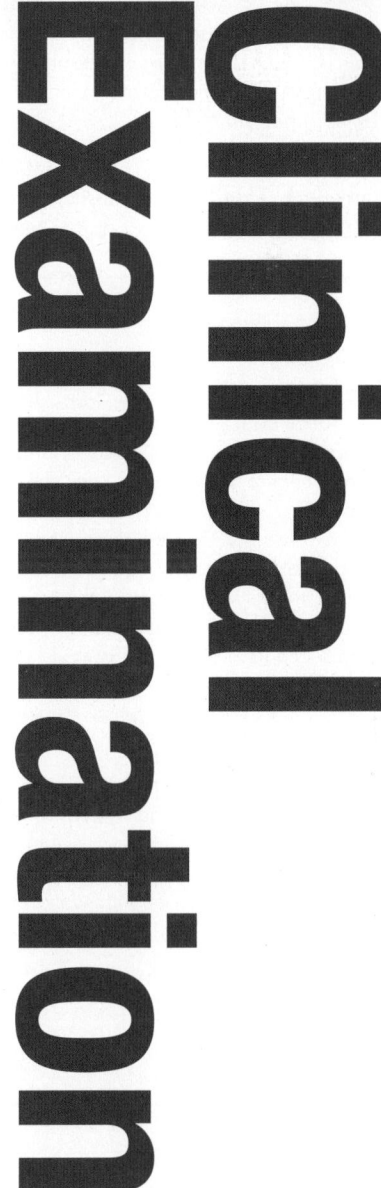

## Clinical Examination

## 15th Edition

Edited by

**Anna R Dover**
MB ChB, PhD, FRCP, SFHEA

Consultant in Diabetes, Endocrinology and General Medicine,
Edinburgh Centre for Endocrinology and Diabetes,
Royal Infirmary of Edinburgh; Honorary Senior Clinical Lecturer,
University of Edinburgh, UK

**J Alastair Innes**
MB ChB, PhD, FRCPE

Consultant Physician (retired), Respiratory Unit,
Western General Hospital, Edinburgh;
Honorary Reader in Respiratory Medicine,
University of Edinburgh, UK

**Karen Fairhurst**
MB BS, PhD

Senior Lecturer, Centre for Population Health Sciences,
University of Edinburgh, UK

Illustrations by Robert Britton, Ethan Danielson
and Wendy Beth Jackelow

ELSEVIER

London   New York   Oxford   Philadelphia   St Louis   Sydney   2024

---

**Notice**

Practitioners and researchers must always rely on their own experience and knowledge in evaluating and using any information, methods, compounds or experiments described herein. Because of rapid advances in the medical sciences, in particular, independent verification of diagnoses and drug dosages should be made. To the fullest extent of the law, no responsibility is assumed by Elsevier, authors, editors or contributors for any injury and/or damage to persons or property as a matter of products liability, negligence or otherwise, or from any use or operation of any methods, products, instructions, or ideas contained in the material herein.

---

*Publisher:* Jeremy Bowes
*Content Development Specialist:* Laura Fisher
*Project Manager:* Thoufiq Mohammed
*Design:* Miles Hitchen
*Graphics Coordinator:* Akshaya Mohan
*Marketing Manager:* Deborah Watkins

Printed in India
Last digit is the print number: 9 8 7 6 5 4 3 2 1

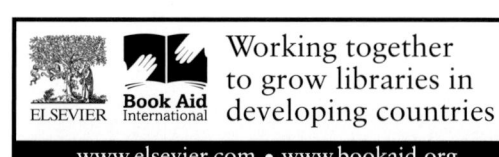

# Contents

Preface     vii

Acknowledgements     ix

How to make the most of this book and associated multimedia     xi

Clinical examination videos     xiii

Contributors     xv

**SECTION 1     PRINCIPLES OF CLINICAL HISTORY AND EXAMINATION     1**

1. **Managing clinical encounters with patients**     3
   Karen Fairhurst, J Alastair Innes, Anna R Dover

2. **General aspects of history taking**     9
   J Alastair Innes, Anna R Dover, Karen Fairhurst

3. **General aspects of examination**     21
   Anna R Dover, Karen Fairhurst, J Alastair Innes

**SECTION 2     SYSTEM-BASED EXAMINATION     41**

4. **The cardiovascular system**     43
   Alan G Japp, Jehangir N Din, Jennifer MJ Robson

5. **The respiratory system**     83
   J Alastair Innes, Peter T Reid

6. **The gastrointestinal system**     105
   John Plevris, Rowan Parks

7. **The nervous system**     133
   Richard Davenport, Hadi Manji

8. **The visual system**     169
   Shyamanga Borooah, Naing Latt Tint

9. **The ear, nose and throat**     193
Iain Hathorn

10. **The endocrine system**     219
Anna R Dover, Nicola Zammitt

11. **The reproductive system**     239
Christina Yip, Colin Duncan, Kirsty Dundas, Alexander Laird

12. **The renal system**     271
Neeraj Dhaun (*Bean*), David Kluth

13. **The musculoskeletal system**     287
Jane Gibson, Phil Walmsley

14. **The skin, hair and nails**     325
Michael J Tidman, Alice SM Tidman

**SECTION 3    APPLYING HISTORY AND EXAMINATION SKILLS IN SPECIFIC SITUATIONS    339**

15. **Babies and children**     341
Ben Stenson, Steve Cunningham

16. **Patients with mental illness and learning disability**     367
Stephen Potts

17. **The frail patient**     379
Andrew Elder, Elizabeth MacDonald

18. **The deteriorating patient**     393
Anna R Dover, Rosaleen Baruah

19. **The dying patient**     405
Kirsty Boyd, Nazir Lone

**SECTION 4    PUTTING HISTORY AND EXAMINATION SKILLS TO USE    413**

20. **Reaching and communicating a diagnosis**     415
Karen Fairhurst, Anna R Dover, J Alastair Innes

21. **Adapting skills for practice**     423
J Alastair Innes, Karen Fairhurst, Anna R Dover

22. **Preparing for assessment**     427
Anna R Dover, J Alastair Innes, Karen Fairhurst

**Index**     435

# Preface

Despite the wealth of diagnostic tools available to the modern clinician, the acquisition of information by direct interaction with the patient through history taking and clinical examination remains the bedrock of clinical practice. An expertly performed history and examination of a patient allow the clinician to reach a differential diagnosis whilst ensuring the patient and their concerns remain central to the process, and avoids potential harm from unnecessary or unjustified tests.

This book aims to assist clinicians in developing the consultation skills required to elicit a clear history and the practical examination skills needed to detect clinical signs of disease. Where possible, the physical basis of clinical signs is explained to aid understanding. Formulation of a differential diagnosis from the information gained is introduced, and the logical initial investigations are included for each system. *Macleod's Clinical Examination* is designed to be used in conjunction with more detailed texts on pathophysiology, differential diagnosis and clinical medicine. It is closely integrated with *Davidson's Principles and Practice of Medicine* and is best read in conjunction with that text.

In this edition, the contents have been updated and diversified by a team of existing and new authors, with the aim of creating an accessible and user-friendly text relevant to clinical practice in the 21st century.

Section 1 addresses the general principles of good interaction with patients, from the basics of taking a history and examining, to the use of pattern recognition to identify spot diagnoses. Section 2 deals with symptoms and signs in specific systems and Section 3 illustrates the application of these skills to specific clinical situations. Section 4 covers the formulation of a diagnosis, the tailored adaptation of clinical skills for everyday practice and preparation for assessments of these skills.

We hope that if young clinicians are encouraged to adopt and adapt these history and examination skills, not only will they serve their patients well as diagnosticians, but also they will continue to develop clinical examination techniques and a better understanding of their mechanisms and diagnostic use.

The 15th edition of *Macleod's Clinical Examination* is accompanied by an expanded set of clinical videos, including eight entirely new topics, which are available in the Elsevier eBooks+ library.

ARD, JAI, KF
Edinburgh, 2023

# Acknowledgements

The editors would like to acknowledge the many distinguished previous editors whose guiding hands have crafted *Macleod's Clinical Examination* over the years into the key resource it has become for clinicians across the globe. Working to update and enhance this book, we are constantly aware of, and grateful for, this unique heritage of clinical skills teaching.

The editors also offer grateful thanks for the input of all previous editions' contributors, without whom this new edition would not have been possible. In particular, we are indebted to those former authors who step down with the arrival of this 15th edition: Anthony Bateman, Ivan Brenkel, Gareth Clegg, Nick Mills, Janet Skinner, James Tiernan and Oliver Young.

We are thankful to the following clinicians from varied professional groups who undertook detailed reviews of the 14th edition and provided us with a wealth of ideas to implement in this new edition: Sunil Bhandari, Iain Hathorn, Ian Lee, Caroline Nicholson, Nathan Oliver and Claire Robertson. Thanks also to the many other students and educators who have provided invaluable feedback on Macleod's via the Student Consult registrant's survey.

Finally, we express our gratitude to the following individuals who helped to create the videos supporting the book. Some created the original videos, others helped us recently to create a series of new videos to augment the range of techniques covered in this particular edition: Omar Ali, Abby Cooke, Eleanor Davidson, Ahmed Eissa, Anas Gomati, Rosemary Hackney, Iain Hennessey, Shiying Hey, Sadiq Jeeyavudeen, Alan Japp, Rachael Lamb, Nick Morley, Dan Pugh, Deepa Rangar, Amy Robb, Colin Robertson, Jenni Wales, Ben Waterson, and the Medical Photography Service, NHS Lothian.

# How to make the most of this book and associated multimedia

This book describes the principles of managing encounters with patients in a systematic and thorough way. In Sections 2 and 3, each of the systems chapters is laid out in the same order:

- Introduction: anatomy and physiology.
- The history: common presenting symptoms, what questions to ask and how to follow them up.
- The physical examination: what and how to examine.
- Investigations: how to select the most relevant and informative initial tests, and how these clarify the diagnosis.
- Objective Structured Clinical Examination (OSCE) examples: a couple of short clinical scenarios included to illustrate the type of problems students may meet in an OSCE assessment of this system.

- Integrated examination sequence: a structured list of steps to be followed when examining the system, intended as a prompt and revision aid.

## Examination sequences

Throughout the book there are outlines of techniques that you should follow when examining a patient. These are identified with a red 'Examination sequence' heading. The bullet-point list provides the exact order in which to undertake the examination. To help your understanding of how to perform these techniques, many of the examination sequences are presented in accompanying videos.

# ▶ Clinical examination videos

Included with your purchase are clinical examination videos, custom-made to accompany this textbook. Filmed with hands-on guidance from the author team, and narrated by experts, these videos offer you the chance to watch specialist doctors performing many of the examination routines described in the book. By helping you to memorise the essential examination steps required for each major system and by demonstrating the proper clinical technique, these videos should act as an important bridge between textbook learning and bedside teaching. The videos will be available for you to view time and again as your clinical skills develop and will prove invaluable as you prepare for your clinical OSCE examinations.

Each examination routine has a detailed explanatory narrative, but for maximum benefit, view the videos in conjunction with the book. See the inside front cover for your access instructions.

## Key points in examinations: photo galleries

Many of the examination sequences are included as photo galleries, illustrating with captions the key stages of the examination routine. These will act as a useful reminder of the main points of each sequence. See the inside front cover for your access instructions.

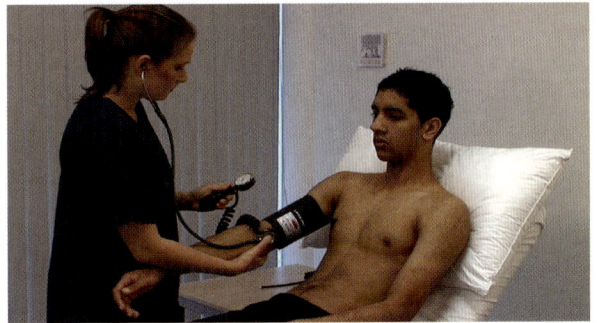

## Video contents

- Video 1: Assessment of fluid balance
- VIdeo 2: Examination of the respiratory system
- Video 3: The cardiovascular system
- Video 4: Measurement of blood pressure
- Video 5: Examination of the peripheral vascular system and diabetic foot
- Video 6: Examination of the gastrointestinal system
- Video 7: Examining for meningeal irritation
- Video 8: Examination of speech
- Video 9: Examination of the trigeminal (V) nerve
- Video 10: Examination of the facial (VII) nerve
- Video 11: Examination of the glossopharyngeal (IX), vagus (X), accessory (XI) and hypoglossal (XII) nerves

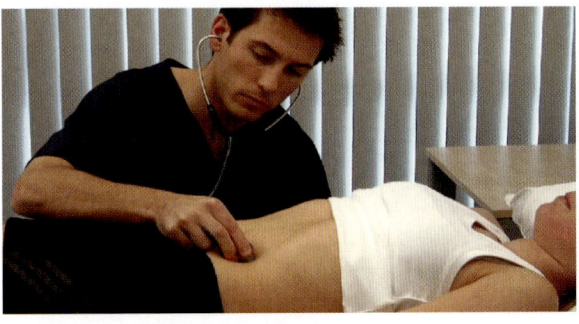

- Video 12: Examination of the motor system of the upper limbs
- Video 13: Examination of the motor system of the lower limbs
- Video 14: Examination of the sensory system of the upper limbs
- Video 15: Examination of the sensory system of the lower limbs
- Video 16: Examination of the motor and sensory systems of the hand
- Video 17: Examination of the optic (II), oculomotor (III), trochlear (IV) and abducens (VI) nerves
- Video 18: Examination of the ear
- Video 19: Examination of the vestibulocochlear (VIII) nerve
- Video 20: Examination of the neck
- Video 21: Examination of the thyroid gland
- Video 22: Gynaecological examination
- Video 23: Obstetric examination
- Video 24: GALS examination
- Video 25: Examination of the cervical spine
- Video 26: Examination of the thoracic and lumbar spine
- Video 27: Examination of the hand and wrist
- Video 28: Examination of the shoulder
- Video 29: Examination of the hip
- Video 30: Examination of the knee
- Video 31: Examination of the ankle and foot
- Video 32: Timed Up and Go

# Contributors

**Rosaleen Baruah MB ChB, FRCPE, FFICM, LL.M**
Consultant in Critical Care and Anaesthesia and Honorary
Clinical Senior Lecturer
Dept of Anaesthesia, Critical Care and Pain Medicine
University of Edinburgh and NHS Lothian
Edinburgh, UK

**Shyamanga Borooah MB BS, PhD, MRCP, MRCSE, FRCOpth**
Assistant Professor
Department of Ophthalmology
University of California San Diego
La Jolla, USA

**Kirsty Boyd MB ChB, PhD, MMedSci, FRCPE**
Reader in Palliative Care
Usher Institute
University of Edinburgh
Edinburgh, UK

**Steve Cunningham MB ChB, PhD**
Professor of Paediatric Respiratory Medicine
Child Life and Health, Centre for Inflammation Research,
University of Edinburgh
Edinburgh, UK

**Richard Davenport BM BS, DM**
Consultant Neurologist
Department of Clinical Neurosciences
University of Edinburgh
Edinburgh, UK

**Anna R Dover MB ChB, PhD, FRCP, SFHEA**
Consultant Physician and Honorary Senior Clinical Lecturer
Edinburgh Centre for Endocrinology and Diabetes
Royal Infirmary of Edinburgh
Edinburgh, UK

**Neeraj Dhaun (*Bean*) MB ChB, PhD**
Senior Clinical Lecturer & Honorary Consultant Nephrologist
Centre for Cardiovascular Science
University of Edinburgh
Edinburgh, UK

**Jehangir N Din MB ChB, MD, FRCP**
Consultant Cardiologist
Cardiology
University Hospitals Dorset
Bournemouth, UK

**Colin Duncan MB ChB, MD, FRCOG**
Professor of Reproductive Medicine and Science
MRC Centre for Reproductive Health
The University of Edinburgh
Edinburgh, UK

**Kirsty Dundas MB ChB, DCH, FRCOG**
Consultant Obstetrician
Royal Infirmary of Edinburgh
Senior Tutor and Honorary Senior Lecturer
University of Edinburgh
Edinburgh, UK

**Andrew Elder PRCP (Edin), MACP**
Honorary Professor
Edinburgh Medical School
Edinburgh, UK

**Karen Fairhurst MB BS, PhD**
Senior Lecturer
Centre for Population Health Sciences
University of Edinburgh
Edinburgh, UK

**Jane Gibson MB ChB, MD, FRCP, FSCP**
Doctor
Fife Rheumatic Diseases Unit
NHS Fife
Kirkcaldy, UK
Senior Lecturer
Bute Medical School
St Andrews University
St Andrews, UK

**Iain Hathorn MB ChB, DOHNS, PGCME, FRCSE (ORL HNS)**
Consultant ENT Surgeon, Honorary Clinical Senior Lecturer
University of Edinburgh ENT Department
Edinburgh, UK

**J Alastair Innes MB ChB, PhD, FRCPE**
Consultant and Honorary Reader in Respiratory Medicine (retired)
Respiratory Unit
Western General Hospital
Edinburgh, UK

**Alan G Japp MB ChB(Hons), PhD, MRCP**
Consultant Cardiologist
Edinburgh Heart Centre
Royal Infirmary of Edinburgh
Edinburgh, UK
Honorary Senior Lecturer
University of Edinburgh
Edinburgh, UK

**David Kluth OBE, MB BS, PhD, FRCP**
Professor of Medical Education & Honorary Consultant Nephrologist
Edinburgh Medical School
University of Edinburgh
Edinburgh, UK

**Alexander Laird MB ChB, PhD, FRCSE(Urol)**
Consultant Urological Surgeon
Department of Urology
Western General Hospital
Edinburgh, UK
Honorary Clinical Senior Lecturer
Institute of Genetics and Cancer
The University of Edinburgh
Edinburgh, UK

**Nazir Lone MB ChB, MSc, PhD, FRCPE, FFICM, FHEA**
Reader in Critical Care
Usher Institute
University of Edinburgh
Edinburgh, UK
Honorary Consultant in Critical Care
Department of Critical Care
Royal Infirmary of Edinburgh
Edinburgh, UK

**Elizabeth MacDonald MB ChB, MRCP, FRCPE, DMCC**
Consultant Physician
Medicine for the Elderly
Western General Hospital
Edinburgh, UK

**Hadi Manji MA, MD, FRCP**
Consultant Neurologist and Honorary Associate Professor
National Hospital for Neurology
Queen Square
London, UK

**Rowan Parks MD, FRCSI, FRCSE**
Professor of Surgical Sciences
Clinical Surgery
University of Edinburgh
Edinburgh, UK

**John Plevris MD, DM, PhD, FRCPE, FEBGH**
Professor
Centre for Liver & Digestive Disorders
The Royal Infirmary
University of Edinburgh
Edinburgh, UK

**Stephen Potts MA, FRCPsych, FRCPE, FRCSE**
Consultant in Transplant Psychiatry
Department of Psychological Medicine
Royal Infirmary of Edinburgh
Edinburgh, UK

**Peter T Reid MD**
Consultant Respiratory Physician
Respiratory Medicine
Lothian University Hospitals
Edinburgh, UK

**Jennifer MJ Robson MB ChB, PhD, FRCSE**
Consultant and Honorary Senior Lecturer
Leeds Vascular Institute
Leeds General Infirmary
Leeds, UK
Honorary Clinical Tutor
University of Edinburgh
Edinburgh, UK

**Ben Stenson MB ChB, MD, FRCPCH, FRCPE**
Consultant Neonatologist
Royal Infirmary of Edinburgh
Hon Professor of Neonatology
University of Edinburgh
Edinburgh, UK

**Alice SM Tidman MBChB, MRCP (Dermatology), PGDipClinDerm**
Consultant Dermatologist
Department of Dermatology
NHS Fife
Kirkcaldy, UK

**Michael J Tidman MD, FRCPE, FRCP**
Consultant Dermatologist
Department of Dermatology
Royal Infirmary of Edinburgh
Edinburgh, UK

**Naing Latt Tint MBChB, PhD, FRCOphth**
Consultant Ophthalmic Surgeon
Princess Alexandra Eye Pavilion
Edinburgh, UK

**Phil Walmsley MD, FFSTE, FRCS(Orth), AFHEA**
Consultant Orthopaedic Surgeon
Orthopaedic Surgery
Victoria Hospital Kirkcaldy
Kirkcaldy, UK
Honorary Senior Lecturer
School of Medicine
University of St Andrews
St Andrews, UK

**Christina Yip MB ChB, MD, FRCS(Plast)**
Consultant Oncoplastic Breast Surgeon
Department of Breast Surgery
East Lancashire Hospitals NHS Trust
Burnley, UK

**Nicola Zammitt MB ChB, MD, FRCPE**
Consultant Physician and Honorary Clinical Senior Lecturer
Edinburgh Centre for Endocrinology and Diabetes
Royal Infirmary of Edinburgh
Edinburgh, UK

# Section 1

## Principles of clinical history and examination

1. Managing clinical encounters with patients  3

2. General aspects of history taking  9

3. General aspects of examination  21

# Managing clinical encounters with patients

**The clinical encounter 4**
Reasons for the encounter 4
The clinical environment 4
Opening the encounter 5
Gathering information 5
Handling sensitive information and third parties 5
Managing patient concerns 5
Showing empathy 6

Showing cultural sensitivity 6
Addressing the problem 6
Concluding the encounter 6
**Professional responsibilities 6**
Confidentiality and consent 7
Social media 7
**Personal responsibilities 7**

## The clinical encounter

The clinical encounter between a patient and doctor lies at the heart of most clinical practice. At its simplest, it is the means by which people who are ill, or believe themselves to be ill, seek the advice of a clinician whom they trust. Traditionally, the clinical encounter is conducted face to face, although non–face-to-face or remote consultation using the telephone, video technology or online is increasingly common. This chapter describes the general principles that underpin clinical interactions with patients.

## Reasons for the encounter

The majority of people who experience symptoms of ill health do not seek professional advice. For the minority who do seek help, the decision to consult is usually based on a complex interplay of physical, psychological and social factors (Box 1.1). The perceived seriousness of the symptoms and the severity of the illness experience can influence whether patients seek help. The perceived severity of symptoms is determined by their intensity, the patient's familiarity with them and their duration and frequency. Beyond this, patients try to understand their symptoms based on their own prior experience and from information they have gathered from a range of sources, including family and friends, print and broadcast media and the internet and social media. Patients who present with a symptom are significantly more likely to believe or worry that their symptom indicates a serious or fatal condition than non-consulters with similar symptoms; for example, a family history of sudden death from heart disease may affect how a person interprets an episode of chest pain. Patients also weigh up the relative costs (financial or other, such as inconvenience) and benefits of consulting. The expectation of benefit from a consultation (e.g. in terms of symptom relief or legitimisation of time off work) is a powerful predictor of consultation. There may also be times when other priorities in patients' lives are more important than their symptoms of ill health and deter or delay consultation. It is important to consider the timing of the consultation. Why has the patient presented now? Sometimes it is not the experience of symptoms themselves that provokes consultation but something else in the patients' lives that triggers them to seek help (Box 1.2).

A range of cultural factors may also influence help-seeking behaviour. Examples of person-specific factors that reduce the propensity to consult include stoicism, self-reliance, guilt, unwillingness to acknowledge psychological distress, and embarrassment about lifestyle factors such as addictions. These factors may vary between patients and also in the same person in different circumstances and may be influenced by gender, education, social class and ethnicity.

## The clinical environment

You should take all reasonable steps to ensure that the consultation is conducted in a calm, private environment. For face-to-face clinic interactions the layout of the consulting room is important and furniture should be arranged to put the patient at ease (Fig. 1.1A) by avoiding confrontational positioning across a table and the incursion of computer screens between patient

A

B

**Fig. 1.1 Seating arrangements.** A In this friendly seating arrangement the clinician sits next to the patient, at an angle. B Barriers to communication are set up by an oppositional/confrontational seating arrangement. The desk acts as a barrier, and the clinician is distracted by looking at a computer screen that is not easily viewable by the patient.

---

### 1.1 Deciding to consult a doctor

- Perceived susceptibility or vulnerability to illness
- Perceived severity of symptoms
- Perceived costs of consulting
- Perceived benefits of consulting

---

### 1.2 Triggers to consultation

- Interpersonal crisis
- Interference with social or personal relations
- Sanctioning or pressure from family or friends
- Interference with work or physical activity
- Reaching the limit of tolerance of symptoms

and clinician (see Fig. 1.1B). Personal mobile devices can also be intrusive if not used judiciously.

For hospital inpatients the environment is a challenge, yet privacy and dignity are always important. There may only be curtains around the bed space, which afford very little by way of privacy for a conversation. If your patient is mobile, try to use a side room or interview room. If there is no alternative to speaking to patients at their bedside, let them know that you understand your conversation may be overheard and give them permission not to answer sensitive questions about which they feel uncomfortable.

## Opening the encounter

At the beginning of any encounter, it is important to start to establish a rapport with the patient. Rapport helps to relax and engage the person in a useful dialogue. This involves greeting the patient, introducing yourself and describing your role clearly. A good reminder is to start any encounter with 'Hello, my name is … '. In face-to-face or video encounters you should wear a name badge that can be read easily. A friendly smile helps to put your patient at ease. The way you dress is important; your dress style and demeanour should never make your patients uncomfortable or distract them. Smart, sensitive and modest dress or scrubs are appropriate. Before examining patients or carrying out procedures, roll up long sleeves, away from your wrists and forearms. Avoid hand jewellery to allow effective hand washing and reduce the risk of cross-infection (see Fig. 3.1). Tie back long hair. You should ensure that the patient is physically comfortable and at ease.

How you address and speak to a patient depends on the person's age, background and cultural environment. Some older people prefer not to be called by their first name, and it is best to ask patients how they would prefer to be addressed. Enquiring about someone's personal gender pronouns (e.g. she/her, he/him, they/them) can help them feel respected and valued and affirms their gender identity. Go on to establish the reason for the encounter: in particular, the problems or issues the patient wishes to address or be addressed. Ask an open question to start with to encourage the patient to talk, such as 'How can I help you today?' or 'What has brought you along to see me today?'

## Gathering information

The next task of the clinician in the clinical encounter is to understand what is causing the patient to be ill or to believe they are ill. To do this you need to establish whether or not the patient is suffering from an identifiable disease or condition, and this requires evaluation of the patient first by history taking and then by physical examination and investigation where appropriate. Chapters 2 and 3 will help you develop a general approach to history taking and physical examination; detailed guidance on history taking and physical examination in specific systems and circumstances is offered in Sections 2 and 3.

Fear of the unknown and of potentially serious illness accompanies many patients as they consult. Reactions to this vary widely, but it can certainly impede clear recall and description. Plain language is essential for all encounters. The use of medical jargon is rarely appropriate because the risk of the clinician and the patient having a different understanding of the same words is simply too great. This also applies to words the patient may use that have multiple possible meanings (e.g. 'indigestion' or 'dizziness'); these terms must always be defined precisely in the course of the discussion.

Clinicians who fill every pause with another specific question will miss the patient's revealing calm reflection, or the hesitant question or aside that reveals an inner concern. Active listening is a core skill in clinical encounters, as it encourages patients to tell their story. It is more than keeping quiet. Encourage the patient to elaborate by making encouraging comments or noises, such as 'Tell me a bit more' or 'Uhuh'. Demonstrate that you understand the meaning of what patients have articulated by reflecting back statements and summarising what you think they have said. Nonverbal communication is also important. Look for nonverbal cues indicating the patient's level of distress and mood. Changes in your patients' demeanour and body language during the consultation can be clues to difficulties that they cannot express verbally. If their body language becomes 'closed' (e.g. if they cross their arms and legs, turn away or avoid eye contact), this may indicate discomfort. Remote consultation increases the chance of miscommunication as nonverbal cues are not so readily apparent (see Chapter 21).

## Handling sensitive information and third parties

Confidentiality is your top priority. Ask your patient's permission if you need to obtain information from someone else: usually a relative but sometimes a friend or a carer. If the patient cannot communicate, you may have to rely on family and carers to understand what has happened to the patient. Third parties may approach you without your patient's knowledge. Find out who they are, their relationship to the patient and whether your patient knows that the third party is talking to you. Tell third parties that you can listen to them but cannot divulge any clinical information without the patient's explicit permission. They may tell you about sensitive matters, such as mental illness, sexual abuse or drug or alcohol addiction. This information needs to be sensitively explored with your patient to confirm the truth.

## Managing patient concerns

Patients are not simply the embodiment of disease but individuals who experience illness in their own unique way. Identifying their disease alone is rarely sufficient to permit full understanding of an individual patient's problems. In most encounters you should therefore also seek a clear understanding of the patient's personal experience of illness. This involves exploring the patients' feelings and ideas about their illness, its impact on their lifestyle and functioning. You should seek to establish what is important to them about their illness, and do not assume that the medical diagnosis is always a patient's main concern; anxiety about an inability to continue to work or to care for a dependent relative may be equally distressing. Find out their expectations of its treatment and course.

Patients may be so fearful of a serious diagnosis that they conceal their concerns; the only sign that a patient fears cancer may be sitting with crossed fingers while the history is taken, hoping inwardly that cancer is not mentioned. The ideas, concerns and expectations that patients have about their illness often derive from their personal belief system, as well as from more widespread social and cultural understandings of illness. These beliefs can influence which symptoms patients choose to present to doctors and when. In some cultures, people derive much of their prior knowledge about health, illness and disease from the media and the internet. Indeed, patients have often sought explanations for their symptoms from the internet (or from other trusted sources) prior to consulting a doctor and may return to these for a second opinion once they have seen a doctor. It is therefore important to establish what a patient already understands about the problem. This allows you and the patient to move towards a mutual understanding of the illness.

## Showing empathy

Being empathic is a powerful way to build your relationship with patients. Empathy is the ability to identify with and understand patients' experiences, thoughts and feelings and to see the world as they do. Being empathic also involves being able to convey that understanding to the patient by making statements such as 'I can understand you must be feeling quite worried about what this might mean'. Empathy is not the same as sympathy, which is about the doctor's own feelings of compassion for or sorrow about the difficulties that the patient is experiencing.

## Showing cultural sensitivity

Patients we treat come from diverse backgrounds and cultures. Miscommunication is a real risk in those for whom English is not their first language, and if in doubt, an interpreter should be used (see Chapter 2). Patients from a culture that is not your own may have different social rules regarding eye contact, touch and personal space. In some cultures, it is normal to maintain eye contact for long periods; however, in most of the world, this is seen as confrontational or rude. Shaking hands with the opposite sex is strictly forbidden in certain cultures. Death may be dealt with differently in terms of what the family's expectations of clinicians may be, which family members will expect information to be shared with them and what rites will be followed. Appreciate and accept differences in your patients' cultures and beliefs. When in doubt, ask them. This lets them know that you are aware of and sensitive to these issues.

## Addressing the problem

Communicating your understanding of the patient's problem to them is crucial and is covered in detail in Chapter 20. It is good practice to ensure privacy for this, particularly if imparting bad news. Ask the patient who else they would like to be present – this may be a relative or partner – and offer a nurse. The telephone should not be used routinely to communicate bad news or sensitive results, as there is limited opportunity to gauge nonverbal reaction or to offer additional support. Check patients' current level of understanding and try to establish what further information they would like. Information should be provided in small chunks and be tailored to the patient's needs. Try to acknowledge and address the patient's ideas, concerns and expectations. Check the patient's understanding and recall of what you have said and encourage questions. After this, you should agree on a management plan together. This might involve discussing and exploring the patient's understanding of the options for their treatment, including the evidence of benefit and risk for particular treatments and the uncertainties around it, or offering recommendations for treatment. Careful thought should also be given to whether it is possible or appropriate to give the patient all the information they need about their condition and treatment options if consulting remotely (see Chapter 21).

## Concluding the encounter

Closing the consultation usually involves summarising the important points that have been discussed during the consultation. This aids patient recall and facilitates adherence to treatment. Any remaining questions that the patient may have should be addressed, and finally you should check that you and the patient have agreed on a plan of action and confirmed arrangements for follow-up.

## Professional responsibilities

Clinical encounters take place within a very specific context configured by the healthcare system within which they occur, the legal, ethical and professional frameworks by which we are bound and by society as a whole.

From your first day as a student, you have professional obligations placed on you by the public, the law and your colleagues, which continue throughout your working life. Patients must be able to trust you with their lives and health, and you will be expected to demonstrate that your practice meets the expected standards (Box 1.3). Furthermore, patients want more from you than merely intellectual and technical proficiency; they will value highly your ability to demonstrate kindness, empathy and compassion.

Fundamentally, patients want clinicians who:

- are knowledgeable
- respect people, healthy or ill, regardless of who they are
- support patients and their loved ones when and where needed
- always ask courteous questions, let people talk and listen to them carefully
- promote health, as well as treat disease
- give unbiased advice and assess each situation carefully

---

### 1.3 The duties of a registered doctor

**Knowledge, skills and performance**

- Make the care of your patient your first concern
- Provide a good standard of practice and care:
  - Keep your professional knowledge and skills up to date
  - Recognise and work within the limits of your competence

**Safety and quality**

- Take prompt action if you think that patient safety, dignity or comfort is being compromised
- Protect and promote the health of patients and the public

**Communication, partnership and teamwork**

- Treat patients as individuals and respect their dignity:
  - Treat patients politely and considerately
  - Respect patients' right to confidentiality
- Work in partnership with patients:
  - Listen and respond to their concerns and preferences
  - Give patients the information they want or need in a way they can understand
  - Respect patients' right to reach decisions with you about their treatment and care
  - Support patients in caring for themselves to improve and maintain their health
- Work with colleagues in the ways that best serve patients' interests

**Maintenance of trust**

- Be honest and open, and act with integrity
- Never discriminate unfairly against patients or colleagues
- Never abuse your patients' trust in you or the public's trust in the profession

*Courtesy General Medical Council (UK).*

---

- use evidence as a tool, not as a determinant of practice
- let people participate actively in all decisions related to their health and healthcare
- humbly accept death as an important part of life, and help people make the best possible choices when death is close
- work cooperatively with other members of the healthcare team
- are advocates for their patients and are ready to learn from others, regardless of their age, role or status.

One way to reconcile these expectations with your inexperience and incomplete knowledge or skills is to put yourself in the situation of the patient and/or relatives. Consider how you would wish to be cared for in the patient's situation, acknowledging that you are different and your preferences may not be the same. Most clinicians approach and care for patients differently once they have had personal experience as a patient or as a relative of a patient. Every healthcare professional involved in caring for patients can have profound influences on how patients experience illness and their sense of dignity. When you are dealing with patients, always consider your:

- A: attitude – How would I feel in this patient's situation?
- B: behaviour – Always treat patients with kindness and respect.
- C: compassion – Recognise the human story that accompanies each illness.
- D: dialogue – Listen to and acknowledge the patient.

## Confidentiality and consent

As a student and as a healthcare professional, you will be given private and intimate information about patients and their families. This information is confidential, even after a patient's death. This is a general rule, although its legal application varies between countries. There are exceptions to the general rules governing patient confidentiality, where failure to disclose information would put the patient or someone else at risk of death or serious harm or where disclosure might assist in the prevention, detection or prosecution of a serious crime. If you find yourself in this situation, contact the senior doctor in charge of the patient's care immediately and inform them of the situation.

Always obtain consent before undertaking any examination or investigation or when providing treatment or involving patients in teaching or research.

## Social media

Through social media, we are able to create and share web-based information. As such, social media has the potential to be a valuable tool in communicating with patients, particularly by facilitating access to information about health and services and by providing invaluable peer support for patients. However, they also have the potential to expose clinicians to risks, especially when there is a blurring of the boundaries between their professional and personal lives. Think carefully about privacy settings on your personal accounts. As a clinician you need to be careful about whom you share your personal information with and, particularly, the type of information you share. You may not intend or wish patients to see your profile and posts, but even with appropriate privacy settings you cannot be sure someone will not share your information, so always bear in mind who you 'friend', 'follow' or allow yourself to be 'followed by'. The obligations on clinicians do not change because they are communicating through social media rather than face to face or through other conventional media. Indeed, using social media creates new circumstances in which the established principles apply.

If patients contact you about their care or other professional matters through your personal profile, you should indicate that you cannot mix social and professional relationships and, where appropriate, direct them to your professional profile.

## Personal responsibilities

You should always be aware that you are in a privileged professional position that you must not abuse. Do not pursue an improper relationship with a patient, and do not give medical care to anyone with whom you have a close personal relationship.

Finally, remember that, to be fit to take care of patients, you must first take care of yourself. If you think you have a medical condition that you could pass on to patients or if your judgement or performance could be affected by a condition or its treatment, consult your general practitioner. Examples might include serious communicable disease, significant psychiatric disease, or drug or alcohol addiction.

J Alastair Innes
Anna R Dover
Karen Fairhurst

2

# General aspects of history taking

**The importance of a clear history 10**

**Gathering information 10**
Beginning the history 10
The history of the presenting symptoms 11
Past medical history 14
Drug history 14
Family history 15
Social history and lifestyle 15

Systematic enquiry 17
Closing the interview 17

**Difficult situations 17**
Patients with communication difficulties 17
Patients with cognitive difficulties 19
Sensitive situations 19
Emotional or angry patients 19

## The importance of a clear history

Understanding the patient's experience of illness by taking a history is central to the practice of all branches of medicine. The process requires patience, empathy and understanding to yield the key information leading to correct diagnosis and treatment.

In a perfect situation a calm, articulate patient would describe clearly their experience of their symptoms in the order of their occurrence, understanding and answering supplementary questions where required to add detail and certainty. In reality, a multitude of factors commonly complicate this encounter and confound the clear communication of information. This chapter is a guide to facilitating the taking of a clear history. Information on specific symptoms and presentations is covered in the following system chapters.

## Gathering information

### Beginning the history

#### Preparation

Read your patient's past records, if they are available, along with any referral, transfer or discharge correspondence before starting.

#### Allowing sufficient time

Consultation length varies. In UK general practice the average appointment is short, but this is usually adequate, provided the doctor knows the patient and the family and social background. In hospital, the similarly brief time allowed for returning out-patients can be challenging for new or temporary staff unfamiliar with the patient. For new and complex problems, a longer appointment is usually scheduled. In all settings, clinicians must learn the skill of managing the pace of the consultation to avoid running late, while not giving any impression that they are short of time. For students, time spent with patients learning and prac-tising history taking is highly valuable; however, learning to communicate efficiently takes time, and patients appreciate advance discussion of the time students need.

#### Starting your consultation

Introduce yourself and anyone who is with you. The appropriate physical greeting depends on both the cultural and infection control context, and since the COVID-19 pandemic, shaking hands is no longer usual in UK practice. Confirm the patient's name and how they wish to be addressed. If you are a student, inform the patient; they are usually happy to help.

#### Using different styles of question

To get the patient's own perspective, begin with open questions that encourage them to think back and report their symptoms in order, such as 'When did you first notice something wrong, and how did it start?' Listen actively, and encourage the patient to talk by looking interested and making encouraging comments,

such as 'Tell me more'. Always give the impression that you have plenty of time. Allow patients to tell their story in their own words, ideally without interruption. You may occasionally need to inter-ject to guide the patient gently back to describing their symp-toms, as anxious patients commonly focus on describing the events or the reactions and opinions of others surrounding an episode of illness rather than what they were feeling. While avoiding unnecessary repetition, it may be helpful occasionally to tell patients what you think they have said and ask if your inter-pretation is correct (reflection).

The way you ask a question is important:

- Open questions are general invitations to talk that avoid anticipating particular answers: for example, 'What was the first thing you noticed when you became ill?' or 'Can you tell me more about that?'
- Closed questions seek specific information and are used for clarification: for example, 'Have you had a cough today?' or 'Did you notice any blood in your bowel motions?'

Both types of question have their place, and normally clinicians move gradually from open to closed questions as the interview progresses.

The following history illustrates the mix of question styles and responses needed to elucidate a clear story:

**When did you first feel unwell, and what did you feel? (Open questioning)**

*Well, I've been getting this funny feeling in my chest over the last few months. It's been getting worse and worse, but it was really awful this morning. My husband called 999. The ambulance came, and the nurse said I was having a heart attack. It was really scary.*

**It does sound scary for you. When you say a 'funny feeling', can you tell me more about what it felt like? (Acknowledging patient's feelings, open questioning, steering away from events and opinions back to symptoms)**

*Well, it was here, across my chest. It was sort of tight, like something heavy sitting on my chest.*

**And did you feel it anywhere else? (Open but clarifying)**

*Well, maybe up here in my neck.*

**What were you doing when it came on? (Clarifying precipitating event)**

*Just sitting in the kitchen, finishing my breakfast.*

**How long was the tightness there? (Closed)**

*About an hour altogether.*

**So, you felt a tightness in your chest this morning that went on for about an hour and you also felt it in your neck? (Reflection)**

*Yes, that's right.*

**Did you feel anything else at the same time? (Open, not overlooking secondary symptoms)**

*I felt a bit sick and sweaty.*

## Showing empathy when taking a history

Being empathic helps your relationship with patients and improves their health outcomes (see Chapter 1, p. 6). Try to see the problem from their point of view and convey that to them in your responses to what they say and your subsequent questions.

Consider a young teacher who has recently had disfiguring facial surgery to remove a benign tumour from her upper jaw. Her wound has healed, but she has a drooping lower eyelid and facial swelling. She returns to work. Imagine how you would feel in this situation. Express empathy through questions that show you can relate to your patient's experience.

**So, it's 3 weeks since your operation. How is your recovery going?**

*OK, but I still have to put drops in my eye.*

**And what about the swelling under your eye?**

*That gets worse during the day, and sometimes by the afternoon I can't see out of this eye.*

**And how are you managing at work?**

*Well, it's really difficult. You know, with the kids and everything. It's all a bit awkward.*

**That must feel pretty uncomfortable and awkward, but hopefully the swelling will settle soon. How do you cope? Has it been a problem when you are with friends or colleagues too?**

## The history of the presenting symptoms

Having established the patient's reason for seeking a consultation, you are now ready to explore the substance of the history.

Listen carefully as they respond to the initial open question inviting them to describe the onset of their symptoms. Pick out the two or three main symptoms they are describing (e.g. pain, cough and shivers); these are the essence of the history of the presenting symptoms. It may help to jot these down as single words, leaving space for associated clarifications by closed questioning as the history progresses.

Experienced clinicians make a diagnosis by recognising patterns of symptoms (see Chapter 20, p. 416). With experience, you will refine your questions according to the presenting symptoms, using a mental list of possible diagnoses (a differential diagnosis) to guide you. Clarify exactly what patients mean by any specific word they use (e.g. catarrh, fits or blackouts); common words can mean different things to different patients and professionals (Box 2.1). Each answer increases or decreases the probability of a particular diagnosis and excludes others.

### 2.1 Examples of terms used by patients that should be clarified

| Patient's term | Common underlying problems | Useful distinguishing features |
|---|---|---|
| Allergy | True allergy (immunoglobulin E–mediated reaction)<br>Intolerance of food or drug, often with nausea or other gastrointestinal upset | Visible rash or swelling, rapid onset<br>Predominantly gastrointestinal symptoms |
| Indigestion | Acid reflux with oesophagitis<br>Abdominal pain due to:<br>　　Peptic ulcer<br>　　Gastritis<br>　　Cholecystitis<br>　　Pancreatitis | Retrosternal burning, acid taste<br>Site and nature of discomfort:<br>　　Epigastric, relieved by eating<br>　　Epigastric, with vomiting<br>　　Right upper quadrant, tender<br>　　Epigastric, severe, tender |
| Arthritis | Joint pain<br>Muscle pain<br>Immobility due to prior skeletal injury | Redness or swelling of joints<br>Muscle tenderness<br>Deformity at site |
| Catarrh | Purulent sputum from bronchitis<br>Infected sinonasal discharge<br>Nasal blockage | Cough, yellow or green sputum<br>Yellow or green nasal discharge<br>Anosmia, prior nasal injury/polyps |
| Fits | Epilepsy<br>Transient syncope from cardiac disease<br>Abnormal involuntary movement | Witnessed tonic/clonic movements; postictal amnesia<br>Witnessed pallor during syncope; known heart disease<br>No loss of consciousness |
| Dizziness | Labyrinthitis<br><br>Syncope from hypotension<br>Cerebrovascular event | Nystagmus, feeling of room spinning, with no other neurological deficit<br>History of palpitation or cardiac disease, postural element<br>Sudden onset, with other neurological deficit |

In the following example, the patient is a 65-year-old male smoker. His age and smoking status increase the probability of certain diagnoses related to smoking. A cough for 2 months increases the likelihood of lung cancer and chronic obstructive pulmonary disease (COPD). Chest pain does not exclude COPD since he could have pulled a muscle on coughing, but the pain may also be pleuritic from underlying infection or thromboembolism. In turn, infection could be caused by obstruction of an airway by lung cancer. Haemoptysis lasting 2 months greatly increases the chance of lung cancer. If the patient also has weight loss, the positive predictive value of all these answers is very high for lung cancer. This will focus your examination and investigation plan.

**What was the first thing you noticed wrong when you became ill? (Open question)**

*I've had a cough that I just can't get rid of. It started after I'd had flu a few weeks ago. I thought it would get better, but it hasn't and it's driving me mad.*

**I'm sorry to hear that. Could you please tell me more about the cough? (Open question)**

*Well, it's bad all the time. I cough and cough and bring up some phlegm. It keeps waking me at night so I feel rough the next day. Sometimes I get pains in my chest because I've been coughing so much.*

**Already you have noted 'Cough', 'Phlegm' and 'Chest pain' as headings for your history. Follow up with key questions to clarify each.**

**Cough: Are you coughing to try to clear something from your chest, or does it come without warning? (Closed question, clarifying)**

*Oh, I can't stop it. Even when I'm asleep it comes.*

**Does it feel as if it starts in your throat or your chest? Can you point to where you feel it first?**

*It's like a tickle here (points to upper sternum).*

**Phlegm: What colour is the phlegm? (Closed question, focusing on the symptom)**

*Clear.*

**Have you ever coughed up any blood? (Closed question)**

*Yes, sometimes.*

**When did it first appear and how often does it come? (Closed questions)**

*Oh, most days. I've noticed it for over a month.*

**How much? A teaspoonful or more? (Closed questions, clarifying the symptom)**

*Just streaks.*

**Is it pure blood or mixed with yellow or green phlegm?**

*Just streaks of blood in clear phlegm.*

**Chest pain: Can you tell me about the chest pains? (Open question)**

*Well, they're here on my side (points) when I cough.*

**Does anything else bring on the pains? (Open, clarifying the symptom)**

*Taking a deep breath, and it really hurts when I cough or sneeze.*

Pain is a very important symptom common to many areas of practice. A general scheme for the detailed characterisation of pain is outlined in Box 2.2.

| 2.2 Characteristics of pain (SOCRATES) |
| --- |
| **Site** |
| • Somatic pain, often well localised (e.g. sprained ankle)<br>• Visceral pain, more diffuse (e.g. angina pectoris) |
| **Onset** |
| • Speed of onset and any associated circumstances |
| **Character** |
| • Described by adjectives (e.g. sharp/dull, burning/tingling, boring/stabbing, crushing/tugging) preferably using the patient's own description rather than offering suggestions |
| **Radiation** |
| • Disease progressing locally<br>• Referred by a shared neuronal pathway to a distant unaffected site (e.g. diaphragmatic pain at the shoulder tip via the phrenic nerve [$C_3$, $C_4$]) |
| **Associated symptoms** |
| • Visual aura accompanying migraine with aura<br>• Numbness in the leg with back pain suggesting nerve root irritation |
| **Timing (duration, course, pattern)** |
| • Since onset<br>• Episodic or continuous:<br>  • If episodic, duration and frequency of attacks<br>  • If continuous, any changes in severity |
| **Exacerbating and relieving factors** |
| • Circumstances in which pain is provoked or exacerbated (e.g. eating, coughing)<br>• Specific activities or postures, and any avoidance measures used to prevent or limit pain<br>• Effects of specific activities or postures, including effects of medication and complementary medical remedies |
| **Severity** |
| • Subjective, but ask patient to rate from 1 (just present) to 10 (worst imaginable)<br>• Sometimes helpful to compare with other common pains (e.g. toothache)<br>• Variation by day or night, during the week or month (e.g. relating to the menstrual cycle) |

Having clarified the presenting symptoms, prompt for any more associated features, using your initial impression of the likely pathology (lung cancer or chronic respiratory infection) to direct relevant questions:

**Do you ever feel short of breath? (relevant for underlying COPD or effusion)**

*A bit.*

**Can you give me an example of something that would make you short of breath? (quantifying the symptom, [see Chapter 5 breathlessness, p. 85])**

*Any time I'm going up a slope or up stairs*

**How has your weight been? (seeking additional confirmation of serious pathology)**

*I've lost about a stone since this started.*

The questions required at this point will vary according to the system involved. A summary of useful starting questions for each system is shown in Box 2.3. Learn to think, as you listen, about the broad categories of disease that may present and how these relate to the history, particularly in relation to the onset and rate of progression of symptoms (Box 2.4).

To complete the history of presenting symptoms, make an initial assessment of how the illness is impacting on the life of your patient. For example, breathlessness on heavy exertion may prevent a 40-year-old builder from working but would have much less impact on a sedentary retired person. 'Can you tell me how far you can walk on a good day?' is a question that can help to clarify the normal level of functioning, and 'How has this changed since you have been unwell?' can reveal disease impact. Ask if the person undertakes sports or regular exercise, and if they have modified these activities because of illness.

While taking the history of the presenting complaint you should also explore the patient's perspective on their symptoms, often referred to as their ideas, concerns and expectations (ICE). These may come up spontaneously or be hinted at (as cues), as the patient responds to open questions, or you may need to ask directly about them (e.g. 'Do you have any ideas about what's happening here?' 'What's your biggest worry when you think about what this might be?' and 'What were you hoping I'd be able to do for you today?').

| 2.3 Questions to ask about common symptoms | |
|---|---|
| **System** | **Question** |
| Cardiovascular | Do you ever have chest pain or tightness?<br>Do you ever wake up during the night feeling short of breath?<br>Have you ever noticed your heart racing or thumping? |
| Respiratory | Are you ever short of breath?<br>Have you had a cough? If so, do you cough anything up?<br>What colour is your phlegm?<br>Have you ever coughed up blood? |
| Gastrointestinal | Are you troubled by indigestion or heartburn?<br>Have you noticed any change in your bowel habits recently?<br>Have you ever seen any blood or slime in your stools? |
| Genitourinary | Do you ever have pain or difficulty passing urine?<br>Do you have to get up at night to pass urine? If so, how often?<br>Have you noticed any dribbling at the end of passing urine?<br>Have your periods been regular? |
| Musculoskeletal | Do you have any pain, stiffness or swelling in your joints?<br>Do you have any difficulty walking or dressing? |
| Endocrine | Do you tend to feel the heat or cold more than you used to?<br>Have you been feeling thirstier or drinking more than usual? |
| Neurological | Have you ever had any fits, faints or blackouts?<br>Have you noticed any numbness, weakness or clumsiness in your arms or legs? |

| 2.4 Typical patterns of symptoms related to disease causation | | | |
|---|---|---|---|
| **Disease causation** | **Onset of symptoms** | **Progression of symptoms** | **Associated symptoms/pattern of symptoms** |
| Infection | Usually hours, unheralded | Usually fairly rapid over hours or days | Fevers, rigors, localising symptoms (e.g. pleuritic pain and cough) |
| Inflammation | May appear acutely | Coming and going over weeks to months | Symptoms may be multifocal, often with local tenderness |
| Metabolic | Variable, hours to months | Steady progression in severity with no remission | Variable, weakness, altered weight |
| Malignant | Gradual, insidious | Steady progression over weeks to months | Weight loss, fatigue |
| Toxic | Abrupt | Rapid | Dramatic onset of symptoms; vomiting often a feature |
| Trauma | Abrupt | Little change from onset | Diagnosis usually clear from history |
| Vascular | Sudden | Stepwise progression with acute episodes | Rapid development of associated physical signs |
| Degenerative | Gradual | Months to years | Gradual worsening with periods of more acute deterioration |

### 2.5 Example of a drug history

| Drug | Dose | Duration | Indication | Side effects/patient concerns |
|---|---|---|---|---|
| Aspirin | 75 mg daily | 5 years | Started after myocardial infarction | Indigestion |
| Atenolol | 50 mg daily | 5 years | Started after myocardial infarction | Cold hands (?adherence) |
| Co-codamol (paracetamol + codeine) | 500 mg paracetamol/8 mg codeine up to 8 tablets daily | 4 weeks | Back pain | Constipation |
| Salbutamol MDI | 2 puffs as necessary | 6 months | Asthma | Palpitation |

*MDI*, Metered-dose inhaler.

## Past medical history

Past medical history may be relevant to the presenting symptoms (e.g. previous migraine in a patient with headache, or haematemesis and multiple minor injuries in a patient with possible excess alcohol intake). It may reveal predisposing past or underlying illness, such as diabetes in a patient with peripheral vascular disease, or childhood whooping cough in someone presenting with bronchiectasis.

The referral letter and case records often contain useful headlines, but the patient is usually the best source. These questions will elicit the key information in most patients:

• What illnesses have you seen a doctor about in the past?
• Have you been in hospital before or attended a clinic?
• Have you had any operations?
• Do you take any medicines regularly?

## Drug history

This follows naturally from asking about past illness. It is good practice to try to reconcile all available sources of information about current medication including the drug list on the referral letter, the hospital record and the patient's own recollection of what they take. Drug history can be complicated by patients' use of brand names, descriptions of tablet number, shape and colour, which should always be translated to generic pharmaceutical names and quantitative doses for the final record. Enquire also about inhalers and topical medications, as patients may assume that you are asking only about tablets. Note all drug names, dosage regimens and duration of treatment, along with any significant adverse effects, in a clear format (Box 2.5). When drugs such as methadone are being prescribed for addiction, ask the community pharmacy to confirm dosage and also to stop dispensing for the duration of any hospital admission.

### Non-prescribed drug use

In addition to prescribed drugs, ask patients if they take any over-the-counter remedies, including herbal and homeopathic remedies and vitamin or mineral supplements. Ask also about recreational drug use. In Britain approximately 30% of the adult population have used illegal recreational drugs (mainly cannabis) at some time. Useful questions are summarised in Box 2.6.

### Concordance and adherence

Half of all patients do not take prescribed medicines as directed. Patients who take their medication as prescribed are said to be adherent. Concordance implies that the patient and doctor have negotiated and reached an agreement on management, and adherence to therapy is likely (although not guaranteed) to improve.

Ask patients to describe how and when they take their medication. Give them permission to admit that they do not take all their medicines by saying, for example, 'That must be difficult to remember'.

### Drug allergies/reactions

Ask if your patient has ever had an allergic reaction to a medication or vaccine. Clarify exactly what patients mean by allergy,

### 2.6 Non-prescribed drug history

• Do you take any drugs that are not prescribed by your doctor?
• What drugs do you take?
• How often and how much?
• How long have you been taking drugs?
• Have you managed to stop at any time? If so, when and why did you start taking the drugs again?
• What symptoms do you have if you cannot get drugs?
• Do you ever inject? If so, where do you get the needles and syringes?
• Do you ever share needles, syringes or other drug-taking equipment?
• Do you see your drug use as a problem?
• Do you want to make changes in your life or change the way you use drugs?
• Have you been checked for infections spread by drug use?

as intolerance (e.g. nausea) is much more common than true allergy. Drug allergies are overreported by patients: for example, only 1 in 7 who report a rash with penicillin will have a positive penicillin skin test. Note other allergies, such as foodstuffs or pollen. Record true allergies prominently in the patient's case records, drug chart and computer records. If patients have had a severe or life-threatening allergic reaction, advise them to wear an alert necklace or bracelet.

## Family history

Start with open questions, such as 'Are there any illnesses that run in your family?' Avoid just asking about a family history of the patient's particular problem. Then follow up the presenting symptoms with a question like 'Have any of your family had heart trouble?' Single-gene inherited diseases are relatively uncommon in clinical practice. Even when present, autosomal recessive diseases such as cystic fibrosis usually arise in patients with healthy parents who are unaffected carriers (although they may have affected siblings). Many other illnesses are associated with a positive family history of the same or related illnesses but are not due to a single-gene disorder. For example, a family history of one autoimmune disease may increase the likelihood of the same or another autoimmune disease in the patient. A further complication is that some illnesses, such as asthma and diseases caused by atheroma, are so common in the UK population

that their presence in family members may not greatly influence the risk to the patient.

Document illness in first-degree relatives (i.e. parents, siblings and children). If you suspect an inherited disorder such as haemophilia, construct a pedigree chart (Fig. 2.1), noting whether any individuals were adopted. Ask about the health of other household members, since this may suggest environmental risks to the patient.

## Social history and lifestyle

No medical assessment is complete without determining the social circumstances of your patient. These may be relevant to the causes of their illness and may also influence the management and outcome. Social deprivation is a powerful predictor of many forms of ill health. Establish who is there to support the patient by asking 'Who is at home with you, or do you live alone?' For those who live alone, establish who is their next of kin and who visits regularly to support them. Check if your patient is a carer for someone vulnerable who may be at risk due to your patient's illness. Enquire sensitively if the patient is bereaved, as this can have profound effects on a patient's health and wellbeing.

Next establish the type and condition of the patient's housing and how well it suits them, given their symptoms. Patients with severe arthritis may, for example, struggle with stairs. Successful

**Fig. 2.1 Symbols used in constructing a pedigree chart, with an example.** The terms 'propositus' and 'proposita' indicate the man or woman identified as the index case, around whom the pedigree chart is constructed.

management of the patient in the community requires these issues to be addressed.

## Smoking

Among other things, tobacco use increases the risk of obstructive lung disease, cardiac and vascular disease, peptic ulceration, intrauterine growth restriction, erectile dysfunction and a range of cancers.

Most patients recognise that smoking harms health, so obtaining an accurate history of tobacco use requires sensitivity. Ask if your patient has ever smoked; if so, enquire at what age they started and whether they still smoke. Patients often play down recent use, so it is often helpful to ask about their average number of cigarettes per day over the years and what form of tobacco they have used (cigarettes, cigars, pipe, chewed). Convert to 'pack-years' (Box 2.7) to estimate the risk of tobacco-related health problems. Ask if they have smoked only tobacco or also cannabis. Never miss the opportunity during history taking to encourage smoking cessation, in a positive and non-judgemental way, as a route to improved health. Do not forget to ask non-smokers about their exposure to environmental tobacco smoke (passive smoking).

## Alcohol

Alcohol causes extensive pathology, including not only hepatic cirrhosis, encephalopathy and peripheral neuropathy but also pancreatitis, cardiomyopathy, erectile dysfunction and injury through accidents. Always ask patients if they drink alcohol but try to avoid appearing critical, as this will lead them to underestimate their intake. If they do drink, ask them to describe how much and what type (beer, wine, spirits) they drink in an average week. The quantity of alcohol consumed each week is best estimated in units; 1 unit (10 mL of ethanol) is contained in one standard measure (25 mL) of spirits or half a pint of 3.8% beer or lager. A small glass (125 mL) of wine contains 1.5 units.

### Alcohol problems

The UK Department of Health now defines hazardous drinking as anything exceeding 14 units per week for both men and women.

Binge drinking, involving a large amount of alcohol causing acute intoxication, is more likely to cause problems than if the same amount is consumed over 4 or 5 days. Most authorities recommend at least two alcohol-free days per week.

Alcohol dependence occurs when alcohol use takes priority over other behaviour that previously had greater value. Warning signs in the history are summarised in Box 2.8.

## Occupational history

Ask all patients about their occupation. Clarify what the person does at work, especially about any chemical or dust exposure. If the patient has worked with harmful materials (e.g. asbestos or stone dust), a detailed employment record is needed, including employer name, timing and extent of exposure, and any workplace protection offered. Unemployment is also associated with increased morbidity and mortality.

Diseases caused by occupational exposure particularly affect the lungs; these are dealt with in Chapter 5 on p. 91. Occupations associated with specific illness are summarised in Box 2.9.

Knowing about the patient's occupation is also vital for assessing how disease may affect lifestyle and livelihood (e.g. arthritis in a manual labourer or obstructive sleep apnoea in a professional driver).

## Travel history

Returning travellers commonly present with illness. They risk unusual or tropical infections, and air travel itself can precipitate certain conditions, such as middle-ear problems or deep vein thrombosis. The incubation period may indicate the likelihood of many illnesses, but some diseases, such as vivax malaria and human immunodeficiency virus, may present a year or more after travel. List the locations visited and dates. Note any travel vaccination and antimalaria prophylaxis taken if affected areas were visited.

---

### 2.7 Calculating pack-years of smoking

A 'pack-year' is smoking 20 cigarettes a day (1 pack) for 1 year

$$\frac{\text{Number of cigarettes smoked per day} \times \text{Number of years smoking}}{20}$$

For example, a smoker of 15 cigarettes a day who has smoked for 40 years would have smoked:

$$\frac{15 \times 40}{20} = 30 \text{ pack-years}$$

---

### 2.8 Features of alcohol dependence in the history

- A strong, often overpowering, desire to take alcohol
- Inability to control starting or stopping drinking and the amount that is drunk
- Drinking alcohol in the morning
- Tolerance, where increased doses are needed to achieve the effects originally produced by lower doses
- A withdrawal state when drinking is stopped or reduced, including tremor, sweating, rapid heart rate, anxiety, insomnia and occasionally seizures, disorientation or hallucinations (delirium tremens); this is relieved by more alcohol
- Neglect of other pleasures and interests
- Continuing to drink in spite of being aware of the harmful consequences

**2.9 Examples of occupational disorders**

| Occupation | Factor | Disorder | Presents |
|---|---|---|---|
| Shipyard workers, marine engineers, plumbers and heating engineers, demolition workers, joiners | Asbestos dust | Pleural plaques<br>Asbestosis<br>Mesothelioma<br>Lung cancer | >15 years later |
| Stonemasons | Silica dust | Silicosis | After years |
| Farmers | Fungus spores on mouldy hay | Farmer's lung (hypersensitivity pneumonitis) | After 4–18 hours |
| Divers | Surfacing from depth too quickly | Decompression sickness<br>Central nervous system, skin, bone and joint symptoms | Immediately, up to 1 week |
| Industrial workers | Chemicals (e.g. chromium) | Dermatitis on hands | Variable |
|  | Excessive noise | Sensorineural hearing loss | Over months |
|  | Vibrating tools | Vibration white finger | Over months |
| Bakery workers | Flour dust | Occupational asthma | Variable |
| Healthcare workers | Cuts, needlestick injuries | Human immunodeficiency virus, hepatitis B and C | Incubation period >3 months |

See also Chapter 5, p. 91

## Sexual history

Take a full sexual history only if the context or pattern of symptoms suggests this is relevant. Ask questions sensitively and objectively (see later). Signal your intentions: 'As part of your medical history, I need to ask you some questions about your relationships. Is this all right?'

## Systematic enquiry

Systematic enquiry uncovers symptoms that may have been forgotten. Start with 'Is there anything else you would like to tell me about?'

Box 2.10 lists common symptoms by system. Asking about all of these is inappropriate and takes too long, so judgement and context are used to select areas to explore in detail. For example:

- With a history of repeated infections, ask about nocturia, thirst and weight loss, which may indicate underlying uncontrolled diabetes.
- In a patient with palpitation are there any symptoms to suggest thyrotoxicosis or is there a family history of thyroid disease? Is the patient anxious or drinking too much coffee?
- If a patient smells of alcohol, ask about related symptoms, such as numbness in the feet due to alcoholic neuropathy.

## Closing the interview

In practice, this normally occurs after any necessary examination has also taken place. Using simple language, explain briefly your

interpretation of the patient's presenting problem and outline the likely possibilities. Be sensitive to any previously expressed concerns and to body language. Always give the patient a final opportunity to raise additional concerns ('Is there anything else you would like to ask?').

Make sure that patients are involved in any decisions by suggesting possible actions and encouraging them to contribute their thoughts. This way, you should be able to negotiate an agreed plan for further investigation and follow-up. Tell them that you will communicate this plan to other professionals involved in their care (p. 419).

# Difficult situations

## Patients with communication difficulties

### Interpreted consultation

Effective communication with patients who do not share your first language may require you to use an interpreter either in person or remotely. However, this will alter the dynamic of the consultation as the interpreter is an additional participant in the consultation. Where possible, use a professional interpreter and not a family member as this is more likely to ensure you get all the appropriate information. It is very easy to accidentally fall into a conversation with the interpreter rather than with the patient. Ask questions of the patient, not the interpreter; for example, ask, 'Can you tell me when the chest pain started?' rather than 'Can you ask her when the chest pain started?' This will help to ensure that the patient feels heard. Be careful to check that the

## 2.10 Systematic enquiry: cardinal symptoms

### General health

- Wellbeing
- Appetite
- Weight change
- Energy
- Sleep
- Mood

### Cardiovascular system

- Chest pain on exertion (angina)
- Breathlessness:
  - Lying flat (orthopnoea)
  - At night (paroxysmal nocturnal dyspnoea)
  - On minimal exertion – record how much
- Palpitation
- Pain in legs on walking (claudication)
- Ankle swelling

### Respiratory system

- Shortness of breath (exercise tolerance)
- Cough
- Wheeze
- Sputum production (colour, amount)
- Blood in sputum (haemoptysis)
- Chest pain (pleuritic or constant)

### Gastrointestinal system

- Mouth (oral ulcers, dental problems)
- Difficulty swallowing (dysphagia – distinguish from pain on swallowing (i.e. odynophagia)
- Nausea and vomiting
- Vomiting blood (haematemesis)
- Indigestion
- Heartburn
- Abdominal pain
- Change in bowel habit
- Change in colour of stools (pale, dark, tarry black, fresh blood)

### Genitourinary system

- Pain passing urine (dysuria)
- Frequency passing urine (at night: nocturia)
- Blood in urine (haematuria)
- Libido
- Incontinence (stress and urge)
- If appropriate: Sexual partners – unprotected intercourse

### Men

If appropriate:
- Prostatic symptoms, including difficulty starting (hesitancy):
- Poor stream or flow
- Terminal dribbling
- Urethral discharge
- Erectile difficulties

### Women

- Last menstrual period (consider pregnancy)
- Timing and regularity of periods
- Length of periods
- Abnormal bleeding
- Vaginal discharge
- Contraception
  If appropriate:
- Pain during intercourse (dyspareunia)

### Nervous system

- Headaches
- Dizziness (vertigo or lightheadedness)
- Faints
- Fits
- Altered sensation
- Weakness
- Visual disturbance
- Hearing problems (deafness, tinnitus)
- Memory and concentration changes

### Musculoskeletal system

- Joint pain, stiffness or swelling
- Mobility
- Falls

### Endocrine system

- Heat or cold intolerance
- Change in sweating
- Excessive thirst (polydipsia)

### Other

- Bleeding or bruising
- Skin rash

interpreter has correctly understood your questions. Non-verbal cues may be harder to pick up in interpreted consultations. It is important to observe the patient when the interpreter is speaking to them or they are replying even if you do not understand what they are saying.

## Hearing or speech difficulties

If your patient has hearing or speech difficulties such as dysphasia or dysarthria, consider the following:

- Write things down for your patient if they can read.
- Involve someone who is used to communicating with your patient.
- Seek a sign language interpreter for a deaf patient skilled in sign language.

## Patients with cognitive difficulties

Be alert for early signs of dementia. Inconsistent or hesitant responses from the patient should always prompt you to suspect and check for memory difficulties. If you do suspect this, ask if they have had any difficulties with their memory, then make a formal assessment using a cognitive rating scale (p. 372). You may have to rely on a history from relatives or carers.

## Sensitive situations

Doctors sometimes need to ask personal or sensitive questions and examine intimate parts. If you are talking to a patient who may be suffering from sexual dysfunction, sexual abuse or sexually transmitted disease, broach the subject sensitively. Indicate that you are going to ask questions in this area, and make sure that the conversation is entirely private. For example:

> *Because of what you're telling me, I need to ask you some rather personal questions. Is that OK?*

*Can I ask if you have a regular sexual partner?*

*Follow this up with:*

**Is your partner male or female?**

*If there is no regular partner, ask sensitively:*

**How many sexual partners have you had in the past year?**

**Have you had any problems with your relationships or in your sex life that you would like to mention?**

## Emotional or angry patients

Ill people feel vulnerable and may become angry and frustrated about how they feel or about their treatment. Staying calm and exploring the reasons for their emotion often defuses the situation. Although their behaviour may be challenging, never respond with anger or irritation and resist passing comment on a patient's account of prior management. Recognise that your patient is upset, show empathy and understanding and ask them to explain why (e.g. 'You seem angry about something' or 'Is there something that is upsetting you?'). If, despite this, their anger escalates, set boundaries on the discussion, withdraw from the room calmly, and seek the assistance and presence of another healthcare worker as a witness and for your own protection.

Talkative patients or those who want to deal with many things at once may respond to 'I only have a short time left with you, so what's the most important thing we need to deal with now?' If patients have a long list of symptoms, suggest 'Of all the things you've raised today, can you tell me which are the most important to you and we'll deal with the rest later?'.

Set professional boundaries if your patient becomes overly familiar: 'Well, it would be inappropriate for me to discuss my personal issues with you. I'm here to help you, so let's focus on your problem.'

Anna R Dover
Karen Fairhurst
J Alastair Innes

# General aspects of examination

General principles of physical examination 22

Preparing for physical examination 22

Sequence for performing a physical examination 23

Initial observations 24
Gait and posture 25
Facial expression and speech 25

Hands 25

Skin 28

Tongue 31

Odours 32

Body habitus and nutrition 32
Weight 32
Stature 33
Hydration 33

Lumps and lymph nodes 34

Spot diagnoses 38
Major chromosomal abnormalities 39

# General principles of physical examination

The process of taking a history and conducting a physical examination is artificially separated in classical medical teaching, to encourage learners to develop a structured approach to information gathering. However, your physical assessment of patients undoubtedly begins as soon as you see them, and the astute clinician may notice signs of disease, such as subtle abnormalities of demeanour, gait or appearance, even before the formal consultation begins. The clinician can be likened to a detective, gathering clues, and the physical assessment of a patient can then be seen as the investigation itself!

Historically, great importance has been placed on the value of empirical observation of patients in the formulation of a differential diagnosis. Modern technological advances have increased the reliance on imaging and laboratory testing for diagnosis, sometimes even at the bedside (such as portable ultrasound or near-patient capillary blood ketone testing), and this has called into question the utility of systematic physical examination in modern practice. Nevertheless, the importance of performing a methodical and accurate physical examination cannot be overstated. The inconstancy of physical signs and the need to monitor patient progress by repeated bedside assessment, often conducted by different clinicians, mean that a standardised approach to physical examination resulting in reproducible findings is crucial. Additionally, the interpretation of many diagnostic investigations (such as detection of interstitial oedema on a chest x-ray in heart failure) is subject to variation between clinicians and is not always more sensitive than the detection of physical signs (such as audible crackles on auscultating the lungs). Furthermore, the utility of many diagnostic investigations relies heavily on the pre-test probability (the likelihood of the disease being present prior to the test being performed; p. 416), which depends on information gathered during the history and examination. Finally, there are a number of conditions, or syndromes, that can be diagnosed only by the detection of a characteristic pattern of physical signs. Thus, by mastering structured skills in physical examination, clinicians can improve the reliability and precision of their clinical assessment, which, together with the appropriate diagnostic investigations, lead to accurate diagnosis.

# Preparing for physical examination

It is important to prepare both yourself and your patient for the physical examination. As a clinician, you must take reasonable steps to ensure that you can give the patient your undivided attention, in an environment free from interruption, noise or distraction. Always introduce yourself to the patient and seek permission to conduct the consultation. Make sure that you have the relevant equipment available (Box 3.1) and that you have

## 3.1 Equipment required for a full examination

- Stethoscope
- Pen torch
- Measuring tape
- Ophthalmoscope
- Otoscope
- Sphygmomanometer
- Tendon hammer
- Tuning fork
- Cotton wool
- Disposable Neurotips
- Wooden spatula
- Thermometer
- Magnifying glass
- Accurate weighing scales and a height-measuring device (preferably a calibrated, wall-mounted stadiometer)
- Personal protective equipment (disposable gloves and apron)
- Facilities for obtaining blood samples and urinalysis

observed local hand hygiene policies (Fig. 3.1). As discussed on page 4, privacy is essential when assessing a patient. At the very least, ensure that screens or curtains are fully closed around a ward bed; where possible, use a separate private room to avoid being overheard. Seek permission from the patient to proceed to examination, and offer a chaperone where appropriate to prevent misunderstandings and to provide support and encouragement for the patient. Regardless of whether the patient is the same gender as the doctor or not, chaperones are always appropriate for intimate (breast, genital or rectal) examination. Chaperones are also advised if the patient is especially anxious or vulnerable, if there have been misunderstandings in the past, or if religious or cultural factors require a different approach to physical examination. Record the chaperone's name and presence. If patients decline the offer, respect their wishes and record this in the notes. Tactfully invite relatives to leave the room before physical examination unless the patient is very apprehensive and requests that they stay. A parent or guardian should always be present when you examine children (p. 343).

The room should be warm and well lit; subtle abnormalities of complexion, such as mild jaundice, are easier to detect in natural light. The height of the examination couch or bed should be adjustable, with a step to enable patients to get up easily. An adjustable backrest is essential, particularly for patients who feel breathless lying flat. It is usual practice to examine a recumbent patient from the right-hand side of the bed. Ensure that the patient is comfortably positioned before commencing the physical examination.

Seek permission and sensitively, but adequately, expose the areas to be examined; cover the rest of the patient with a blanket or sheet to ensure that they do not become cold. Avoid unnecessary exposure and embarrassment; a patient may appreciate the opportunity to replace their top after examination of the chest before exposing the abdomen. Remain gentle towards the patient at all times, and be vigilant during aspects of the examination that may cause distress or discomfort. Acknowledge any anxiety or concerns raised by the patient during the consultation.

**How to hand-rub with alcohol-based hand-rub**

1. Apply a palmful of the product and cover all hand surfaces

**How to hand-wash with soap and water**

1. Wet hands and apply enough soap to cover all hand surfaces

2. Rub hands palm to palm

3. Right palm over the back of the other hand with interlaced fingers and vice versa

4. Palm to palm with fingers interlaced

5. Backs of fingers to opposing palms with fingers interlocked

6. Rotational rubbing of left thumb clasped in right palm and vice versa

7. Rotational rubbing, backwards and forwards with clasped fingers of right hand in left palm and vice versa

8. Rinse hands with water

9. Dry thoroughly with towel

10. Use elbow to turn off tap

8. Steps 2–7 should take at least 15 seconds

11. Steps 2–7 should take at least 15 seconds

**Fig. 3.1** Techniques for hand hygiene. *From WHO Guidelines on Hand Hygiene in Health Care First Global Patient Safety Challenge Clean Care is Safer Care;* http://www.who.int/gpsc/clean_hands_protection/en/ © World Health Organization 2009. All rights reserved.

## Sequence for performing a physical examination

The purpose of the physical examination is to look for the presence, or absence, of physical signs that confirm or refute the differential diagnoses you have obtained from the history. The extent of the examination will depend on the symptoms that you are investigating and the circumstances of the encounter. Often, in a brief, focused consultation (such as a patient presenting to a general practitioner with headache), a single system (the nervous system in this case) will be examined. In other circumstances, however, a full integrated physical examination will be required, and this is described in detail on page 424.

There is no single correct way to perform a physical examination, but standardised systematic approaches help to ensure that nothing is omitted. With experience, you will develop your own style and sequence of physical examination. Broadly speaking, any systematic examination involves looking at the patient (for skin changes, scars, abnormal patterns of breathing or pulsation, for example), laying hands on the patient to palpate (feel) and percuss (tapping on the body), and, finally, using a stethoscope, where appropriate, to listen to the relevant system (auscultate). This structured approach to the examination of the system can be summarised as:

- inspection
- palpation
- percussion
- auscultation.

## Initial observations

The physical examination begins as soon as you see the patient. Start with a rapid assessment of how unwell the patient is, since the clinical assessment may have to be adjusted for a deteriorating or dying patient, and any abnormal physiology may need to be addressed urgently before the actual diagnosis is found (see Chapter 18, p. 395). Early warning scoring systems (which include assessment of vital signs: pulse, blood pressure, respiratory rate and oxygen saturations, temperature, conscious level and pain score) are used routinely to assess unwell patients, and these clinical measurements aid decisions about illness severity and urgency of assessment (see Chapter 18, p. 394). If your patient is distressed or in pain, giving effective analgesia may take priority before undertaking a more structured evaluation, although a concurrent evaluation for the cause of the pain is clearly important.

For the stable or generally well patient, a more measured assessment can begin. Observe the patient before the consultation begins. Do they look generally well or unwell? What is their demeanour? Are they sitting up comfortably reading or on the telephone to a relative, or do they seem withdrawn, distressed or confused?

Notice the patient's attire. Are they dressed appropriately? Clothing gives clues about personality, state of mind and social circumstances, as well as a patient's physical state. Patients with recent weight loss may be wearing clothes that look baggy and loose. Are there signs of self-neglect (which may be underpinned by other factors, such as cognitive impairment, immobility, or drug or alcohol dependence) or inappropriate attire? For example, a patient with thyrotoxicosis may come to see you dressed for summer in the depths of winter due to heat intolerance.

Often, there will be clues to the patient's underlying medical condition given by the person's effects (e.g. they may be wearing a subcutaneous insulin pump to treat their type 1 diabetes, or carrying a portable oxygen cylinder if they have pulmonary fibrosis). If they are in bed, look on the bedside table for a hearing aid, peak flow meter or inhaler device, and note any walking aid, commode and wheelchair, which provide clues to the patient's functional status. Patients may be wearing a medical identity bracelet or other jewellery alerting you to an underlying medical condition or life-sustaining treatment. Note any tattoos or piercings; as well as alerting you to possible associated infections, these can provide important background information (Fig. 3.2). Be sure to look for any venepuncture marks of intravenous drug use (Fig .3.3) or linear (usually transverse) scars from recent or previous deliberate self-harm (Fig. 3.4).

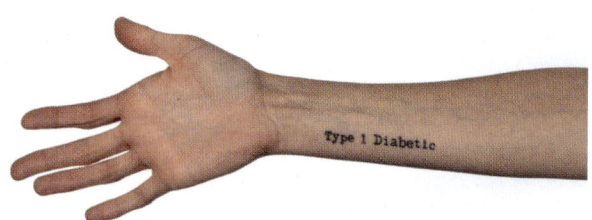

**Fig. 3.2** Tattoos can be revealing.

**Fig. 3.3** The linear marks of intravenous injection at the right antecubital fossa.

**Fig. 3.4** Scars from deliberate self-harm (cutting).

## Gait and posture

If patients are ambulant, watch how they rise from a chair and walk towards you. Are they using a walking aid? Is the gait normal or is there evidence of pain, immobility or weakness? Abnormalities of gait can be pathognomonic signs of neurological or musculoskeletal disease: for example, the hemiplegic gait after stroke, the ataxic gait of cerebellar disease or the *marche à petits pas* ('walk of little steps') gait in a patient with diffuse cerebrovascular disease or Parkinsonism (see Fig. 7.17, p. 152). Note any abnormal movements, such as tremor (in alcohol withdrawal, for example), dystonia (often a side effect of neuroleptic therapy), or chorea (jerky, involuntary movements, characteristic of Huntington's disease). Abnormalities of posture and movement can also be a clue to the patient's overall wellbeing and may represent pain, weakness, or psychological or emotional disturbance.

## Facial expression and speech

As with gait and posture, a patient's facial expression and how they interact with you can provide clues to their physical and psychological wellbeing (Box 3.2). Reluctance to engage in the consultation may indicate underlying depression, anxiety, fear, anger or grief, and it is important to recognise these emotions to ensure that both the physical and the emotional needs of the patient are addressed. Some people conceal anxieties and depression with inappropriate cheerfulness. Illness itself may alter demeanour: frontal lobe disease or bipolar disorders may lead to animated disinhibition, whereas poverty of expression may occur in depression or Parkinson's disease. Physical signs in the face that are associated with specific diagnoses are covered later (Box 3.7, p. 38).

Listen for abnormalities in the character of speech, such as slurring (due to alcohol, for example, or dysarthria caused by motor neurone disease; p. 369), hoarseness (which can represent recurrent laryngeal nerve damage; p. 215), or abnormality of speech cadence (which could be caused by pressure of speech in hyperthyroidism or slowing of speech in myxoedema; p. 222).

### 3.2 Facial expression as a guide to diagnosis

| Features | Diagnosis |
| --- | --- |
| Poverty of expression | Parkinsonism |
| Startled expression | Hyperthyroidism |
| Apathy, with poverty of expression and poor eye contact | Depression |
| Apathy, with pale and puffy skin | Hypothyroidism |
| Agitated expression | Anxiety, hyperthyroidism, hypomania |

## Hands

Some conditions are associated with pathognomonic signs. For example, the rare disease myotonic dystrophy (which is over-represented in candidate assessments) causes a patient to fail to release a handgrip (due to delayed muscle relaxation). A patient with neurological disease may be unable to move their hand or may have signs of muscle wasting or tremor. Detailed examination of the hands is described on page 303, but even a brief inspection and palpation may be very revealing.

### Deformity

Deformity in the hands may indicate nerve palsies or arthritic changes (such as ulnar deviation at the metacarpophalangeal joints in longstanding rheumatoid arthritis; see Fig. 13.22, p. 266). Arthritis frequently involves the small joints of the hands. Rheumatoid arthritis typically affects metacarpophalangeal and proximal interphalangeal joints (Fig. 13.22, p. 266), and osteoarthritis and psoriatic arthropathy affect the distal interphalangeal joints (Fig. 13.8, p. 295). Small-muscle wasting of the hands is common in rheumatoid arthritis, producing 'dorsal guttering' of the hands, and also occurs in cervical spondylosis with nerve root entrapment. In carpal tunnel syndrome, median nerve compression leads to wasting of the thenar muscles, also seen in damage affecting the T1 nerve root (Fig. 13.23, p. 305).

Dupuytren's contracture is a thickening of the palmar fascia causing fixed flexion deformity, and it usually affects the little and ring fingers (Fig. 3.5). Arachnodactyly (long, thin fingers) is typical of Marfan's syndrome (Fig. 3.21B). Trauma is the most common cause of hand deformity.

### Colour

Look for peripheral cyanosis in the nail bed and tobacco staining of the fingers (see Fig. 5.7, p. 94). Examine the skin creases for pigmentation, although pigmentation is normal in many non-Caucasian races (Fig. 3.6).

**Fig. 3.5** Dupuytren's contracture.

**Fig. 3.6 Normal palms.** African (*left*) and European (*right*).

## Temperature

The temperature of the patient's hand is a good guide to peripheral perfusion. In chronic obstructive pulmonary disease, the hands may be cyanosed due to reduced arterial oxygen saturation but warm due to vasodilatation from elevated arterial carbon dioxide levels. In heart failure the hands are often cold and cyanosed because of vasoconstriction in response to a low cardiac output. If they are warm, heart failure may be due to a high-output state, such as hyperthyroidism.

## Skin

Skin changes in the hands can indicate systemic disease, as in the coarse skin and broad hands of a patient with acromegaly (see Fig. 10.8, p. 228), or the tight, contracted skin (scleroderma) and calcium deposits associated with systemic sclerosis (Figs 3.30C and 13.6, p. 294). Clues about lifestyle can also be seen in the hands: manual workers may have specific callosities due to pressure at characteristic sites, while disuse results in soft, smooth skin.

## Nails

Nail changes occur in a wide variety of systemic diseases. Box 3.3 and Fig. 3.7 summarise nail changes seen on general examination that may indicate underlying systemic disease.

Finger clubbing describes painless soft tissue swelling of the terminal phalanges and increased convexity of the nail (Fig. 3.8). Clubbing usually affects the fingers symmetrically. It may also involve the toes and can be unilateral if caused by a proximal vascular condition, such as arteriovenous shunts for dialysis. It is sometimes congenital, but, in over 90% of patients it accompanies a serious underlying disorder (Box 3.4). Clubbing may recede if the underlying condition resolves.

## Examination sequence

- Look across the nail bed from the side of each finger. Observe the distal phalanges, nail and nail bed:
  - Estimate the interphalangeal depth at the level of the distal interphalangeal joint (this is the anteroposterior thickness of the digit rather than the width). Repeat at the level of the nail bed.
  - Assess the nail bed (hyponychial) angle (Fig. 3.9A).

| 3.3 The nails in systemic disease | | |
|---|---|---|
| **Nail changes** | **Description of nail** | **Differential diagnosis** |
| Beau's lines | Transverse grooves (Fig. 3.7B) | Sequela of any severe systemic illness that affects growth of the nail matrix |
| Clubbing | Loss of angle between nail fold and nail plate (Fig. 3.8) | Serious cardiac, respiratory or gastrointestinal disease (Box 3.4) |
| Leuconychia | White spots, ridges or complete discoloration of nail (Fig. 3.7C) | Trauma, infection, poisoning, chemotherapy, vitamin deficiency |
| Lindsay's nails | White/brown 'half-and-half' nails (see Fig. 12.7, p. 278) | Chronic kidney disease |
| Koilonychia | Spoon-shaped depression of nail plate (Fig. 3.7D) | Iron deficiency anaemia, lichen planus, repeated exposure to detergents |
| Muehrcke's lines | Narrow, white transverse lines (see Fig. 12.6, p. 278) | Decreased protein synthesis or protein loss |
| Nail-fold telangiectasia | Dilated capillaries and erythema at nail fold (see 14.17B, p. 335) | Connective tissue disorders, including systemic sclerosis, systemic lupus erythematosus, dermatomyositis |
| Onycholysis | Nail separates from nail bed (Fig. 3.7A) | Psoriasis, fungal infection, trauma, thyrotoxicosis, tetracyclines (photo-onycholysis) |
| Onychomycosis | Thickening of nail plate with white, yellow or brown discoloration | Fungal infection |
| Pitting | Fine or coarse pits in nail (Fig. 3.7A) | Psoriasis (onycholysis, thickening and ridging may also be present), eczema, alopecia areata, lichen planus |
| Splinter haemorrhages | Small red streaks that lie longitudinally in nail plate (Fig. 4.5B, p. 51) | Trauma, infective endocarditis |
| Yellow nails | Yellow discoloration and thickening (Fig. 14.18, p. 336) | Yellow nail syndrome |

**3**

**Fig. 3.7 Nail abnormalities in systemic disease.** [A] Onycholysis with pitting in psoriasis. [B] Beau's lines seen after acute severe illness. [C] Leuconychia. [D] Koilonychia. *(A) From Innes JA. Davidson's Essentials of Medicine. 2nd ed. Edinburgh: Churchill Livingstone; 2016.*

**Fig. 3.8 Clubbing.** [A] Anterior view. [B] Lateral view.

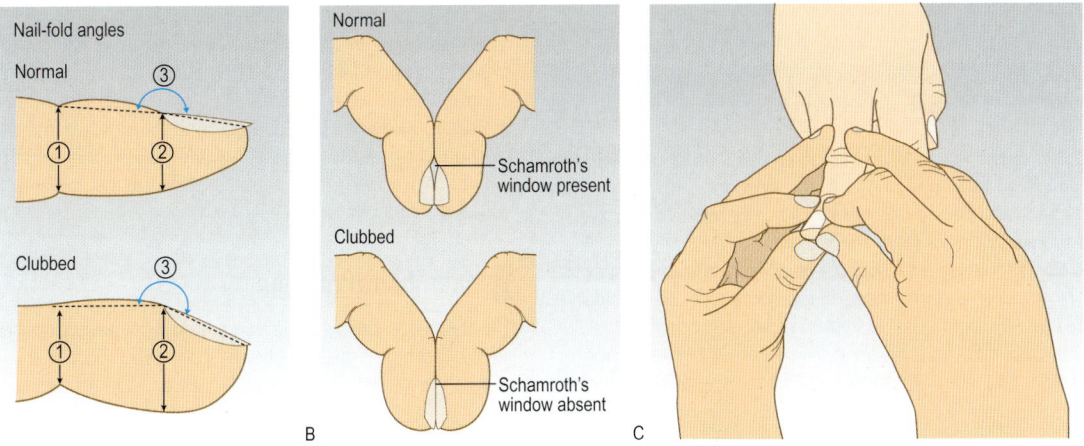

**Fig. 3.9 Examining for finger clubbing.** [A] Assessing interphalangeal depth at (**1**) interphalangeal joint and (**2**) nail bed, and nail-bed angle (**3**). [B] Schamroth's window sign. [C] Assessing nail-bed fluctuation.

## 3.4 Causes of clubbing

**Congenital or familial (5%–10%)**

*Acquired*
- Thoracic (~70%):
  - Lung cancer
  - Pulmonary fibrosis, including asbestosis
  - Chronic suppurative conditions: pulmonary tuberculosis, bronchiectasis, cystic fibrosis, lung abscess, empyema
  - Mesothelioma
- Cardiovascular:
  - Cyanotic congenital heart disease
  - Infective endocarditis
  - Arteriovenous shunts and aneurysms
- Gastrointestinal:
  - Cirrhosis
  - Inflammatory bowel disease
  - Coeliac disease
- Others:
  - Thyrotoxicosis (thyroid acropachy)
  - Primary hypertrophic osteoarthropathy

- Ask the patient to place the nails of corresponding (ring) fingers back-to-back and look for the normal 'diamond-shaped' gap between the nail beds (Schamroth's window sign; Fig. 3.9B).
- Place your thumbs under the pulp of the distal phalanx and use your index fingers alternately to see if there is fluctuant movement of the nail on the nail bed (Fig. 3.9C).
  Finger clubbing is likely if:
- the interphalangeal depth ratio is >1 (that is, the digit is thicker at the level of the nail bed than the level of the distal interphalangeal joint; Fig. 3.9A),
- the nail fold angle is >190 degrees (Fig. 3.9A), or
- Schamroth's window sign is absent (Fig. 3.9B).
  Increased nail-bed fluctuation may be present and may support the finding of clubbing, but its presence is subjective and less discriminatory than the above features.

# Skin

A detailed approach to examination of the skin is described in Chapter 14. In everyday practice, the skin can provide insights into present and past medical disorders, as well as information about the patient's social or mental status.

The skin should be exposed where appropriate and inspected carefully for any abnormalities of pigmentation. Skin colour is determined by pigments – melanin, an endogenous brown pigment, and carotene, an exogenous yellow pigment (derived mainly from ingestion of carrots and other vegetables) – as well

**Fig. 3.10** Vitiligo.

as by the amount of oxyhaemoglobin (red) and deoxyhaemoglobin (dusky blue) circulating in the dermis.

The autoimmune condition vitiligo causes irregular pale patches of skin depigmentation (Fig. 3.10), commonly on the face, neck, hands and extensor aspects of the limbs. It can be symmetrical, but often is not. It is associated with other autoimmune diseases, such as diabetes mellitus, thyroid and adrenal disorders and pernicious anaemia. Hypopituitarism also results in pale skin due to reduced production of melanotrophic peptides. Albinism is an inherited disorder in which patients have little or no melanin in their skin or hair. The amount of pigment in the iris varies; some individuals have reddish eyes, but most have blue.

Hyperpigmentation can be due to excess of the pituitary hormone adrenocorticotrophic hormone (ACTH), as in adrenal insufficiency (or the very rare condition Nelson's syndrome, in which there is ACTH overproduction following bilateral adrenalectomy for pituitary Cushing's disease). Excess ACTH produces brown pigmentation, particularly in skin creases, recent scars, sites overlying bony prominences, areas exposed to pressure, such as belts and bra straps, and the mucous membranes of the lips and mouth, where it results in muddy brown patches (see Fig 10.9B, p. 229). Pregnancy and oral contraceptives may also cause blotchy hyperpigmentation on the face, known as chloasma, and pregnancy may increase pigmentation of the areolae, axillae, genital skin and linea alba (producing a dark line in the midline of the lower abdomen, called a 'linea nigra').

## Haemochromatosis

This inherited condition of excessive iron absorption results in skin hyperpigmentation due to iron deposition and increased melanin production (Fig. 3.11). When iron deposition in the

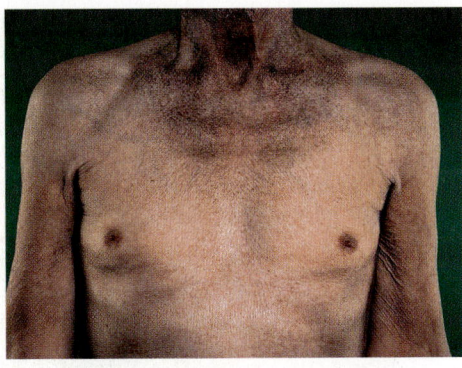

**Fig. 3.11** Haemochromatosis with increased skin pigmentation.

**Fig. 3.13** Hypercarotenaemia. A control normal hand is shown on the right for comparison.

pancreas also causes diabetes mellitus, this is called 'bronze diabetes'.

## Haemosiderin

This product of haemoglobin breakdown is deposited in the skin of the lower legs following subcutaneous extravasation of blood due to venous insufficiency. Local deposition of haemosiderin (erythema ab igne or 'granny's tartan') occurs with heat damage to the skin from sitting too close to a fire or from applying local heat, such as a hot water bottle, to a site of pain (Fig. 3.12).

## Easy bruising

Easy bruising can be a reflection of skin and connective tissue fragility due to advancing age or glucocorticoid usage, or a more serious coagulopathy.

## Hypercarotenaemia

Hypercarotenaemia occurs due to excessive ingestion of carotene-containing vegetables or in situations of impaired metabolism, such as hypothyroidism or anorexia nervosa. A yellowish discolouration is seen on the face, palms and soles but not the sclera or conjunctiva, and this distinguishes it from jaundice (Fig. 3.13).

## Discolouration

Skin discolouration can also occur due to abnormal pigments, such as the sallow yellow-brownish tinge in chronic kidney disease. A bluish tinge is produced by abnormal haemoglobins, such as sulphaemoglobin or methaemoglobin (see the section on cyanosis later), or by drugs, such as dapsone. Some drug metabolites cause strikingly abnormal colouration of the skin, particularly in areas exposed to light: for example, mepacrine (yellow), amiodarone (bluish-grey), clofazimine (brownish-black) and phenothiazines (slate-grey; Fig. 3.14).

### Jaundice

Jaundice is an abnormal yellow discoloration of the skin, sclera and mucous membranes. It is usually detectable when serum bilirubin concentration rises above 50 μmol/L (3 mg/dL) as a result of parenchymal liver disease, biliary obstruction or haemolysis (see Fig. 6.8, p. 115).

### Pallor

Pallor can result from anaemia, in which there is a reduction in circulating oxyhaemoglobin in the dermal and subconjunctival capillaries, or from vasoconstriction due to cold exposure or sympathetic activation. The best sites to assess for the pallor of anaemia are the conjunctiva (specifically the anterior rim; Fig. 3.15), the palmar skin creases and the face, in general, although absence of pallor does not exclude anaemia. Nail-bed pallor lacks diagnostic value for predicting anaemia. In significant iron deficiency anaemia, there may be additional findings of angular stomatitis, glossitis (Fig. 3.16), koilonychia (spoonshaped nails) and blue sclerae.

**Fig. 3.12** Erythema ab igne.

**Fig. 3.14** Phenothiazine-induced pigmentation.

**Fig. 3.15** Conjunctival pallor.

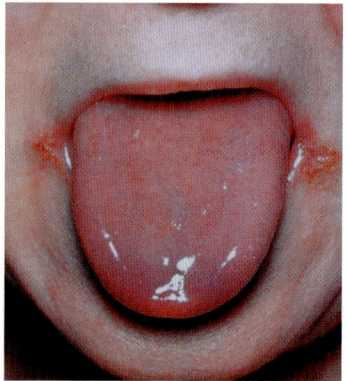

**Fig. 3.16** Smooth red tongue (glossitis) and angular stomatitis of iron deficiency.

A

B

**Fig. 3.17** Flushing due to carcinoid syndrome. **A** Acute carcinoid flush. **B** Chronic telangiectasia.

Conversely, vasodilatation, or flushing, may produce a pink complexion, even in anaemia, and may be due to fever, heat, exercise, food, drugs and other neurological or hormonal disturbances (Fig. 3.17 and Box 3.5). Facial plethora is caused by raised haemoglobin concentration with elevated haematocrit (polycythaemia). Polycythaemia may be primary or may indicate an underlying disease causing chronic hypoxia or excess erythropoietin production. Plethora of the head and neck only may indicate superior vena cava obstruction (see Fig. 5.9, p. 96).

## Cyanosis

Cyanosis is a blue discoloration of the skin and mucous membranes that occurs when the absolute concentration of deoxygenated haemoglobin is increased. It can be difficult to detect,

## 3.5 Conditions associated with facial flushing

**Physiological**

- Fever
- Exercise
- Heat exposure
- Emotional

**Drugs (e.g. glyceryl trinitrate, calcium channel blockers, nicotinic acid)**

Anaphylaxis

**Endocrine**

- Menopause
- Androgen deficiency (in men)
- Carcinoid syndrome
- Medullary thyroid cancer

**Others**

- Serotonin syndrome
- Food/alcohol ingestion
- Neurological (e.g. Frey's syndrome)
- Rosacea
- Mastocytoses

particularly in black and Asian patients, but is most easily seen where the subepidermal vessels are close to the skin surface, as in the lips, mucous membranes, nose, cheeks, ears, hands and feet. Rarely, cyanosis can be due to excessive circulating methaemoglobin (which can be congenital or acquired, most often due to drug therapy) or sulphaemoglobin (usually due to drug therapy), and typically does not resolve with oxygen administration.

### Central cyanosis

Central cyanosis can be seen in the lips, tongue and buccal or sublingual mucosa (Figs 3.18 and 5.11) and can accompany any disease (usually cardiac or respiratory) that results in hypoxia sufficient to raise the capillary deoxyhaemoglobin concentration above 50 g/L (5 g/dL). Since the detection of cyanosis relies on the absolute quantity of deoxyhaemoglobin present in the skin or mucous membrane, it may be absent in anaemic or hypovolaemic patients despite the presence of hypoxia. Conversely, cyanosis may appear at relatively mild levels of hypoxia in polycythaemic patients.

### Peripheral cyanosis

Peripheral cyanosis is seen in the distal extremities and may simply be a result of cold exposure, when prolonged peripheral capillary flow allows greater oxygen extraction and, hence, increased levels of deoxyhaemoglobin. As the patient is warmed, and the circulation improves, so does the cyanosis. Pathological causes of peripheral cyanosis include low cardiac output states, arterial disease and venous stasis or obstruction.

## Characteristic skin changes

Characteristic skin changes also occur in other conditions, such as scurvy (Fig. 3.19), neurofibromatosis (Fig. 3.20) and acanthosis nigricans (Fig. 10.13A, p. 236).

## Tongue

In addition to revealing central cyanosis, examination may uncover the smooth tongue of iron deficiency (Fig. 3.16), enlargement in acromegaly, or wasting and fasciculation in motor neurone disease.

A

B

**Fig. 3.19 Scurvy.** **A** Bleeding gums. **B** Bruising and perifollicular haemorrhages.

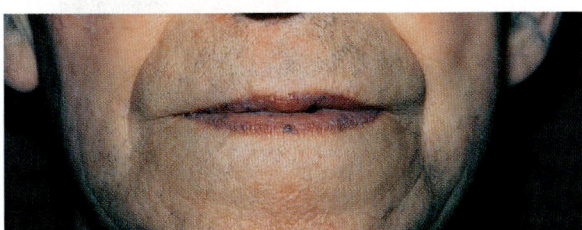

**Fig. 3.18 Central cyanosis of the lips.**

**Fig. 3.20** Neurofibromatosis.

| 3.6 The relationship between body mass index (BMI), nutritional status and ethnic group | | |
|---|---|---|
| Nutritional status | BMI non-Asian | BMI Asian |
| Underweight | <18.5 | <18.5 |
| Normal | 18.5–24.9 | 18.5–22.9 |
| Overweight | 25–29.9 | 23–24.9 |
| Obese | 30–39.9 | 25–29.9 |
| Morbidly obese | ≥40 | ≥30 |

more useful than weight alone, as it allows for differing height. Normal values for different ethnicities are available (Box 3.6).

## Obesity

Obesity is associated with an increased risk of malignancy, particularly oesophageal and renal cancer in both sexes, thyroid and colon cancer in men, and endometrial and gallbladder cancer in women, as well as hypertension, hyperlipidaemia, type 2 diabetes mellitus, gastro-oesophageal reflux, gallbladder disease, osteoarthritis and sleep apnoea. While it is usually the result of excessive calorie intake relative to calories expended, it can rarely be secondary to hypothyroidism, Cushing's syndrome, hypothalamic disease or drugs such as oral hypoglycaemic agents, insulin and antipsychotics.

Note the distribution of fat, since central obesity (as judged by the waist circumference: the maximum abdominal girth at the midpoint between the lower costal margin and the iliac crest) correlates with increased visceral adiposity and has worse health outcomes due to its association with hypertension, insulin resistance, type 2 diabetes mellitus and coronary artery disease. Waist-to-hip ratio can also be a useful assessment of adipose distribution: gluteal–femoral obesity or the 'pear shape' (waist:hip ratio of ≤0.8 in females or <0.9 in males) has a better prognosis, whereas 'apple-shaped' patients with a greater waist:hip ratio have an increased risk of coronary artery disease and the 'metabolic syndrome'.

## Weight loss

Weight loss or malnutrition (p. 106) may be due to inadequate energy consumption or utilisation (such as malabsorption, anorexia, glycosuria) or to conditions in which nutritional demand is increased (such as fever, infection, thyrotoxicosis, malignancy, surgery). Psychiatric disease and alcohol or drug dependency may also result in weight loss. Useful markers of malnutrition include arm muscle circumference and grip strength. Malnutrition may also be associated with biochemical and physical evidence of hypoproteinaemia and/or vitamin deficiencies. Malnutrition lengthens recovery time from illness and surgery, as well as delays wound healing.

## Odours

Odours can provide clues to a patient's social or behavioural habits; the smell of alcohol, tobacco or cannabis may be readily apparent. Stale urine and anaerobic skin infections also produce distinctive smells. Halitosis (bad breath) can be due to poor dental hygiene, gingivitis, stomatitis, atrophic rhinitis, tumours of the nasal passages, or suppurative lung conditions, such as lung abscess or bronchiectasis.

Other characteristic odours include:

- ketones: a sweet smell (such as nail varnish remover) due to acetone in diabetic ketoacidosis or starvation
- fetor hepaticus: the stale, 'mousy' smell of the volatile amine dimethylsulphide in patients with liver failure
- uraemic fetor: a fishy or ammoniacal smell on the breath in uraemia
- foul-smelling belching in patients with gastric outlet obstruction
- a faecal smell in patients with gastrocolic fistula.

## Body habitus and nutrition

### Weight

Weight is an important indicator of general health and nutrition, and serial weight measurements can be useful in monitoring both acute and chronic disease. The body mass index (BMI; calculated from the formula weight (kg)/height (m)$^2$) is

## Stature

### Short stature

Short stature may reflect general nutritional state or significant illness during childhood, although it may be familial (ask about the height of the patient's parents and siblings; p. 310). Loss of height is part of normal ageing but is accentuated by compression fractures of the spine due to osteoporosis, particularly in women. In postmenopausal women, loss of >5 cm height is an indication to investigate for osteoporosis.

### Tall stature

Tall stature is less common than short stature and is usually familial. Most individuals with heights above the 95th centile are not abnormal, so ask about the height of close relatives. Pathological causes of increased height include Marfan's syndrome, prepubertal hypogonadism and gigantism. In Marfan's syndrome, the limbs are long in relation to the length of the trunk, and the arm span exceeds height (Fig. 3.21A). Additional features include long, slender fingers (arachnodactyly; Fig. 3.21B), narrow feet, a high-arched palate (Fig. 3.21C), upward dislocation of the lenses of the eyes (Fig. 3.21D), cardiovascular abnormalities, such as mitral valve prolapse, and dilatation of the aortic root with aortic regurgitation.

During puberty, the epiphyses close in response to stimulation from the sex hormones, so, in some patients with hypogonadism, the limbs continue to grow for longer than usual (as in Klinefelter's syndrome). Gigantism is a very rare cause of tall stature due to excessive growth hormone secretion (from a pituitary adenoma) before epiphyseal fusion has occurred.

## Hydration (Video 1)

Assessment of a patient's hydration is particularly important, especially in the acutely unwell patient. Look for evidence of dehydration or generalised oedema (p. 385).

A

C

B

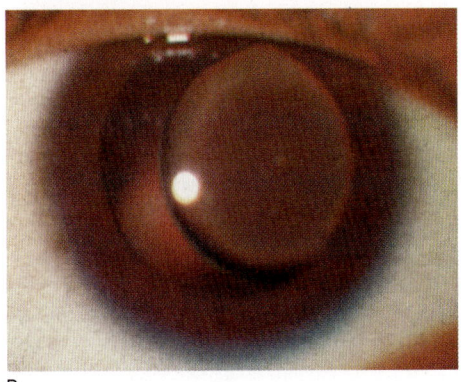

D

**Fig. 3.21 Marfan's syndrome, an autosomal dominant condition.** [A] Tall stature, with the torso shorter than the legs (note surgery for aortic dissection). [B] Long fingers. [C] High-arched palate. [D] Dislocation of the lens in the eye. *(A–D) From Forbes CD, Jackson WF. Color Atlas of Clinical Medicine. 3rd ed. Edinburgh: Mosby; 2003.*

**Fig. 3.22** Swollen right leg, suggesting deep vein thrombosis or inflammation. Causes include soft tissue infection or a ruptured Baker's cyst.

## Localised oedema

Localised oedema (an excess of interstitial fluid) is most commonly caused by venous disease but may also develop in lymphatic, inflammatory or allergic disorders.

### Venous causes

Increased venous pressure raises hydrostatic pressure within capillaries, producing oedema in the area drained by that vein. Venous causes include deep vein thrombosis, external pressure from a tumour or pregnancy, or venous valvular incompetence from previous thrombosis or surgery (Fig. 3.22). Conditions that impair the normal muscle pumping action, such as hemiparesis and forced immobility, increase venous pressure by impairing venous return. As a result, oedema may occur in immobile, bedridden patients, in a paralysed limb, or in a healthy person sitting for long periods, such as during travel.

### Lymphatic causes

Normally, interstitial fluid returns to the central circulation via the lymphatic system. Any obstruction to lymphatic flow may produce localised oedema (lymphoedema; Fig. 3.23). If the condition persists, fibrous tissue proliferates in the interstitial space, and the affected area becomes hard and no longer pits on pressure. In the UK, the most common cause of chronic leg lymphoedema is congenital hypoplasia of leg lymphatics (Milroy's disease); in the arm, lymphoedema usually follows radical mastectomy and/or irradiation for breast cancer. Lymphoedema is common in some tropical countries because of lymphatic obstruction by filarial worms (elephantiasis).

**Fig. 3.23** Lymphoedema of the right arm following right-sided mastectomy and radiotherapy.

### Inflammatory causes

Any cause of tissue inflammation, including infection or injury, liberates mediators, such as histamine, bradykinin and cytokines, which cause vasodilatation and increase capillary permeability. Inflammatory oedema is accompanied by the other features of inflammation (redness, tenderness and warmth) and is, therefore, painful.

### Allergic causes

Increased capillary permeability occurs in acute allergic conditions, for example, an insect bite in an allergic individual. The affected area is usually red and pruritic (itchy) because of local release of histamine and other inflammatory mediators but, in contrast to inflammation, is not painful.

Angio-oedema is a severe form of allergic oedema affecting the face, lips and mouth, most commonly caused by insect bites, food allergy or drug reactions (Fig. 3.24). Swelling may develop rapidly and become life-threatening if the upper airway is involved.

## Lumps and lymph nodes

Patients often present with a lump or enlarged lymph nodes (lymphadenopathy), which, while usually benign, can herald a serious underlying infective or malignant process. Alternatively, when examining a patient you may find a lump of which they were unaware.

## Lumps

Ask about the rapidity of onset of the lump and the presence of any associated pain, tenderness, or colour change. Document the following features (mnemonic: SPACESPIT):

Fig. 3.24 Angio-oedema following a wasp sting.

Fig. 3.25 Blister on a leg.

### Size

Measure the size of any lump (preferably using callipers).

### Position

The source of some lumps may be obvious from position, such as in the breast, thyroid or parotid gland; in other sites, such as the abdomen, this is less clear. Multiple lumps may occur in neurofibromatosis (see Fig. 3.20), skin metastases, lipomatosis and lymphomas.

### Attachment

Malignant masses commonly infiltrate adjacent tissues, causing them to feel fixed and immobile.

Lymphatic obstruction may cause skin swelling with fine dimpling where the skin is tethered by hair follicles, giving it an 'orange peel' appearance (*peau d'orange*; Fig. 11.6, p. 242). This is common in malignant disease when attachment to deeper structures, such as underlying muscle, may also occur.

### Consistency

The consistency of a lump can vary from soft to 'stony' hard. Very hard swellings are usually malignant, calcified or dense fibrous tissue. Fluctuation occurs in the presence of fluid, as in an abscess, cyst, or blister (Fig. 3.25), or in soft, encapsulated tumours, such as lipoma.

### Edge

The margin may be well delineated or ill defined, regular or irregular, and sharp or rounded. The margins of enlarged organs, such as the thyroid gland, liver, spleen, or kidney, can usually be defined more clearly than those of inflammatory or malignant masses. An indefinite margin suggests infiltrating malignancy, in contrast to the clearly defined edge of a benign tumour.

### Surface and shape

The surface and shape of a swelling can be characteristic. In the abdomen, examples include an enlarged spleen or liver, a distended bladder, or the uterine fundus in pregnancy. The surface may be smooth or irregular: for example, the surface of the liver is smooth in acute hepatitis but is often nodular in metastatic disease.

### Pulsations, thrills and bruits

Arterial swellings (aneurysms) and highly vascular tumours are pulsatile, expanding in time with the arterial pulse. Other swellings may transmit pulsation if they lie over a major artery. If the blood flow through a lump is increased, a systolic murmur (bruit) may be auscultated; occasionally, with sufficient flow, a thrill may be palpable. Bruits are also heard over arterial aneurysms and arteriovenous malformations due to turbulent flow.

### Inflammation

Redness, tenderness and warmth suggest inflammation:

- Redness (erythema): the skin over acute inflammatory lesions is usually red due to vasodilatation. In haematomas, the pigment from extravasated blood may produce the range of colours in a bruise (ecchymosis).
- Tenderness: inflammatory lumps, such as boils or abscesses, are usually tender or painful, while non-inflamed swellings, such as lipomas, skin metastases and neurofibromas, are characteristically painless.
- Warmth: inflammatory lumps and some tumours, especially if rapidly growing, may feel warm due to increased blood flow.

### Transillumination

In a darkened room, press the lighted end of a pen torch onto one side of the swelling. A cystic swelling, such as a testicular hydrocoele, will light up if the fluid is translucent, providing the covering tissues are not too thick (see Fig. 15.9, p. 349).

## Examination sequence

- Inspect the lump, noting any change in the colour or texture of the overlying skin.
- Define the site and shape of the lump.
- Measure its size and record the findings diagrammatically.
- Gently palpate for tenderness or change in skin temperature.
- Feel the lump for a few seconds to determine if it is pulsatile.
- Assess the consistency, surface texture and margins of the lump.
- Try to pick up an overlying fold of skin to assess whether the lump is fixed to the skin.
- Try to move the lump in different planes relative to the surrounding tissues to see if it is fixed to deeper structures.
- Compress the lump on one side; see and feel if a bulge occurs on the opposite side (fluctuation). Confirm the fluctuation in two planes. Fluctuation usually indicates that the lump contains fluid, although some soft lipomas can feel fluctuant.
- Auscultate for vascular bruits.
- Transilluminate.

## Lymph nodes

Palpable lymphadenopathy (enlarged peripheral lymph nodes) may be local or generalised, and it is of diagnostic and prognostic significance in the staging of lymphoproliferative and other malignancies. Lymph nodes may also be palpable in normal people, especially in the submandibular, axilla and groin regions (Fig. 3.26).

As with any lump, note the size and position of the nodes (normal nodes in adults are < 0.5 cm in diameter) and assess fixation to deeper structures (lymph nodes fixed to deep structures or skin suggest malignancy). Assess consistency: normal nodes feel soft. In Hodgkin's lymphoma, they are characteristically 'rubbery', in tuberculosis they may be 'matted', and, in metastatic

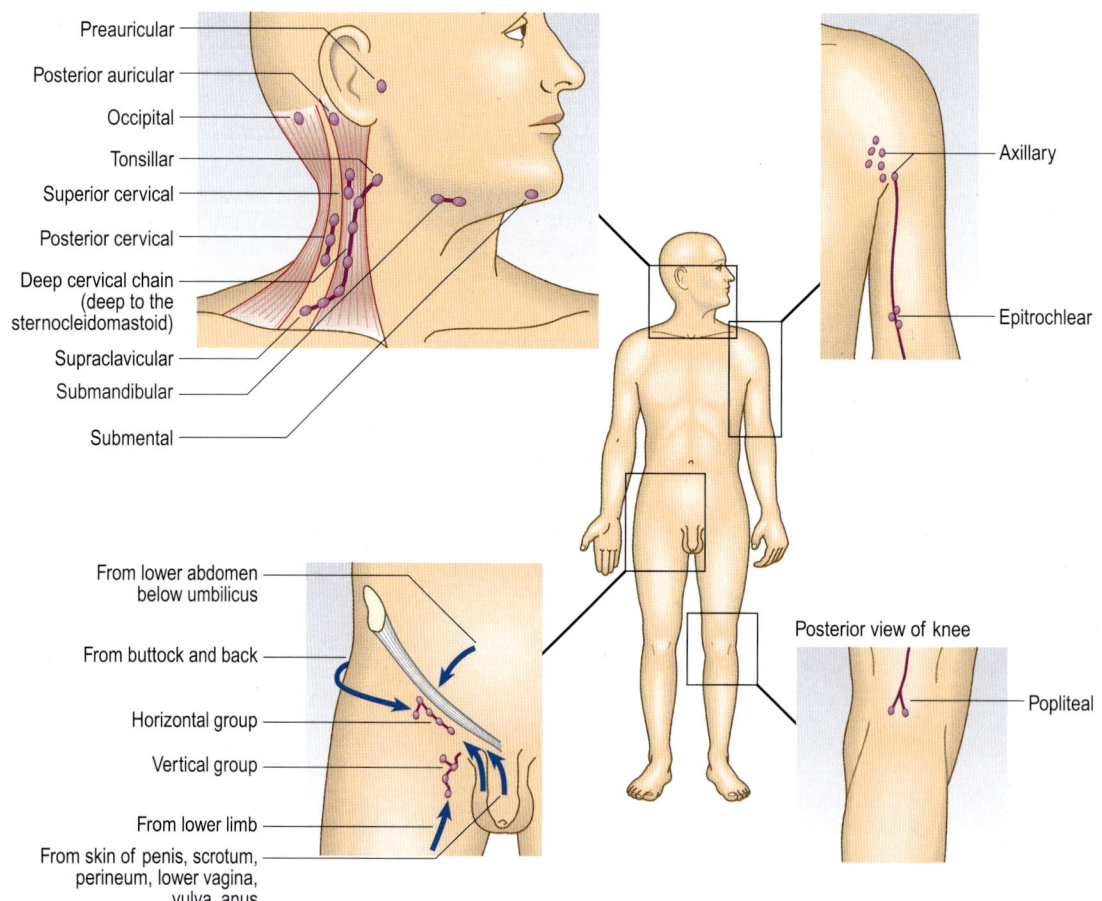

**Fig. 3.26** Distribution of palpable lymph glands.

cancer, they feel hard. Acute viral or bacterial infections, including infectious mononucleosis, dental sepsis and tonsillitis, cause tender, variably enlarged lymph nodes.

## Examination sequence (Video 2A)

### General principles

- Inspect for visible lymphadenopathy.
- Palpate one side at a time, using the fingers of each hand, in turn.
- Compare with the nodes on the contralateral side.
- Assess:
  - Site;
  - Size.
- Determine whether the node is fixed to:
  - Surrounding and deep structures
  - Skin.
- Check consistency.
- Check for tenderness.

### Cervical nodes

- Examine the cervical and axillary nodes with the patient sitting.
- From behind, examine the submental, submandibular, pre-auricular, tonsillar, supraclavicular and deep cervical nodes in the anterior triangle of the neck (Fig. 3.27A).
- Palpate for the scalene nodes by placing your index finger between the sternocleidomastoid muscle and clavicle. Ask the patient to tilt their head to the same side and press firmly down towards the first rib (Fig. 3.27B).
- From the front of the patient, palpate the posterior triangles, up the back of the neck and the posterior auricular and occipital nodes (Fig. 3.27C).

### Axillary nodes

- To palpate the right axilla, support the patient's right arm with your right arm to relax their shoulder muscles and explore the axilla with your left hand (Fig. 3.28A; follow a mirror image for other side).

A    B    C

**Fig. 3.27 Palpation of the cervical glands.** **A** Examine the glands of the anterior triangle from behind, using both hands. **B** Examine for the scalene nodes from behind with your index finger in the angle between the sternocleidomastoid muscle and the clavicle. **C** Examine the glands in the posterior triangle from the front.

A    B    C

**Fig. 3.28 Palpation of the axillary, epitrochlear and inguinal glands.** **A** Examination for right axillary lymphadenopathy. **B** Examination of the left epitrochlear glands. **C** Examination of the left inguinal glands.

- Gently place your fingertips into the apex of the axilla and then draw them downwards, feeling the medial, anterior and posterior axillary walls, in turn.

## Epitrochlear nodes

- Support the patient's right wrist with your left hand, hold their partially flexed elbow with your right hand, and use your thumb to feel for the epitrochlear node. Examine the left epitrochlear node with your left thumb (Fig. 3.28B).

## Inguinal nodes

- Examine for the inguinal and popliteal nodes with the patient lying down.
- Palpate over the horizontal chain, which lies just below the inguinal ligament, and then over the vertical chain along the line of the saphenous vein (Fig. 3.28C).

If you find localised lymphadenopathy, examine the areas that drain to that site. Infection commonly causes lymphadenitis (localised tender lymphadenopathy); in acute tonsillitis, for example, the submandibular nodes are involved. If the lymphadenopathy is non-tender, look for a malignant cause, tuberculosis, or features of human immunodeficiency virus (HIV) infection. Generalised lymphadenopathy occurs in a number of conditions, including lymphoma, tuberculosis, HIV and systemic inflammatory disorders, such as sarcoidosis. Examine for enlargement of the liver and spleen, and for other haematological features, such as purpura (bruising under the skin), which can be large (ecchymoses) or pinpoint (petechiae; Fig. 3.29).

**Fig. 3.29** Petechiae.

## Spot diagnoses

Several disorders have characteristic physical or facial features (Box 3.7) that allow a diagnosis to be made by observation alone. These conditions, together with those that have a more generalised distinctive physical phenotype, are often over-represented in candidate assessments, where they are referred to as 'spot diagnoses'.

Osteogenesis imperfecta is a rare autosomal dominant condition causing fragile and brittle bones; the sclerae (Fig. 3.30A) are blue due to abnormal collagen formation. Hereditary haemorrhagic telangiectasia is an autosomal dominant condition associated with small, dilated capillaries or terminal arteries

| 3.7 Conditions with characteristic facial appearances | |
|---|---|
| Diagnosis | Facial features |
| Hypothyroidism (Fig. 10.5, p. 224) | Sparse, coarse hair and eyebrows; periorbital puffiness; dry, waxy skin; apathetic expression; macroglossia |
| Graves disease (autoimmune thyrotoxicosis) (Fig. 10.2A, p. 221) | Staring appearance due to lid retraction, proptosis, evidence of weight loss |
| Hypopituitarism | Pale, often unwrinkled skin with loss of hair |
| Acromegaly (Fig. 10.8A, p. 228) | Thickened, coarse skin with enlarged nose and frontal bones, prognathism (lower jaw protrusion), widely spaced teeth, macroglossia |
| Cushing's syndrome (Fig. 10.10A, p. 230) | Moon-shaped plethoric facies |
| Osteogenesis imperfecta (Fig. 3.30A) | Blue sclerae |
| Hereditary haemorrhagic telangiectasia (Fig. 3.30B) | Telangiectasia on and around lips |
| Systemic sclerosis (Fig. 3.30C) | Tight skin constricting mouth, 'beaking' of nose, loss of nasolabial folds |
| Myotonic dystrophy (Fig. 3.30D) | Frontal balding, paucity of expression, bilateral ptosis |
| Down's syndrome (Fig. 3.31) | Flat facial profile, up-slanting palpebral fissures, small, low-set ears, macroglossia, Brushfield spots in iris |
| Systemic lupus erythematosus | 'Butterfly' erythematous rash on cheeks |

**Fig. 3.30** Characteristic facial features of some disorders. **A** Blue sclerae of osteogenesis imperfecta. **B** Telangiectasia around the mouth, typical of hereditary haemorrhagic telangiectasia. **C** Systemic sclerosis with 'beaking' of the nose and taut skin around the mouth. **D** Myotonic dystrophy with frontal balding and bilateral ptosis.

(telangiectasia), most commonly on the lips and tongue (Fig. 3.30B). In systemic sclerosis, the skin is thickened and tight, causing loss of the normal wrinkles and skin folds, 'beaking' of the nose, and narrowing and puckering of the mouth (Fig. 3.30C). Myotonic dystrophy, mentioned previously in the context of delayed relaxation of handgrip, is an autosomal dominant condition with characteristic features of frontal balding and bilateral ptosis (Fig. 3.30D).

## Major chromosomal abnormalities

There are several genetic or chromosomal syndromes that are easily identified on first contact with the patient.

### Down's syndrome (trisomy 21 − 47XX/XY + 21)

Down's syndrome is characterised by typical physical features, including short stature, a small head with flat occiput, up-slanting palpebral fissures, epicanthic folds, a small nose with a poorly developed bridge, and small, low-set ears (Fig. 3.31A). Grey–white areas of depigmentation are seen in the iris (Brushfield spots; Fig. 3.31B). The hands are broad with a single palmar crease (Fig. 3.31C), the fingers are short and the little finger is curved. Trisomy 21 is also associated with characteristic cognitive, cardiac, gastrointestinal, ophthalmic, ocular, endocrine and haematological disorders, for which patients should be screened.

### Turner's syndrome (45XO)

Turner's syndrome (Fig. 3.32) is due to loss of an X chromosome. It occurs in 1:2500 live female births and is a cause of delayed puberty in girls. Typical features include short stature, webbing of the neck, small chin, low-set ears, low hairline, short fourth finger, increased carrying angle at the elbows and widely spaced nipples ('shield-like chest').

A                    B                    C

**Fig. 3.31 Down's syndrome.** **A** Typical facial appearance. **B** Brushfield spots: grey–white areas of depigmentation in the iris. **C** Single palmar crease. *(A) From Phelps K, Hassed C. Genetic conditions. In General Practice: The Integrative Approach. 1st ed. Churchill Livingstone; 2011.*

**Fig. 3.32 Turner's syndrome.** *From Seidel HM, Ball J, Dain J, Benedict GW. Growth and measurement. In: Mosby's Guide to Physical Examination. 6th ed. 2006.*

## Klinefelter's syndrome (47XXY)

This chromosomal abnormality results in tall stature, gynaeco-mastia, reduced pubic hair and small testes. It is the most common cause of primary hypogonadism in men.

## Achondroplasia

This is an autosomal dominant disease of cartilage caused by mutation of the fibroblast growth factor gene. Although the trunk

**Fig. 3.33 Child with achondroplasia.** *From Moore KL, Persaud TVN. Congenital anatomic anomalies or human birth defects. In: Developing Human: Clinically Oriented Embryology. 8th ed. 2008.*

is of normal length, the limbs are very short and broad (Fig. 3.33). The vault of the skull is enlarged, the face is small and the bridge of the nose is flat.

# Section 2

## System-based examination

4. The cardiovascular system  43

5. The respiratory system  83

6. The gastrointestinal system  105

7. The nervous system  133

8. The visual system  169

9. The ear, nose and throat  193

10. The endocrine system  219

11. The reproductive system  239

12. The renal system  271

13. The musculoskeletal system  287

14. The skin, hair and nails  325

Alan G Japp
Jehangir N Din
Jennifer MJ Robson

**4**

# The cardiovascular system

**Heart 44**

**Anatomy and physiology 44**

**The history 44**
Common presenting symptoms 44
Past medical history 49
Drug history 49
Family history 49
Social history 50

**The physical examination  50**
General examination 51
Arterial pulses 52
Blood pressure 55
Jugular venous pressure and waveform 57
Precordium 58

**Interpretation of the findings 66**

**Investigations 67**

**Peripheral arterial system 70**

**Anatomy and physiology 70**

**The history 70**

Common presenting symptoms 70
Past medical history 74
Drug history 74
Family history 74
Social history 74

**The physical examination 74**

**Investigations 77**

**Peripheral venous system 77**

**Anatomy and physiology 77**

**The history 78**
Common presenting symptoms 78
Past history 80

**The physical examination 80**

**Investigations 81**

**OSCE example 1: Chest pain history 81**

**OSCE example 2: Cardiac examination 81**

**Integrated examination sequence for the cardiovascular system 82**

# HEART

## Anatomy and physiology

The heart comprises two muscular pumps working in a series, covered in a serous sac (pericardium) that allows free movement with each heart beat and respiration (Fig. 4.1). The right heart (right atrium and ventricle) pumps deoxygenated blood returning from the systemic veins into the pulmonary circulation at relatively low pressures. The left heart (left atrium and ventricle) receives blood from the lungs and pumps it round the body to the tissues at higher pressures (Fig. 4.2). Atrioventricular valves (tricuspid on the right side, mitral on the left) separate the atria from the ventricles. The pulmonary valve on the right side of the heart and

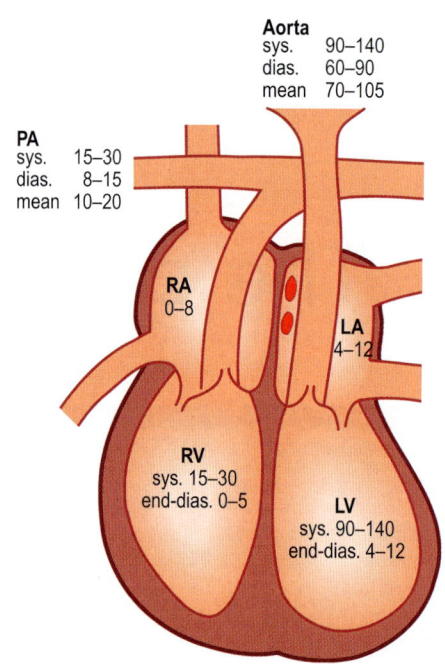

**Aorta**
sys. 90–140
dias. 60–90
mean 70–105

**PA**
sys. 15–30
dias. 8–15
mean 10–20

**RA** 0–8

**LA** 4–12

**RV**
sys. 15–30
end-dias. 0–5

**LV**
sys. 90–140
end-dias. 4–12

**Fig. 4.2** Normal resting pressures (mmHg) in the heart and great vessels. *dias.*, Diastolic; *LA*, left atrium; *LV*, left ventricle; *PA*, pulmonary artery; *RA*, right atrium; *RV*, right ventricle; *sys.*, systolic.

Superior vena cava
Ascending aorta
Pulmonary trunk
Right atrium
Pulmonary valve
Tricuspid valve
Right ventricle
Papillary muscle
Inferior vena cava

Left atrium
Left pulmonary veins
Aortic valve
Mitral valve
Chordae tendineae
Left ventricle

**Fig. 4.1** The heart chambers and valves.

the aortic valve on the left separate the ventricles from the pulmonary and systemic arterial systems, respectively. Cardiac contraction is coordinated by specialised groups of cells. The cells in the sinoatrial node normally act as the cardiac pacemaker. Subsequent spread of impulses through the heart ensures that atrial contraction is complete before ventricular contraction (systole) begins. At the end of systole the ventricles relax and the atrioventricular valves open, allowing them to refill with blood from the atria (diastole).

## The history

### Common presenting symptoms

Cardiovascular disease may present with a number of diverse symptoms; non-cardiac causes must also be considered (Box 4.1).

### 4.1 Common symptoms of heart disease

| Symptom | Cardiovascular causes | Other causes |
|---------|----------------------|--------------|
| Chest discomfort | Myocardial infarction<br>Angina<br>Pericarditis<br>Aortic dissection | Oesophageal spasm<br>Pneumothorax<br>Musculoskeletal pain |
| Breathlessness | Heart failure<br>Valvular disease<br>Angina<br>Pulmonary embolism<br>Pulmonary hypertension | Respiratory disease<br>Anaemia<br>Obesity<br>Anxiety |
| Palpitation | Tachyarrhythmias<br>Ectopic beats | Anxiety<br>Hyperthyroidism<br>Drugs |
| Syncope/presyncope | Arrhythmias<br>Postural hypotension<br>Aortic stenosis<br>Hypertrophic cardiomyopathy<br>Atrial myxoma | Simple faints<br>Epilepsy<br>Anxiety |
| Oedema | Heart failure<br>Constrictive pericarditis<br>Venous stasis<br>Lymphoedema | Nephrotic syndrome<br>Liver disease<br>Drugs<br>Immobility |

## Chest pain

### Intermittent chest pain

Chest pain due to intermittent myocardial ischaemia (angina pectoris) is typically a dull discomfort, often described as a tight or pressing 'band-like' sensation akin to a heavy weight. It tends to be felt diffusely across the anterior chest and may radiate down one or both arms and into the throat, jaw or teeth. In stable angina (caused by chronic narrowing in one or more coronary arteries), episodes of pain are precipitated by exertion and may occur more readily when walking in cold or windy weather, after a large meal or while carrying a heavy load; the pain is promptly relieved by rest and/or sublingual glyceryl nitrate (GTN) spray, and typically lasts for less than 10 minutes. The degree of physical exertion required to precipitate symptoms is a better guide to disease severity than the intensity of discomfort (Box 4.2). Chest pain can be classified into typical angina, atypical angina and non-anginal chest pain (Box 4.3). A history of typical angina significantly increases the likelihood of obstructive coronary heart disease. In unstable angina (caused by a sudden severe narrowing in a coronary artery), there is usually an abrupt onset or a worsening of chest pain episode that may occur on minimal exertion or at rest. It may be difficult to distinguish between angina and non-cardiac causes of episodic chest pain, such as oesophageal pain or musculoskeletal problems (Box 4.4). The latter may occur at any site over the chest, often vary with posture or specific movements (such as twisting or turning) and may be associated with tenderness to palpation.

Ask about:

- site, onset, severity and character of the pain, and whether the pain radiates anywhere
- associated symptoms such as breathlessness
- aggravating and relieving factors, especially their relationship to exertion
- frequency and duration of symptoms, and any recent change in pattern
- degree of limitation caused by symptoms.

### 4.2 Canadian Cardiovascular Society: functional classification of stable angina

| Grade | Description |
|-------|-------------|
| 1 | Ordinary physical activity, such as walking and climbing stairs, does not cause angina. Angina with strenuous, rapid or prolonged exertion at work or during recreation |
| 2 | Slight limitation of ordinary activity. Walking or climbing stairs rapidly, walking uphill, walking or climbing stairs after meals, in cold, in wind, or when under emotional stress, or only during the few hours after awakening |
| 3 | Marked limitation of ordinary physical activity. Walking one to two blocks on the level and climbing less than one flight in normal conditions |
| 4 | Inability to carry on any physical activity without discomfort; angina may be present at rest |

### 4.3 Nature of chest pain and likelihood of obstructive coronary heart disease

| Type | Characteristics | Likelihood of obstructive coronary heart disease |
|------|-----------------|--------------------------------------------------|
| Typical angina | Meets all three of the following characteristics:<br>• retrosternal chest discomfort of characteristic quality and duration;<br>• provoked by exertion or emotional stress;<br>• relieved by rest and/or nitrates within minutes. | ++++ |
| Atypical angina | Meets two of these characteristics. | ++ |
| Non-anginal chest pain | Meets only one or none of the characteristics. | – |

### Acute chest pain

Myocardial infarction causes symptoms that are similar to, but more severe and prolonged than, those of angina pectoris. Associated features include restlessness, breathlessness and a feeling of impending death (*angor animi*). Radiation to one or both arms/shoulders, an association with exertion, sweating, nausea or vomiting and similarity to previous myocardial infarction all increase the likelihood of acute myocardial infarction. Pain that is pleuritic, positional, sharp, or reproduced with palpation is unlikely to be due to myocardial infarction.

Pericardial pain is typically a constant anterior central chest pain that may radiate to the shoulders. It tends to be sharp or stabbing in character, exacerbated by inspiration or lying down, and relieved by sitting forwards. It is caused by inflammation of the pericardium secondary to viral infection, connective tissue disease or myocardial infarction, or after surgery, catheter ablation or radiotherapy.

Aortic dissection (a tear in the intima of the thoracic aorta) is a life-threatening condition which is often missed. It is associated with abrupt onset of very severe, tearing chest pain that can radiate to the back (typically the interscapular region) and may be associated with profound autonomic stimulation. Over 90% of patients report the pain as severe or their 'worst ever', and the onset is sudden in 85% of cases; the absence of abrupt onset makes the diagnosis less likely. If the tear involves the cranial or upper limb arteries, there may be associated syncope, stroke or upper limb pulse asymmetry. Predisposing factors include connective tissue disorders, such as Marfan's syndrome (see Fig. 3.21A–D), family history of aortic disease, known aortic valve disease, previous aortic manipulation and known thoracic aortic aneurysm.

As with intermittent chest pain, explore the characteristics of the pain, and ask specifically about associated symptoms that

## 4.4 Cardiovascular causes of chest pain and their characteristics

|  | Angina | Myocardial infarction | Aortic dissection | Pericardial pain | Oesophageal pain |
|---|---|---|---|---|---|
| Site | Retrosternal | Retrosternal | Interscapular/retrosternal | Retrosternal or left-sided | Retrosternal or epigastric |
| Onset | Progressive increase in intensity over 1–2 minutes | Rapid over a few minutes | Very sudden | Gradual; postural change may suddenly aggravate | Over 1–2 minutes; can be sudden (spasm) |
| Character | Constricting, heavy | Constricting, heavy | Tearing or ripping | Sharp, 'stabbing', pleuritic | Gripping, tight or burning |
| Radiation | Sometimes arm(s), neck epigastrium | Often to arm(s), neck, jaw sometimes epigastrium | Back, between shoulders | Left shoulder or back | Often to back sometimes to arms |
| Associated features | Breathlessness | Sweating, nausea, vomiting, breathlessness, feeling of impending death (angor animi) | Sweating, syncope, focal neurological signs, signs of limb ischaemia, mesenteric ischaemia | Flu-like prodrome, breathlessness, fever | Heartburn, acid reflux |
| Timing | Intermittent, with episodes lasting 2–10 minutes | Acute presentation; prolonged duration | Acute presentation; prolonged duration | Acute presentation; variable duration | Intermittent, often at night-time; variable duration |
| Exacerbating/relieving factors | Triggered by emotion, exertion, especially if cold, windy Relieved by rest, nitrates | 'Stress' and exercise are rare triggers, usually spontaneous Not relieved by rest or nitrates | SpontaneousNo manoeuvres relieve pain | Sitting up/lying down may affect intensity NSAIDs help | Lying flat/some foods may trigger Not relieved by rest; nitrates sometimes relieve |
| Severity | Mild to moderate | Usually severe | Very severe | Can be severe | Usually mild but oesophageal spasm can mimic myocardial infarction |
| Cause | Coronary atherosclerosis, aortic stenosis, hypertrophic cardiomyopathy | Plaque rupture and coronary artery occlusion | Thoracic aortic dissection rupture | Pericarditis (usually viral, also post myocardial infarction) | Oesophageal spasm, reflux, hiatus hernia |

*NSAIDs,* Non-steroidal anti-inflammatory drugs.

may guide you to a likely diagnosis, such as interscapular pain, sweating, nausea, vomiting, syncope or neurological features (see Box 4.4).

## Dyspnoea (breathlessness)

Heart failure is the most common cardiovascular cause of both acute and chronic dyspnoea (Box 4.5). Other cardiovascular causes of acute breathlessness include valvular heart disease, pulmonary embolism and arrhythmia, whilst non-cardiac dyspnoea may be due to pulmonary disease, obesity, anaemia, neuromuscular disease, chest wall disorders, pregnancy, hyperventilation syndrome and anxiety disorders.

Patients with acute heart failure and pulmonary oedema (accumulation of fluid in the alveoli) usually prefer to be upright, while patients with massive pulmonary embolism are often more comfortable lying flat and may faint (syncope) if made to sit upright.

Exertional dyspnoea is the symptomatic hallmark of chronic heart failure. The New York Heart Association grading system is used to assess the degree of symptomatic limitation caused by the exertional breathlessness of heart failure (Box 4.6). Dyspnoea

## 4.5 Some mechanisms and causes of heart failure

| Mechanism | Cause |
|---|---|
| Reduced ventricular contractility (systolic dysfunction) | Myocardial infarction Dilated cardiomyopathy, e.g. genetic, idiopathic, alcohol excess, cytotoxic drugs, peripartum cardiomyopathy Myocarditis |
| Impaired ventricular filling (diastolic dysfunction) | Left ventricular hypertrophy Constrictive pericarditis Hypertrophic or restrictive cardiomyopathy |
| Increased metabolic and cardiac demand (rare) | Thyrotoxicosis Arteriovenous fistulae Paget's disease |
| Valvular or congenital lesions | Mitral and/or aortic valve disease Tricuspid and/or pulmonary valve disease (rare) Ventricular septal defect Patent ductus arteriosus |

| Class | Description |
|-------|-------------|
| I | No limitations. Ordinary physical activity does not cause undue fatigue, dyspnoea or palpitation (asymptomatic left ventricular dysfunction) |
| II | Slight limitation of physical activity. Such patients are comfortable at rest. Ordinary physical activity results in fatigue, palpitation, dyspnoea or angina pectoris (symptomatically 'mild' heart failure) |
| III | Marked limitation of physical activity. Less than ordinary physical activity will lead to symptoms (symptomatically 'moderate' heart failure) |
| IV | Symptoms of congestive heart failure are present, even at rest. With any physical activity, increased discomfort is experienced (symptomatically 'severe' heart failure) |

**4.6 New York Heart Association classification of heart failure symptom severity**

caused by myocardial ischaemia is known as 'angina equivalent'. It may occur instead of, or with, chest discomfort, especially in patients who are elderly or who have diabetes. It has identical precipitants to angina and may be relieved by GTN.

Orthopnoea, dyspnoea on lying flat, may occur in patients with heart failure, where it signifies advanced disease or incipient decompensation. Lying flat increases venous return and in patients with left ventricular impairment may precipitate pulmonary oedema. The severity can be graded by the number of pillows used at night: 'three-pillow orthopnoea', for example. Paroxysmal nocturnal dyspnoea is caused by the same mechanism, resulting in sudden breathlessness that wakes the patient from sleep (Fig. 4.3). Patients may choke or gasp for air, sit on the edge of the bed and open windows in an attempt to relieve their distress. It may be confused with asthma, which can also cause night-time dyspnoea, chest tightness, cough and wheeze, but patients with heart failure may also produce frothy white or blood-stained sputum.

Bendopnoea is a symptom of dyspnoea when bending forward at the waist and is associated with increased cardiac filling pressures. Whilst common (18–49%) in patients with heart failure, it is not diagnostic and may occur in other conditions.

In acute dyspnoea, ask about:

- duration of onset
- background symptoms of exertional dyspnoea and usual exercise tolerance
- associated symptoms: chest pain, syncope, palpitation or respiratory symptoms (such as cough, sputum, wheeze or haemoptysis; p. 87).

In patients with chronic symptoms, ask about:

- relationship between symptoms and exertion
- degree of limitation caused by symptoms and their impact on everyday activities
- effect of posture on symptoms and/or episodes of nocturnal breathlessness
- associated symptoms: ankle swelling, cough, wheeze or sputum.

## Palpitation

Palpitation is an unexpected or unpleasant awareness of the heart beating in the chest. Detailed history-taking can help to distinguish the different types of palpitation (Box 4.7).

Ask about:

- nature of the palpitation: is the heart beat rapid, forceful or irregular? Can the patient tap it out?
- timing of symptoms: speed of onset and offset; frequency and duration of episodes
- precipitants for symptoms or relieving factors
- associated symptoms: presyncope, syncope or chest pain
- history of underlying cardiac disease.

Healthy people are occasionally aware of their heart beating with normal (sinus) rhythm, especially after exercise or in stressful situations such as when waiting for an interview or examination. The sensation is often more common in bed at night and slim people may notice it when lying on their left side.

Ectopic beats (extrasystoles) are a benign cause of palpitation at rest and are abolished by exercise. The premature ectopic beat produces a small stroke volume and an impalpable impulse due to incomplete left ventricular filling. The subsequent compensatory pause leads to ventricular overfilling and a forceful contraction with the next beat. Accordingly, patients often

**Mechanism**

Fluid redistributed into lungs

Reabsorption of fluid from tissues into plasma

Rise in left atrial pressure and fall in $PaO_2$ during sleep

Increased venous return to heart

**Features**

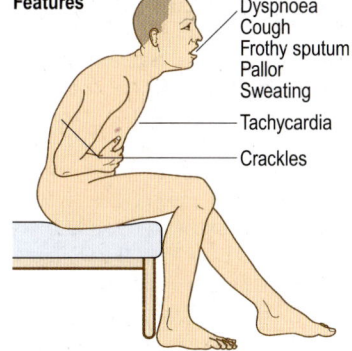

Dyspnoea
Cough
Frothy sputum
Pallor
Sweating
Tachycardia
Crackles

**Fig. 4.3 Paroxysmal nocturnal dyspnoea.**

## 4.7 Descriptions of arrhythmias

| | Extrasystoles | Sinus tachycardia | Supraventricular tachycardia | Atrial fibrillation | Ventricular tachycardia |
|---|---|---|---|---|---|
| Site | – | – | – | – | – |
| Onset | Sudden | Gradual | Sudden, with 'jump' | Sudden | Sudden |
| Character | 'Jump', missed beat or flutter | Regular, fast, 'pounding' | Regular, fast | Irregular, usually fast; slower in elderly | Regular, fast |
| Radiation | – | – | – | – | – |
| Associated features | Nil | Anxiety | Polyuria, lightheadedness, chest tightness | Polyuria, breathlessness Syncope uncommon | Presyncope, syncope, chest tightness |
| Timing | Brief | A few minutes | Minutes to hours | Variable | Variable |
| Exacerbating/relieving factors | Fatigue, caffeine, alcohol may trigger, often relieved by walking (increases sinus rate) | Exercise or anxiety may trigger | Usually at rest, trivial movements, e.g. bending, may trigger Vagal manoeuvres may relieve | Exercise or alcohol may trigger; often spontaneous | Exercise may trigger; often spontaneous |
| Severity | Mild (usually) | Mild to moderate | Moderate to severe | Very variable, may be asymptomatic | Often severe |

describe 'missed beats', sometimes followed by a particularly strong heart beat ('jolt' or 'thump').

Supraventricular tachycardia produces sudden paroxysms of rapid, regular palpitation that can sometimes be terminated with vagal stimulation using Valsalva breathing manoeuvres or carotid sinus pressure. It often affects young patients with no other underlying cardiac disease. Ventricular tachycardia can produce similar symptoms but is more commonly associated with presyncope or syncope, and tends to affect patients with cardiomyopathy or previous myocardial infarction.

High-risk features that increase the likelihood of a life-threatening arrhythmia such as ventricular tachycardia include:

- previous myocardial infarction or cardiac surgery
- associated syncope or severe chest pain
- family history of sudden death
- Wolff–Parkinson–White syndrome
- significant structural heart disease such as hypertrophic cardiomyopathy or aortic stenosis.

## Syncope and presyncope

Syncope is a transient loss of consciousness due to transient cerebral hypoperfusion and episodes are typically characterised by rapid onset, short duration, and spontaneous complete recovery. Causes include postural hypotension, neurocardiogenic syncope, arrhythmias and mechanical obstruction to cardiac output. The same mechanisms may lead to a sensation of lightheadedness and impending loss of consciousness without progressing to actual loss of consciousness (presyncope). The main differential diagnosis of syncope is seizure (p. 136), while lightheadedness and presyncope must be distinguished from dizziness or vertigo due to non-cardiovascular causes (p. 44).

In patients who present with syncope, ask about:

- circumstances of the event and any preceding symptoms: palpitation, chest pain, lightheadedness, nausea, tinnitus, sweating or visual disturbance
- duration of loss of consciousness, appearance of the patient while unconscious and any injuries sustained (a detailed witness history is extremely helpful)
- time to recovery of full consciousness and normal cognition
- current driving status, including occupational driving.

In patients with presyncopal symptoms of lightheadedness or dizziness, ask about:

- exact nature of symptoms and associated features such as palpitation
- precipitants for symptoms, such as postural change, prolonged standing, intense emotion or exertion
- frequency of episodes and impact on lifestyle
- possible contributing medications, such as antihypertensive agents (Box 4.8).

Postural hypotension, a fall of more than 20 mmHg in systolic blood pressure on standing, may lead to syncope or presyncope. It can be caused by hypovolaemia, drugs (see Box 4.8) or autonomic neuropathy and is common in the elderly, affecting up to one-third of individuals over 65 years.

Reflex or neurocardiogenic syncope results from excessive autonomic reflexes which produce sudden bradycardia) and/or vasodilatation. Vasovagal syncope is the most common form of reflex syncope and may be triggered in healthy people following a period of prolonged standing or a painful or emotional stimulus, such as the sight of blood. There is typically a prodrome of lightheadedness, tinnitus, nausea, sweating and facial pallor, and a darkening of vision before loss of consciousness. When laid flat to aid cerebral circulation the individual wakes up, often flushing from vasodilatation and nauseated or even vomiting due to vagal overactivity. If the person is held upright by misguided

**4.8 Symptoms related to medication**

| Symptom | Medication |
|---|---|
| Angina | Aggravated by thyroxine or drug-induced anaemia, e.g. aspirin or NSAIDs |
| Dyspnoea | Beta-blockers in patients with asthma<br>Exacerbation of heart failure by beta-blockers, some calcium channel antagonists (verapamil, diltiazem), NSAIDs |
| Palpitation | Tachycardia and/or arrhythmia from thyroxine, $\beta_2$ stimulants, e.g. salbutamol, digoxin toxicity, hypokalaemia from diuretics, tricyclic antidepressants |
| Syncope/ presyncope | Vasodilators, e.g. nitrates, alpha-blockers, ACE inhibitors and angiotensin II receptor antagonists<br>Bradycardia from rate-limiting agents, e.g. beta-blockers, some calcium channel antagonists (verapamil, diltiazem), digoxin, amiodarone |
| Oedema | Glucocorticoids, NSAIDs, some calcium channel antagonists, e.g. nifedipine, amlodipine |

*ACE,* Angiotensin-converting enzyme; *NSAIDs,* non-steroidal anti-inflammatory drugs.

bystanders, continued cerebral hypoperfusion delays recovery and may lead to a seizure and a mistaken diagnosis of epilepsy. In patients presenting with transient loss of consciousness, predictors of vasovagal syncope include a history of syncope or presyncope with pain or medical procedures, an age less than 35 at first syncopal episode, prodrome of sweating, warmth or abdominal discomfort or a postdrome of nausea.

In patients with hypersensitive carotid sinus syndrome, pressure over the carotid sinus may lead to reflex bradycardia and syncope.

Arrhythmias can cause syncope or presyncope. The most common cause is bradyarrhythmia caused by sinoatrial disease or atrioventricular block: Stokes–Adams attacks. Rate-limiting drugs are a common cause of bradyarrhythmia. Supraventricular tachyarrhythmias, like atrial fibrillation, rarely cause syncope whereas ventricular tachycardia often causes syncope or presyncope, especially in patients with impaired left ventricular function.

Mechanical obstruction to left ventricular outflow, including severe aortic stenosis and hypertrophic cardiomyopathy, can cause syncope or presyncope, especially on exertion, when cardiac output cannot meet the increased metabolic demand. Massive pulmonary embolism can lead to syncope by obstructing outflow from the right ventricle; associated features are usually apparent and include acute dyspnoea, chest pain and hypoxia. Cardiac tumours, such as atrial myxoma, and thrombosis, or failure of prosthetic heart valves are rare causes of syncope.

## Oedema

Excess fluid in the interstitial space causes oedema (tissue swelling). It is usually gravity-dependent and so is seen especially around the ankles, or over the sacrum in patients lying in bed. Unilateral lower limb oedema may occur in deep vein thrombosis (DVT) (p. 77). Heart failure is a common cause of bilateral lower limb oedema, but other causes include chronic venous disease, vasodilating calcium channel antagonists (such as amlodipine) and hypoalbuminaemia.

## Other symptoms of cardiac disease

Infective endocarditis, microbial infection of a heart valve, frequently presents with non-specific symptoms, including weight loss, tiredness, fever and night sweats.

Embolisation of intracardiac thrombus, tumour (such as atrial myxoma) or infective 'vegetations' (Fig. 4.4) may produce symptoms of stroke (p. 74), acute limb ischaemia (p. XXX) or acute mesenteric ischaemia (p. 73).

Advanced heart failure may result in either abdominal distension due to ascites, or weight loss and muscle wasting ('cardiac cachexia') due to a prolonged catabolic state.

## Past medical history

Obtaining a detailed record of any previous cardiac disease, investigations and interventions is essential (Box 4.9). You may need to consult the patient, family members and electronic case records.

Also ask about:

- conditions associated with increased risk of vascular disease such as hypertension, diabetes mellitus and hyperlipidaemia
- rheumatic fever or heart murmurs during childhood
- potential causes of bacteraemia in patients with suspected infective endocarditis, such as skin infection, recent dental work, intravenous drug use or penetrating trauma
- systemic disorders with cardiovascular manifestations such as connective tissue diseases (pericarditis and Raynaud's phenomenon), Marfan's syndrome (aortic dissection) and myotonic dystrophy (atrioventricular block).

## Drug history

Drugs may cause or aggravate symptoms such as breathlessness, chest pain, oedema, palpitation or syncope (see Box 4.8). Ask about 'over-the-counter' purchases, such as non-steroidal anti-inflammatory drugs (NSAIDs) and alternative and herbal medicines, as these may have cardiovascular actions.

## Family history

Many cardiac disorders such as cardiomyopathies have a genetic component. Ask about premature coronary artery disease in first-degree relatives (<60 years in a female or <55 years in a male); sudden unexplained death at a young age may raise the possibility of a cardiomyopathy or inherited arrhythmia. Patients with venous thrombosis may have inherited thrombophilia, such as a factor V Leiden mutation. Familial hypercholesterolaemia is associated with premature arterial disease. Aortic disease can be

A          B          C

**Fig. 4.4** **Cardiac sources of systemic embolism: echocardiographic images.** [A] A large apical thrombus in the left ventricle *(arrow)*. [B] An atrial myxoma attached to the interatrial septum *(arrow)*. [C] A vegetation on the mitral valve *(arrow)* in infective endocarditis. Because all of these lesions are located within the left side of the heart, emboli would flow to the systemic (or coronary) circulation. Conversely, emboli from the right side of the heart would flow to the pulmonary circulation.

inherited, and a family history of aortic aneurysm or dissection may be relevant.

## Social history

Smoking is the strongest risk factor for coronary and peripheral arterial disease (PAD). Take a detailed smoking history (p. 16). Alcohol can induce atrial fibrillation and, in excess, is associated with obesity, hypertension and dilated cardiomyopathy. Recreational drugs such as cocaine and amphetamines can cause arrhythmias, chest pain, occlusive and aneurysmal PAD and even myocardial infarction. Heart disease may have important consequences for employment. Patients with limiting exertional symptoms may struggle to perform jobs that entail a high degree

of physical activity. In addition, some diagnoses such as ischaemic heart disease or cardiac arrhythmia may impact on eligibility for certain occupations that have implications for public safety, such as commercial drivers and pilots. Finally, ask about undue stress or anxiety as these are commonly associated with cardiac-type symptoms including chest pain, dyspnoea and palpitation.

## The physical examination (Video 3)

Tailor the sequence and extent of examination to the patient's condition. If you suspect that the person may be unstable, deteriorating or critically unwell (breathless, distressed, cyanosed

### 4.9 Key elements of the past cardiac history

|  | Ischaemic heart disease | Heart failure | Valvular disease |
|---|---|---|---|
| Baseline symptoms | Exertional angina? If so, ascertain functional limitation (see Box 4.2) / response to GTN spray | Dyspnoea, fatigue, ankle swelling Record usual functional status (see Box 4.6) | Often asymptomatic Exertional dyspnoea (common), chest pain or syncope |
| Major events | Previous myocardial infarction/unstable angina | Hospitalisation for decompensated heart failure Ventricular arrhythmias | Infective endocarditis Previous rheumatic fever |
| Investigations | Coronary angiography (invasive or computed tomography): presence, extent and severity of coronary artery disease, Exercise electrocardiogram (or other stress test): evidence of inducible ischaemia? Exercise capacity and symptoms | Echocardiogram (± cardiac magnetic resonance imaging): left ventricular size, wall thickness and systolic function; valvular disease; right ventricular function | Echocardiogram (transthoracic ± transoesophageal): nature and severity of valve lesion; ventricular size and function |
| Procedures | Percutaneous coronary intervention (angioplasty and stenting) Coronary artery bypass graft surgery | Implantable cardioverter–defibrillator Cardiac resynchronisation therapy | Surgical valve repair or replacement (note whether mechanical or bioprosthetic) Transcatheter valve procedures |

*GTN*, Glyceryl trinitrate.

or obtunded, for example), adopt an ABCDE approach initially (p. 395) and defer detailed examination until stabilised. In stable patients, perform a detailed and comprehensive physical examination.

## General examination

Look at the patient's general appearance. Do they look unwell, frightened or distressed? Are there any signs of breathlessness or cyanosis? Is the patient overweight or cachectic? Are there any features of conditions associated with cardiovascular disease such as Marfan's (p. 33), Down's (p. 39) or Turner's syndrome (p. 106), or ankylosing spondylitis (p. 300)?

Conclude by examining the entire skin surface for petechiae, checking the temperature (p. 345) and performing urinalysis (p. 281). Fever is a feature of infective endocarditis and pericarditis, and may occur after myocardial infarction. Urinalysis is necessary to check for haematuria (endocarditis, vasculitis), glucosuria (diabetes) and proteinuria (hypertension and renal disease).

## Hands

### Examination sequence (Video 3A) ▶

- Feel the temperature of the hands and measure capillary refill time (p. 396).
- Examine the hands for tobacco staining (see Fig. 5.7), skin crease pallor (anaemia) or peripheral cyanosis.
- Look at the nails for finger clubbing (p. 326) and for splinter haemorrhages: linear, reddish-brown marks along the axis of the fingernails and toenails (Fig. 4.5B).
- Examine the extensor surface of the hands for tendon xanthomata: hard, slightly yellowish masses over the extensor tendons of the hand from lipid deposits (see Fig. 4.6B).
- Examine the palmar aspect of the hands for:
  - Janeway lesions: painless, blanching red macules on the thenar/hypothenar eminences (see Fig. 4.5A)
  - Osler's nodes: painful raised erythematous lesions, typically on the pads of the fingers (see Fig. 4.5C).

The hands usually feel dry and warm at ambient temperature. Normal capillary refill time is 2 seconds or less. Cool extremities and prolonged capillary refill time signify impaired peripheral perfusion, which may occur in shock (p. 57) or chronic conditions associated with a low cardiac output state (as in severe aortic stenosis, mitral stenosis or pulmonary hypertension).

One or two isolated splinter haemorrhages from trauma are common in healthy individuals, especially in manual workers. Splinter haemorrhages (see Fig. 4.5B) are found in infective endocarditis and some vasculitic disorders. A petechial rash (caused by vasculitis), most often present on the legs and conjunctivae (see Fig. 4.5E), is a transient finding in endocarditis and can be confused with the rash of meningococcal disease. Janeway lesions and Osler's nodes (see Fig. 4.5A and C) are features of endocarditis but are rare in the modern era.

Tendon xanthomata (Fig. 4.6) are a sign of familial hypercholesterolaemia, a genetic disorder associated with severe

**Fig. 4.5 Peripheral signs that may be present in infective endocarditis.** **A** Janeway lesions on the hypothenar eminence *(arrows)*. **B** Splinter haemorrhages. **C** Osler's nodes. **D** Roth's spot on fundoscopy. **E** Petechial haemorrhages on the conjunctiva. *(B and E) From Walker BR, Colledge NR, Ralston SR, et al., eds. Davidson's Principles and Practice of Medicine. 22nd ed. Edinburgh: Churchill Livingstone; 2014. (D) From Forbes CD, Jackson WF. Color Atlas of Clinical Medicine. 3rd ed. Edinburgh: Mosby; 2003.*

elevations in serum cholesterol and premature coronary artery disease.

## Face

### Examination sequence (Video 3B) ▶

- Look in the mouth for central cyanosis: a purplish blue discoloration of the lips and underside of the tongue (see Fig. 5.11).
- Examine the eyelids for xanthelasmata: soft, yellowish plaques found periorbitally and on the medial aspect of the eyelids (Fig. 4.6A).
- Look at the iris for corneal arcus: a creamy yellow discoloration at the boundary of the iris and cornea (Fig. 4.6C).
- Examine the fundi (p. 184) for features of hypertension (p. 189), diabetes (p. 188) or Roth's spots (flame-shaped retinal haemorrhages with a 'cotton-wool' centre; Fig. 4.5D).

Cardiac causes of central cyanosis include heart failure sufficient to cause pulmonary congestion and oedema impairing gas

A

B

C

**Fig. 4.6 Features of hyperlipidaemia.** A Xanthelasmata. B Tendon xanthomata. C Corneal arcus. *(B) From Swartz M. Textbook of Physical Diagnosis. 6th ed. Philadelphia: Saunders; 2009. (C) From Kanski J. Clinical Diagnosis in Ophthalmology. London: Mosby; 2006.*

exchange, or, rarely, congenital heart disease, in which case it is associated with right-to-left shunting and finger clubbing (p. 326).

Xanthelasmata and corneal arcus (see Fig. 4.6A and C) are associated with hyperlipidaemia but also occur frequently in normolipidaemic patients. The presence of xanthelasma is an independent risk factor for coronary heart disease and

myocardial infarction but corneal arcus has no independent prognostic value.

## Arterial pulses

The palpable pulse in an artery reflects the pressure wave generated by the ejection of blood into the circulation from the left ventricle.

When taking a pulse, assess:

- rate: the number of pulses occurring per minute
- rhythm: the pattern or regularity of pulses
- volume: the perceived degree of pulsation
- character: an impression of the pulse waveform or shape.

The rate and rhythm of the pulse are usually determined at the radial artery; use the larger pulses (brachial, carotid or femoral) to assess the pulse volume and character.

## Examination sequence

### Radial pulse (Video 3C)
- Place the pads of your index and middle fingers over the right wrist, just lateral to the flexor carpi radialis tendon (Fig. 4.7A).
- Assess the rhythm of the pulse and count the number over 15 seconds; multiply by 4 to obtain the rate in beats per minute (bpm).
- To detect a collapsing pulse: first, check that the patient has no shoulder or arm pain or restriction on movement; next, feel the pulse with the base of your fingers, then raise the patient's arm vertically above their head (see Fig. 4.7B).
- Palpate both radial pulses simultaneously, assessing any delay between the two.

### Brachial pulse
- Cup your hand under the elbow and use your thumb to palpate the pulse in the antecubital fossa, just medial to the biceps tendon (see Fig. 4.7C). Use your right thumb for the patient's right arm and your left thumb for the patient's left arm. Assess the character and volume of the pulse.

### Carotid pulse (Video 3D)
- Explain what you are going to do.
- With the patient semi-recumbent, place the tips of your fingers between the larynx and the anterior border of the sternocleidomastoid muscle (see Fig. 4.7D).
- Palpate the pulse gently to avoid a vagal reflex, and never assess both carotids simultaneously.
- Listen for bruits over both carotid arteries, using the diaphragm of your stethoscope in held inspiration.

## Rate and rhythm

Resting heart rate is normally 50–95 bpm but should be considered in the clinical context. A pulse rate of 40 bpm can be normal in a fit young adult, whereas a pulse rate of 65 bpm may be abnormally low in acute heart failure. Bradycardia is defined as a pulse rate of less than 60 bpm; tachycardia is a rate of greater than 100 bpm. The most common causes of bradycardia are medication, athletic conditioning and sinoatrial or

4

**Fig. 4.7 The radial, brachial and carotid pulses.** A Locating and palpating the radial pulse. B Feeling for a collapsing radial pulse. C Assessing the brachial pulse. D Locating the right carotid pulse with the fingers.

atrioventricular node dysfunction. The most common cause of tachycardia is sinus tachycardia (Box 4.10).

The pulse may be regular or irregular (see Box 4.10). Sinus rhythm is regular (Fig. 4.8A) but heart rate varies with the respiratory cycle, particularly in children, young adults or athletes (sinus arrhythmia). During inspiration, parasympathetic tone falls and the heart rate increases; on expiration, the heart rate decreases (Box 4.11). With intermittent extrasystoles (see Fig. 4.8B) or second-degree atrioventricular block, there may be an underlying regularity to the pulse, interspersed with periods of irregularity (sometimes referred to as 'regularly irregular'). In atrial fibrillation the pulse has no appreciable pattern and is often described as 'irregularly irregular' (see Fig. 4.8C). The rate in atrial fibrillation depends on the number of beats conducted by the atrioventricular node. Untreated, the ventricular rate may be very fast (up to 200 bpm). The variability of the pulse rate (and therefore ventricular filling) explains why the pulse volume varies

**Fig. 4.8 Electrocardiogram rhythm strips.** A Sinus rhythm. B Ventricular ectopic beat. C Atrial fibrillation with 'controlled' ventricular response. D Atrial flutter: note the regular 'saw-toothed' atrial flutter waves at about 300/min. E Ventricular tachycardia, with a ventricular rate of about 200/min.

### 4.10 Causes of abnormal pulse rate or rhythm

| Abnormality | Sinus rhythm | Arrhythmia |
|---|---|---|
| Fast rate (tachycardia, >100 bpm) | Exercise<br>Pain<br>Excitement/anxiety<br>Fever<br>Hyperthyroidism<br>Medication:<br>  Sympathomimetics,<br>  e.g. salbutamol<br>  Vasodilators | Atrial fibrillation<br>Atrial flutter<br>Supraventricular tachycardia<br>Ventricular tachycardia |
| Slow rate (bradycardia, <60 bpm) | Sleep<br>Athletic training<br>Hypothyroidism<br>Medication:<br>  Beta-blockers<br>  Digoxin<br>  Verapamil, diltiazem | Carotid sinus hypersensitivity<br>Sick sinus syndrome<br>Second-degree heart block<br>Complete heart block |
| Irregular pulse | Sinus arrhythmia<br>Atrial extrasystoles<br>Ventricular extrasystoles | Atrial fibrillation<br>Atrial flutter with variable response<br>Second-degree heart block with variable response |

### 4.11 Haemodynamic effects of respiration

|  | Inspiration | Expiration |
|---|---|---|
| Pulse/heart rate | Accelerates | Slows |
| Systolic blood pressure | Falls (up to 10 mmHg) | Rises |
| Jugular venous pressure | Falls | Rises |
| Second heart sound | Splits | Fuses |

and there may be a pulse deficit, with some cycles not felt at the radial artery. The pulse deficit can be calculated by counting the radial pulse rate and subtracting this from the apical heart rate, assessed by auscultation.

## Volume and character

The ventricles fill during diastole. Longer diastolic intervals are associated with increased stroke volume, which is reflected by increased pulse volume on examination. Abnormalities of pulse volume and character are highly subjective, however, and tend to have poor inter-observer agreement.

A large pulse volume is a reflection of a large pulse pressure, which can occur in physiological states such as exercise or pregnancy, or in pathological conditions such as anaemia, thyrotoxicosis or aortic regurgitation.

Low pulse volume may result from severe heart failure and conditions associated with inadequate ventricular filling such as hypovolaemia, cardiac tamponade and mitral stenosis. Asymmetric pulses may represent occlusive PAD or stenosis and, rarely, aortic dissection. Coarctation is a congenital narrowing of the aorta, usually distal to the left subclavian artery (Fig. 4.9); it may produce reduced-volume lower limb pulses, which are also delayed relative to the upper limb pulses (radiofemoral delay). In adults, coarctation usually presents with hypertension and heart failure.

A slow-rising pulse has a gradual upstroke with a reduced peak occurring late in systole, and is a feature of severe aortic stenosis (Fig. 4.10).

A collapsing pulse may occur with severe aortic regurgitation. The peak of the pulse wave arrives early and is followed by a rapid fall in pressure (see Fig. 4.10) as blood flows back into the left ventricle, resulting in a wide pulse pressure (systolic – diastolic blood pressure >80 mmHg). This rapid fall imparts the 'collapsing' sensation, and is exaggerated by raising the patient's arm above the level of the heart (see Fig. 4.7B).

Pulsus bisferiens, an increased pulse with a double systolic peak separated by a distinct mid-systolic dip, is classically produced by concomitant aortic stenosis and regurgitation. Pulsus alternans, beat-to-beat variation in pulse volume with a normal rhythm, may occur in advanced heart failure. Both of these signs are rare, however, and of limited relevance in contemporary practice.

Pulsus paradoxus is an exaggeration of the normal variability of pulse volume with breathing. Pulse volume normally increases in

**Fig. 4.9** Coarctation of the aorta. Magnetic resonance image showing the typical site of aortic coarctation, just distal to the origin of the left subclavian artery *(arrow)*. This explains why there is synchrony of the radial pulses but radiofemoral delay.

**Fig. 4.10** Pulse waveforms.

expiration and decreases during inspiration due to intrathoracic pressure changes affecting venous return to the heart. This variability is exaggerated when ventricular diastolic filling is impeded by elevated intrapericardial pressure. This is usually due to accumulation of pericardial fluid (cardiac tamponade; Fig. 4.11) but can occur to a lesser extent with pericardial constriction and in acute severe asthma. If suspected, pulsus paradoxus can be confirmed using a blood pressure (BP) cuff (see later and Fig. 4.12); a fall of greater than 10 mmHg between the cuff pressure at which Korotkoff sounds appear in expiration only and the cuff pressure at which Korotkoff sounds persist throughout the respiratory cycle is diagnostic.

## Blood pressure

BP is a measure of the pressure that the circulating blood exerts against the arterial walls. Systolic pressure is the maximal pressure that occurs during ventricular contraction (systole). During ventricular filling (diastole), arterial pressure is maintained at a lower level by the elasticity and compliance of the vessel wall. The lowest value (diastolic pressure) occurs immediately before the next cycle.

BP is usually measured using a sphygmomanometer (see Fig. 4.12). In certain situations, such as the intensive care unit, it is measured invasively using an indwelling intra-arterial catheter connected to a pressure sensor.

BP is measured in mmHg and recorded as systolic pressure/ diastolic pressure, together with a note of where and how the reading was taken: for example, BP 146/92 mmHg, right arm, supine.

BP provides vital information on the haemodynamic condition of acutely ill or injured patients. Over the longer term it is also an important guide to cardiovascular risk. BP constantly varies and rises with stress, excitement and environment. 'White coat hypertension' refers to a transient increase in BP caused by the stress of being in a healthcare setting. Ambulatory BP measurement, using a portable device at intervals during normal daytime activity and at night, is better at determining cardiovascular risk.

## Hypertension

Although any threshold for distinguishing abnormal elevation of BP from normal BP is somewhat arbitrary, hypertension is widely defined as a systolic pressure of ≥140 mmHg and/or a diastolic pressure ≥90 mmHg (Box 4.12). Hypertension is associated with significant morbidity and mortality from vascular disease (heart failure, coronary artery disease, cerebrovascular disease

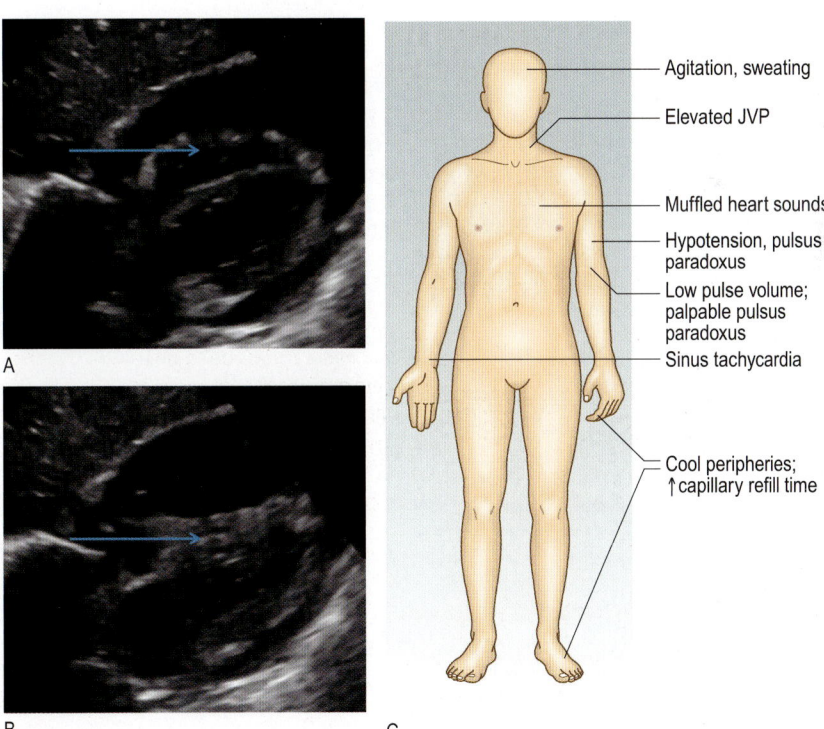

A

B

C

- Agitation, sweating
- Elevated JVP
- Muffled heart sounds
- Hypotension, pulsus paradoxus
- Low pulse volume; palpable pulsus paradoxus
- Sinus tachycardia
- Cool peripheries; ↑capillary refill time

**Fig. 4.11 Clinical and echocardiographic features of cardiac tamponade.** [A] and [B] Echocardiographic images taken from the subcostal position at the onset of systole (A) and in early diastole (B). The right ventricle *(arrows)* is collapsed in the early phase of diastole due to the elevated intrapericardial pressure; this is an important echo finding in tamponade. In both images there is a large pericardial effusion adjacent to the right ventricle. [C] Clinical features. *JVP,* jugular venous pressure.

**Fig. 4.12** Measuring the blood pressure.

and chronic kidney disease). It is almost invariably asymptomatic, although, rarely and in severe hypertension, headaches and visual disturbances can occur. In most hypertensive patients there is no identifiable cause – so-called 'essential hypertension'. Secondary hypertension is rare, occurring in less than 1% of the hypertensive population (Box 4.13).

| 4.12 European Society of Cardiology/European Society of Hypertension classification of blood pressure[a] and definitions of hypertension grade | | |
|---|---|---|
| **BP** | **Systolic BP (mmHg)** | **Diastolic BP (mmHg)** |
| Optimal | <120 | <80 |
| Normal | <130 | <85 |
| High normal | 130–139 | 85–89 |
| **Hypertension**<br>Grade 1 (mild) | 140–159 | 90–99 |
| Grade 2 (moderate) | 160–179 | 100–109 |
| Grade 3 (severe) | >180 | >110 |
| **Isolated systolic hypertension[b]** | 140–159 | <90 |

[a]BP category is defined according to seated clinic BP and by the highest level of BP, whether systolic or diastolic.
[b]Isolated systolic hypertension is graded 1, 2, or 3 according to SBP values in the ranges indicated.

*BP,* Blood pressure.

From Williams B, Mancia G, Spiering W, et al. 2018 ESC/ESH Guidelines for the management of arterial hypertension: The Task Force for the management of arterial hypertension of the European Society of Cardiology (ESC) and the European Society of Hypertension (ESH). *Eur Heart J*. 2018;39(33):3021–3104.

| 4.13 Clinical clues to secondary hypertension | |
|---|---|
| **Clinical feature** | **Cause** |
| Widespread vascular disease Renal bruit | Renovascular disease, including renal artery stenosis |
| Episodes of sweating, headache and palpitation | Phaeochromocytoma |
| Hypokalaemia | Primary aldosteronism |
| Cushingoid facies, central obesity, abdominal striae, proximal muscle weaknessChronic glucocorticoid use | Cushing's syndrome |
| Low-volume femoral pulses with radiofemoral delay | Coarctation of the aorta |
| Bilateral palpable kidneys | Adult polycystic kidney disease (p. 277) |

Assess the hypertensive patient for:

- potential underlying causes (see Box 4.13)
- end-organ damage:
  - cardiac: heart failure
  - renal: chronic kidney disease, proteinuria
  - eye: hypertensive retinopathy (see Fig. 8.18).

## Korotkoff sounds

These sounds are produced when the cuff pressure is between systolic and diastolic because the artery collapses completely and reopens with each heart beat, producing a snapping or knocking sound (Fig. 4.13). The first appearance of sounds (phase 1) during cuff deflation indicates systole. As pressure is

| Phase | Korotkoff sounds | |
|---|---|---|
| | | 120 mmHg systolic |
| 1 | A thud | |
| | | 110 mmHg |
| 2 | A blowing noise | |
| | | 100 mmHg |
| 3 | A softer thud | |
| | | 90 mmHg diastolic (1st) |
| 4 | A disappearing blowing noise | |
| | | 80 mmHg diastolic (2nd) |
| 5 | Nothing | |

**Fig. 4.13** Korotkoff sounds.

gradually reduced, the sounds muffle (phase 4) and then disappear (phase 5).

## Examination sequence (Video 4)

- Rest the patient for 5 minutes.
- Ideally, measure BP in both arms (brachial arteries); the higher of the two is closest to central aortic pressure and should be used to determine treatment.
- With the patient seated or lying down, support their arm comfortably at about heart level, with no tight clothing constricting the upper arm.
- Apply an appropriately sized cuff to the upper arm, with the centre of the bladder over the brachial artery.
- Palpate the brachial pulse.
- Inflate the cuff until the pulse is impalpable. Note the pressure on the manometer; this is a rough estimate of systolic pressure.
- Inflate the cuff another 30 mmHg and listen through the diaphragm of the stethoscope placed over the brachial artery.
- Deflate the cuff slowly (2–3 mmHg/s) until you hear a regular tapping sound (phase 1 Korotkoff sounds). Record the reading to the nearest 2 mmHg. This is the systolic pressure.
- Continue to deflate the cuff slowly until the sounds disappear.
- Record the pressure at which the sounds completely disappear as the diastolic pressure (phase 5). If muffled sounds persist (phase 4) and do not disappear, use the point of muffling as the diastolic pressure.

### Common problems in blood pressure (bp) measurement

- Different BP in each arm: a difference of greater than 10 mmHg on repeated measurements suggests the presence of aortic or subclavian artery disease. Record the highest pressure and use this to guide management.
- Wrong cuff size: the bladder should be approximately 80% of the length and 40% of the width of the upper arm circumference. A standard adult cuff has a bladder that measures approximately 13 × 30 cm and suits an arm circumference of 22–26 cm. In obese patients a standard adult cuff will overestimate BP, so use a large adult (bladder 16 × 38 cm) or thigh cuff (20 × 42 cm).
- Auscultatory gap: up to 20% of elderly hypertensive patients have Korotkoff sounds that appear at systolic pressure and disappear for an interval between systolic and diastolic pressure. If the first appearance of the sound is missed, the systolic pressure will be recorded at a falsely low level. Avoid this by palpating the systolic pressure first.
- Patient's arm at the wrong level: the patient's elbow should be level with the heart. Hydrostatic pressure causes a change of approximately 5 mmHg in recorded systolic and diastolic BP for a 7 cm change in arm elevation.
- Postural change: the pulse increases by about 11 bpm, systolic BP falls by 3–4 mmHg and diastolic BP rises by 5–6 mmHg when a healthy person stands. The BP stabilises after 1–2 minutes. Check the BP after a patient has been standing for 2 minutes; a drop of greater than 20 mmHg on standing is postural hypotension.
- Atrial fibrillation: in this condition, stroke volume and BP vary from beat to beat, making accurate measurement challenging, so extra care is needed. Reducing cuff pressure slowly and repeating the measurement more than once will allow an acceptable average value of BP to be obtained.

## Jugular venous pressure and waveform

Estimate the jugular venous pressure (JVP) by observing the level of pulsation in the internal jugular vein. The vein runs deep to the sternomastoid muscle and enters the thorax between the sternal and clavicular heads. The normal JVP waveform has two main peaks per cycle, which helps to distinguish it from the carotid arterial pulse (Box 4.14). Although the right internal jugular vein is traditionally used, studies using the left internal jugular vein have yielded similarly accurate results. The external jugular vein is more superficial, prominent and easier to see. It can be kinked or obstructed as it traverses the deep fascia of the neck but, when visible and pulsatile, can be used to estimate the JVP in difficult cases.

The JVP level reflects right atrial pressure (normally <7 mmHg/ 9–10 cmH$_2$O). If right atrial pressure is low, the patient may have to lie flat for the JVP to be seen; if high, the patient may need to sit upright (Fig. 4.14).

## Examination sequence (Video 3E)

- Position the patient supine, reclined at 45 degrees, with the head resting on a pillow and turned slightly to the left. The jugular venous pressure (JVP) is seen best if the sternocleidomastoid muscles and overlying skin are relaxed, so ensure the head is supported and avoid excessive head turning or elevation of the chin.
- Look across the patient's neck from the right side (Fig. 4.15A). Use oblique lighting if the JVP is difficult to see.

### 4.14 Differences between carotid artery and jugular venous pulsation

| Carotid | Jugular |
|---|---|
| Rapid outward movement | Rapid inward movement |
| One peak per heart beat | Two peaks per heart beat (in sinus rhythm) |
| Palpable | Impalpable |
| Pulsation unaffected by pressure at the root of the neck | Pulsation diminished by pressure at the root of the neck |
| Independent of respiration | Height of pulsation varies with respiration |
| Independent of the position of the patient | Varies with the position of the patient |
| Independent of abdominal pressure | Rises with abdominal pressure |

A                                   B                                   C

**Fig. 4.14 Jugular venous pressure in a healthy subject.** [A] Supine: jugular vein distended, pulsation not visible. [B] Reclining at 45 degrees: the point of transition between the distended and the collapsed vein can usually be seen to pulsate just above the clavicle. [C] Upright: the upper part of the vein is collapsed and the transition point obscured.

- Identify the jugular vein pulsation behind the sternocleido-mastoid muscle (usually just above the clavicle, unless it is elevated).
- If a pulsation is visualised, use the abdominojugular test and/or occlusion to help confirm that it is the JVP.
- The JVP is the vertical height in centimetres between the upper limit of the venous pulsation and the sternal angle (junction of the manubrium and sternum at the level of the second costal cartilages; Fig. 4.15B).
- Identify the timing and waveform of the pulsation and note any abnormality.

It can be difficult to differentiate the jugular venous waveform from arterial pulsation (see Box 4.14). If that is the case, the following may help:
- Abdominojugular test: press firmly over the abdomen. This increases venous return to the right side of the heart temporarily and the JVP normally rises.
- Changes with respiration: the JVP normally falls with inspiration due to decreased intrathoracic pressure.
- Waveform: the normal JVP waveform has two distinct peaks per cardiac cycle (see Fig. 4.15C):
  - The 'a' wave corresponds to right atrial contraction and occurs just before the first heart sound. In atrial fibrillation the 'a' wave is absent.
  - The 'v' wave is caused by atrial filling during ventricular systole when the tricuspid valve is closed.
  - Rarely, a third peak ('c' wave) may be seen due to closure of the tricuspid valve.
- Occlusion: the JVP waveform is obliterated by gently occluding the vein at the base of the neck with your finger.
- Changes with position: the JVP will vary with the position of the patient (see Fig. 4.14).

The JVP provides a reasonably accurate guide to central venous pressure, though it is better to estimate whether this is high, normal or low rather than attempting to measure a specific value. A JVP greater than 3 cm above the sternal angle strongly suggests elevated central venous pressure which occurs in states of volume overload (particularly heart failure). It is also elevated in any condition that leads to high right ventricular filling pressures, such as pulmonary embolism, chronic pulmonary hypertension, cardiac tamponade (see Fig. 4.11) or pericardial constriction (Box 4.15).

In patients presenting with dyspnoea, an elevated JVP is a very valuable sign for diagnosing heart failure; examine the patient for pulmonary oedema or pleural effusions (p. 85), ascites (p. 123) and/or peripheral oedema (p. 280).

Mechanical obstruction of the superior vena cava (most often caused by lung cancer) may cause extreme, non-pulsatile elevation of the JVP. In this case the JVP no longer reflects right atrial pressure and the abdominojugular test will be negative.

Kussmaul's sign is a paradoxical rise of JVP on inspiration that is seen in pericardial constriction, severe right ventricular failure and restrictive cardiomyopathy.

Prominent 'a' waves are caused by delayed or restricted right ventricular filling, as in pulmonary hypertension or tricuspid stenosis.

Cannon waves (giant 'a' waves) occur when the right atrium contracts against a closed tricuspid valve. Irregular cannon waves are seen in complete heart block and are due to atrio-ventricular dissociation. Regular cannon waves occur during junctional rhythm and with some ventricular and supraventricular tachycardias.

Tricuspid regurgitation results in prominent systolic 'v' waves, which can fuse with the 'c' waves to produce 'cv' waves; there may be an associated pulsatile liver.

## Precordium

The precordium is the anterior chest surface overlying the heart and great vessels.

Learn the surface anatomy and basic physiology of the heart to understand the basis and timing of the heart sounds and murmurs, and why they are heard best in different locations and radiate in a particular direction (Fig. 4.16).

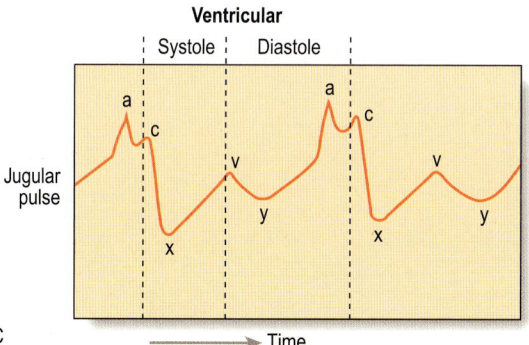

**Fig. 4.15 Jugular venous pressure.** [A] Inspecting the jugular venous pressure from the side (the internal jugular vein lies deep to the sternocleidomastoid muscle). [B] Measuring the height of the jugular venous pressure. [C] Form of the venous pulse wave tracing from the internal jugular vein: *a*, atrial systole; *c*, closure of the tricuspid valve; *v*, peak pressure in the right atrium immediately prior to opening of the tricuspid valve; *a–x*, descent, due to right atrial relaxation followed by downward displacement of the tricuspid ring during systole; *v–y*, descent at the commencement of ventricular filling.

**4.15 Abnormalities of the jugular venous pulse**

| Condition | Abnormalities |
|---|---|
| Heart failure | Elevation, sustained abdominojugular reflux >10 seconds |
| Pulmonary embolism | Elevation |
| Pericardial effusion | Elevation, prominent 'y' descent |
| Pericardial constriction | Elevation, Kussmaul's sign |
| Superior vena cava obstruction | Elevation, loss of pulsation |
| Atrial fibrillation | Absent 'a' waves |
| Tricuspid stenosis | Giant 'a' waves |
| Tricuspid regurgitation | Giant 'v' or 'cv' waves |
| Complete heart block | 'Cannon' waves |

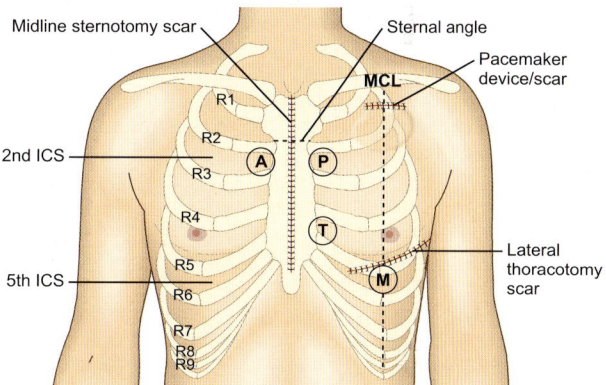

**Fig. 4.16** Surface anatomy of the praecordium with common scars, anatomical landmarks and areas for auscultation. *A*, Aortic area; *M*, mitral area; *P*, pulmonary area; *T*, tricuspid area; *R*, rib; *ICS*, intercostal space; *MCL*, mid-clavicular line.

## Inspection

Pectus excavatum (funnel chest; see Fig. 5.5D), a posterior displacement of the lower sternum, and pectus carinatum (pigeon chest; see Fig. 5.5C) may displace the heart and affect palpation and auscultation. Scars or visible bulges on the chest may indicate previous cardiac surgery or device implantation, e.g. cardiac pacemaker.

## Palpation

The cardiac impulse results from the left ventricle moving forwards and striking the chest wall during systole and may be visible on inspection. The apex beat is defined as the most lateral and inferior position at which the cardiac impulse can be felt. A heave is a palpable impulse that noticeably lifts your hand. A thrill is the tactile equivalent of a murmur and is a palpable vibration.

## Examination sequence (Video 3F) ▶

- Explain that you wish to examine the chest and ask the patient to remove all clothing above the waist. Keep a female patient's chest covered with a sheet as far as possible.
- Inspect the precordium with the patient sitting at a 45-degree angle with shoulders horizontal. Look for surgical scars, visible pulsations and chest deformity.
- Place your right hand flat over the precordium to obtain a general impression of the cardiac impulse (Fig. 4.17A) then lay your fingers on the chest parallel to the rib spaces to locate the most inferior and lateral position at which the impulse is palpable (the apex beat); if you cannot feel it, ask the patient to roll onto their left side (see Fig. 4.17B).
- Assess the character of the apex beat and note its position by counting down the intercostal spaces from the second, which is just below the sternal angle.
- Apply the heel of your right hand firmly to the left parasternal area and feel for a right ventricular heave. Ask the patient to hold their breath in expiration (see Fig. 4.17C).
- Palpate for thrills at the apex and on both sides of the sternum using the flat of your fingers.

A midline sternotomy scar usually indicates previous valve replacement or coronary artery bypass surgery, in which case it may be accompanied by the saphenous vein or radial artery graft harvest scars. A left submammary scar is usually the result of mitral valvotomy or transapical-transcatheter aortic-valve implantation. Infraclavicular scars are seen after pacemaker or defibrillator implantation, and the bulge of the device may be obvious in this position.

A normal apical impulse briefly lifts your fingers and is localised, but it may be impalpable, particularly in overweight or muscular people, or in patients with hyperinflated lungs due to obstructive airways disease (see Fig. 5.4).

The apex beat is normally in the fifth left intercostal space at, or just medial to, the mid-clavicular line (see Fig. 4.16). It may be displaced laterally, to the anterior or mid-axillary line, or inferiorly to the sixth or seventh intercostal space when the left ventricle is dilated e.g. in patients with heart failure or severe aortic regurgitation. When detected, a displaced apex beat is one of the most helpful clinical signs for identifying patients with left ventricular systolic dysfunction, although it is important to note that a non-displaced apex beat does not help to rule out heart disease. In dextrocardia the cardiac apex is palpable on the right side but this condition is uncommon, with a prevalence of 1:10,000.

A sustained and forceful but undisplaced apical impulse, known as an apical 'heave' is sometimes detected in patients with left ventricular hypertrophy due to hypertension or severe aortic stenosis, whilst a diffuse and less forceful impulse is more characteristic of left ventricular dilatation. Pulsation over the left parasternal area (right ventricular heave) indicates right ventricular hypertrophy or dilatation, most often accompanying pulmonary hypertension. The 'tapping' apex beat in mitral stenosis represents a palpable first heart sound and is not usually displaced.

The most common thrill is that of aortic stenosis, which is usually palpable over the upper right sternal border. The thrill caused by a ventricular septal defect is best felt at the left and right sternal edges. Diastolic thrills are very rare.

## ▍Auscultation

Use auscultation to identify and characterise the heart sounds and any added sounds and/or murmurs. The optimal sites for auscultation do not correspond with the location of cardiac structures but are where the transmitted sounds and murmurs are best heard (Box 4.16).

The diaphragm accentuates high-frequency sounds and is better for hearing normal heart sounds and high-pitched sounds, such as the early diastolic murmur of aortic regurgitation. The bell is better for hearing low pitched sounds, particularly the diastolic murmur of mitral stenosis and third and fourth heart sounds.

**Fig. 4.17 Palpating the heart.** [A] Use your hand to palpate the cardiac impulse. [B] Localise the apex beat with your finger (if necessary, roll the patient into the left lateral position). [C] Palpate with the heel of your hand in the left parasternal area.

**4.16 Cardiac auscultation: the best sites for hearing an abnormality**

| Site | Sound |
|---|---|
| Cardiac apex (mitral area) | First heart sound<br>Third and fourth heart sounds<br>Mid-diastolic murmur of mitral stenosis<br>Opening snap of mitral stenosis |
| Lower left sternal border (tricuspid area) | Early diastolic murmur of aortic regurgitation and pansystolic murmur of tricuspid regurgitation<br>Pansystolic murmur of ventricular septal defect |
| Upper left sternal border (pulmonary area) | Second heart sound<br>Pulmonary valve murmurs |
| Upper right sternal border (aortic area) | Systolic ejection (outflow) murmurs, e.g. aortic stenosis, hypertrophic cardiomyopathy |
| Left axilla | Radiation of the pansystolic murmur of mitral regurgitation |
| Below left clavicle | Continuous 'machinery' murmur of a persistent patent ductus arteriosus |

## Examination sequence (Video 3G) ▶

Minimise external noise as far as possible when you auscultate. Your stethoscope should fit comfortably with the earpieces angled slightly forwards. The tubing should be approximately 25 cm long and thick enough to reduce external sound.

Follow the same approach at each site that you auscultate:

- Identify the first and second heart sounds ($S_1$ and $S_2$) by simultaneously palpating the carotid pulse; the $S_1$ immediately precedes the upstroke of the pulse, while the $S_2$ follows well after.
  - Assess the character and intensity of $S_1$ and $S_2$; note any splitting of $S_2$ and how it varies with respiration.
- Next, concentrate in turn on systole (the interval between $S_1$ and $S_2$) and diastole (the interval between $S_2$ and $S_1$). Listen specifically for:
  - Added heart sounds ($S_3$ and $S_4$)
  - Additional sounds such as clicks, snaps and pericardial rubs
  - Murmurs (see below)

Follow a regular sequence for auscultation:

- Listen with your stethoscope diaphragm at the:
  - apex
  - lower left sternal border
  - upper right and left sternal borders.
- Listen with your stethoscope bell at the:
  - apex
  - lower left sternal border.
- Listen over the carotid arteries (ejection systolic murmur of aortic stenosis and carotid bruits) and in the left axilla (pansystolic murmur of mitral regurgitation).
- Roll the patient on to their left side. Listen at the apex using light pressure with the bell to detect the mid-diastolic murmur of mitral stenosis (Fig. 4.18A).

A

B

**Fig. 4.18 Auscultating the heart.** **A** Listen for the murmur of mitral stenosis using the bell lightly applied with the patient in the left lateral position. **B** Listen for the murmur of aortic regurgitation using the diaphragm with the patient leaning forwards.

- Ask the patient to sit up and lean forwards, then to breathe out fully and hold their breath (see Fig. 4.18B). Listen over the right second intercostal space and over the left sternal edge with the diaphragm for the murmur of aortic regurgitation.

Integrate the findings from the different sites you have auscultated to characterise any murmurs detected.

- Timing and duration. Ask yourself if the murmur is systolic (interval between $S_1$ and $S_2$) or diastolic (interval between $S_2$ and $S_1$).
- If the murmur is systolic, does it:
  - persist throughout the whole of systole with no distinct gap between the murmur and either $S_1$ or $S_2$ ('pansystolic' or 'holosystolic')?
  - occur from the onset of systole (no gap between $S_1$ and murmur) but with a distinct gap between the end of the murmur and $S_2$ (typical of 'ejection systolic' murmur)?
  - begin later in systole with a distinct gap between $S_1$ and the onset of the murmur (mid/late systolic murmur)?
- If the murmur is diastolic does it:
  - persist throughout the whole of diastole with no distinct gap between the murmur and either $S_1$ or $S_2$ ('holodiastolic')?

- occur from the onset of diastole (no gap between $S_2$ and murmur) but with a distinct gap between the end of the murmur and $S_1$ (early diastolic murmur)
  - begin later in diastole with a distinct gap between $S_2$ and the onset of the murmur (mid-diastolic murmur)?
- Quality and pitch. This is somewhat subjective but ask yourself whether the murmur is:
  - a coarse or harsh sound akin to noises generated from the back of the mouth such as clearing the throat (typical of ejection systolic murmurs)?
  - a blowing sound akin to noises generated from the front of the mouth with lips parted such as an unsuccessful whistle (typical of regurgitant systolic murmurs)
  - a low-pitched, rumbling sound akin to noises generated from the back of the mouth with lips closed like a gentle growl (typical of mitral stenosis)?
- Intensity. Ask yourself how easily the murmur is heard and whether there is an associated thrill then grade according to Box 4.17.
- Location and radiation. Ask yourself the following questions:
  - At what sites on the precordium is the murmur audible?
  - At what site is the murmur most easily heard/loudest?
  - Is the murmur audible at any other site, e.g. over the carotids or in the axilla?

### Heart sounds

#### First heart sound

The first heart sound ($S_1$), 'lub', is caused by closure of the mitral and tricuspid valves at the onset of ventricular systole. It is best heard at the apex. In mitral stenosis the intensity of $S_1$ is increased due to elevated left atrial pressure (Box 4.18).

#### Second heart sound

The second heart sound ($S_2$), 'dub', is caused by closure of the pulmonary and aortic valves at the end of ventricular systole and is best heard at the left sternal edge. It is louder and higher-pitched than the $S_1$ 'lub', and the aortic component is normally louder than the pulmonary component.

Physiological splitting of $S_2$ occurs because left ventricular contraction ends slightly before that of the right ventricle so that the aortic valve closes before the pulmonary valve. This splitting increases on inspiration ('lub d-dub') because increased venous filling of the right ventricle further delays pulmonary valve closure. The separation disappears on expiration ('lub dub'; Fig. 4.19).

#### 4.17 Grades of intensity of murmur

| Grade | Description |
|---|---|
| 1 | Heard by an expert in optimum conditions |
| 2 | Heard by a non-expert in optimum conditions |
| 3 | Easily heard; no thrill |
| 4 | A loud murmur, with a thrill |
| 5 | Very loud, often heard over a wide area, with thrill |
| 6 | Extremely loud, heard without a stethoscope |

#### 4.18 Abnormalities of intensity of the first heart sound

**Quiet**
- Low cardiac output
- Poor left ventricular function
- Rheumatic mitral regurgitation
- Long P–R interval (first-degree heart block)

**Loud**
- Increased cardiac output
- Large stroke volume
- Mitral stenosis
- Short P–R interval
- Atrial myxoma (rare)

**Variable**
- Atrial fibrillation
- Extrasystoles
- Complete heart block

Wide splitting of $S_2$, but with normal respiratory variation, occurs in conditions that delay right ventricular emptying, such as right bundle branch block or pulmonary hypertension. Wide and fixed splitting of $S_2$, with no variation in respiration, is almost always due to an atrial septal defect (Fig. 4.20). In this condition, shunting of blood from the left atrium to the right atrium causes

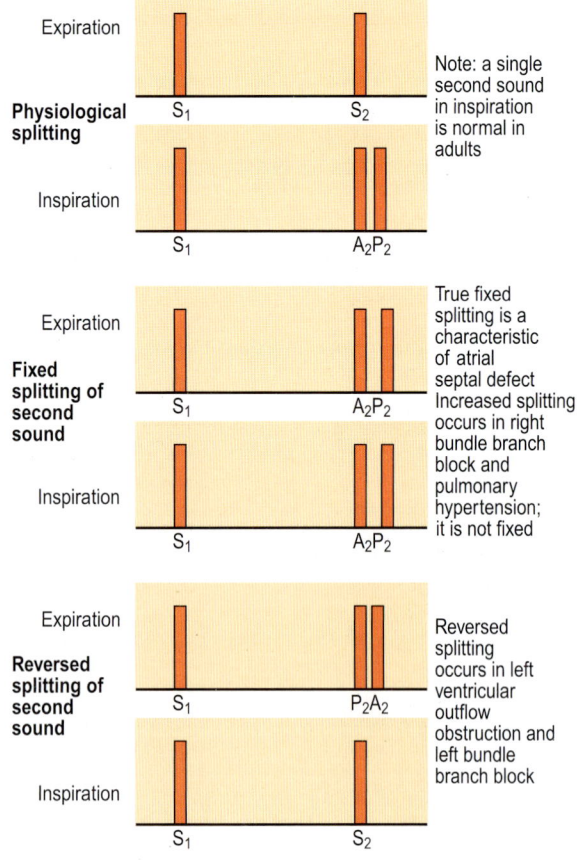

Fig. 4.19 Physiological and pathological splitting of the second heart sound.

Ejection systolic murmur
(pulmonary flow murmur) with
fixed splitting of second sound

$S_1$ $A_2P_2$

**Additional clinical findings**

Right parasternal heave*
Loud pulmonary component of
second heart sound*

*If pulmonary hypertension
has developed

4

**Fig. 4.20** Atrial septal defect. The increased blood flow through the right heart resulting from the left to right shunt produces a pulmonary flow murmur, best heard in the pulmonary area (left parasternal edge, second intercostal space).

right ventricular stroke volume to be significantly larger than the left throughout the respiratory cycle.

Reversed splitting of $S_2$ ('lub dub' on inspiration; 'lub d-dub' on expiration; Fig. 4.19) occurs when left ventricular emptying is delayed so that the aortic valve closes after the pulmonary valve. Examples include left bundle branch block and severe aortic stenosis.

The aortic component of $S_2$ is sometimes quiet or absent in calcific aortic stenosis. A loud pulmonary component of $S_2$ is an important sign of pulmonary hypertension.

### Third heart sound

The third heart sound ($S_3$) is a low-pitched early diastolic sound best heard with the bell at the apex. It results from a brief period of rapid ventricular filling immediately after opening of the atrioventricular valves and is therefore heard after the second heart sound as 'lub dub-dum'. It may be a normal physiological finding in children and young adults or during fever or pregnancy. However, after the age of 40 years, it is usually due to left ventricular failure or mitral regurgitation, with the rapid ventricular filling a consequence of high left atrial pressure at the onset of diastole. In patients presenting to hospital with acute breathlessness, the presence of an $S_3$, on examination, strongly increases the likelihood of heart failure but its absence does not help to rule out heart failure. In the context of heart failure, $S_3$ is typically accompanied by a tachycardia and referred to as a 'gallop' rhythm.

### Fourth heart sound

A fourth heart sound ($S_4$) is less common than an $S_3$ and less useful in modern clinical practice. It is soft and low-pitched, best heard with the bell at the apex. It occurs just before $S_1$ (da-lub-dub). It is caused by forceful atrial contraction against a non-compliant or stiff ventricle, most often with left ventricular hypertrophy due to hypertension, aortic stenosis or hypertrophic cardiomyopathy. It cannot occur when there is atrial fibrillation.

### Additional sounds

An opening snap is commonly heard in mitral (rarely, tricuspid) stenosis. It results from sudden opening of a stenosed valve and

occurs early in diastole, just after the $S_2$ (Fig. 4.21A). It is best heard with the diaphragm at the apex.

Ejection clicks are high-pitched sounds best heard with the diaphragm. They occur early in systole just after the $S_1$, in

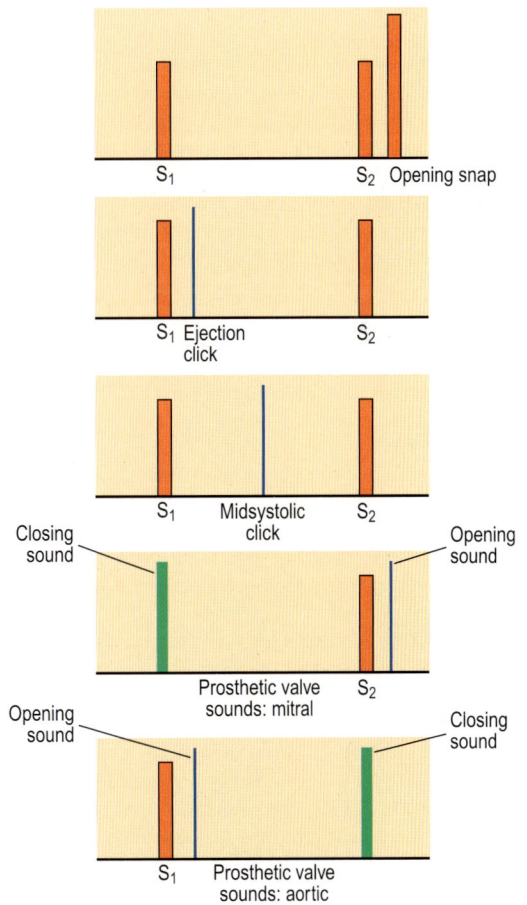

$S_1$                    $S_2$  Opening snap

$S_1$ Ejection          $S_2$
click

$S_1$  Midsystolic      $S_2$
       click

Closing                          Opening
sound                            sound

Prosthetic valve        $S_2$
sounds: mitral

Opening                          Closing
sound                            sound

$S_1$  Prosthetic valve
       sounds: aortic

**Fig. 4.21** 'Added sounds' on auscultation.

patients with congenital pulmonary or aortic stenosis (see Fig. 4.21B). The mechanism is similar to that of an opening snap. Ejection clicks do not occur in calcific aortic stenosis because the cusps are rigid.

Mid-systolic clicks are high-pitched and best heard at the apex with the diaphragm. They occur in mitral valve prolapse (see Fig. 4.21C) where they are often associated with a late systolic murmur.

A pericardial (friction) rub is a coarse scratching sound that is typically biphasic, with both systolic and diastolic components. It is best heard using the diaphragm with the patient holding their breath in expiration. It may be audible over any part of the pre-cordium but is often localised, varying in intensity over time and with the position of the patient. It is highly specific for pericarditis and present in 35–85% of cases. It is an important sign in contemporary practice because it is one of four criteria (along with characteristic chest pain, suggestive electrocardiogram (ECG) changes and new or worsening pericardial effusion) used to diagnose acute pericarditis; at least two of the four criteria need to be present.

### Prosthetic valve sounds

Mechanical heart valves can make a sound when they close or open. The closure sound is normally louder, especially with modern valves. The sounds are high-pitched, with a 'metallic' quality, are often heard without a stethoscope, and may even be palpable. A mechanical mitral valve replacement makes a metallic $S_1$ and a sound like a loud opening snap early in diastole (see Fig. 4.21D). Mechanical aortic valves have a loud, metallic $S_2$ and an opening sound like an ejection click at the start of systole (see Fig. 4.21E); they are normally associated with a flow murmur.

Heart sounds arising from bioprosthetic valves usually sound similar to those of normal valves.

### Murmurs

Heart murmurs are produced by increased velocity of flow through a normal valve or by turbulent flow across an abnormal valve, septal defect or outflow obstruction.

#### Systolic murmurs

Causes of systolic murmurs are shown in Box 4.19.

'Innocent' murmurs occur when stroke volume is increased, as in pregnant women, athletes with resting bradycardia or pa-tients with fever or anaemia. They tend to be low in intensity (grade 2), short in duration and best heard at the left sternal edge with no radiation.

The murmur of aortic stenosis is often audible all over the precordium with radiation to the suprasternal notch and carotid arteries (Fig. 4.22). It is a harsh, ejection systolic murmur that is usually loud and there may be a thrill. The absence of an ejection systolic murmur makes clinically significant aortic stenosis extremely unlikely. In the presence of an ejection systolic murmur, several clinical signs support the diagnosis (see Fig. 4.22) and moderate to severe stenosis is highly likely if three or more of these are present.

Aortic sclerosis (thickening and calcification of the aortic valve without obstruction) produces a similar quality of murmur but it is

---

**4.19 Causes of systolic murmurs**

**Ejection systolic murmurs**

- High cardiac output state: severe anaemia, fever, athletes (bradycardia → large stroke volume), pregnancy, thyrotoxicosis, liver cirrhosis, arteriovenous fistula.
- Pulmonary flow murmur from increased RV stroke volume: atrial septal defect; pulmonary regurgitation
- Aortic flow murmur from increased LV stroke volume: aortic regurgitation
- Valvular stenosis: aortic stenosis; pulmonary stenosis
- Other valve abnormalities: mechanical aortic or pulmonary valve; aortic sclerosis (turbulent flow without significant pressure gradient)
- Subvalvular obstruction: hypertrophic obstructive cardiomyopathy; subaortic membrane

**Pansystolic murmurs**

- Mitral regurgitation
- Tricuspid regurgitation
- Ventricular septal defect

**Late systolic murmurs**

- Mitral valve prolapse

---

less likely to radiate and is not associated with a thrill or other signs of aortic stenosis.

Mitral regurgitation is the most common cause of a pansystolic murmur and tends to have a 'blowing' quality. The most helpful feature in distinguishing it from other causes is its location (Fig. 4.23): a murmur that extends from the apex to the anterior axillary line – but is only audible below the third intercostal space – strongly suggests mitral regurgitation. With mitral valve pro-lapse, regurgitation begins in mid-systole, producing a late sys-tolic murmur (see Fig. 4.23).

The murmur of tricuspid regurgitation is another common cause of a pansystolic murmur. Localisation to the lower left sternal edge (only audible below the third intercostal space or lateral to the mid-clavicular line (Fig. 4.24), strongly supports the diagnosis, as does an increase in its intensity with inspiration, which increases blood flow through the right heart. Notably, the absence of a murmur does not exclude tricuspid regurgitation.

Ventricular septal defects also cause a pansystolic murmur. Small congenital defects produce a loud murmur audible at the left sternal border, radiating to the right sternal border and often associated with a thrill. Rupture of the interventricular septum can complicate myocardial infarction, producing a harsh pan-systolic murmur, typically accompanied by major haemodynamic compromise.

#### Diastolic murmurs

The murmur of aortic regurgitation (Fig. 4.25) may last throughout most, or even all of diastole, but is usually termed an 'early diastolic murmur' because it is loudest in early diastole. It is best heard at the left sternal edge with the patient leaning for-wards in held expiration. Significant aortic regurgitation increases

**4**

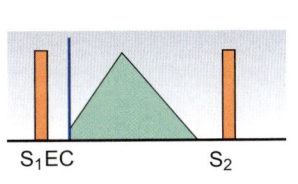

S₁EC          S₂

Lean patient forward with
breath held in expiration to feel
thrill and hear murmur best

**Additional clinical findings**

Slow rising pulse*
Reduced pulse volume*
Narrow pulse pressure
Apical heave
Thrill in aortic region
Reduced or absent second
heart sound over aortic area*
Radiation of murmur to
carotid artery*

*In patients with an ESM, 3 or more
of these features make moderate to
severe aortic stenosis highly likely

**Fig. 4.22** Aortic stenosis. There is a systolic pressure gradient across the stenosed aortic valve. The resultant high-velocity jet tends to be widely audible throughout the praecordium, though it is best heard with the diaphragm in the aortic area. Alternatively, the bell may be placed in the suprasternal notch. In patients with bicuspid aortic valve, the ejection systolic murmur follows an ejection click (EC).

Apical pansystolic murmur
radiates to axilla

S₁          S₂ S₃

Variant:  mid-systolic click/
late systolic murmur
(mitral valve prolapse)

S₁  MSC    S₂ S₃

**Additional clinical findings**

Displaced apex beat
Third heart sound

**Fig. 4.23** Mitral regurgitation. The murmur is best heard at the apex with radiation to the axilla and is usually audible only below the third intercostal space. It typically begins at the moment of valve closure and may obscure the first heart sound. It varies little in intensity throughout systole. In mitral valve prolapse the murmur begins in mid- or late systole and there is often a mid-systolic click (MSC).

S₁          S₂

Pansystolic murmur.
The murmur intensity
increases with inspiration.

**Additional clinical findings**

Elevated JVP with systolic
cv wave
Pulsatile hepatomegaly
Right parasternal heave*
Loud pulmonary component of
second heart sound*

*If pulmonary hypertension
has developed

**Fig. 4.24** Tricuspid regurgitation. The murmur is usually heard only in the tricuspid area (left sternal edge, fourth intercostal space) and not at the other common sites of auscultation. It typically begins at the moment of valve closure and varies little in intensity throughout systole. *JVP*, Jugular venous pressure.

Lean patient forward with
breath in held expiration
to hear murmur best

$S_1$  $S_2$

**Additional clinical findings**

Large volume pulse
Collapsing pulse
Wide pulse pressure
Prominent carotid pulsations
(Corrigan's sign)
Displaced apex beat

**Fig. 4.25** Aortic regurgitation. There is an early diastolic murmur, best heard along the left sternal edge, with the diaphragm during held expiration. An associated systolic murmur is common because of the increased flow through the aortic valve in systole.

left ventricular stroke volume so there is usually an associated systolic flow murmur – which may be more obvious than the diastolic murmur. Rarely, impingement of the regurgitant jet on the anterior mitral valve leaflet can produce a mid-diastolic murmur akin to that of mitral stenosis ('Austin Flint' murmur), but this sign has negligible value in contemporary practice.

Pulmonary regurgitation produces a similar murmur to aortic regurgitation but is far less common.

Mitral stenosis causes a low-pitched, rumbling mid-diastolic murmur that may follow an opening snap (Fig. 4.26). The cadence sounds like 'lup-ta-ta-rru': 'lup' is the $S_1$ (typically loud), 'ta-ta' the $S_2$ and opening snap, and 'rru' the mid-diastolic murmur. If the patient is in sinus rhythm, left atrial contraction causes presystolic accentuation of the murmur. The murmur is often difficult to hear but is best appreciated with the bell (using light pressure) at the apex with the patient positioned on their left side; it can be accentuated by exercise such as touching the toes or raising the legs up and down on the bed several times.

The murmur of tricuspid stenosis is similar but very rare.

## Continuous murmurs

Continuous murmurs are rare in adults. The most common cause is a patent ductus arteriosus. In the fetus this connects the upper descending aorta and pulmonary artery, and normally closes just after birth. The murmur is best heard at the upper left sternal border and radiates over the left scapula. Its continuous character is 'machinery-like'; as aortic pressure always exceeds pulmonary pressure, there is continuous ductal flow, with the greatest pressure difference in systole, resulting in a louder systolic component.

## Interpretation of the findings

Serious cardiac pathology such as ischaemic heart disease can occur in the absence of any clinical signs, so a clear history (combined with ECG and other basic tests) is vital to accurate diagnosis.

Loud  $S_2$  Loud
$S_1$  OS  $S_2$

Roll patient towards left
to hear murmur best

**Additional clinical findings**

Low volume pulse
Tapping apex beat
Loud S1
Opening snap
Right parasternal heave*
Loud pulmonary component
of second heart sound*

*If pulmonary hypertension
has developed

**Fig. 4.26** Mitral stenosis. There is a pressure gradient across the mitral valve, giving rise to a low-pitched mid-diastolic murmur that is heard best with the bell at the apex. Occasionally, an opening snap (OS) can arise due to the sharp movement of the tethered anterior cusp of the mitral valve at the time when the flow commences.

Identifying clinical signs of cardiac congestion – most notably an elevated JVP – is critical to the diagnosis, assessment, monitoring and treatment of cardiac failure, as well as other conditions such as cardiac tamponade.

Despite the availability of echocardiography, auscultation remains an important clinical skill: the detection of abnormal signs is required to guide appropriate investigation, and some diagnostically useful auscultatory signs, such as a pericardial friction rub, have no direct equivalent on echocardiography.

Clinical examination also permits opportunistic detection of asymptomatic but potentially important cardiovascular disease, such as atrial fibrillation, valvular heart disease, and abdominal aortic aneurysm (AAA), which can then be assessed further by appropriate investigation.

# Investigations

## Haematology and clinical chemistry

As anaemia can unmask angina or exacerbate heart failure, a full blood count is useful and helps guide the safe use of antiplatelet therapies and anticoagulants. Thyroid function should be assessed since thyroid disorders can cause or exacerbate most cardiac conditions. Urea and electrolytes are measured and liver function tests performed prior to starting therapies that may have impact upon renal function or cause hepatotoxicity.

Blood glucose and a lipid profile help identify patients with diabetes mellitus and assess cardiovascular risk. In patients with acute chest pain, cardiac troponin is measured to determine whether there is myocardial injury or infarction.

## Electrocardiography

In performing a standard 12-lead electrocardiogram (ECG; Fig. 4.27), the patient must be resting supine and relaxed to avoid muscle tremor. Good contact between the electrode and skin is important and it may be necessary to shave the chest. The electrodes must be positioned correctly to obtain recordings made from the six precordial electrodes ($V_1$–$V_6$) and six recordings from the limb electrodes (left arm, right arm and left leg). The right leg electrode is used as a reference. Confirm that the ECG is calibrated using a 1 mV signal prior to recording. The ECG plays an indispensable role in the diagnosis of acute coronary syndromes (most notably, ST segment-elevation myocardial infarction; Fig 4.27C), cardiac arrhythmias, acute pericarditis and inherited heart conditions such as cardiomyopathies or congenital long QT syndrome.

### Ambulatory ECG monitoring

Continuous ECG recording over 24–48 hours can be used to identify symptomatic or asymptomatic rhythm disturbances in patients with palpitation or syncope. If symptoms are less frequent, it may be necessary to use patient-activated recorders that record the heart rhythm only when the patient is symptomatic; the device is activated by the patient (Fig. 4.28).

### Exercise ECG

An exercise ECG is useful in the diagnosis and functional assessment of patients with suspected coronary artery disease. Down-sloping ST segment depression, particularly when it occurs during minor exertion, or ST segment elevation, is of prognostic significance and helps inform the need for invasive investigation with coronary angiography.

## Ambulatory blood pressure monitoring

A portable device can be worn by the patient at home that takes at least two BP measurements per hour. It is used to confirm the diagnosis of hypertension and provide a more reliable assessment of response to treatment.

## Chest X-ray

The maximum width of the heart divided by the maximum width of the thorax on a posteroanterior chest x-ray (the cardiothoracic ratio) should normally be less than 0.5. An increased cardiothoracic ratio is common in heart failure and some valvular lesions. In the former this is often accompanied by distension of the upper lobe pulmonary veins, diffuse shadowing within the lungs due to pulmonary oedema, and Kerley B lines (horizontal, engorged lymphatics at the periphery of the lower lobes; Fig. 4.29A). A widened mediastinum may indicate a thoracic aortic aneurysm.

## Echocardiography

Echocardiography uses high-frequency sound waves to evaluate cardiac structure and function. It permits measurements of chamber size and wall thickness, assessment of regional and global ventricular systolic function and detection of abnormal valve morphology or motion. In addition, Doppler echocardiography, through visualisation of blood flow and measurement of blood velocity, enables detection and quantification of valvular stenosis or regurgitation and other lesions such as intracardiac shunts. Most echocardiography scans are performed through the anterior chest wall (transthoracic; Fig. 4.29B). Transoesophageal echocardiography requires sedation but gives high resolution of posterior structures such as the left atrium, mitral valve and descending aorta, and is useful in detecting valvular vegetations in infective endocarditis.

## Radionuclide studies

Technetium-99 is injected intravenously and detected using a gamma camera to assess left ventricular function. Thallium and sestamibi are taken up by myocardial cells and indicate myocardial perfusion at rest and exercise.

A

B

C

**Fig. 4.27 Electrocardiography (ECG).** **A** 12-lead ECG lead placement. **B** Normal PQRST complex. **C** Acute anterior myocardial infarction. Note the ST elevation in leads $V_1$–$V_6$ and $aV_L$, and 'reciprocal' ST depression in leads II, III and $aV_F$.

**4**

**Fig. 4.28** Printout from a 24-hour ambulatory electrocardiogram recording, showing complete heart block. Arrows indicate visible P waves. At times, these are masked by the QRS complex or T wave (*).

**Fig. 4.29 Cardiovascular imaging.** A Chest X-ray in heart failure. This shows cardiomegaly with patchy alveolar shadowing of pulmonary oedema and Kerley B lines (engorged lymphatics, *arrow*) at the periphery of both lungs. B Transthoracic echocardiogram in an apical two-chamber view, showing thinning of the left ventricular apex. This is the site of a recent anterior myocardial infarct. *LA,* Left atrium; *LV,* left ventricle. C Coronary angiography. The *arrow* indicates an abrupt occlusion of the proximal left anterior descending artery. *CX,* circumflex; *LAD,* left anterior descending; *LM,* left main. D Cardiac magnetic resonance imaging. Gadolinium enhancement image demonstrates regional uptake of gadolinium *(white arrows)* consistent with myocardial fibrosis in the territory of the LAD.

## Cardiac catheterisation

A fine catheter is introduced under local anaesthetic via a peripheral artery (usually the radial or femoral) and advanced to the heart under x-ray guidance. Although measurements of intracardiac pressures, and therefore estimates of valvular and cardiac function, are possible, the primary application of this technique is imaging of the coronary circulation using contrast medium. This is performed to inform and guide revascularisation, either by coronary angioplasty or bypass grafting (see Fig. 4.29C).

## Computed tomography and magnetic resonance imaging

Computed tomography (CT), combined with cardiac gating permits high resolution imaging of the coronary arteries including coronary atheroma and calcification. CT is particularly useful for ruling out obstructive coronary artery disease (and thereby angina) in patients with chest pain who are deemed to be at low to moderate risk of coronary disease. It can also reduce the need for invasive investigation in patients with a low probability of occlusive coronary disease who require valve surgery. Magnetic resonance imaging (MRI; Fig. 4.29D) provides superior spatial resolution to echocardiography, together with an unrestricted viewing plane. It is the most accurate method of measuring cardiac volumes and ventricular ejection fraction and is the imaging modality of choice for investigating the aetiology of heart muscle diseases (cardiomyopathy).

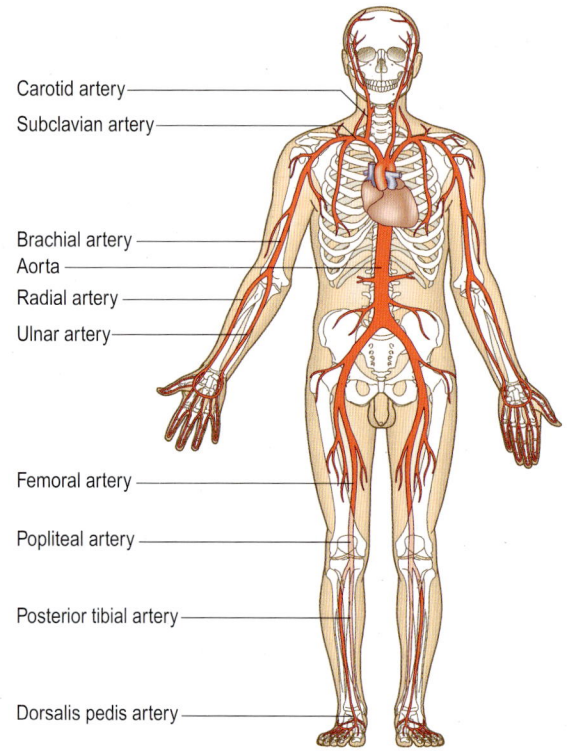

Carotid artery
Subclavian artery

Brachial artery
Aorta
Radial artery
Ulnar artery

Femoral artery

Popliteal artery

Posterior tibial artery

Dorsalis pedis artery

**Fig. 4.30** The arterial system.

# PERIPHERAL ARTERIAL SYSTEM

## Anatomy and physiology

See Fig. 4.30.

## The history

## Common presenting symptoms

### Leg pain

#### Asymptomatic ischaemia

PAD is recognised as a worldwide public health challenge with a concerning increase in prevalence over recent decades in both high- and low- income countries. Studies from Scotland suggest around 5% of men and women over 55 years of age experience intermittent claudication and a further 25% had evidence of asymptomatic PAD. The underlying pathology is usually atherosclerosis affecting large and medium-sized vessels. PAD affects the legs eight times more commonly than the arms. This is partly because the lower limb arteries are more frequently affected by atherosclerosis, but also because the arterial supply to the legs is less well developed in relation to the muscle mass. Haemodynamically significant lower limb ischaemia is defined as an ankle-to-brachial pressure index (ABPI) of less than 0.9 at rest (p. 76). The Fontaine classification describes the progression of symptoms that occurs as the atherosclerotic burden increases and the blood supply to the limb diminishes (Box 4.20).

| 4.20 Fontaine classification of lower limb ischaemia | |
|---|---|
| **Stage** | **Description** |
| I | Asymptomatic |
| II | Intermittent claudication |
| III | Night/rest pain |
| IV | Tissue loss (ulceration/gangrene) |

Whilst the risk of limb loss is low even in patients with intermittent claudication (1–2% per year), PAD carries additional clinical importance because it has a very strong association with coronary and cerebrovascular atherosclerotic disease. There is an elevated risk of major adverse cardiovascular events in both symptomatic and asymptomatic patients with PAD, and the mortality is double that of the age-matched population. Atherosclerosis is a systemic disease, and it is therefore important that patients with PAD are identified and treated similarly to those patients presenting with coronary and cerebrovascular events.

Remember that many patients with PAD may be asymptomatic either because they choose not to walk very far, or because their exercise tolerance is limited by other comorbidities such as cardiac disease.

### Intermittent claudication

Intermittent claudication is pain felt in the legs on walking due to arterial insufficiency and is the most common symptom of PAD. It is important to distinguish claudication due to arterial insufficiency from other causes of lower limb pain, which include osteoarthritis, neurogenic claudication and venous claudication (Box 4.21).

Patients with intermittent claudication describe tightness or 'cramp-like' pain that develops after a relatively constant distance; the distance is often shorter if walking uphill. The pain disappears completely within a few minutes of rest but recurs on walking. The 'claudication distance' is how far patients say they can walk before the pain comes on. The 'total walking distance' is how far they can walk before the pain is so bad that they have to stop.

The pain is felt in major muscle groups and its location depends on the level at which the arteries are diseased. The calf muscle is most commonly affected due to femoropopliteal disease, while pain in the thigh or buttock suggests common femoral or aortoiliac obstruction. Male patients who have bilateral common iliac or internal iliac artery occlusion may develop Leriche's syndrome, involving buttock claudication and erectile dysfunction.

Claudication is not in itself limb-threatening, although it is a marker for widespread atherosclerotic disease. With best medical therapy and supervised exercise programmes, 50% will improve, 30% will remain stable and only 20% will deteriorate further.

Any intervention for claudication is performed purely for the purpose of symptomatic relief, since only a small minority of patient's progress to critical limb ischaemia. The patient's age, occupation and comorbidities are important in determining the extent to which claudication limits their lifestyle. A postal worker who is only able to walk 100 metres is seriously limited, but an elderly person who simply wants to cross the road to the shops may cope well. While absolute distances are important, it may be more helpful to ask specific questions about how symptoms affect the patient's lifestyle:

- Can you walk to the clinic from the bus stop or car park without stopping?
- Can you do your own shopping?
- What are you unable to do because of the pain?

| 4.21 The clinical features of arterial, neurogenic and venous claudication | | | |
|---|---|---|---|
| | Arterial | Neurogenic | Venous |
| Pathology | Stenosis or occlusion of major lower limb arteries | Lumbar nerve root or cauda equina compression (spinal stenosis) | Obstruction to the venous outflow of the leg due to iliofemoral venous occlusion |
| Site of pain | Muscles, usually the calf but may involve thigh and buttocks | Ill-defined Whole leg May be associated with numbness and tingling | Whole leg 'Bursting' in nature |
| Laterality | Unilateral or bilateral | Often bilateral | Nearly always unilateral |
| Onset | Gradual after walking the 'claudication distance' | Often immediate on walking or standing up | Gradual, from the moment walking starts |
| Relieving features | On stopping walking, the pain disappears completely in 1–2 minutes | Bending forwards and stopping walking Patient may sit down for full relief | Leg elevation |
| Colour | Normal or pale | Normal | Cyanosed Often visible varicose veins |
| Temperature | Normal or cool | Normal | Normal or increased |
| Oedema | Absent | Absent | Always present |
| Pulses | Reduced or absent | Normal | Present but may be difficult to feel owing to oedema |
| Straight-leg raising | Normal | May be limited | Normal |

## Night pain

The patient is woken with pain or numbness in the affected foot due to poor perfusion. Night pain develops because on lying, the beneficial effects of gravity on perfusion are lost, and in addition, heart rate, BP and cardiac output are reduced during sleep. Patients may find relief by hanging the leg out of bed or by getting up and walking around. On return to bed, however, the pain recurs and patients often choose to sleep in a chair. This leads to dependent oedema, increased interstitial tissue pressure, a further reduction in tissue perfusion and ultimately a worsening of the pain.

## Rest pain

Rest pain occurs when blood flow is insufficient to meet the metabolic demands of the tissues, even at rest. Critical ischaemia is defined as rest pain (persisting for more than 2 weeks and requiring opiate analgesia) or tissue loss associated with an ankle pressure of less than 50 mmHg or a toe pressure of less than 30 mmHg.

Rest or night pain indicates severe, multilevel, lower limb PAD and requires urgent referral to a vascular surgeon, as failure to revascularise the leg usually leads to the development of tissue loss (gangrene, ulceration) and amputation.

In patients with diabetes it may be difficult to differentiate between rest pain and diabetic neuropathy, as both may be worse at night. Neuropathic pain may not be confined to the foot, is associated with burning and tingling, is not relieved by dependency and is accompanied by dysaesthesia (pain or uncomfortable sensations, sometimes described as burning, tingling or numbness). Many patients with neuropathy cannot even bear the pressure of bedclothes on their feet.

## Tissue loss (ulceration and/or gangrene)

In patients with severe lower limb PAD, perfusion is inadequate to support the tissues, and areas of tissue loss (gangrene) develop at the tips of the digits, gradually spreading proximally. Furthermore, even trivial injuries do not heal and cause ulceration. Tissue loss often progresses rapidly and, without revascularisation, leads to amputation and/or death.

## Tissue loss in the diabetic patient

Tissue loss in the diabetic patient (see p. 208) can progress rapidly and represent a surgical emergency, even if outward signs are relatively few. There are often a number of factors at play. These include poor perfusion at the major vessel and microcirculatory levels, sensory and motor neuropathy, loss of foot architecture, concomitant renal dysfunction, increased susceptibility to infection and even delayed identification of the problem due to visual and sensory impairment.

## Acute limb ischaemia

The classical features of acute limb ischaemia are the 'six Ps' (Box 4.22). Pallor, pain, pulselessness and perishing cold are relatively early signs. Paralysis (inability to move the toes/fingers) and paraesthesia (numbness or tingling over the forefoot or dorsum of the hand) are the most important and indicate severe ischaemia affecting nerve and muscle function. Muscle

| 4.22 Signs of acute limb ischaemia |
| --- |
| • Pallor |
| • Pulselessness |
| • Perishing cold |
| • Paraesthesia |
| • Pain (worse when muscle squeezed) |
| • Paralysis |

tenderness is a grave sign indicating actual or impending muscle infarction. A limb with these features will usually become irreversibly damaged unless the circulation is restored within a few hours.

It is important to consider the most likely underlying cause:

- Thromboembolism: usually from the left atrium in association with atrial fibrillation or myocardial infarction. There is usually no history of claudication.
- Thrombosis in situ: thrombotic occlusion of an already narrowed atherosclerotic arterial segment (Box 4.23). In this situation the patient is likely to have a past history of claudication.

Reperfusion of the acutely ischaemic limb is time critical and patients often proceed to the operating theatre on the basis of high-quality clinical evaluation, without undergoing any further investigations.

## Compartment syndrome

The perfusion pressure of a muscle is the difference between the mean arterial pressure and the pressure within the fascial compartment within which it lies. Compartment syndrome occurs where there is increased pressure within the fascial compartments of the limb that compromises the perfusion and viability of muscle and nerves. The calf is most commonly

| 4.23 Acute limb ischaemia: embolus versus thrombosis in situ | | |
| --- | --- | --- |
| | **Embolus** | **Thrombosis** |
| Onset and severity | Acute (seconds or minutes), ischaemia profound (no pre-existing collaterals) | Insidious (hours or days), ischaemia less severe (pre-existing collaterals) |
| Embolic source | Present | Absent |
| Previous claudication | Absent | Present |
| Pulses in contralateral leg | Present | Often absent, reflecting widespread peripheral arterial disease |
| Diagnosis | Clinical | Angiography |
| Treatment | Embolectomy and anticoagulation | Medical, bypass surgery, catheter-directed thrombolysis |

affected and the two leading causes are lower limb trauma (such as fractured tibia or crush injury) and reperfusion injury following treatment of acute lower limb ischaemia. A high index of suspicion is required since failure to recognise and treat compartment syndrome may result in limb amputation. The key symptom is severe pain that is often unrelieved by opioids and exacerbated by active or passive movement. It is worth remembering that peripheral pulses are usually present, since the major arteries lie outside the fascial compartments and are not affected by increased compartment pressure. Compartment monitors can be used as an adjunct to measure compartment pressure with high or rising pressures indicating the need for fasciotomies.

## Abdominal pain

### Mesenteric ischaemia

Because of the rich collateral circulation of the gut, usually two of the three major visceral arteries (coeliac trunk, superior and inferior mesenteric arteries) must be critically stenosed or occluded before symptoms and signs of chronic mesenteric arterial insufficiency occur. Severe central abdominal pain typically develops 10–15 minutes after eating. The patient becomes scared of eating and significant weight loss is a universal finding. Diarrhoea may also be present and the non-specific nature of symptoms may result in misdiagnosis; the patient may have had numerous investigations before the diagnosis is made.

Acute mesenteric ischaemia is a surgical emergency. It is most commonly caused by an embolus from the heart or by thrombosis in situ of a pre-existing atherosclerotic plaque in one of the mesenteric vessels. It is often hard to diagnose in the early stages, as patients typically present initially with severe abdominal pain that is out of proportion to often unimpressive abdominal signs. Presentation with severe abdominal pain, shock, bloody diarrhoea and profound metabolic acidosis indicates infarction of the bowel, which carries a high mortality rate. Rarely, renal angle pain occurs from renal infarction or ischaemia, and is associated with visible or non-visible haematuria.

Any patient suspected of having visceral ischaemia should undergo urgent CT angiography.

### Abdominal aortic aneurysm

AAA is an abnormal focal dilatation of the aorta to at least 150% of its normal diameter (Fig. 4.31). It is often diagnosed incidentally during a CT scan or alternative imaging for other reasons.

Patients may present with abdominal and/or back pain, or occasionally with more subtle signs such as an awareness of abdominal pulsation or the observation of ripples in the water when they are in the bath (Richards' wave sign). However, most patients are asymptomatic until the aneurysm ruptures.

The classical features of AAA rupture include abdominal/back pain, pulsatile abdominal mass, syncope and shock (hypotension), but these are not always present, and it is important to have a low threshold of suspicion and consider early referral and/or CT imaging.

A

B

C

**Fig. 4.31 Abdominal aortic aneurysm.** [A] Abdominal x-ray showing calcification *(arrow)*. [B] Computed tomogram of the abdomen showing an abdominal aortic aneurysm *(arrow)*. [C] At laparotomy the aorta is seen to be grossly and irregularly dilated.

## Digital ischaemia

### Blue toes

Blue toe syndrome occurs when there is atheroembolism from an AAA or alternative proximal embolic source (such as popliteal aneurysm or atherosclerotic plaque). Patchy bluish discoloration appears over the toes and forefoot of one or both feet. There is usually a full set of pedal pulses. Although seemingly innocuous, this symptom should be taken seriously, as small emboli may herald the risk of a major embolus leading to acute limb ischaemia and even limb loss.

### Vasospastic symptoms

Raynaud's phenomenon is digital ischaemia induced by cold and emotion. It has three phases (Fig. 4.32):

- pallor: due to digital artery spasm and/or obstruction
- cyanosis: due to deoxygenation of static venous blood (this phase may be absent)
- redness: due to reactive hyperaemia.

Raynaud's phenomenon may be primary (Raynaud's disease) and caused by idiopathic digital artery vasospasm, or secondary to other conditions (Raynaud's syndrome) such as drugs, connective tissue disease, hyperviscosity syndromes or use of power tools (vibration white finger). While for most patients this is a self-limiting condition, a small minority develop tissue loss.

Patients over 40 years old presenting with unilateral Raynaud's phenomenon should be investigated for underlying PAD, especially if they have cardiovascular risk factors, diabetes or a smoking habit.

## Stroke

Stroke is a focal neurological deficit that has a vascular cause and is discussed on p. 137.

## Past medical history

Is the patient known to have established peripheral vascular disease? Ask about previous investigations, operations or procedures. Is there a history of other atherosclerotic conditions such as coronary artery disease or cerebrovascular disease? Ask about risk factors for atherosclerotic disease, including hypertension, hypercholesterolaemia and diabetes mellitus. Are there any other comorbidities (such as severe cardiac or lung disease) that would make any potential operative intervention high-risk or futile? Enquire about general health status since symptoms of vascular disease may be precipitated by another medical condition. For example, the new onset of rest pain may result from poor cardiac output or anaemia.

## Drug history

Enquire about medication used for secondary prevention and adherence to these: antiplatelet, lipid-lowering, antihypertensive and diabetes therapies. Patients may be taking vasoactive drugs for claudication (naftidrofuryl or cilostazol, for example), although their efficacy in this setting is not clear. Enquire about other cardiac medications, as these may make symptoms of rest pain worse through their BP-lowering or negatively inotropic effects. Anticoagulants and drugs that impair the immune system or wound healing are relevant when considering invasive investigations or procedures.

## Family history

Ask about a family history of premature coronary or other vascular disease (p. 49). There is a strong familial association for AAAs so, where relevant, a family history should be sought.

## Social history

Take a smoking history (p. 16). Enquire about occupation and activities of daily living. How are the patient's symptoms impacting on quality of life or employment?

## The physical examination

Follow the routine described for the heart, looking for evidence of anaemia or cyanosis, signs of heart failure, and direct or indirect evidence of PAD. Box 4.24 lists some of the direct and indirect signs of PAD.

A

B

**Fig. 4.32 Raynaud's syndrome.** A The acute phase, showing severe blanching of the tip of one finger. B Raynaud's syndrome occasionally progresses to fingertip ulceration or even gangrene. *(A and B) From Forbes CD, Jackson WF. Color Atlas of Clinical Medicine. 3rd ed. Edinburgh: Mosby; 2003.*

## 4.24 Signs suggesting vascular disease

| Sign | Implication |
|---|---|
| **Hands and arms** | |
| Tobacco stains | Smoking |
| Purple discoloration of the fingertips | Atheroembolism from a proximal subclavian aneurysm |
| Pits and healed scars in the finger pulps | Secondary Raynaud's syndrome |
| Calcinosis and visible nail-fold capillary loops | Systemic sclerosis and CREST (calcinosis, Raynaud's phenomenon, oesophageal dysfunction, sclerodactyly, telangiectasia) |
| Wasting of the small muscles of the hand | Thoracic outlet syndrome |
| **Face and neck** | |
| Corneal arcus and xanthelasma | Hypercholesterolaemia |
| Horner's syndrome | Carotid artery dissection or aneurysm |
| Hoarseness of the voice and 'bovine' cough | Recurrent laryngeal nerve palsy from a thoracic aortic aneurysm |
| Prominent veins in the neck, shoulder and anterior chest | Axillary/subclavian vein occlusion |
| **Abdomen** | |
| Epigastric/umbilical pulsation | Aortoiliac aneurysm |
| Mottling of the abdomen | Ruptured abdominal aortic aneurysm or saddle embolism occluding aortic bifurcation |
| Evidence of weight loss | Visceral ischaemia |

Perform a detailed examination of the arterial pulses.

## Examination sequence (Video 5)

Work down the body, starting with the hands, and using the sequence and principles of inspection, palpation and auscultation for each area.

### Arms
- Examine the radial and brachial pulses (p. 52 and see Fig. 4.7).
- Measure the BP in both arms (p. 77 and see Fig. 4.12).

### Neck
- Examine the carotid pulses (p. 52 and see Fig. 4.7).

### Abdomen
- Inspect from the side for obvious pulsation.
- Palpate over the abdominal aorta. The aortic bifurcation is at the level of the umbilicus, so feel in the epigastrium for a palpable AAA.
- If you feel a pulsatile mass, try to gauge its approximate size by placing the fingers of each hand on either side of it. If the fingers move apart with each pulsation, the mass is expansile.

- Listen over the aorta for a bruit due to a stenosis, and for renal artery bruits bilaterally; absence of bruits does not exclude significant stenosis.

Aortic palpation is highly dependent on body habitus. In thin patients a tortuous but normal-diameter aorta can be palpable; an aneurysm tends to be expansile rather than just pulsatile. Conversely, even a large aneurysm may be impalpable in an obese patient due to its posterior position. The finding of an expansile mass in the epigastrium strongly suggests the presence of an AAA but, importantly, its absence does not exclude AAA. Accordingly, referral for further imaging should depend on overall clinical suspicion, not solely examination findings. If there is no evidence of pulsatile expansion, there may be a mass anterior to the aorta through which the aortic pulsation is felt.

A pulsatile mass below the umbilicus suggests an iliac aneurysm.

### Legs
- Inspect and feel the legs and feet for changes of ischaemia, including temperature and colour changes (see Box 4.24), thin skin, brittle nails and absence of hair.
- Note scars from previous vascular or non-vascular surgery.
- Note the position, margin, depth and colour of any ulceration.
- Look for tissue loss, including specifically between the toes for ulcers and at the heels for ischaemic changes (the most common site of 'pressure sores').

### Femoral pulse
- Ask the patient to lie down and explain what you are going to do.
- Place the pads of your index and middle fingers over the femoral artery. If you are having trouble feeling it (in an obese patient, for example), remember that the femoral artery lies at the mid-inguinal point, halfway between the anterior superior iliac spine and the pubic symphysis (Fig. 4.33).
- Remember that, while it is possible to listen for femoral bruits using the stethoscope diaphragm, the presence or absence of a bruit is of little value in assessing the severity of aortoiliac disease.
- Palpate the femoral and radial pulses simultaneously to assess for radiofemoral delay (Fig. 4.34A).

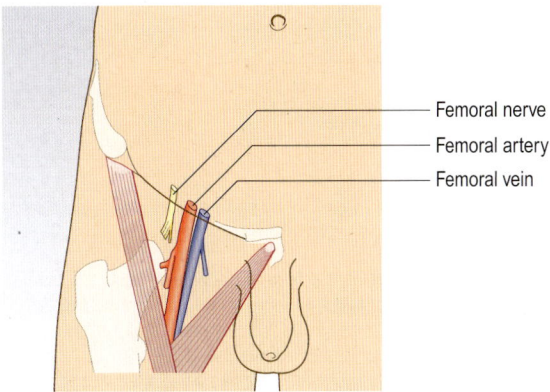

Femoral nerve
Femoral artery
Femoral vein

**Fig. 4.33 Femoral triangle: vessels and nerves.**

**Fig. 4.34 Examination of the femoral, popliteal, posterior tibial and dorsalis pedis arteries.** **A** Examine the femoral artery, while simultaneously checking for radiofemoral delay. **B** Feel the popliteal artery with your fingertips, having curled the fingers into the popliteal fossa. **C** Examine the posterior tibial artery. **D** Examine the dorsalis pedis artery.

## Popliteal pulse

- With the patient lying down, flex their knee to 30 degrees.
- With your thumbs on the tibial tuberosity and your fingers in the midline posteriorly (2–3 cm below the skin crease), try to compress the artery against the back of the tibia (see Fig. 4.34B).

The popliteal artery is usually hard to feel, so if it is readily palpable consider that there may be a popliteal artery aneurysm.

## Posterior tibial pulse

- Place the pads of your middle three fingers along the line between the medial malleolus and the tip of the heel (see Fig. 4.34C).

## Dorsalis pedis pulse

- Using the pads of your middle three fingers, feel at the origin of the first web space just lateral to the tendon of extensor hallucis longus (see Fig. 4.34D).

The presence of foot pulses does not completely exclude significant lower limb PAD, but they are almost always diminished or absent. If the history is convincing but pulses are felt, ask the patient to walk on a treadmill until pain develops (exercise ABPI). If they have flow-limiting PAD, their APBI will fall (see below).

## Buerger's test

Buerger's test is performed to aid assessment of arterial insufficiency.

### Examination sequence (Video 3H)

- With the patient lying supine, stand at the foot of the bed. Raise the patient's feet and support the legs at 45 degrees to the horizontal for 2–3 minutes.
- Watch for developing pallor with emptying and 'guttering' of the superficial veins.
- Ask the patient to sit up and hang their legs over the edge of the bed.
- Watch for reactive hyperaemia – the foot becomes red on dependency due to accumulation of vasoactive metabolites; the loss of pallor and spreading redness make a positive test. This is also known as 'sunset foot'.
- The test is positive if the foot becomes pale on elevation and red when lowered.
- If you see a patient with rest pain symptoms, do not be falsely reassured by a warm, red foot!

## Ankle: brachial pressure index

Assessing pulse status can be unreliable in patients with obesity or oedema. Routinely measure the ABPI whenever there is difficulty palpating lower limb pulses or when PAD is suspected on the basis of the history.

## Examination sequence

- Use a hand-held Doppler probe and a sphygmomanometer.
- Hold the probe over the posterior tibial artery at an angle of 45 degrees.
- Inflate a BP cuff round the ankle.
- Note the pressure at which the Doppler signal disappears. This is the systolic pressure in that artery as it passes under the cuff.
- Repeat, holding the probe over the dorsalis pedis artery.
- Measure the brachial BP in both arms, holding the Doppler probe over the brachial artery at the elbow or the radial artery at the wrist.

The ratio of the pedal artery pressure to the highest brachial artery pressure gives the ABPI in each limb. In health, the ABPI is greater than 1.0–1.2 when the patient is supine. An ABPI of less than 0.9 would be consistent with intermittent claudication, and a value less than 0.4 may indicate critical limb ischaemia. Patients with critical limb ischaemia (rest pain, tissue loss) typically have an ankle BP of less than 50 mmHg and a positive Buerger's test.

Patients with lower limb PAD, particularly those with diabetes mellitus, often have incompressible, calcified crural arteries that give falsely reassuring pedal pressures and ABPI. If the ABPI is greater than 1.2 you should be suspicious that this is the case. Toe pressures may be more accurate in these patients and can be measured using a cuff round the base of the hallux with a laser Doppler probe at the tip of the toe.

## Investigations

Further investigations must be carefully selected to provide the most information with the least risk to the patient and at least expense. Duplex ultrasound is often the first-line investigation of choice for unilateral disease, while bilateral symptoms can be investigated using a CT or MR angiogram (Box 4.25).

There is an increasing use of bedside ultrasound to assess patients presenting acutely with PVD.

# PERIPHERAL VENOUS SYSTEM

## Anatomy and physiology

Blood is returned to the heart from the peripheries by a network of deep (90%) and superficial (10%) veins. Venous return from the head and neck is passive, while blood from the legs must be pumped actively back up to the heart against gravity. Pressure on the sole of the foot on walking, together with a contraction of muscles in the calf (the 'calf muscle pump') and, to a lesser extent, in the thighs and buttocks, drives blood back up through the veins. Backward flow (reflux) is prevented by valves that divide the long column of blood from the foot to the right atrium into a series of short, low-pressure segments. As a result, the 'ambulatory venous pressure' in the feet in health is usually less than 20 mmHg.

Deep veins follow the course of the main arteries. Valvular insufficiency causing venous reflux may be primary or post-thrombotic (following DVT). Following DVT, the vein may remain occluded or recanalised; however, even in recanalised veins valve function is usually compromised. Post-thrombotic syndrome results from deep venous incompetence due to either occlusion, valvular dysfunction or a combination. Symptoms include pain, venous claudication, blue discoloration, swelling, dilated superficial veins, skin changes and ulceration; it can be difficult to treat.

The long and short saphenous veins are the superficial veins of the lower limb and may also be affected by primary valvular failure and by valvular failure secondary to superficial thrombophlebitis. The long (great) saphenous vein passes anterior to the medial malleolus at the ankle, then up the medial aspect of the calf and thigh to join the common femoral vein in the groin at the saphenofemoral junction (Fig. 4.35).

The short (lesser) saphenous vein passes behind the lateral malleolus at the ankle and up the posterior aspect of the calf. It commonly joins the popliteal vein at the saphenopopliteal junction, which usually lies 2 cm above the posterior knee crease.

There are numerous intercommunications between the long and short saphenous veins, and between the deep and superficial venous systems, via perforator or communicating veins. The venous anatomy of the lower limb is highly variable.

Superficial venous incompetence is characterised by varicose veins, aching and skin changes consistent with chronic venous insufficiency (see Fig. 4.36A).

| 4.25 Investigations in peripheral arterial disease | |
|---|---|
| **Investigation** | **Indication/comment** |
| Duplex ultrasound | Carotid artery stenosis, abdominal aortic aneurysm surveillance, peripheral arterial disease |
| Computed tomography | Abdominal aortic aneurysm, peripheral arterial disease, carotid artery stenosis |
| Magnetic resonance imaging | Peripheral arterial disease, carotid artery stenosis, arteriovenous malformations |
| Angiography | Acute and chronic limb ischaemia, carotid artery stenosisInvasive angiography has largely been replaced by computed tomography/magnetic resonance angiography as a diagnostic test |

Femoral vein

Profunda
femoris vein

Long saphenous
vein

Popliteal vein

Venae comitantes
of posterior and
anterior tibial
arteries

Short
saphenous vein

Great saphenous
vein

Dorsal
venous arch

**Fig. 4.35** Veins of the lower limb.

# The history

## Common presenting symptoms

Lower limb venous disease presents in four ways:

- varicose veins
- deep venous thrombosis
- chronic venous insufficiency and ulceration
- superficial thrombophlebitis.

The severity of symptoms may bear little relationship to the severity of the underlying pathology and the physical signs. Life-threatening DVT may be asymptomatic, while apparently trivial varicose veins may be associated with significant symptoms.

## Pain

Patients with uncomplicated varicose (dilated, tortuous, superficial) veins often complain of aching leg discomfort, itching and a feeling of swelling (see Fig. 4.36A). Symptoms are aggravated by prolonged standing and are often worse towards the end of the day. Once established, DVT causes pain and tenderness in the affected part (usually the calf). Superficial thrombophlebitis produces a red, painful area on the skin overlying the vein involved, and the vein may be palpable as a tender cord. Varicose ulceration may be surprisingly painless. If there is pain, this may be relieved by limb elevation, but it is extremely important to exclude coexisting arterial disease (Box 4.26). Graduated compression bandaging is the mainstay of treatment for a venous leg ulcer, but is contraindicated unless there is documented evidence of adequate arterial circulation, which is assessed by feeling the pulses or by measuring the ABPI (see earlier).

## Limb swelling

Swelling, or a feeling of swelling, even in the absence of visible signs, may be associated with lower limb venous disease. Enquire about risk factors for DVT (Box 4.27).

In upper limb DVT the arm is swollen and the skin is cyanosed and mottled, especially when dependent. Look for superficial distended veins (acting as collaterals) in the upper arm, over the shoulder region and on the anterior chest wall (Fig. 4.37). Symptoms are often exacerbated by activity, especially when holding the arm overhead.

There may be a history of repetitive trauma at the thoracic outlet due to vigorous, repetitive exercise (e.g. swimming, weight lifting, or racquet sports). Upper limb DVT may also complicate indwelling subclavian/jugular venous catheters.

## Skin changes

Chronic venous insufficiency is often associated with bluish discoloration of the distal extremity. A range of skin changes may be observed (see Fig. 4.36A). Varicose eczema leads to red, itchy, dry areas of skin over the lower leg. Venous hypertension causes extravasation of blood components into surrounding tissues, leading to haemosiderin deposition, which is seen as a brown discoloration of the skin, primarily around the medial aspect of the lower third of the leg. Lipodermatosclerosis occurs when there is an inflammatory response to the haemosiderin and causes red/purple discoloration and induration of the skin. The thickened, fibrotic skin forms a tight band around the lower leg, giving the appearance of an inverted champagne bottle. In *atrophie blanche*, there are multiple, small, white, scarred areas within the affected skin.

### Chronic venous ulceration

In developed countries, about 70–80% of lower limb ulceration is primarily due to venous disease. In addition to arterial disease and neuropathic ulceration, other rare causes include pyoderma gangrenosum, syphilis, tuberculosis, leprosy (Hansen's disease),

4

A                                                                          B

**Fig. 4.36 Lower limb venous disease.** A Varicose veins and associated haemosiderin deposition. B Venous ulcer. *(A) From Metcalfe M, Baker D. Varicose veins. Surgery (Oxford). 2008;26(1):4–7.*

## 4.26 Clinical features of venous and arterial ulceration

| Clinical feature | Venous ulceration | Arterial ulceration | Neuropathic ulceration |
|---|---|---|---|
| Sex | More common in women | More common in men | Equal in men and women |
| Risk factors | Thrombophilia, family history, previous deep vein thrombosis, varicose veins | Known peripheral vascular disease or risk factors for atherosclerotic disease, e.g. smoking, diabetes, dyslipidaemia, hypertension | Diabetes or other peripheral neuropathy (loss of sensation, loss of intrinsic foot muscle function, autonomic dysregulation) |
| Pain | Often painless but some patients have some pain that improves with elevating the leg | Severe pain, except in diabetics with neuropathy; improves on dependency | Painless or neuropathic pain |
| Site | Gaiter areas; 80% medial (long saphenous vein), 20% lateral (short saphenous vein) | Pressure areas (malleoli, heel, fifth metatarsal base, metatarsal heads and toes) | Pressure areas, sole of foot, tips of toes |
| Appearance | Shallow, irregular margin Slough on granulating base | Regular, 'punched out' Sloughy or necrotic base | Macerated, moist white skin surrounded by callus, often on load-bearing aspects (motor neuropathy) |
| Surrounding skin | Lipodermatosclerosis always present Oedema | Shiny, hairless, trophic changes | Dry due to reduced sweating (autonomic neuropathy) |
| Veins | Full and usually varicose | Empty with 'guttering' on elevation | Normal |
| Temperature | Warm Palpable pulses | Cold Absent pulses | Warm or cold due to autonomic neuropathy Palpable pulses |

### 4.27 Risk factors for deep vein thrombosis

- Obesity
- Smoking
- Recent bed rest or operations (especially to the leg, pelvis or abdomen)
- Recent travel, especially long flights
- Previous trauma to the leg, especially long-bone fractures, plaster of Paris splintage and immobilisation
- Pregnancy or features suggesting pelvic disease
- Malignant disease
- Previous deep vein thrombosis
- Family history of thrombosis
- Inherited thrombophilia, e.g. factor V Leiden
- Recent central venous catheterisation, injection of drug
- Use of oral contraceptive or hormone replacement therapy

A

B

**Fig. 4.37 Axillary vein thrombosis.** [A] Angiogram. *Single arrow* shows site of thrombosis. *Double arrows* show dilated collateral vessels. [B] Clinical appearance with swollen left arm and dilated superficial veins.

sickle cell disease and tropical conditions. Chronic venous ulceration (see Fig. 4.36B) usually affects the gaiter area of the calf, most commonly on the medial aspect. Ulcers are shallow and pink (granulation tissue) or yellow/green (slough) in colour, with an irregular margin, and are usually associated with other skin changes of chronic venous insufficiency (varicose eczema, lipodermatosclerosis).

It can be useful to append photographs to clinical records to enable the progress of ulcer healing or deterioration to be monitored. Furthermore, photographs taken in the community can be used to enable consultations with hospital specialists to be undertaken remotely for certain patients.

## Superficial venous thrombophlebitis

This condition affects up to 10% of patients with severe varicose veins and is more common during pregnancy. Recurrent superficial venous thrombophlebitis, especially that affecting different areas sequentially, and non-varicose veins, may be associated with underlying malignancy. It may propagate into the deep system, leading to DVT and pulmonary embolism.

### Past history

Enquire about previous varicose vein surgery and risk factors for DVT (see Box 4.27).

## The physical examination

### Examination sequence

Expose the patient's legs and examine them with the patient standing and then lying supine.
- Are there any skin changes consistent with chronic venous hypertension, such as haemosiderin deposition, varicose eczema, lipodermatosclerosis, atrophie blanche (scars from healed ulcers), or champagne bottle deformity?
- Are there any ulcers? Venous ulcers typically appear shallow, lie in the gaiter area of the calf and are non-painful.
- Are there varicosities and if so where on the leg are they? Varicosities on the medial side of the thigh or calf are likely to originate from the long saphenous vein, whilst those on the lateral side are likely to come from the short saphenous vein.
- Feel for any temperature difference.
- Press gently with your fingertip over the tibia above the ankle for a few seconds and then see if your finger has left a pit (pitting oedema). Remember to avoid areas that might be tender such as around ulcers.
- If the leg is grossly swollen, press at a higher level to establish how far the oedema extends.
- If you find oedema, check the JVP (p. 57). If the JVP is raised, this suggests cardiac disease or pulmonary hypertension as a cause, especially if both legs are oedematous.
- A positive Homan's sign (calf pain on passive dorsiflexion of the ankle) may be present in DVT, but is neither sensitive nor specific and therefore cannot be relied upon to rule in or rule

out DVT. If you suspect DVT, the patient should have a Duplex ultrasound.

## Investigations

Tests such as the tourniquet and the Trendelenburg tests, to assess for saphenofemoral valve incompetence, are now obsolete and have been replaced by hand-held Doppler. With the patient standing, ask them to put their weight on the contralateral foot and position the hand-held Doppler probe over the long saphenous vein or saphenofemoral junction (2 cm below and medial to the mid-inguinal point). Squeeze the calf muscle and listen for blood flowing up through the long saphenous vein. If the valves are competent, you will hear only very brief backflow of blood (<0.5 second) only when you release the calf muscle, which is physiological as the valves close. If the valves are incompetent, you will hear the prolonged sound of blood refluxing back down the vein.

4

### OSCE example 1: Chest pain history

Mrs. Khan, 62 years old, presents to you with intermittent chest pain.

#### Please take a history

- Introduce yourself and clean your hands.
- Invite the patient to describe the presenting symptoms, using open questioning.
- Take a detailed history of the presenting symptoms, including the onset, duration, site, quality and severity of the pain, and any aggravating or relieving factors, in particular the relationship to exertion. Determine the functional consequences and any change in the pattern of symptoms.
- Ask about relevant past history and vascular risk factors, including hypertension, diabetes and hyperlipidaemia.
- Enquire about drug history or intolerances, including preventative therapies.
- Ask about premature coronary artery disease in first-degree relatives.
- Take a social history, including occupation, smoking and alcohol.
- Conduct a systematic inquiry. In particular, is there associated palpitation, breathlessness, orthopnoea and ankle swelling, or has there been any bleeding?
- Ask about any other patient concerns.
- Thank the patient and clean your hands.

#### Summarise your findings

Mrs. Khan gives a 6-week history of intermittent chest discomfort. She reports a dull central ache that does not radiate to the arms or jaw. It occurs predominantly with effort, is worse on inclines or walking on cold mornings, and resolves at rest after a few minutes. These symptoms make her work as a carer challenging. She has no previous cardiac problems but is known to have hypertension and type 2 diabetes; she takes metformin for the latter. There is no family history of premature coronary artery disease and she has never been a smoker.

#### Suggest a likely diagnosis

The likely diagnosis is stable angina pectoris.

#### Suggest further evaluation

Full cardiovascular examination, blood glucose and lipid profile, and a 12-lead electrocardiogram. Consider referral for an exercise tolerance test or coronary angiogram.

### OSCE example 2: Cardiac examination

Mr. Munro, 82 years old, presents with progressive breathlessness and lightheadedness on exertion.

#### Please examine his cardiovascular system

- Introduce yourself and clean your hands.
- Carry out general observations. Is the patient tachypnoeic or distressed at rest? Are his hands cool?
- Measure the pulse, blood pressure and jugular venous pressure. Are the pulse volume and systolic pressure reduced? Is the jugular venous pressure elevated?
- Palpate the precordium. Is the apex more forceful or displaced?
- Auscultate over the apex and lower left, upper right and upper left sternal borders for the character of the first and second heart sounds, and the presence and characteristics of any added sounds or murmurs. If a murmur is heard, is there any radiation?
- Examine the chest, sacrum and lower limbs for signs of heart failure.
- Thank the patient and clean your hands.

*Continued*

## OSCE example 2: Cardiac examination—cont'd

### Summarise your findings

Mr. Munro appears comfortable. His heart rate is 80 bpm with a low-volume, slow-rising pulse. His blood pressure is 110/60 mmHg. The jugular venous pressure is not raised. There is an apical heave, but the apex is not displaced. The first heart sound is normal but the second is diminished. There is a grade 3 ejection systolic murmur, loudest over the aortic area but heard widely, radiating to the carotids. There are fine end-inspiratory crackles at the lung bases.

### Suggest a likely diagnosis

The likely diagnosis is aortic stenosis with left ventricular decompensation and heart failure.

### Suggest initial investigations

Twelve-lead electrocardiogram, chest x-ray and transthoracic echocardiogram.

## Integrated examination sequence for the cardiovascular system

- Position the patient: supine and reclined at 45 degrees, with the head resting on a pillow.
- Examine the general appearance:
  - Is the patient breathless, cyanosed, sweating or distressed?
  - Note body habitus (overweight or cachectic), Marfanoid features and the presence of radial or saphenous vein harvest scars.
- Check the hands, pulse and blood pressure, face and neck:
  - Hands: colour and temperature, tobacco staining, clubbing, splinter haemorrhages, Janeway lesions or Osler's nodes, tendon xanthomata.
  - Pulse: rate, rhythm, character and synchronicity of radial pulse, collapsing pulse, volume and character of brachial or carotid pulse.
  - Blood pressure: systolic and diastolic pressure at the brachial artery.
  - Face: central cyanosis, xanthelasmata, corneal arcus, petechiae.
  - Neck: timing, waveform and abnormalities of the jugular venous pressure, carotid bruits.
- Examine the precordium:
  - Inspection: look for midline sternotomy or left submammary scars, pacemaker site, visible pulsation.
  - Palpation: define the character and position of the apex beat, parasternal heave, thrills.
  - Auscultation: listen over the apex, lower left sternal border, upper right and left sternal borders, over the carotid arteries and left axilla. Listen with the patient on their left side and leaning forward during expiration.
    - Heart sounds: identify first and second heart sounds ($S_1$ and $S_2$), and any extra heart sounds ($S_3$ or $S_4$).
    - Additional sounds: clicks and snaps.
    - Murmurs in systole and/or diastole (timing, duration, character, pitch, intensity, location and radiation).
  - Pericardial rub.
- Other:
  - Listen for fine end-inspiratory crackles or pleural effusion at the lung bases.
  - Examine the abdomen for hepatomegaly or pulsatile liver.
  - Check for ankle and sacral oedema.

### Peripheral arterial and venous system

- Inspection of the lower limbs:
  - Check temperature and colour, capillary refill time, skin discoloration, ulceration, varicosities, scars.
- Palpation:
  - Examine the abdomen for expansile aortic aneurysm.
  - Identify the femoral, popliteal, posterior tibial and dorsalis pedis pulses.
  - Identify pitting oedema.
  - Perform Buerger's test.
- Auscultation:
  - Listen for bruits over the abdomen and over the femoral arteries.

# 5

# The respiratory system

J Alastair Innes
Peter T Reid

Anatomy and physiology 84

The history 84
Common presenting symptoms 85
Past medical history 90
Drug and allergy history 90
Family history 90
Social history 91
Systematic enquiry 92

The physical examination 92
Inspection 92

Palpation 96
Percussion 97
Auscultation 98

Interpretation of the findings 99

Investigations 99

OSCE example 1: Respiratory history 101

OSCE example 2: Respiratory examination 102

Integrated examination sequence for the respiratory system 103

## Anatomy and physiology

Understanding the surface anatomy of the lungs (Fig. 5.1) and their relation to adjacent structures is essential for the practice of respiratory medicine. At the end of tidal expiration, the dome of the diaphragm extends high into the thorax, level with the anterior end of the fifth rib, slightly lower on the left. The lower lateral ribs therefore overlie the liver on the right and the stomach and spleen on the left, with the parietal pleura extending lower than the lungs on the lateral chest wall. Posteriorly, the lungs extend much lower, approaching the 12th rib on full inspiration.

The lung apex lies immediately beneath the brachial plexus, so apical lung tumours commonly disrupt T1 root fibres, causing pain and numbness in the inner aspect of the upper arm and wasting of the small hand muscles. The upper thoracic sympathetic outflow to the eye may also be compromised, leading to a constricted pupil and ptosis. In the mid and lower mediastinum, tumours can invade and compromise the pericardium, atria and oesophagus.

In health, the lungs optimise gas exchange by close matching of regional ventilation and perfusion. Airway and parenchymal lung diseases disrupt this matching, causing hypoxia and cyanosis, and commonly stimulate breathing through lung afferent nerves, leading to a history of breathlessness and tachypnoea upon examination.

## The history

The key features of the history are summarised in Box 5.1.

| 1 Pleural markings | 4 Oblique fissure |
| 2 Lung markings | 5 Horizontal fissure |
| 3 Cardiac notch | 6 Trachea |

A

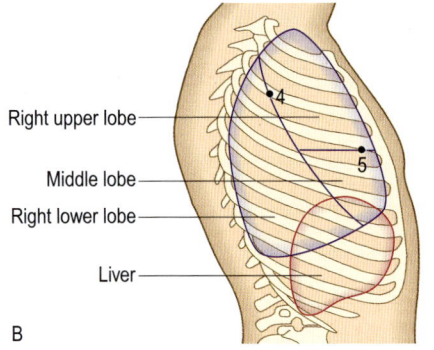

Right upper lobe

Middle lobe

Right lower lobe

Liver

B

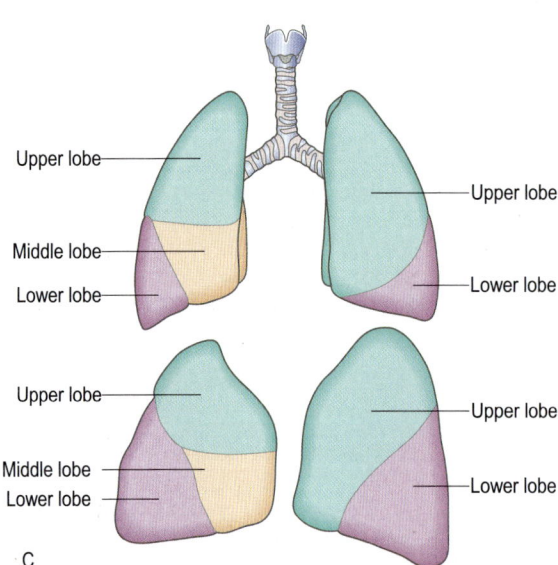

Upper lobe

Middle lobe

Lower lobe

Upper lobe

Lower lobe

Upper lobe

Middle lobe

Lower lobe

Upper lobe

Lower lobe

C

**Fig. 5.1** Surface anatomy of the thorax. **A** Anterior view. **B** Right lateral view. **C** Lobar anatomy of the lung surfaces: anterior view (*upper*), lateral view (*lower*).

### 5.1 Respiratory history-taking/documentation framework

**History of presenting symptoms**

***Specific respiratory symptoms***
- Breathlessness
- Wheeze
- Cough
- Sputum/haemoptysis
- Chest pain
- Fever/rigors/night sweats
- Weight loss
- Sleepiness

**Past medical history**
- Respiratory disease
- Other illness/hospital encounters

**Drug and allergy history**
- Drugs causing or relieving respiratory symptoms
- Allergies to pollens/pets/dust; anaphylaxis

**Social and family history**
- Family history of respiratory disease
- Home circumstances/effect of and on disease
- Smoking
- Occupational history

**Systematic review**
- Systemic diseases involving the lung
- Risk factors for lung disease

# Common presenting symptoms

## Breathlessness

Breathlessness (dyspnoea) denotes the feeling of an 'uncomfortable need to breathe' and is the most commonly reported respiratory symptom. It is also one of the most challenging to quantify, being inherently subjective. Breathlessness may be caused by respiratory or cardiac disease and also occurs in anaemia or as a manifestation of psychological distress.

Respiratory disease can cause breathlessness through a range of mechanisms:

- stimulation of intrapulmonary afferent nerves by interstitial inflammation or thromboembolism
- mechanical loading of respiratory muscles by airflow obstruction or reduced lung compliance in fibrosis
- hypoxia due to ventilation/perfusion mismatch, stimulating chemoreceptors.

The Medical Research Council (MRC) breathlessness scale (Box 5.2) is a useful and validated way to document formally the patient's level of dyspnoea.

Specific questions may help to distinguish the causes of breathlessness. Ask in particular:

- *How did the breathlessness start?* If the onset was instantaneous, think of pneumothorax, pulmonary embolus or anaphylaxis. Paroxysmal nocturnal dyspnoea (p. 47) may wake a sleeping patient with breathlessness. Onset over hours is typical in asthma, acute pulmonary oedema, lobar pneumonia, or acute hypersensitivity pneumonitis, while an insidious onset is more typical of an evolving pleural effusion, chronic obstructive pulmonary disease (COPD), interstitial lung disease and lung tumours.
- *How is your breathing at rest and overnight?* Asthma commonly wakes patients, while most patients with COPD are comfortable at rest and when asleep but struggle with exertion. Breathlessness provoked by lying down (orthopnoea) is a feature of heart failure (p. 47) but also occurs frequently in patients with severe airflow obstruction or diaphragmatic

weakness because the weight of the abdomen displaces the diaphragm cranially on lying down, compromising the vital capacity.

- *Does your breathlessness vary from day to day or week to week?* Variable breathlessness is typical of asthma, whereas patients with COPD or interstitial lung disease usually report consistent daily limitation.
- *Can you tell me something you do that would make you breathless?* and *How far can you walk on a good day?* These questions reveal the disability caused by respiratory disease. Record restrictions on normal activity or work and the corresponding MRC breathlessness score. Enquiring about hobbies and daily activities reveals the time course of breathlessness; for example, '*When was the last time you could walk to the shops / play a full round of golf?*'
- *When does the breathlessness start?* Asthma induced by exercise frequently appears only after exercise during early recovery, because sympathetic drive during exercise defends airway patency.

Certain phrases in the history strongly suggest a psychological aetiology of breathlessness, particularly 'I feel I can't get enough air (or oxygen) into my chest.' In patients with hyperventilation due to anxiety, this symptom is frequently accompanied by a normal measured vital capacity. Associated symptoms induced by hypocapnia in hyperventilation include digital and perioral paraesthesia, light-headedness and chest tightness.

Fig. 5.2 summarises how to use the history and examination findings to distinguish some common causes of breathlessness. Remember that patients do not always report exactly what textbooks describe.

## Wheeze

Wheeze describes the high-pitched musical or 'whistling' sounds produced by turbulent air flow through small airways narrowed by bronchospasm and/or airway secretions. It is heard mostly during expiration, which additionally narrows the airways. Wheeze must be distinguished from the rattling inspiratory and expiratory sounds caused by loose, mobile secretions in the upper airways, and from the louder, dramatic croak of stridor (see below) caused by obstruction in the trachea or large airways. Patients may be unaware of nocturnal wheeze, which may be noticed only by their bed partner.

Wheeze is most commonly associated with asthma and COPD but can also occur with acute bronchitis, exacerbations of bronchiectasis or congestive cardiac failure ('cardiac wheeze').

Ask:

- *Is the wheeze worse during or after exercise?* If it occurs during exercise and limits it, this suggests COPD; in asthma, wheeze and tightness usually appear after exercise.
- *Do you wake with wheeze during the night?* This suggests asthma.
- *Do you have hay fever or other allergies?* Atopy is common in allergic asthma. A family history of wheeze or asthma is common.

### 5.2 Medical Research Council breathlessness scale

| Grade | Degree of breathlessness related to activities |
|---|---|
| 1 | Not troubled by breathlessness except on strenuous exercise |
| 2 | Short of breath when hurrying on the level or walking up a slight hill |
| 3 | Walks slower than most people on the level, stops after a mile or so, or stops after 15 min walking at own pace |
| 4 | Stops for breath after walking about 100 yards or after a few minutes on level ground |
| 5 | Too breathless to leave the house, or breathless when undressing |

Used with the permission of the Medical Research Council.

**Fig. 5.2** Common causes of breathlessness: distinguishing features on history and examination. *COPD,* Chronic obstructive pulmonary disease; *JVP,* jugular venous pressure; *MI,* myocardial infarction.

- *Is it worse on waking in the morning and relieved by clearing sputum?* This is common in COPD and bronchiectasis.

## Cough

The cough reflex has evolved to dislodge foreign material and secretions from the central airways and may be triggered by pathology at any level of the bronchial tree. Inspiration is followed by an expiratory effort against a closed glottis. Subsequent sudden opening of the glottis with rapid expiratory flow produces the characteristic sound.

Cough is most commonly a symptom of acute viral bronchitis, which is usually self-limiting over days to weeks. A cough that fails to settle within 3 weeks should prompt consideration of underlying respiratory disease. Causes of chronic cough and features in the history that may indicate the underlying cause are summarised in Box 5.3.

Ask about:

- Duration of the cough.
- Whether it is present every day.
- If it is intrusive/irresistible or whether the patient coughs deliberately to clear a perceived obstruction (throat clearing).
- Whether it produces sputum. If so, how much, and what colour?
- Any haemoptysis?
- Any triggers (such as swallowing, cold air, during or after exercise, allergens).

## 5.3 Causes of chronic cough and accompanying clues in the history

| Pathophysiology | Suggestive features in history/ examination |
|---|---|
| Airways inflammation | |
| • Asthma – 'cough-variant asthma' | Affects children and some adults<br>Often present at night<br>Associated wheezing, atopy |
| • Chronic obstructive pulmonary disease | History of smoking and intermittent sputum |
| • Persisting airway reactivity following acute bronchitis | Cough persisting after recent infection |
| • Bronchiectasis | Daily purulent sputum for long periods<br>Pneumonia or whooping cough in childhood<br>Recurrent haemoptysis |
| Lung cancer | Persistent cough, especially in smokers<br>Any haemoptysis<br>Pneumonia that fails to clear in 4–6 weeks |
| Rhinitis with postnasal drip | Chronic sneezing, nasal blockage/discharge |
| Oesophageal reflux | Heartburn or acid reflux after eating, bending or lying<br>Nocturnal and daytime cough |
| Drug effects | Angiotensin-converting enzyme inhibitors |
| Interstitial lung diseases | Persistent dry cough<br>Fine inspiratory crackles at bases |
| Idiopathic cough | Long history with no signs and negative investigations – diagnosis of exclusion |

- Smoking. This increases the likelihood of chronic bronchitis or lung cancer.
- Associated clinical features:
  - Wheeze: may signal cough-variant asthma.
  - Heartburn or reflux: gastro-oesophageal reflux commonly triggers cough.
  - Altered voice or swallowing: consider laryngeal causes.
- Drug history, especially angiotensin-converting enzyme (ACE) inhibitors.

Cough that produces green or yellow sputum suggests bronchial infection. Large volumes of sputum over long periods suggest bronchiectasis.

In patients with malignancy at the left hilum, damage to the left recurrent laryngeal nerve may paralyse the left vocal cord, making it impossible for the patient to close the glottis and generate a normal explosive cough. The resulting hoarse forced expiration without the initial explosive glottal opening is called a 'bovine cough.'

## Sputum

In health, the airway lining fluid coating the tracheobronchial tree ascends the mucociliary escalator to the larynx, where it mixes with upper respiratory tract secretions and saliva and is swallowed. In disease, the accumulation of inflammatory cells, mucus and proteinaceous secretions in the airways results in cough with expectoration of sputum. Ask the patient about the colour, volume and consistency of sputum. Direct examination of the sputum is useful to verify the account (Fig. 5.3).

In acute or chronic airway infection, the characteristics of sputum help to clarify the pathology. A change in colour or consistency, or an increase in volume may indicate a new infection in chronic disease.

### Colour

- Clear (mucoid): COPD/bronchiectasis without current infection.
- Yellow (mucopurulent): acute lower respiratory tract infection/asthma.
- Green (purulent): current infection – acute disease or exacerbation of chronic disease, such as COPD. In bronchiectasis (and COPD), the colour and volume of sputum may be used to guide the need for antibiotics (see Fig. 5.3A) whereas in asthma, mucopurulent sputum may be the result of sputum eosinophilia.
- Red/brown (rusty): pneumococcal pneumonia (see Fig. 5.3B). Try to distinguish between rusty and frank red blood (see below).
- Pink (serous/frothy): acute pulmonary oedema.

### Volume

- Establish the volume produced over 24 hours: small amounts into a tissue or enough to fill a spoon(s), eggcup(s) or cup(s).
- Compare the current volume with the patient's baseline volume.

### Consistency

- An increase in stickiness (viscosity) may indicate exacerbation in bronchiectasis.
- Occasionally, sputum is produced as firm 'plugs' by patients with asthma (see Fig. 5.3C), sometimes indicating underlying allergic bronchopulmonary aspergillosis.
- Large volumes of frothy secretions over weeks/months are a feature of the uncommon bronchoalveolar cell carcinoma.

## Haemoptysis

Haemoptysis means coughing up blood from the respiratory tract. Whilst it can complicate any severe forceful cough, never assume haemoptysis has a benign cause, particularly in a smoker, until underlying pathology has been excluded.

Enquire about these features:

- *Was the blood coughed up from the chest?* Blood in the mouth may be vomited, may have come from the nose in epistaxis, or may appear on chewing or tooth brushing in patients with gum disease.
- *When did blood appear, how much blood, were there associated symptoms and over what time period was it present?*

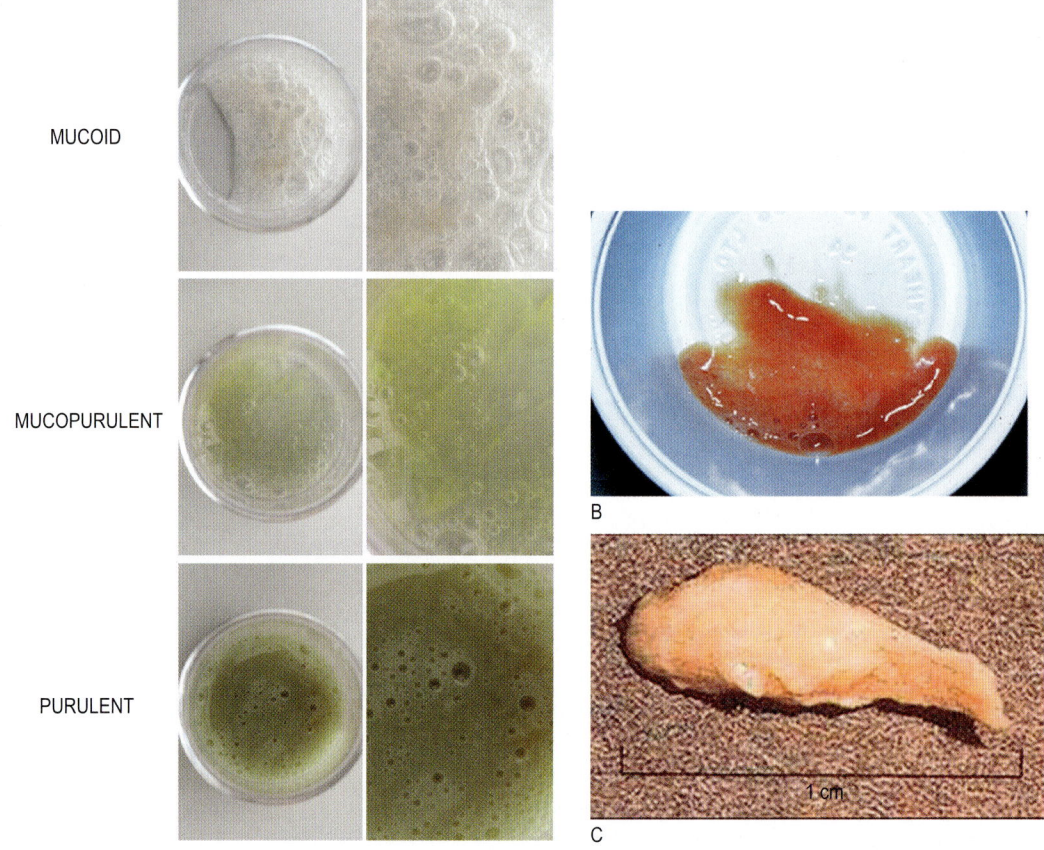

MUCOID

MUCOPURULENT

PURULENT

A

B

C

**Fig. 5.3** Sputum appearance in disease. [A] Colour chart of sputum purulence used in bronchiectasis. [B] Rusty red sputum of pneumococcal pneumonia. [C] Mucus plug from a patient with asthma. *(A, Courtesy Medical Photography, NHS Lothian.)*

- Any fever/symptoms of infection? Acute or chronic bronchial infections, including tuberculosis, often trigger haemoptysis.
- Recurrent blood streaks in clear sputum should prompt a search for lung cancer.
- Recurrent blood streaks in purulent sputum over years suggests bronchiectasis.
- A sudden episode of haemoptysis with pleuritic pain and breathlessness suggests pulmonary embolism.
- Large volumes of haemoptysis (> 20 mL) suggest specific causes:
  - lung cancer eroding a pulmonary vessel
  - bronchiectasis (such as in cystic fibrosis)
  - cavitary disease (e.g., complicating an aspergilloma or cavitary pulmonary tuberculosis).
  - pulmonary vasculitis
  - pulmonary arteriovenous malformation.

## Stridor

This harsh, grating respiratory sound is caused by vibration of the tracheal walls or major bronchi when the airway lumen is critically narrowed by compression, tumour or inhaled foreign material. Inspiration lowers the pressure inside the extrathoracic trachea, so critical narrowing here leads to inspiratory stridor. In contrast, the intrathoracic large airways are compressed during expiration by positive pressure in the surrounding lung, leading to fixed expiratory wheeze or stridor. Large airway narrowing at the thoracic inlet (e.g., tracheal compression by a large goitre) may cause both inspiratory and expiratory stridor. Rapid investigation and treatment are vital when this sign is present.

## Chest pain

Chest pain can arise from the chest wall, parietal pleura, mediastinal structures, tracheobronchial tree, pericardium, oesophagus and subdiaphragmatic organs (liver and gallbladder). Pain does not originate in the lung parenchyma or visceral pleura, as they have only an autonomic nerve supply.

Establish:

- Site and severity.
- Character: sharp suggests pleural pain.
- Onset: gradual or rapid?

- Exacerbating or relieving factors: worsening with cough or deep breaths suggests pleural disease.
- Associated symptoms: breathlessness, fever and cough suggest an infective cause.

A large pulmonary embolus can cause angina-like chest pain (p. 85), due to increase of right ventricular work together with reduced coronary oxygen delivery caused by hypotension and hypoxaemia, resulting in right ventricular ischaemia.

Pleuritic pain is worse on inspiration and coughing, and is usually described as sharp, stabbing or knife-like. It is usually sited away from the midline and may be localised or affect a wide area of chest wall. Disease causes parietal pleural pain in several ways:

- pneumonia and pulmonary infarcts: either direct pleural inflammation or adhesions with pleural traction on respiratory movement
- pneumothorax: mechanical distortion of pleura with lung collapse
- lung cancer: pleural distortion by infiltration, although constant pain is more typical

Musculoskeletal chest pain is common and may occur with chest trauma, forceful coughing or connective tissue disease. The chest is characteristically tender to palpation, and the pain can be reproduced by respiratory movements and/or movement of the spine or shoulder muscles. There may be associated soft tissue injury or rib fractures. A detailed history of events preceding the onset is vital, as injury is easily overlooked.

Two other uncommon conditions can cause acute chest pain. Bornholm disease is an infection with an enterovirus (Coxsackie B). This causes acute but self-limiting inflammation of intercostal muscles, with episodes of severe unilateral intercostal myalgia lasting a few days. Costochondritis (called Tietze's syndrome when costochondral swelling is present) is idiopathic inflammation of the costochondral cartilages adjoining the sternum, with acute localised pain and tenderness. The pain is eased by simple analgesia and settles spontaneously in both conditions.

Herpes zoster infection (shingles) may start with superficial itch or burning pain in a thoracic dermatome, followed by the appearance of a vesicular rash (a 'belt of roses from hell'). Pain and altered sensation may persist long after the rash has resolved, often with scarring in the affected dermatome.

Burning retrosternal pain may indicate oesophagitis but also occurs with myocardial ischaemia. Worsening of oesophageal discomfort after eating or relief after antacids helps to distinguish it from cardiac pain.

Cardiac pain is described on page 45.

Central, constant, progressive, non-pleuritic chest pain may represent mediastinal disease, particularly malignancy. Similarly, chest wall pain (without trauma) that is constant, progressive and non-pleuritic suggests chest wall invasion by malignancy. Sleep disturbance is a feature of such malignant pains.

## Fevers/rigors/night sweats

These symptoms are not specific but are commonly reported by patients with respiratory illnesses. Infection (acute or chronic) is the usual cause, but other aetiologies such as lung cancer, lymphoma or vasculitis should also be considered.

Patients use many different terms to describe fever (e.g., shivers, chills, shakes), so take care to clarify their actual symptoms.

Rigors are generalised, uncontrollable episodes of vigorous body shaking lasting a few minutes. Despite high fever, the patient may complain of feeling cold and seek extra clothing. Rigors usually indicate bacterial sepsis; lobar pneumonia and acute pyelonephritis are the most common causes.

Night sweats, particularly if persistent, are associated with chronic infection such as tuberculosis or malignancy, particularly lymphoma. Occasional episodes are inconclusive, but if patients report having to change their nightclothes or sheets frequently due to profuse nocturnal sweating over several weeks, this suggests underlying disease.

## Weight loss

Weight loss is a common feature of respiratory diseases, including lung cancer, COPD, interstitial lung disease, and chronic infections such as tuberculosis and bronchiectasis. The pathophysiology is complex; however, breathlessness is associated with diminished appetite, and the systemic inflammatory response is also thought to contribute to weight loss.

Weight loss also occurs in acute infection with loss of appetite, particularly during hospitalisation. Ask the patient to estimate the extent and duration of weight loss and enquire about appetite and dietary intake.

## Sleepiness

Excessive daytime sleepiness may be a symptom of an underlying sleep-related breathing disorder – obstructive sleep apnoea (OSA) or OSA/sleep hypopnoea (OSASH). In these conditions, the upper airway collapses intermittently and repeatedly during sleep. Partial obstruction results in snoring, but complete collapse stimulates increased respiratory effort resulting in transient wakening. Repeated episodes of sleep disturbance cause excessive daytime sleepiness and poor concentration. OSASH is more common in men; particularly if obese and with a large neck (collar sizes >17 inches) and can be aggravated by alcohol.

Ask about:

- Normal sleeping habit: does the patient keep hours that allow reasonable rest?
- Shift or night work: this can disrupt and prevent healthy sleep patterns.
- Does the person wake refreshed or exhausted? Sleep apnoea patients are exhausted in the morning.
- Have they struggled to stay awake in the day: for example, at work or when driving?

It is vital to advise cessation of driving pending investigation if OSA is suspected.

Ideally, seek a description of any night-time breathing disturbance from a bed partner. In OSA, the partner may observe periodic cessation of breathing, accompanied by increasing respiratory efforts, followed by a sudden and loud resumption of breathing, often with postural repositioning, then repetition of this cycle.

Validated sleepiness scores (such as the Epworth Sleepiness Scale: http://epworthsleepinessscale.com/) can be used to quantify daytime somnolence and are helpful if considering referral to a sleep clinic.

## Past medical history

Past illnesses relevant to respiratory disease are summarised in Box 5.4. These include respiratory disease that may recur or cause long-term symptoms, and disease in other systems that may cause, complicate or present with respiratory symptoms, including thromboembolic, cardiovascular, haematological, malignant and connective tissue diseases.

Note prior respiratory treatments (including need for critical care) and the degree of chronic symptoms, such as usual exacerbation frequency, prescription rate and hospitalisation.

| 5.4 Previous illness relevant to respiratory history | |
|---|---|
| **History** | **Current implications** |
| Eczema, hay fever | Allergic tendency relevant to asthma |
| Childhood asthma | Many wheezy children do not have asthma as adults, yet many adults with asthma had childhood wheeze |
| Whooping cough, inhaled foreign body, measles | Recognised causes of bronchiectasis, especially if complicated by pneumonia |
| Pneumonia, pleurisy | Recurrent episodes may be a manifestation of bronchiectasis. Some pneumonias may cause bronchiectasis |
| Tuberculosis | Reactivation if not previously treated effectively Post-tuberculous bronchiectasis – sputum, haemoptysis. Aspergilloma in lung cavity may present with haemoptysis |
| Connective tissue disorders, e.g., rheumatoid arthritis | Many have respiratory manifestations, e.g., pulmonary fibrosis, effusions, bronchiectasis Immunomodulatory treatments for rheumatological diseases may cause pulmonary toxicity or make patients susceptible to respiratory infection |
| Previous malignancy | Recurrence, metastatic/pleural disease Chemotherapy can cause pulmonary fibrosis (e.g., bleomycin) Radiotherapy-induced pulmonary fibrosis |
| Cancer, recent travel, surgery or immobility | Pulmonary thromboembolism |
| Recent surgery, loss of consciousness | Aspiration of foreign body, gastric contents leading to pneumonia, lung abscess |
| Neuromuscular disorders | Respiratory failure Aspiration |

## Drug and allergy history

Note all drugs that the patient is currently using, including inhalers, nebulised therapy, domiciliary oxygen, non-prescription remedies and recreational drugs. Cross-check the drug names and doses with a separate source such as the general practitioner's records.

Drugs given for other problems commonly cause respiratory side effects; these are summarised in Box 5.5.

Ask whether the patient has allergies such as hay fever, as allergic asthma is far more common in those with a history of atopy.

## Family history

Respiratory diseases with a known genetic cause are relatively rare. Patients with autosomal recessive conditions such as cystic fibrosis usually have unaffected carrier parents but may have affected siblings. A family history of venous thromboembolism should prompt investigation of inherited thrombophilias such as Factor V Leiden or protein C or protein S deficiency. In rare cases, idiopathic pulmonary fibrosis and primary pulmonary hypertension may be familial.

| 5.5 Respiratory problems caused by drugs | |
|---|---|
| **Respiratory condition** | **Drug** |
| Bronchoconstriction | Beta-blockers (including eye drops) Opioids Nonsteroidal anti-inflammatory drugs |
| Cough | Angiotensin-converting enzyme inhibitors |
| Bronchiolitis obliterans | Penicillamine |
| Diffuse parenchymal lung disease | Cytotoxic agents: bleomycin, methotrexate Anti-inflammatory agents: sulfasalazine, penicillamine, gold salts, aspirin Cardiovascular drugs: amiodarone, hydralazine Antibiotics: nitrofurantoin |
| Pulmonary thromboembolism | Oestrogens |
| Pulmonary hypertension | Oestrogens Dexfenfluramine, fenfluramine |
| Pleural effusion | Amiodarone Nitrofurantoin Phenytoin Methotrexate Pergolide |
| Respiratory depression | Opioids Benzodiazepines |
| Tuberculosis | Reactivation by glucocorticoids or disease modifying antirheumatic drugs (DMARDs)/ biological immunomodulators given for rheumatic disease |

## Social history

Exposures at home may cause or aggravate respiratory disease. Passive smoking increases the risk of respiratory infection and burning biomass fuels in confined spaces increases the risk of bronchitis and COPD. Domestic pets, especially cats and rodents, may be the cause of suboptimal asthma control. A pet bird, feather duvet or an infestation of mould may cause hypersensitivity pneumonitis or suboptimal asthma control.

The home circumstances may reveal the impact of respiratory disability, for example if the patient has relocated to ground-floor accommodations or relies on others for shopping.

### Smoking

Obtaining an accurate history of tobacco use is difficult and is covered on page 16 (Chapter 2). Ask if any cohabitees smoke; this can be a major obstacle to cessation. Remember also to ask about cannabis, waterpipes and e-cigarettes. Cannabis may be smoked without tobacco; for example using a bong; or cut with tobacco as an unfiltered joint. Waterpipes ('narghileh', 'shisha' or 'hookah') are used to smoke tobacco, cannabis or flavoured tobacco (maassel). E-cigarettes are used increasingly to assist with smoking cessation.

### Occupational history

Many respiratory diseases are caused by occupational exposure to inhaled substances; these are summarised in Box 5.6. Ask the patient about their work history, starting with their first job documenting the employers' names, the dates and duration of exposure, and whether any protective masks were offered or used.

Occupational asthma should be considered if symptoms improve on days away from work.

### 5.6 Occupational factors in respiratory disease

| Respiratory disease | Toxic agent(s) | Affected occupations |
| --- | --- | --- |
| Asthma<br>Rhino-conjunctivitis | Isocyanates<br>Flour, grain dust, enzymes<br>Animal dander/urine<br>Wood dust | Spray painters<br>Baking industry<br>Laboratory and veterinary workers<br>Joiners |
| Chronic obstructive pulmonary disease | Cadmium fumes<br>Coal dust<br>Silica<br><br>Coke dust | Solderers<br>Underground miners<br>Stone cutting, masonry, tunnelling, quarrying, pottery, metal ore mining, siliceous abrasive users, foundry workers<br>Coke oven workers |
| Byssinosis | Cotton dust | Flax workers |
| Pneumoconiosis | Coal (Coal Miners Pneumoconiosis)<br>Silica (Silicosis)<br>Asbestos (Asbestosis)<br><br>Iron (Siderosis)<br>Tin (Stannosis) | Miners<br>see above<br>Former laggers, asbestos textile manufacture; asbestos insulation work including marine engineering, shipbreaking.<br>Iron ore miners, welders, iron foundry fettlers<br>Tin smelters |
| Hypersensitivity pneumonitis | Thermophilic bacteria:<br>• Mouldy hay<br>• Mouldy grain<br>• Mushroom compost<br>• Mouldy sugar cane (Bagassosis)<br>Avian serum/excreta<br>Metal working fluids | Farmers<br>Grain workers<br>Mushroom pickers<br>Sugar workers<br>Bird fanciers<br>Machinists |
| Pneumonia | Strep. pneumonia<br>Q fever (Cox.burnetii)<br>Psittacosis (C. psittaci)<br>Leptospirosis (Leptospira) | Welders<br>Dairy farmers, abattoir workers<br>Poultry workers<br>Sewage workers, animal handlers, vets |
| Tuberculosis | Silica (silicotuberculosis) | See above |
| Granulomatous disease | Beryllium (Berylliosis) | Aerospace industry, nuclear industry, oil/gas drilling, dental technicians |
| Pleural disease | Asbestos: pleural plaques, diffuse pleural thickening, mesothelioma | See above |
| Lung cancer | Asbestos<br>Silica<br>Coke dust | See above |
| Connective tissue disease | Silica increases the risk of scleroderma. | See above |

Inhalation of organic dusts may trigger hypersensitivity pneumonitis. Whilst the cause is often unknown, contact with birds, bird droppings or feathers, metal working fluids, hay and mould remain common causes.

Inhalation of inorganic dusts such as asbestos, coal or silica cause pneumoconiosis, with gradual onset of cough and breathlessness, often years after exposure. Despite improved controls, asbestos and silica exposure remain important causes of ill health.

Certain occupations increase the risk of respiratory infection, for example Q fever in abattoir workers and leptospirosis in sewage workers and animal handlers.

## Systematic enquiry

Systematic enquiry may reveal extrapulmonary symptoms linked to underlying respiratory disease. For example, morning headaches can indicate an elevated $PaCO_2$ in respiratory failure, dysphagia following stroke can increase the risk of aspiration pneumonia, and joint pains may indicate connective tissue disease underlying pleural or parenchymal lung disease.

## The physical examination

Observations made during history taking can be valuable. For example, how easily did the patient converse? Did they cough repeatedly?

It is often easiest to examine the patient reclining on the bed or an examination couch at about 45 degrees, with the thorax exposed and the head supported by a pillow.

## Inspection

Much can be learned about the respiratory system by careful inspection from the end of the bed. The normal shape and respiratory movements of the chest wall are significantly altered by the hyperinflation that accompanies chronic airflow obstruction (Fig. 5.4). Such obstruction also causes prolonged expiration relative to inspiration, and sometimes 'pursed-lip' breathing on expiration. Forceful inspiration at these very high lung volumes may cause indrawing of the intercostal spaces during mid-inspiration and the recruitment of muscles not normally involved in breathing ('accessory muscles'). These include the sternocleidomastoid muscles lifting the sternum, and the trapezius and the scalenes lifting the shoulder girdle. Patients sometime sit forwards and brace their arms on a surface, allowing them to use the pectoralis major to pull the ribs outwards during inspiration. In contrast to the hyperinflation of obstructive disease, interstitial disease causes small, stiff lungs, diminishes thoracic volume and raises resting respiratory rate.

Chest deformity (Fig. 5.5) may be congenital, as in pectus excavatum, or acquired, as in pectus carinatum. The latter is an inward displacement of the lower ribs with a prominent sternum, caused by severe airflow obstruction in early childhood, during rib cage development. Asymmetry of the chest may be

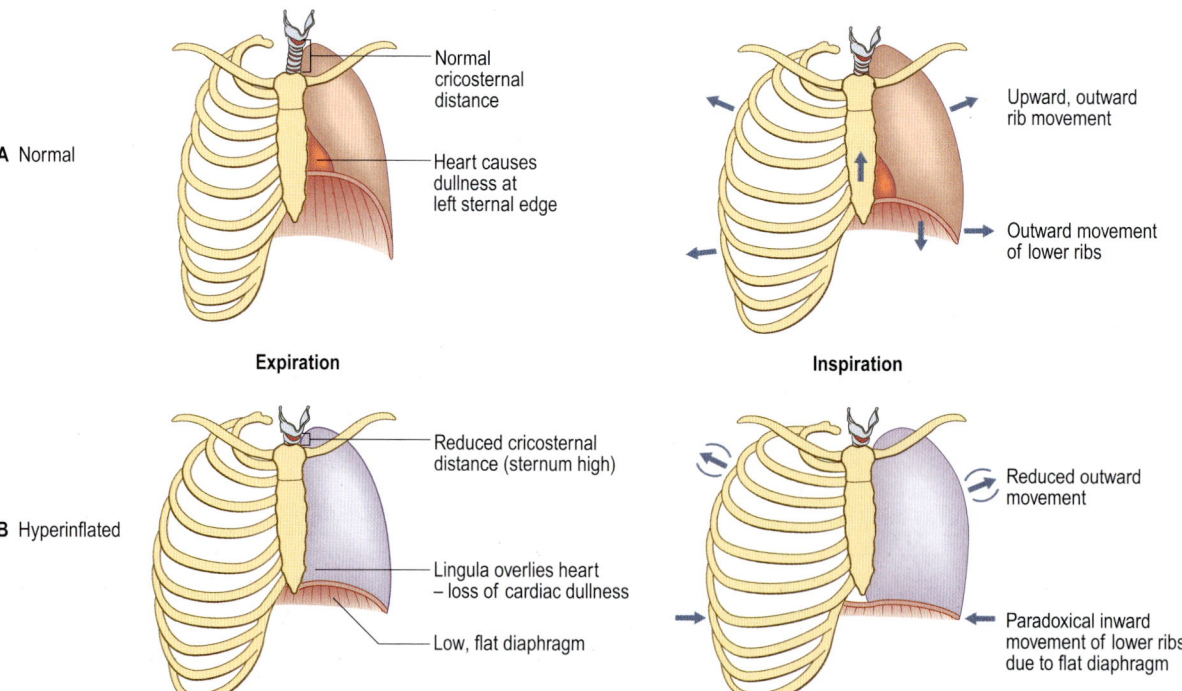

**A** Normal

Normal cricosternal distance

Heart causes dullness at left sternal edge

Expiration

Upward, outward rib movement

Outward movement of lower ribs

Inspiration

**B** Hyperinflated

Reduced cricosternal distance (sternum high)

Lingula overlies heart – loss of cardiac dullness

Low, flat diaphragm

Reduced outward movement

Paradoxical inward movement of lower ribs due to flat diaphragm

**Fig. 5.4** Respiratory movement of the ribs, sternum and diaphragm. **A** In normal adults. **B** In chronic hyperinflation due to obstructive lung disease. Hyperinflation causes upward displacement of the sternum and clavicles, increased anteroposterior thoracic diameter, loss of cardiac dullness at the lower left sternal edge, and a low flat diaphragm that pulls the lower ribs in during inspiration.

5

**Fig. 5.5** Abnormalities in the shape of the chest. **A** Hyperinflated chest with raised sternum and shoulder girdle. **B** Kyphoscoliosis. **C** Pectus carinatum with Harrison's sulcus *(arrow).* **D** Pectus excavatum.

secondary to scoliosis, shrinkage of scarred lung following tuberculosis, or prior surgical resection of the lung and/or ribs.

## Examination sequence (Videos 2 and 2B) ▶

- Note the presence of nebulisers or inhalers (indicating obstructive lung disease), oxygen therapy and cyanosis; check sputum pots, noting the colour and viscosity of the sputum and whether any blood is present. Foul-smelling sputum may indicate anaerobic infection.
- Look for asymmetry of the chest, deformities, surgical scars and chest drains, remembering that thoracotomy scars may be visible only from the side or behind.
- Quietly observe and time respiratory rate (for example, breaths in 15 s × 4) without drawing the patient's attention to

it, as this may cause it to change. Feeling the radial pulse, while timing breathing, is a common solution to this problem.
- Inspect the remaining skin for relevant abnormalities (Fig. 5.6).

At rest, the respiratory rate is normally 12 to 15 breaths/min; anxious patients may breathe at 15 to 20 breaths/min but a rate of over 20 breaths/min is abnormal for an adult.

In healthy adults at altitude, elderly people and patients with heart failure, or during the final stages of dying, a distinctive pattern of alternating periods of deep and shallow breathing may be seen. This is known as Cheyne–Stokes respiration and is thought to represent abnormal feedback from the carotid chemoreceptors to the respiratory centre.

A

B

**Fig. 5.6** Skin lesions associated with respiratory conditions. $\boxed{A}$ Metastatic nodules of lung cancer. $\boxed{B}$ Erythema nodosum on the shins in sarcoidosis.

Subcutaneous metastases from lung tumours (see Fig. 5.6A) may be seen and offer the chance for rapid biopsy and diagnosis. In the legs, the painful dusky red lesions of erythema nodosum (see Fig. 5.6B) may indicate underlying sarcoidosis, or asymmetrical swelling may signal venous thrombosis.

## Hands and arms

Finger clubbing is due to overgrowth of soft tissue in the terminal phalanx, which increases the lateral and longitudinal curvature of the nail (Fig. 3.8), raising the nail bed of the underlying bone. It is palpable as a boggy fluctuation of the nail when pressure is applied just proximal to the nail (Fig. 3.9C). Finding this in an adult patient should prompt consideration of lung cancer or pulmonary fibrosis. In younger patients, chronic suppurative lung disease such as cystic fibrosis should be considered (Box 3.4). In some cases of lung cancer, finger clubbing is accompanied by hypertrophic pulmonary osteoarthropathy, with painful, tender swelling of the wrists and ankles. X-rays of the distal forearm and lower legs show subperiosteal new bone formation overlying the cortex of the long bones.

Other important signs of respiratory disease in the hands include:

- cyanosis
- tar staining of fingers from tobacco use (Fig. 5.7)

**Fig. 5.7** Tobacco 'tar'-stained finger.

- small-muscle wasting (Fig. 13.23), which may indicate T1 root damage by an apical lung tumour
- rarely, yellow-brown discoloration of nails in yellow nail syndrome (Fig. 14.13C) or vasculitis in nail bed or finger pulp (Fig. 14.13B).

## Examination sequence (Video 2C) ▶

- Examine the hands for finger clubbing (Fig. 3.8), tar staining, nail discoloration and cyanosis.
- Ask the patient to hold their arms out straight with the wrists extended (Fig. 5.8).
- Measure the respiratory rate while feeling the pulse.
- Check for any tenderness in the distal forearm.

Fine tremor of the outstretched hands is common in respiratory patients and usually due to the direct effect of high-dose beta-agonist bronchodilators on skeletal muscle. Respiratory failure with carbon dioxide retention is one of the causes of a coarse flapping tremor of the outstretched hands (asterixis).

**Fig. 5.8** Hand position for testing for the coarse tremor of $CO_2$ retention.

## Face

Superior vena cava obstruction causes dusky, generalised swelling of the head, neck and face (Fig. 5.9) with subconjunctival oedema (looking like a tear inside the lower lid, but not mobile); this usually indicates tumour invasion of the upper mediastinum.

Tumours at the root of the neck may disrupt the sympathetic nerves to the eye, which run from the upper thoracic spinal segments via ganglia in the neck to join the carotid artery sheath. This causes unilateral ptosis, hypohydrosis, pupillary constriction and apparent enophthalmos (Horner's syndrome, Fig. 5.10).

**Fig. 5.9** Superior vena cava obstruction. Dusky, swollen face and neck, and distended superficial collateral veins on the chest wall. *(From Midthun DE, Jett JR. Clinical presentation of lung cancer. In: Pass HI, Mitchel JB, Johnson DH, et al., eds. Lung Cancer: Principles and Practice. Philadelphia, PA: Lippincott–Raven; 1996;421.)*

## Examination sequence

- Check the conjunctiva of one eye for pallor of anaemia, and the colour of the tongue for the blue-grey discolouration of central cyanosis (Fig. 5.11).
- Check for ptosis and pupil asymmetry.
- Check the jaw and mouth for abnormalities, which may obstruct the airway (e.g., macroglossia, small mandible, large tonsils).

Central cyanosis only becomes visible when enough deoxy-haemoglobin is circulating. This makes cyanosis harder to detect in anaemia compared to polycythaemia at the same level of tissue hypoxia. Methaemoglobinaemia may also cause cyanosis, which persists despite oxygen treatment.

**Fig. 5.11** Central cyanosis of the tongue.

## Neck

Jugular venous pressure (JVP) is raised in many patients with pulmonary hypertension and may be acutely raised in those with tension pneumothorax or large pulmonary embolism. In superior vena cava obstruction, the JVP may be raised above the angle of

**Fig. 5.10** Horner's syndrome showing ptosis and meiosis on the right. (From Rempell JS, Harris NS, Brown DFM, et al. *J Emerg Med.* 2009;36[4]:395–399.)

**Fig. 5.12** Examining for tracheal deviation.

the jaw, making pulsatility invisible. In those who are using the sternocleidomastoids as accessory muscles (see above), it is frequently impossible to see the JVP, as the internal jugular vein lies deep in the active muscle.

## Examination sequence (Video 2D)

- Support the patient's head with a pillow to facilitate relaxation of the sternocleidomastoid muscles.
- Using a tangential light source, examine the jugular venous pressure (p. 52).
- Check for tracheal deviation by gently advancing a single finger resting in the sternal notch in the midline (Fig. 5.12). The trachea should be equidistant from the two sternomastoid heads.
- Check the cricosternal distance (the vertical distance between the sternal notch and the cricoid cartilage, the first prominent ridge felt above the tracheal rings). In health, three average fingers fit between the sternal notch and the cricoid.
- Examine the cervical lymph nodes from behind with the patient sitting forward, as described on page 36.

Tracheal deviation away from the affected side is seen acutely in tension pneumothorax. Chronic tracheal deviation towards the affected side occurs with loss of lung volume in upper lobe fibrotic scarring or collapse and following lobectomy or pneumonectomy.

Reduction in cricosternal distance is a sign of hyperinflation and reflects upward displacement of the sternum (see Fig. 5.4B). Upward movement of the sternum and downward movement of the trachea on inspiration are normal but may become more obvious with forceful inspiratory efforts in respiratory disease. Rarely, systolic downward movement of the trachea is felt in patients with aortic aneurysm (sometimes called 'tracheal tug').

Palpable cervical lymph nodes may be a sign of metastatic disease from lung cancer. They are also a common presentation of lymph node tuberculosis and lymphoma.

## Thorax

First, inspect the chest closely again, in case abnormalities were missed from the end of the bed. Look carefully for any scars,

particularly under the pectoral fold for a thoracotomy scar and on the lateral and posterior chest wall for scars from pleural biopsies and drains. In patients with a thin chest wall and increased respiratory drive (as in exacerbation of COPD), forced, rapid inspiration often causes visible indrawing of the skin in the intercostal spaces during inspiration, seen more easily with tangential light (see Fig. 5.5A).

## Palpation

### Examination sequence

- Locate the apex beat, the most inferior and lateral place where the finger is lifted by the twisting systolic movement of the cardiac apex. This is normally in the fifth intercostal space in the mid-clavicular line. Count down the intercostal spaces; the second is below the second rib, which attaches at the manubriosternal junction.
- Palpate for a right ventricular heave using a straight arm, with the palm over the lower sternum (see Fig. 4.18C).

The apex beat is displaced laterally by dilatation of the ventricles or leftward displacement of the mediastinum. In patients with significant hyperinflation, the apex beat may be impalpable because the lingula expands between the heart and the chest wall (see Fig. 5.4B). In this situation, the heart sounds are often barely audible and may be heard better by auscultating in the epigastrium.

In pulmonary hypertension, the lower sternum is lifted by the cardiac cycle (right ventricular heave) and a finger gently placed over the pulmonary area may detect closure of the pulmonary valve: a so-called palpable P2.

Next, assess thoracic expansion in both the upper and lower anterior chest wall.

### Examination sequence (Video 2E)

- First, place the palms of your hands over the pectoral region overlying both upper lobes and oppose the elevated thumbs over the midline. Ask the patient to take a deep breath using the thumbs as pointers to judge how much each hand moves outwards. Then, cup your hands, with fingers spread, around the patient's lower anterior chest wall overlying the lingula and right middle lobe, pressing the fingertips firmly in the mid-axillary line. Pull your hands medially towards each other to tighten any loose skin, and once again use your thumbs (off the skin) as pointers to judge how much each hand moves outwards when the patient is instructed to take a full breath in (Fig. 5.13). In a healthy thorax, the ribs move out and up with inspiration.
- Check for any asymmetry. This is more important than the absolute degree of expansion, which will vary between individuals.

In COPD with hyperinflation, the normal outward movement of the lower ribs on inspiration is replaced by paradoxical inward movement ('Hoover's sign'), caused by contraction of the abnormally low, flat diaphragm (see Fig. 5.4). This important sign may be missed if expansion is assessed only in the upper chest or from behind.

Palpation of the chest wall may rarely reveal surgical emphysema, indicating air trapped in the subcutaneous tissues (Fig. 5.14). This most commonly complicates pneumothorax with chest drainage or rib fracture and feels like a palpable crackling under the skin of the upper thorax, supraclavicular fossae and neck.

Finally, examine carefully for any tumour deposits (see Fig. 5.6A). Mesothelioma may grow down the track left from a pleural biopsy or chest drain and present as a firm lump at the scar site.

**Fig. 5.13** Assessing chest expansion from the front. **A** Expiration. **B** Inspiration.

## Percussion

Correctly performed, percussion should generate a hollow, ringing sound accompanied by a palpable resonance over air-filled lungs, but a dull thud lacking resonance over consolidation or fluid. Percussion is most valuable when detecting asymmetry of resonance between mirror image positions on the right and left sides. The absolute quality and volume of the percussed sound vary widely between individuals with differing chest wall thickness, muscularity and subcutaneous fat, and is of little value.

### Examination sequence (Videos 2F and 2G) ▶

- To percuss the chest, apply the middle finger of your non-dominant hand firmly to an intercostal space, parallel to the ribs, and drum the middle phalanx with the flexed tip of your dominant index or middle finger (Fig. 5.15A). The movement should come from the wrist and not the elbow.
- Starting in the supraclavicular fossae, compare percussion at mirror image sites on right and left before moving to the next level (see Fig. 5.15B).
- Posteriorly, the scapular and spinal muscles obstruct percussion, so position the patient sitting forwards with their arms folded in front to move the scapulae laterally. Percuss a few centimetres lateral to the spinal muscles, taking care to compare positions the same distance from the midline on right and left (see Fig. 5.15C).
- Remember to percuss the lateral chest wall in the mid-axillary line, comparing both sides.

In healthy people, anterior chest percussion is symmetrical except for the area immediately lateral to the lower left sternal edge, where the right ventricle causes dullness; this 'cardiac

**Fig. 5.14** Subcutaneous air (surgical emphysema) seen in the neck and chest wall on chest X-ray *(arrows)*.

**Fig. 5.15** Percussion of the chest. **A** Technique. **B** Anterior and lateral sites. **C** Posterior sites.

dullness' is lost in hyperinflated patients in whom the lingula overlies the heart (see Fig. 5.4). Clear resonance ('hyper-resonance') is the usual finding over a pneumothorax, although the difference between a normal lung and the pneumothorax may be quite subtle because normal lung is almost all air. Resonance on percussion together with unilateral absent breath sounds indicates pneumothorax.

## Auscultation

To understand chest auscultation, it is necessary to understand the origin of breath sounds. The tracheobronchial tree branches 23 times between the trachea and the alveoli. This results in an exponential rise in the number of airways and their combined cross-sectional area moving towards the alveoli. During a maximal breath in and out, the same vital capacity (about 5 L of air in healthy adults) passes through each generation of airway. In the larynx and trachea, this volume must all pass through a cross-sectional area of only a few square centimetres and therefore flow rate is fast, causing turbulence with vibration of the airway wall, generating sound. In the distal airway, the large combined cross-sectional area of the multitude of bronchioles means that 5 L can easily pass at slow flow rates, so flow is normally virtually silent. The harsh 'bronchial' sound generated by the major airways can be appreciated by listening with the diaphragm of the stethoscope applied to the larynx (try this on yourself).

Most of the sound heard when auscultating the chest wall originates in the large central airways but is muffled and deadened by passage through overlying air-filled alveolar tissue; this, together with a small contribution from medium-sized airways, results in 'normal' breath sounds at the chest wall, sometimes termed 've-sicular'. When healthy, air-filled lungs become consolidated by pneumonia or thickened and stiffened by fibrotic scarring (e.g., post-tuberculous scarring), sound conduction is improved, and the centrally generated 'bronchial' breath sounds may be auscultated clearly and loudly on the overlying chest wall. In the same way, with soft speech ('say one, one, one'), the laryngeal sounds are muffled by healthy lung but heard clearly and loudly at the chest wall overlying consolidation and fibrotic scarring, due to improved conduction of major airway sounds through diseased lung.

When there is lobar collapse caused by a proximal bronchial obstruction, the signs are different from those in simple consol-idation. The usual findings are diminished expansion, sometimes with chest asymmetry due to loss of volume, dullness to per-cussion over the collapsed lobe, and reduced breath sounds and vocal resonance.

When the lung tissue is physically separated from the chest wall by intervening air (pneumothorax) or fluid (pleural effusion), sound conduction is greatly impaired and the breath sounds are usually very quiet or absent. These two causes are readily distinguished by percussion, which will be resonant with pneu-mothorax and dull over pleural fluid.

## Use of the stethoscope

Remember to wear the stethoscope with the earpieces facing forwards to align them with your auditory canal. Normal breath sounds are relatively quiet, so the greater area of contact offered

by the diaphragm is usually well-adapted to chest auscultation. The two common exceptions are in patients with:

- A cachectic chest wall with sunken intercostal spaces, where it may be impossible to achieve flat skin contact with the diaphragm.
- A hairy chest wall, where movement of chest hairs against the diaphragm is easily mistaken for lung crackles. In these situations, use the stethoscope bell instead to listen to the breath sounds.

### Breath sounds

As with percussion, the absolute volume and character of breath sounds in individuals are greatly affected by the thickness, muscularity and fat content of the chest wall. The symmetry of sounds is therefore the key feature.

## Examination sequence (Videos 2H and 2I)

- Auscultate the apices, comparing right with left, and changing to the bell if you cannot achieve flat skin contact with the diaphragm.
- Ask the patient to take repeated slow, deep breaths in and out through their open mouth. Auscultate the anterior chest wall from top to bottom, always comparing mirror image positions on right and left before moving down.
- Use the same sequence of sites as for percussion (see Fig. 5.15B and C).
- Note whether the breath sounds are soft and muffled, absent, or loud and harsh (bronchial, like those heard over the larynx). Seek and note any asymmetry and added sounds (see later), deciding which side is abnormal.
- Auscultate the lateral chest wall in the mid-axillary line, again comparing right with left before changing level.

### Added sounds

The three common added sounds are wheezes, crackles and rubs.

Wheeze is a musical whistling sound accompanying airflow and usually originates in narrowed small airways. It is most commonly expiratory, due to dynamic airway narrowing on expiration, but can also occur on inspiration. Usually, multiple wheezing sounds are heard together (polyphonic wheeze); this sign is common in asthma, bronchitis and exacerbation of COPD. A single (monophonic) wheeze that is present consis-tently with each breath and does not clear with coughing is consistent with a fixed bronchial obstruction and may indicate an underlying cancer partially obstructing a bronchus.

Crackles are brief non-musical sounds that are most often heard on inspiration but may occur in any phase of breathing. They are thought to represent the sudden opening of small airways but sometimes indicate secretions in the airways or underlying interstitial fibrosis. In healthy people, gravitational compression of the dependent lung bases may cause a few crackles on the first few deep breaths; these should clear with a deliberate cough and are of no pathological significance. Crackles that persist after several breaths and a cough are pathological. They are graded as 'fine', meaning soft, multiple crackles, to 'coarse,' indicating loud, scanty crackles that tend to change with each breath. Showers of fine crackles during inspiration, resem-bling the sound made by peeling a Velcro fastener, are characteristic of interstitial pulmonary fibrosis, and are commonly heard at the lung bases posteriorly and laterally. Fine crackles also occur in pulmonary oedema and some viral pneumonias. Coarse crackles are generally heard in patients with significant purulent airway secretions such as those with bronchopneumonia or bronchiectasis. Inspiratory crackles may also be heard over incompletely inflated lung immediately above a pleural effusion.

A pleural rub is a rasping, grating sound occurring with each breath and sounding superficial, just under the stethoscope, like two sheets of sandpaper rubbing together. It indicates pleural inflammation, usually due to infection or infarction of the lung, and is often accompanied by pleuritic chest pain. In pneumonia, a pleural rub and the associated pain may disappear if a para-pneumonic effusion or empyema develops.

Very rarely, a clicking or crunching sound may be heard synchronous with the heartbeat; this can indicate a pneumomediastinum.

### Vocal resonance

Breath sounds normally reveal the presence of consolidation or fibrotic scarring (bronchial breath sounds) or pleural air or fluid (diminished or absent breath sounds). These signs can be confirmed by asking the patient to generate laryngeal sounds deliberately ('Please say "one, one, one" each time I move my stethoscope') and listening on the chest wall in the same sequence of sites used for breath sounds. Through the stethoscope, the spoken sound is muffled and deadened over healthy lung but is heard loudly and clearly over consolidated or fibrotic scarred lung. As with breath sounds, vocal resonance is absent or greatly diminished over pneumothorax and pleural effusion.

'Whispering pectoriloquy' may be used to confirm the same changes in sound conduction. Whispered speech is muffled to silence by normal lung but may be heard over consolidated or scarred lung.

## Interpretation of the findings

Review your findings and collate the positive features. Upon completing the history and examination, you should have a broad idea of the respiratory illness category with which you are dealing. Consistent groups of signs may even be diagnostic; for example, unilateral absent breath sounds, resonant percussion, and tracheal deviation to the opposite side in a collapsed patient indicate a likely tension pneumothorax.

As with any system, consider as you go the likely disease categories and how these affect presentation. This approach is summarised in Box 5.7.

## Investigations

Selecting the relevant investigation depends on the clinical problem revealed on history and examination. Investigations are costly and many carry risks, so choose tests capable of distinguishing the likely diagnoses and prioritise the most decisive ones. In respiratory disease, imaging of the lungs is fundamental, but respiratory function testing is equally important to distinguish obstructive disease of the airways from the restrictive pattern seen in many parenchymal diseases, and to quantify the degree of abnormality. A summary of the appropriate initial investigations according to the type of respiratory presentation is shown in Box 5.8.

### 5.7 Categories of respiratory disease and associated features upon history and examination

| Category of problem | Suggestive features on history | Suggestive features on examination |
|---|---|---|
| Infection<br>• Acute bronchitis<br>• Exacerbation of COPD<br>• Pneumonia | Cough, sputum, wheeze, Acute-on-chronic dyspnoea<br>Cough, mucopurulent sputum, ankle swelling ('cor pulmonale'), headache (hypercapnia)<br>Fever, rigors, pleuritic pain, rusty sputum, loss of appetite | Polyphonic wheeze<br>Hyperinflation, quiet breath sounds, polyphonic wheeze, flapping tremor ($CO_2$ retention), ankle oedema ('cor pulmonale')<br>If lobar, dull percussion, bronchial breathing and increased vocal resonance |
| Malignancy | Insidious onset, weight loss, cough, haemoptysis persisting pain | Cervical lymphadenopathy, finger clubbing, signs of lobar/lung collapse ± effusion |
| Pulmonary fibrosis | Progressive dyspnoea, cough | Tachypnoea, finger clubbing, central cyanosis, inspiratory fine crackles at bases |
| Pleural effusion | Progressive dyspnoea | Unilateral basal dullness and reduced breath sounds |
| Pulmonary embolism:<br>• Large<br>• Medium<br>• Multiple small | Sudden severe dyspnoea<br>Episodes of pleuritic pain, haemoptysis<br>Progressive dyspnoea | Normal breath sounds<br>Pleural rub, crackles if infarct<br>Raised JVP, Residual Volume heave, loud P2 |
| Asthma | Atopy, hay fever, pet ownership, variable wheeze, disturbance of sleep | Polyphonic expiratory wheeze, eczema |

*COPD*, Chronic obstructive pulmonary disease; *JVP*, jugular venous pressure.

## 5.8 Selecting investigations for different respiratory presentations

| Problem from history and examination | Appropriate initial investigations | Diagnostic value |
|---|---|---|
| Infection (e.g., acute bronchitis, exacerbation of COPD and pneumonia) | Chest X-ray<br>$O_2$ saturation, ABG<br>Sputum/blood culture<br>WCC, CRP | Consolidation in pneumonia<br>Assessment of respiratory failure<br>Identify causal infection<br>Degree of inflammation |
| Malignancy | Chest X-ray<br>CT thorax + abdomen<br>Bronchoscopy if central<br>Endobronchial ultrasound (EBUS)<br>CT-guided biopsy if peripheral<br>Respiratory function | Identification of lesion<br>Tumour stage<br>Diagnostic pathology<br>Allows lymph node sampling<br><br>Diagnostic pathology<br>Fitness for surgery and radical radiotherapy |
| Pulmonary fibrosis/interstitial lung disease | Chest X-ray<br>High-resolution CT thorax<br>Respiratory function<br><br><br>Autoantibodies | Bi-basal reticular shadows<br>Extent and pattern of disease<br>Quantification; identification of restrictive pattern; impaired gas transfer<br>Exercise test (6 min walk or incremental) – functional capacity<br>Identification of any associated connective tissue disease |
| Pleural effusion | Chest X-ray<br>Ultrasound-guided aspiration<br><br><br><br><br><br>CT thorax + abdomen | Dense basal fluid pool<br>Culture for infection<br>pH low in empyema<br>Glucose low in infection<br>Cytology to identify malignancy<br>Protein and LDH in pleural fluid and serum to distinguish exudate from transudate (Light's criteria)<br>Identification of underlying tumour |
| Pulmonary embolism | d-Dimer<br>CT pulmonary angiogram<br><br>Echocardiogram<br>$O_2$ saturation or ABG | High negative predictive value<br>Detection of emboli<br>Right heart strain<br>Detection of right ventricular strain<br>Assessment of respiratory failure |
| Asthma | Respiratory function:<br>Peak flow diary<br>$FEV_1$ /reversibility<br>FeNO<br>$O_2$ saturation or ABG<br>IgE, allergen skin tests<br>FBC – eosinophils | <br>Variable obstruction<br>Reversible obstruction<br>Often raised in asthma<br>Assessment of respiratory failure<br>Detection of allergic stimuli<br>Common in allergic patients |
| Emphysema | Chest X-ray<br>CT thorax<br>Respiratory function<br><br><br>FBC<br>Serum $\alpha_1$ antitrypsin | Hyperinflation/reduced lung markings<br>Emphysema<br>Reduced $FEV_1$/VC ratio, no reversibility<br>Raised Total Lung Capacity, RV<br>Reduced Kco<br>$2°$ polycythaemia<br>Reduced with abnormal phenotype (rare, in premature disease) |

*ABG,* Arterial blood gas; *COPD,* chronic obstructive pulmonary disease; *CRP,* C-reactive protein; *CT,* computed tomography; *FEV₁,* forced expiratory volume in 1 second; *IgE,* immunoglobulin E; *WCC,* white cell count.

5

## OSCE example 1: Respiratory history

Mrs. Walker, 55 years old, presents to the respiratory clinic with coughing and wheezing.

### Please take a history

- Introduce yourself and clean your hands.
- Ask an open question about why this person has come to the clinic.
- Explore each presenting symptom:
  - Cough:
    - Onset, duration?
    - Productive? If so, characterise sputum volume and colour, and any blood.
    - Triggers? Did it start with an upper respiratory tract infection? Is it provoked by exercise or environment?
    - Time pattern – nocturnal? (Suggests asthma or reflux)
    - On angiotensin-converting enzyme inhibitors?
  - Wheeze:
    - What exactly does the patient mean by 'wheeze'?
    - When does it occur – at night? During or after exercise?
    - Provoking factors – infection, environment, contact with animals, dust, beta-blockers?
    - Any relieving factors – inhalers?
    - Associated respiratory symptoms – breathlessness, chest pain, fevers/rigors, weight loss.
- Ask about past respiratory diagnoses, particularly childhood wheeze or asthma, rhinitis/hay fever and prior respiratory treatments/admissions.
- Explore past non-respiratory illness: for example, eczema (suggests atopy), hypertension or angina (on beta-blockers?), other prior illnesses.
- Take a drug history – prescribed medications, including inhalers/nebulisers and recreational drugs.
- Ask about any known allergies.
- Take a social history: smoking, occupation, contact with animals.
- Establish whether there is a family history of respiratory disease (including asthma).
- Ask about any other patient concerns.
- Thank the patient and clean your hands.

### Summarise your findings

Mrs. Walker is a 55-year-old cook who gives a 6-month history of wheezing disturbing her sleep, associated with an unproductive cough. Her symptoms vary from day to day and sometimes make climbing stairs difficult. She smokes 10 cigarettes a day and has a 20-pack-year smoking history.

### Suggest a differential diagnosis

The most likely diagnosis is asthma (variable, nocturnal symptoms) and the differential is chronic obstructive pulmonary disease.

### Suggest initial investigations

Spirometry and reversibility, peak-flow diary, chest X-ray, blood count for eosinophils, serum immunoglobulin E, and skin tests to common allergens.

## OSCE example 2: Respiratory examination

Mr. Tate, 87 years old, reports increasing breathlessness over several weeks.

### Please examine his respiratory system:

- Introduce yourself and clean your hands.
- Note clues around the patient, such as oxygen, nebulisers, inhalers or sputum pots.
- Observe from the end of the bed:
  - Scars, chest shape, asymmetry, pattern of breathing, accessory muscle use.
  - Chest wall movement, paradoxical rib movement, intercostal indrawing.
- Examine the hands: clubbing, tar staining, muscle wasting.
- Check for tremor and flap.
- Measure respiratory rate unobtrusively.
- Examine the face: anaemia, cyanosis, Horner's syndrome and superior vena cava obstruction.
- Examine the neck: jugular venous pressure, tracheal deviation, cricosternal distance.
- Examine the anterior chest wall:
  - Palpate: apex beat, right ventricular heave, expansion of the upper and lower chest.
  - Percuss: compare right with left, from top with bottom, then axillae.
  - Auscultate: deep breaths; compare right with left, from top with bottom, then axillae. Repeat, checking vocal resonance.
- Examine the posterior chest wall (commonly in OSCEs, you may be directed to examine either anterior or posterior):
  - Ask the patient to sit forwards.
  - Inspect the back for scars, asymmetry and so on.
  - Palpate:
    - Cervical lymph nodes.
    - Chest expansion of the upper and lower chest.
  - Percuss: ask the patient to fold his arms at the front to part the scapulae; compare right with left, from top to bottom.
  - Auscultate: deep breaths; compare right with left, from top to bottom, then axillae. Repeat, checking vocal resonance.
- Check for pitting oedema over the sacrum and lumbar spine.
- Thank the patient and clean your hands.

### Summarise your findings

The patient has finger clubbing, a raised respiratory rate, and diminished expansion with dullness to percussion and loss of breath sounds at the right base. A small scar suggests prior pleural aspiration.

### Suggest a differential diagnosis

Signs suggest a large right pleural effusion.
*(Away from patient's bedside)* A large unilateral effusion with finger clubbing suggests an underlying neoplasm. Alternatives include chronic empyema and tuberculous effusion.

### Suggest initial investigations

Chest X-ray to confirm effusion and possibly show an underlying tumour. Ultrasound to reveal pleural disease and loculation, and guide aspiration. Pleural aspiration for cytology, culture and biochemical analysis. CT scan for staging.

5

## Integrated examination sequence for the respiratory system

- Introduce yourself and seek the patient's consent to chest examination.
- Position the patient: resting comfortably, with the chest supported at about 45 degrees and the head resting on a pillow.
- Carry out general observations: note any clues around the patient, such as oxygen, nebulisers, inhalers, sputum pots, etc.
- Observe from the end of the bed:
  - Scars.
  - Chest shape, asymmetry.
  - Pattern of breathing:
    - Respiratory rate.
    - Time spent in inspiration and expiration.
    - Pursed-lip breathing.
  - Chest wall movement, paradoxical rib movement, intercostal indrawing.
  - Accessory muscle use.
- Examine the hands:
  - Clubbing, tar staining, muscle wasting.
  - Check for tremor and flap.
  - Measure respiratory rate unobtrusively.
- Examine the face:
  - Check for anaemia, cyanosis, Horner's syndrome and signs of superior vena cava obstruction.
- Examine the neck:
  - Jugular venous pressure, tracheal deviation and cricosternal distance.
- Examine the anterior chest wall:
  - Palpate: apex beat, right ventricular heave, expansion of upper and lower chest.
  - Percuss: compare right with left, from top to bottom, then axillae.
  - Auscultate: deep breaths; compare right with left, from top to bottom, then axillae. Repeat positions, asking the patient to say 'one, one, one' for vocal resonance.
- Examine the posterior chest wall: ask the patient to sit forwards so that you can:
  - Inspect the back for scars, asymmetry and so on.
  - Palpate:
    - Cervical lymph nodes.
    - Expansion of the upper and lower chest.
  - Percuss: ask the patient to fold their arms at the front to part the scapulae. Compare right with left, from top to bottom (see Fig. 5.15 for positions).
  - Auscultate: deep breaths; compare right with left, from top to bottom, then axillae. Repeat positions, asking the patient to say 'one, one, one' for vocal resonance.
- Check for pitting oedema over the sacrum and lumbar spine.

John Plevris
Rowan Parks

# The gastrointestinal system

**Anatomy and physiology 106**

**The history 106**
Common presenting symptoms 106
Past medical history 116
Drug history 116
Family history 116
Social history 116

**The physical examination 116**
General examination 117

Abdominal examination 118
Hernias 125
Rectal examination 126
Proctoscopy 128

**Investigations 128**

**OSCE example 1: Abdominal pain and diarrhoea 131**

**OSCE example 2: Jaundice 132**

**Integrated examination sequence for the gastrointestinal system 132**

# Anatomy and physiology

The gastrointestinal system comprises the alimentary tract, liver, biliary system, pancreas and spleen. The alimentary tract extends from the mouth to the anus and includes the oesophagus, stomach, small intestine or small bowel (comprising the duodenum, jejunum and ileum), colon (large intestine or large bowel) and rectum (Figs 6.1–6.2 and Box 6.1).

The abdominal surface can be divided into nine regions by the intersection of two horizontal and two vertical planes (Fig. 6.1C).

# The history

Gastrointestinal symptoms are common and are often caused by functional dyspepsia and irritable bowel syndrome. Alarm symptoms, indicating a more serious alternative or coexistent diagnosis, include persistent vomiting, dysphagia, gastrointestinal bleeding, weight loss, painless, watery, high-volume diarrhoea, nocturnal symptoms, fever and anaemia. The risk of serious disease increases with age. Always explore the patient's ideas, concerns and expectations about the symptoms (p. 5) to understand the clinical context.

## Common presenting symptoms

### Mouth symptoms

Bad breath (halitosis) due to gingival, dental or pharyngeal infection and dry mouth (xerostomia) are common mouth symptoms. Rarely patients complain of altered taste sensation (dysgeusia) or a foul taste in the mouth (cacogeusia).

### Anorexia and weight loss

Anorexia is a loss of appetite and/or a lack of interest in food. In addition to enquiring about appetite, ask 'Do you still enjoy your food?'

Weight loss, in isolation, is rarely associated with serious organic disease. Ask how much weight has been lost, over what time. Loss of less than 3 kg in the previous 6 months is rarely significant. Weight loss is usually the result of reduced energy intake, not increased energy expenditure. It does not specifically indicate gastrointestinal disease, although it is common in many gastrointestinal disorders, including malignancy and liver disease. Energy requirements average 2500 kcal/day for males and 2000 kcal/day for females. Reduced energy intake arises from dieting, loss of appetite, malabsorption or malnutrition. Increased energy expenditure occurs in hyperthyroidism, fever or with the adoption of a more energetic lifestyle. A net calorie deficit of 1000 kcal/day results in weight loss of approximately 1 kg/week (7000 kcal ≅ 1 kg of fat). Greater weight loss during the initial stages of energy restriction arises from salt and water loss and depletion of hepatic glycogen stores, not from fat loss. Rapid weight loss over days suggests loss of body fluid as a result of vomiting, diarrhoea or diuretics (1 L of water = 1 kg). Check

**A**

1 Liver     3 Spleen
2 Gallbladder     4 Pancreas

**B**

| 1 Oesophagus | 7 Caecum |
|---|---|
| 2 Stomach | 8 Appendix (in pelvic position) |
| 3 Pyloric antrum | 9 Ascending colon |
| 4 Duodenum | 10 Transverse colon |
| 5 Duodenojejunal flexure | 11 Descending colon |
| 6 Terminal ileum | 12 Sigmoid colon |

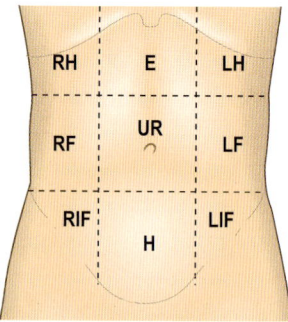

**C**

**Fig. 6.1 Surface anatomy.** A Abdominal surface markings of non-alimentary tract viscera. B Surface markings of the alimentary tract. C Regions of the abdomen. *E*, epigastrium; *H*, hypogastrium or suprapubic region; *LF*, left flank or lumbar region; *LH*, left hypochondrium; *LIF*, left iliac fossa; *RF*, right flank or lumbar region; *RH*, right hypochondrium; *RIF*, right iliac fossa; *UR*, umbilical region.

Fig. 6.2 Normal computed tomogram (CT) of the abdomen at L1 level.

### 6.1 Surface markings of the main non-alimentary tract abdominal organs

| Structure | Position |
|---|---|
| Liver | Upper border: fifth right intercostal space on full expiration. Lower border: at the costal margin in the mid-clavicular line on full inspiration |
| Spleen | Underlies left ribs 9–11, posterior to the mid-axillary line |
| Gallbladder | At the intersection of the right lateral vertical plane and the costal margin, i.e. tip of the ninth costal cartilage |
| Pancreas | The neck of the pancreas lies at the level of L1; the head lies below and right; the tail lies above and left |
| Kidneys | Upper pole lies deep to the 12th rib posteriorly, 7 cm from the midline; the right is 2–3 cm lower than the left |

A

B

Fig. 6.3 Some causes of a painful mouth. A Lichen planus. B Small, 'punched-out' aphthous ulcer (arrow).

current and previous weight records to confirm apparent weight loss on examination (loose-fitting clothes, for example).

## Pain

### Painful mouth

Causes of sore lips, tongue or buccal mucosa include:

- deficiencies, including iron, folate, vitamin B$_{12}$ or C
- dermatological disorders, including lichen planus (Fig. 6.3A)
- chemotherapy
- aphthous ulcers (Fig. 6.3B)
- infective stomatitis
- inflammatory bowel disease and coeliac disease, associated with mouth ulcers.

### Heartburn and reflux

Heartburn is a hot, burning retrosternal discomfort.

To differentiate heartburn from cardiac chest pain, ask about associated features:

- character of pain: burning
- radiation: upward
- precipitating factors: lying flat or bending forward
- associated symptoms:
  - waterbrash (sudden appearance of fluid in the mouth due to reflex salivation as a result of gastro-oesophageal reflux disease (GORD) or, rarely, peptic ulcer disease)
  - the taste of acid appearing in the mouth due to reflux/regurgitation.

When heartburn is the principal symptom, GORD is the most likely diagnosis.

## Dyspepsia

Dyspepsia is pain or discomfort centred in the upper abdomen. In contrast, 'indigestion' is a term commonly used by patients for ill-defined symptoms from the upper gastrointestinal tract.

Ask about:

- site of pain
- character of pain
- exacerbating and relieving factors, such as food and antacid
- associated symptoms, such as nausea, belching, bloating and premature fullness (early satiety).

Clusters of symptoms are used to classify dyspepsia:

- reflux-like dyspepsia (heartburn-predominant dyspepsia)
- ulcer-like dyspepsia (epigastric pain relieved by food or antacids)
- dysmotility-like dyspepsia (nausea, belching, bloating and premature fullness (early satiety).

Often there is no structural cause and the dyspepsia is functional. Patients below the age of 55 without alarm symptoms and with a negative *Helicobacter pylori* test can be positively diagnosed as having functional dyspepsia thus avoiding unnecessary investigations but if symptoms persist then further investigations should be considered. However, in patients over the age of 55 organic pathology should always be excluded by upper gastrointestinal (GI) endoscopy.

Dyspepsia that is worse with an empty stomach and eased by eating is typical of peptic ulceration. The patient may indicate a single localised point in the epigastrium (pointing sign) and complain of nausea and abdominal fullness that is worse after fatty or spicy meals. 'Fat intolerance' is common with all causes of dyspepsia, including gallbladder disease.

## Odynophagia

Odynophagia is pain from swallowing, often precipitated by drinking hot liquids. It can be present with or without dysphagia (see below) and may indicate oesophageal ulceration or oesophagitis from gastro-oesophageal reflux or oesophageal candidiasis. It implies intact mucosal sensation, making oesophageal cancer unlikely.

## Abdominal pain

Characterise the pain using the acronym SOCRATES (see Box 2.2). Ask about the characteristics described here.

### Site

Visceral abdominal pain from distension of hollow organs, mesenteric traction or excessive smooth-muscle contraction is deep and poorly localised in the midline. The pain is conducted via sympathetic splanchnic nerves. Somatic pain from the parietal peritoneum and abdominal wall is lateralised and localised to the inflamed area. It is conducted via intercostal nerves.

Pain arising from foregut structures (stomach, pancreas, liver and biliary system) is localised above the umbilicus (Fig. 6.4). Central abdominal pain arises from midgut structures, such as the small bowel and appendix. Lower abdominal pain arises from hindgut structures, such as the colon. Inflammation may cause localised pain: for example, left iliac fossa pain due to diverticular disease of the sigmoid colon.

Pain from an unpaired structure, such as the pancreas, is midline and radiates through to the back. Pain from paired structures, such as renal colic, is felt on, and radiates to, the affected side (Fig. 6.5). Torsion of the testis may present with abdominal pain (p. 267). In females, consider gynaecological causes such as ruptured ovarian cyst, pelvic inflammatory disease, endometriosis or ectopic pregnancy (p. 247).

### Onset

Sudden onset of severe abdominal pain, rapidly progressing to become generalised and constant, suggests a hollow viscus perforation (usually due to peptic ulceration, diverticular disease or colorectal cancer), a ruptured abdominal aortic aneurysm or mesenteric infarction.

Torsion of the caecum or sigmoid colon (volvulus) presents with sudden abdominal pain associated with acute intestinal obstruction.

**Fig. 6.4 Abdominal pain.** Perception of visceral pain is localised to the epigastric, umbilical or suprapubic region, according to the embryological origin of the affected organ.

Foregut – pain localises to epigastric area

Midgut – pain localises to periumbilical area

Hindgut – pain localises to suprapubic area

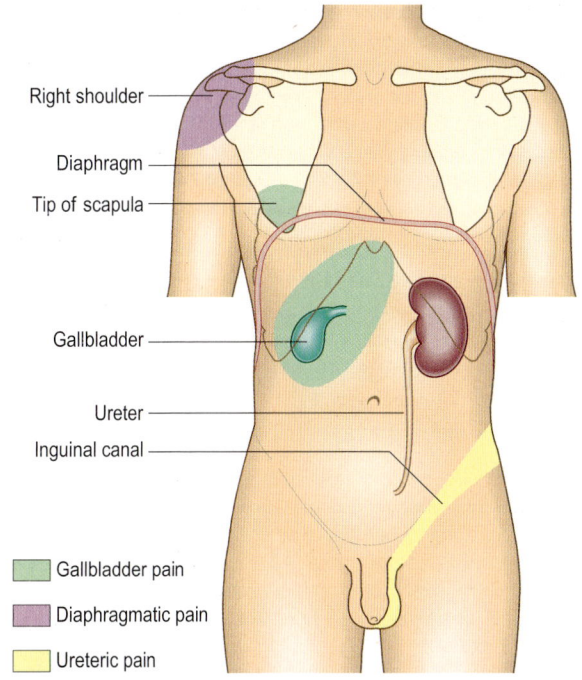

Right shoulder

Diaphragm

Tip of scapula

Gallbladder

Ureter

Inguinal canal

■ Gallbladder pain

■ Diaphragmatic pain

■ Ureteric pain

**Fig. 6.5** Characteristic radiation of pain from the gallbladder, diaphragm and ureters.

**6**

## Character

Colicky pain lasts for a short time (seconds or minutes), eases off and then returns. It arises from hollow structures, as in small or large bowel obstruction, or the uterus during labour.

Biliary and renal 'colic' are misnamed, as the pain is rarely colicky; pain rapidly increases to a peak and persists over several hours before gradually resolving. Dull, constant, vague and poorly localised pain is more typical of an inflammatory process or infection, such as pelvic inflammatory disease, appendicitis or diverticulitis (Box 6.2).

## Radiation

Pain radiating from the right hypochondrium to the shoulder or interscapular region may reflect diaphragmatic irritation, as in acute cholecystitis (Fig. 6.5). Pain radiating from the loin to the groin and genitalia is typical of renal colic. Central upper abdominal pain radiating through to the back, partially relieved by sitting forward, suggests pancreatitis. Central abdominal pain that later shifts into the right iliac fossa occurs in acute appendicitis. The combination of severe back and abdominal pain may indicate a ruptured or dissecting abdominal aortic aneurysm.

## Associated symptoms

Anorexia, nausea and vomiting are common but non-specific symptoms. They may accompany any very severe pain but conversely may be absent, even in advanced intra-abdominal disease. Abdominal pain due to irritable bowel syndrome,

| 6.2 Diagnosing abdominal pain | | | | |
|---|---|---|---|---|
| | **Disorder** | | | |
| | **Peptic ulcer** | **Biliary colic** | **Acute pancreatitis** | **Renal colic** |
| Site | Epigastrium | Epigastrium/right hypochondrium | Epigastrium/left hypochondrium | Loin |
| Onset | Gradual | Rapidly increasing | Sudden | Rapidly increasing |
| Character | Gnawing | Constant | Constant | Constant |
| Radiation | Into back | Below right scapula | Into back | Into genitalia and inner thigh |
| Associated symptoms | Non-specific | Non-specific | Non-specific | Non-specific |
| Timing | | | | |
|   Frequency/ periodicity | Remission for weeks/months | Attacks can be enumerated | Attacks can be enumerated | Usually a discrete episode |
|   Special times | Nocturnal and especially when hungry | Unpredictable | After heavy drinking | Following periods of dehydration |
|   Duration | 1/2–2 hours | 4–24 hours | >24 hours | 4–24 hours |
| Exacerbating factors | Stress, spicy foods, alcohol, non-steroidal anti-inflammatory drugs | Eating – unable to eat during bouts | Alcohol Eating – unable to eat during bouts | – |
| Relieving factors | Food, antacids, vomiting | – | Sitting upright | – |
| Severity | Mild to moderate | Severe | Severe | Severe |

diverticular disease or colorectal cancer is usually accompanied by altered bowel habit. Other features such as breathlessness or palpitation suggest non-alimentary causes (Box 6.3).

Hypotension and tachycardia following the onset of pain suggest intra-abdominal sepsis or bleeding: for example, from a peptic ulcer, a ruptured aortic aneurysm or an ectopic pregnancy.

### Timing

During the first 1–2 hours after perforation, a 'silent interval' may occur when abdominal pain resolves transiently. The initial chemical peritonitis may subside before bacterial peritonitis becomes established. For example, in acute appendicitis, pain is initially periumbilical (visceral pain) and moves to the right iliac fossa (somatic pain) when localised inflammation of the parietal peritoneum becomes established. If the appendix ruptures, generalised peritonitis may develop. Occasionally, a localised appendix abscess develops, with a palpable mass and localised pain in the right iliac fossa.

| 6.3 Non-alimentary causes of abdominal pain | |
|---|---|
| **Disorder** | **Clinical features** |
| Myocardial infarction | Epigastric pain without tenderness<br>*Angor animi* (feeling of impending death)<br>Hypotension<br>Cardiac arrhythmias |
| Dissecting aortic aneurysm | Tearing interscapular pain<br>*Angor animi*<br>Hypotension<br>Asymmetry of femoral pulses |
| Acute vertebral collapse | Lateralised pain restricting movement<br>Tenderness overlying involved vertebra |
| Cord compression | Pain on percussion of thoracic spine<br>Hyperaesthesia at affected dermatome with sensory loss below<br>Spinal cord signs |
| Pleurisy | Lateralised pain on coughing<br>Chest signs (e.g. pleural rub) |
| Herpes zoster | Hyperaesthesia in dermatomal distribution<br>Vesicular eruption |
| Diabetic ketoacidosis | Cramp-like pain<br>Vomiting<br>Air hunger<br>Tachycardia<br>Ketotic breath |
| Pelvic inflammatory disease or tubal pregnancy | Suprapubic and iliac fossa pain, localised tenderness<br>Nausea, vomiting<br>Fever |
| Torsion of testis/ovary | Lower abdominal pain<br>Nausea, vomiting<br>Localised tenderness |

A change in the pattern of symptoms suggests either that the initial diagnosis was wrong or that complications have developed. In acute small bowel obstruction, a change from typical intestinal colic to persistent pain with abdominal tenderness suggests intestinal ischaemia, as in strangulated hernia, and is an indication for urgent surgical intervention.

Abdominal pain persisting for hours or days suggests an inflammatory disorder, such as acute appendicitis, cholecystitis or diverticulitis.

### Exacerbating and relieving factors

Pain exacerbated by movement or coughing suggests inflammation. Patients tend to lie still to avoid exacerbating the pain. People with colic typically move around or draw their knees up towards the chest during spasms.

### Severity

Excruciating pain, poorly relieved by opioid analgesia, suggests an ischaemic vascular event, such as bowel infarction or ruptured abdominal aortic aneurysm. Severe pain rapidly eased by potent analgesia is more typical of acute pancreatitis or peritonitis secondary to a ruptured viscus.

Features of the pain can help distinguish between possible causes (Box 6.3).

### The acute abdomen

The majority of general surgical emergencies are patients with sudden severe abdominal pain (an 'acute abdomen'). Patients may be so occupied by recent and severe symptoms that they forget important details of their history unless asked directly. Seek additional information from family or friends if severe pain, shock or altered consciousness makes it difficult to obtain a history from the patient. Note any relevant past history, such as known diverticular disease in a patient with a possible acute perforation. Causes range from self-limiting to severe life-threatening diseases (Box 6.4). Evaluate patients rapidly, and then resuscitate critically ill patients immediately before undertaking further assessment and surgical intervention. Parenteral opioid analgesia to alleviate severe abdominal pain will help, not hinder, clinical assessment. In patients with undiagnosed acute abdominal pain, reassess their clinical state regularly, undertake urgent investigations and consider surgical intervention in a timely fashion.

## ▌Dysphagia

Patients with dysphagia complain that food or drink sticks when they swallow.

Ask about:

- onset: recent or longstanding
- nature: intermittent or progressive
- difficulty swallowing solids, liquids or both
- the level where food is felt to stick
- any regurgitation or reflux of food or fluid
- any associated pain (odynophagia) or heartburn
- any recent weight loss.
- past history of food bolus obstruction

### 6.4 Typical clinical features in patients with an 'acute abdomen'

| Condition | History | Examination |
|---|---|---|
| Acute appendicitis | Nausea, vomiting, central abdominal pain that later shifts to the right iliac fossa | Fever, tenderness, guarding or palpable mass in the right iliac fossa, pelvic peritonitis on rectal examination |
| Perforated peptic ulcer with acute peritonitis | Vomiting at onset associated with severe acute-onset abdominal pain, previous history of dyspepsia, ulcer disease, non-steroidal anti-inflammatory drugs or glucocorticoid therapy | Shallow breathing with minimal abdominal wall movement, abdominal tenderness and guarding, board-like rigidity, abdominal distension and absent bowel sounds |
| Acute pancreatitis | Anorexia, nausea, vomiting, constant severe epigastric pain, previous alcohol abuse/cholelithiasis | Fever, periumbilical or loin bruising, epigastric tenderness, variable guarding, reduced or absent bowel sounds |
| Ruptured aortic aneurysm | Sudden onset of severe, tearing back/loin/abdominal pain, hypotension and past history of vascular disease and/or high blood pressure | Shock and hypotension, pulsatile, tender, abdominal mass, asymmetrical femoral pulses |
| Acute mesenteric ischaemia | Anorexia, nausea, vomiting, bloody diarrhoea, constant abdominal pain, previous history of vascular disease and/or high blood pressure | Atrial fibrillation, heart failure, asymmetrical peripheral pulses, absent bowel sounds, variable tenderness and guarding |
| Intestinal obstruction | Colicky central abdominal pain, nausea, vomiting and constipation | Surgical scars, hernias, mass, distension, visible peristalsis, increased bowel sounds |
| Ruptured ectopic pregnancy | Premenopausal female, delayed or missed menstrual period, hypotension, unilateral iliac fossa pain, pleuritic shoulder-tip pain, 'prune juice'-like vaginal discharge | Suprapubic tenderness, periumbilical bruising, pain and tenderness on vaginal examination (cervical excitation), swelling/fullness in fornix on vaginal examination |
| Pelvic inflammatory disease | Sexually active young female, previous history of sexually transmitted infection, recent gynaecological procedure, pregnancy or use of intrauterine contraceptive device, irregular menstruation, dyspareunia, lower or central abdominal pain, backache, pleuritic right upper quadrant pain (Fitz-Hugh–Curtis syndrome) | Fever, vaginal discharge, pelvic peritonitis causing tenderness on rectal examination, right upper quadrant tenderness (perihepatitis), pain/tenderness on vaginal examination (cervical excitation), swelling/fullness in fornix on vaginal examination |

6

Do not confuse dysphagia with early satiety, the inability to complete a full meal because of premature fullness, or with globus, which is a feeling of a lump in the throat. Globus does not interfere with swallowing and is not related to eating.

Neurological dysphagia resulting from bulbar or pseudobulbar palsy (p. 140) is worse for liquids than solids and may be accompanied by choking, spluttering and fluid regurgitating from the nose.

Neuromuscular dysphagia, or oesophageal dysmotility, presents in middle age, is worse for solids and may be helped by liquids and sitting upright. Achalasia, when the lower oesophageal sphincter fails to relax normally, typically results in dysphagia for both solids and liquids and leads to progressive oesophageal dilatation above the sphincter. Overflow of secretions and food into the respiratory tract may then occur, especially at night when the patient lies down, causing aspiration pneumonia. Oesophageal dysmotility and acid reflux can provoke oesophageal spasms and central chest pain, which may be confused with cardiac pain.

A pharyngeal pouch may cause food to stick or be regurgitated undigested from previous days and may lead to recurrent chest infections due to chronic silent aspiration.

'Mechanical' dysphagia is often due to oesophageal stricture but can be caused by external compression. With weight loss, a short history and no reflux symptoms, suspect oesophageal cancer. Longstanding dysphagia without weight loss but accompanied by heartburn is more likely to be due to benign peptic stricture. Eosinophilic oesophagitis is the most common cause of food bolus obstruction and should be considered in younger patients with dysphagia; it is associated with atopy and food allergy. Record the site at which the patient feels the food sticking; although this is not an entirely reliable guide to the site of obstruction. If dysphagia is experienced high in the neck, consider tumours of the pharynx or larynx or extrinsic compression from a mass lesion such as a thyroid goitre.

## Nausea and vomiting

Nausea is the sensation of feeling sick. Vomiting is the expulsion of gastric contents via the mouth. Both are associated with pallor, sweating and hyperventilation.

Ask about:

- relation to meals and timing, such as early morning or late evening
- associated symptoms, such as dyspepsia and abdominal pain, and whether they are relieved by vomiting
- whether the vomit is bile-stained (green), blood-stained or faeculent
- associated weight loss
- the patient's medications.

Nausea and vomiting, particularly with abdominal pain or discomfort, suggest upper gastrointestinal disorders. Dyspepsia causes nausea without vomiting. Peptic ulcers seldom cause painless vomiting unless they are complicated by pyloric stenosis, which causes projectile vomiting of large volumes of gastric content that is not bile-stained. Obstruction distal to the pylorus produces bile-stained vomit. Severe vomiting without significant pain suggests gastric outlet or proximal small bowel obstruction. Faeculent vomiting of small bowel contents (not faeces) is a late feature of distal small bowel or colonic obstruction. In peritonitis, the vomitus is usually small in volume but persistent. The more distal the level of intestinal obstruction, the more marked the accompanying abdominal distension and colic.

Vomiting is common in gastroenteritis, cholecystitis, pancreatitis and hepatitis. It is typically preceded by nausea but raised intracranial pressure may occur without warning. Severe pain may precipitate vomiting, as in renal or biliary colic or myocardial infarction.

Anorexia nervosa and bulimia are eating disorders characterised by undisclosed, self-induced vomiting. In bulimia, weight is maintained or increased, unlike in anorexia nervosa, where profound weight loss is common.

Other non-gastrointestinal causes of nausea and vomiting include:

- drugs, such as opioids, theophyllines, digoxin, cytotoxic agents, antidepressants or alcohol
- pregnancy
- diabetic ketoacidosis
- renal or liver failure
- hypercalcaemia
- Addison's disease
- raised intracranial pressure (meningitis, brain tumour)
- vestibular disorders (labyrinthitis and Ménière's disease).

## Wind and flatulence

Belching, excessive or offensive flatus, abdominal distension and borborygmi (audible bowel sounds) are often called 'wind' or flatulence. Clarify exactly what the patient means. Belching is due to air swallowing (aerophagy) and has no medical significance. It may indicate anxiety but sometimes occurs in an attempt to relieve abdominal pain or discomfort and accompanies GORD.

Normally, 200–2000 mL of flatus is passed each day. Flatus is a mixture of gases derived from swallowed air and colonic bacterial fermentation of poorly absorbed carbohydrates. Excessive flatus occurs particularly in lactase deficiency and intestinal malabsorption.

Borborygmi result from the movement of fluid and gas along the bowel. Loud borborygmi, particularly if associated with colicky discomfort, suggest small bowel obstruction or dysmotility.

## Abdominal distension

Abdominal girth slowly increasing over months or years is usually due to obesity but in a patient with weight loss, it suggests intra-

abdominal disease. The most common causes of abdominal distension are:

- fat due to obesity
- flatus due to pseudo-obstruction or bowel obstruction
- faeces due to subacute obstruction or constipation
- fluid due to ascites (accumulation of fluid in the peritoneal cavity; Fig. 6.6), tumours (especially ovarian) or a distended bladder
- fetus
- functional bloating (fluctuating abdominal distension that develops during the day and resolves overnight, usually occurring in irritable bowel syndrome).

## Altered bowel habit

### Diarrhoea

Clarify what patients mean by diarrhoea. They may complain of frequent stools or a change in the consistency of the stools. Normal frequency ranges from three bowel movements daily to once every 3 days. Diarrhoea is the frequent passage of loose stools. Steatorrhoea is diarrhoea associated with fat malabsorption. The stools are greasy, pale and bulky, and they float, making them difficult to flush away.

Ask about:

- onset of diarrhoea: acute, chronic or intermittent
- stool:
  - frequency
  - volume
  - colour
  - consistency: watery, unformed or semisolid
  - contents: red blood, mucus or pus

**Fig. 6.6** Abdominal distension due to ascites.

- associated features: urgency, faecal incontinence or tenesmus (the sensation of needing to defecate, although the rectum is empty), abdominal pain, vomiting, sleep disturbance
- recent travel and where to
- recent medication, in particular any antibiotics.

High-volume diarrhoea (>1 L/day) occurs when the stool water content is increased (the principal site of physiological water absorption being the colon) and may be:

- secretory, due to intestinal inflammation, as in infection or inflammatory bowel disease
- osmotic, due to malabsorption, drugs (as in laxative abuse) or motility disorders (autonomic neuropathy, particularly in diabetes).

If the patient fasts, osmotic diarrhoea stops but secretory diarrhoea persists. The most common cause of acute diarrhoea is infective gastroenteritis due to norovirus, *Salmonella* species or *Clostridium difficile*. Infective diarrhoea can become chronic (>4 weeks) in cases of parasitic infestations (such as giardiasis (*Giardia lamblia*), amoebiasis or cryptosporidiosis). Steatorrhoea is common in coeliac disease, chronic pancreatitis and pancreatic insufficiency due to cystic fibrosis. Bloody diarrhoea may be caused by inflammatory bowel disease, colonic ischaemia or infective gastroenteritis. Change in the bowel habit towards diarrhoea can be a manifestation of colon cancer, in particular, cancer of the right side of the colon and in patients over 50 years. Thyrotoxicosis is often accompanied by secretory diarrhoea or steatorrhoea and weight loss.

Low-volume diarrhoea is associated with irritable bowel syndrome. Abdominal pain, bloating, dyspepsia and non-alimentary symptoms commonly accompany irritable bowel symptoms. Criteria have been developed to define irritable bowel syndrome more precisely, taking into account the duration of symptoms, the presence of abdominal pain and its relationship to defecation, and the frequency and consistency of stools (see Rome IV criteria for irritable bowel syndrome).

## Constipation

Clarify what the patient means by constipation. Use the Bristol stool form scale (Fig. 6.7) to describe the stools. Constipation is the infrequent passage of hard stools.

Ask about:

- onset: lifelong or of recent onset
- stool frequency: how often the patient moves their bowels each week and how much time is spent straining at stool
- shape of the stool: for example, pellet-like
- associated symptoms, such as abdominal pain, anal pain on defecation or rectal bleeding
- drugs that may cause constipation.

Constipation may be due to lack of dietary fibre, impaired colonic motility, mechanical intestinal obstruction, impaired rectal sensation or anorectal dysfunction impairing the process of defecation. Constipation is common in irritable bowel syndrome. Other important causes include colorectal cancer, hypothyroidism, hypercalcaemia, drugs (opiates, iron) and immobility (Parkinson's disease, stroke). Absolute constipation (no flatus or

**THE BRISTOL STOOL FORM SCALE**

| Type 1 | Separate hard lumps, like nuts (hard to pass) |
| Type 2 | Sausage-shaped but lumpy |
| Type 3 | Like a sausage but with cracks on its surface |
| Type 4 | Like a sausage or snake, smooth and soft |
| Type 5 | Soft blobs with clear-cut edges (passed easily) |
| Type 6 | Fluffy pieces with ragged edges, a mushy stool |
| Type 7 | Watery, no solid pieces ENTIRELY LIQUID |

Reproduced by kind permission of Dr KW Heaton,
Formerly Reader in Medicine at the University of Bristol.
©2000 Produced by Norgine Pharmaceuticals Limited.

**Fig. 6.7** Bristol stool form scale. *Reproduced with kind permission of Dr KW Heaton, formerly Reader in Medicine at the University of Bristol. ©2000, Norgine group of companies.*

bowel movements) suggests intestinal obstruction and is usually associated with pain, vomiting and distension. Tenesmus suggests rectal inflammation or tumour. Faecal impaction can occasionally present as overflow diarrhoea.

## Bleeding

### Haematemesis

Haematemesis is the vomiting of blood.
Ask about:

- Colour: is the vomitus fresh red blood or dark brown, resembling coffee grounds?
- Onset: was haematemesis preceded by intense retching or was blood staining apparent in the first vomit?
- History of dyspepsia, peptic ulceration, gastrointestinal bleeding or liver disease.
- Alcohol, non-steroidal anti-inflammatory drugs (NSAIDs) and glucocorticoid ingestion.

If the source of bleeding is above the gastro-oesophageal sphincter, as with oesophageal varices, fresh blood may well up in the mouth, as well as being actively vomited. With a lower oesophageal mucosal tear due to the trauma of forceful retching (Mallory–Weiss syndrome), fresh blood appears only after the patient has vomited forcefully several times.

## Melaena

Melaena is the passage of tarry, shiny black stools with a characteristic odour and results from upper gastrointestinal bleeding. Distinguish this from the matt black stools associated with oral iron or bismuth therapy.

Peptic ulceration (gastric or duodenal) is the most common cause of upper gastrointestinal bleeding and can manifest with melaena, haematemesis or both. Excessive alcohol ingestion may cause haematemesis from erosive gastritis, Mallory–Weiss tear or bleeding oesophagogastric varices in cirrhotic patients. Oesophageal or gastric cancer, gastric angioectasias (Dieulafoy lesion when localised in the fundus) and portal hypertensive gastropathy due to splenic vein thrombosis are rare causes of upper gastrointestinal bleeding.

The Rockall and Blatchford scores are used to assess the risk of gastrointestinal bleeding (Boxes 6.5 and 6.6). A profound upper gastrointestinal bleed may lead to the passage of purple stool or, rarely, fresh blood.

## Rectal bleeding

Establish whether the blood is mixed with stool, coats the surface of the otherwise normal stool or is seen on the toilet paper or in the pan. Fresh rectal bleeding (haematochezia) usually indicates a disorder in the anal canal, rectum or colon. During severe upper gastrointestinal bleeding, however, blood may pass through the intestine unaltered, causing fresh rectal

---

### 6.5 Prediction of the risk of mortality in patients with upper gastrointestinal bleeding: Rockall score

| Criterion | Score |
|---|---|
| **Age** | |
| <60 years | 0 |
| 60–79 years | 1 |
| >80 years | 2 |
| **Shock** | |
| None | 0 |
| Pulse >100 beats per minute and systolic blood pressure >100 mmHg | 1 |
| Systolic blood pressure <100 mmHg | 2 |
| **Comorbidity** | |
| None | 0 |
| Heart failure, ischaemic heart disease or other major illness | 2 |
| Renal failure or disseminated malignancy | 3 |
| **Endoscopic findings** | |
| Mallory–Weiss tear and no visible bleeding | 0 |
| All other diagnoses | 1 |
| Upper gastrointestinal malignancy | 2 |
| **Major stigmata of recent haemorrhage** | |
| None | 0 |
| Visible bleeding vessel/adherent clot | 2 |
| Total score | |
| Pre-endoscopy (maximum score = 7) | Score 4 = 14% mortality pre-endoscopy |
| Post-endoscopy (maximum score = 11) | Score 8+ = 25% mortality post-endoscopy |

*Reproduced from Rockall TA, Logan RF, Devlin HB, et al. Risk assessment after acute upper gastrointestinal haemorrhage. Journal of the British Society of Gastroenterology 1996; 38(3):316, with permission from BMJ Publishing Group Ltd.*

---

### 6.6 Prediction of need to have a medical intervention (e.g. blood transfusion or endoscopy) in patients with upper gastrointestinal bleeding: The Glasgow-Blatchford bleeding score

| Admission risk marker | Score component value |
|---|---|
| **Blood urea (mmol/L)** | |
| >6–5 <8–0 | 2 |
| >8–0 <10–0 | 3 |
| <1–0 <25–0 | 4 |
| >25 | 6 |
| **Haemoglobin (g/L) for men** | |
| >120 <130 | 1 |
| >100 <120 | 3 |
| <10–0 | 6 |
| **Haemoglobin (g/L) for women** | |
| ≥100<120 | 1 |
| <100 | 6 |
| **Systolic blood pressure (mmHg)** | |
| <100–109 | 1 |
| 90–99 | 2 |
| <90 | 3 |
| **Other markers** | |
| Pulse >100 (per min) | 1 |
| Presentation with melaena | 1 |
| Presentation with synoope | 2 |
| Hepatic disease | 2 |
| Cardiac failure | 2 |

Score of 0 no interventions needed; patient can be treated as an outpatient

Scores of 6 >50% risk of needing an intervention.

*Reprinted with permission from Elsevier, Blatchford O, Murray WR, Blatchford M. A risk score to predict need for treatment for upper-gastrointestinal haemorrhage. Lancet 2000;356:1318–21.*

bleeding. Common causes of rectal bleeding include haemorrhoids, anal fissures (blood on the toilet paper or in the pan), complicated diverticular disease, colorectal cancer or colonic polyps, inflammatory bowel disease, ischaemic colitis and colonic angioectasias.

## Jaundice

Jaundice is a yellowish discolouration of the skin, sclerae (Fig. 6.8) and mucous membranes caused by hyperbilirubinaemia (Box 6.7). There is no absolute level at which jaundice is clinically detected but, in good light, most clinicians will recognise jaundice when bilirubin levels exceed 50 μmol/L (2.92 mg/dL).

Ask about:

- associated symptoms: abdominal pain, fever, weight loss, itching
- colour of stools (normal or pale) and urine (normal or dark)
- alcohol intake
- travel history and immunisations
- use of illicit or intravenous drugs
- sexual history
- previous blood transfusions
- recently prescribed drugs.

Unconjugated bilirubin is insoluble and binds to plasma albumin; it is therefore not filtered by the renal glomeruli. In jaundice from unconjugated hyperbilirubinaemia, the urine is a normal colour (acholuric jaundice; Box 6.8).

Bilirubin is conjugated to form bilirubin diglucuronide in the liver and excreted in bile, producing its characteristic green colour. In conjugated hyperbilirubinaemia, the urine is dark brown due to the presence of bilirubin diglucuronide. In the colon, conjugated bilirubin is metabolised by bacteria to stercobilinogen and stercobilin, which contribute to the brown colour of stool. Stercobilinogen is absorbed from the bowel and excreted in the urine as urobilinogen, a colourless, water-soluble compound.

### Prehepatic jaundice

In haemolytic disorders, anaemic pallor combined with jaundice may produce a pale lemon complexion. The stools and urine are

| 6.7 Common causes of jaundice | | |
|---|---|---|
| **Increased bilirubin production** | | |
| - Haemolysis (unconjugated hyperbilirubinaemia) | | |
| **Impaired bilirubin excretion** | | |
| - Congenital: | | - Intrahepatic cholestasis: |
|   - Gilbert's syndrome (unconjugated) | |   - Drugs |
| - Hepatocellular: | |   - Primary biliary cirrhosis |
|   - Viral hepatitis | | - Extrahepatic cholestasis: |
|   - Cirrhosis | |   - Gallstones |
|   - Drugs | |   - Cancer: pancreas, cholangiocarcinoma |
|   - Autoimmune hepatitis | | |

normal in colour. Gilbert's syndrome is common and causes unconjugated hyperbilirubinaemia. Serum liver enzyme concentrations are normal and jaundice is mild (plasma bilirubin <100 μmol/L (5.85 mg/dL)) but increases during prolonged fasting or intercurrent febrile illness.

### Hepatic jaundice

Hepatocellular disease causes hyperbilirubinaemia that is both unconjugated and conjugated. Conjugated bilirubin leads to dark brown urine. The stools are normal in colour.

### Posthepatic/cholestatic jaundice

In biliary obstruction, conjugated bilirubin in the bile does not reach the intestine, so the stools are pale. Obstructive jaundice may be accompanied by pruritus (generalised itch) due to skin deposition of bile salts. Obstructive jaundice with abdominal pain is usually due to gallstones; if fever or rigours also occur (Charcot's triad), ascending cholangitis is likely. Painless obstructive jaundice suggests malignant biliary obstruction, as in cholangiocarcinoma or cancer of the head of the pancreas. Obstructive jaundice can be due to intrahepatic as well as extrahepatic cholestasis, as in primary biliary cirrhosis, certain hepatotoxic drug reactions (Box 6.9) and profound hepatocellular injury.

## Groin swellings and lumps

Ask about:

- associated pain

**Fig. 6.8** Yellow sclera of jaundice.

| 6.8 Urine and stool analysis in jaundice | | | | |
|---|---|---|---|---|
| | **Urine** | | | **Stools** |
| | Colour | Bilirubin | Urobilinogen | Colour |
| Unconjugated | Normal | – | ++++ | Normal |
| Hepatocellular | Dark | ++ | ++ | Normal |
| Obstructive | Dark | ++++ | – | Pale |

## 6.9 Examples of drug-induced gastrointestinal conditions

| Symptom | Drug |
| --- | --- |
| Weight gain | Oral glucocorticoids |
| Dyspepsia and gastrointestinal bleeding | Aspirin<br>Non-steroidal anti-inflammatory drugs |
| Nausea | Many drugs, including selective serotonin reuptake inhibitor antidepressants |
| Diarrhoea (pseudomembranous colitis) | Antibiotics<br>Proton pump inhibitors |
| Constipation | Opioids |
| Jaundice: hepatitis | Paracetamol (overdose)<br>Pyrazinamide<br>Rifampicin<br>Isoniazid |
| Jaundice: cholestatic | Flucloxacillin<br>Chlorpromazine<br>Co-amoxiclav |
| Liver fibrosis | Methotrexate |

- precipitating/exacerbating factors, such as straining due to chronic constipation, chronic cough, heavy manual labour and relationship with micturition
- timing: when the symptoms are worse

Hernias are common causes of groin lumps and frequently present with dull, dragging discomfort (rather than acute pain), which is often exacerbated by straining and after long periods of standing or activity. Patients can often manually reduce the hernia by applying gentle pressure over the swelling or by lying flat. Other causes of groin swellings include lymph nodes, skin and subcutaneous lumps and, less commonly, saphena varix (a varicosity of the long saphenous vein), hydrocoele of the spermatic cord, undescended testis, femoral aneurysm or a psoas abscess.

## Past medical history

History of a similar problem may suggest the diagnosis: for example, pancreatitis, bleeding peptic ulcer or inflammatory bowel disease. Coexisting peripheral vascular disease, hypertension, heart failure or atrial fibrillation may suggest aortic aneurysm or mesenteric ischaemia as the cause of acute abdominal pain. Primary biliary cirrhosis and autoimmune hepatitis are associated with thyroid disease, and non-alcoholic fatty liver disease (NAFLD) is associated with diabetes and obesity. Ask about previous abdominal surgery.

## Drug history

Ask about all prescribed medications, over-the-counter medicines and herbal preparations. Many drugs affect the gastrointestinal tract (Box 6.9) and are hepatotoxic.

## Family history

Inflammatory bowel disease is more common in patients with a family history of either Crohn's disease or ulcerative colitis. Colorectal cancer in a first-degree relative increases the risk of colorectal cancer and polyps. Peptic ulcer disease may be familial but is mainly due to environmental factors, such as the transmission of *H. pylori* infection. Gilbert's syndrome is an autosomal dominant condition; haemochromatosis and Wilson's disease are autosomal recessive disorders. Autoimmune diseases, particularly thyroid disease, are common in relatives of those with primary biliary cirrhosis and autoimmune hepatitis. A family history of diabetes is frequently seen in the context of NAFLD.

## Social history

Ask about:

- Dietary history: assess the intake of calories and sources of essential nutrients. For guidance, there are 9 kcal per g of fat and 4 kcal per g of carbohydrates and protein.
- Food intolerances: patients with irritable bowel syndrome often report specific food intolerances, including wheat, dairy products and others. Painless diarrhoea may indicate high alcohol intake, lactose intolerance or coeliac disease.
- Alcohol consumption: calculate the patient's intake in units (p. 75).
- Smoking: this increases the risk of oesophageal cancer, colorectal cancer, Crohn's disease and peptic ulcer, while patients with ulcerative colitis are less likely to smoke.
- Stress: many disorders, particularly irritable bowel syndrome and dyspepsia, are exacerbated by stress and mental disorders.
- Foreign travel: this is particularly relevant in liver disease and diarrhoea.
- Risk factors for liver disease: these include intravenous drug use, tattoos, foreign travel, blood transfusions, and sex between men or with prostitutes and multiple sexual partners. Hepatitis B and C may present with chronic liver disease or cancer decades after the primary infection, so enquire about risk factors in the distant as well as the recent past.

## The physical examination

Examination of the gastrointestinal system includes intimate examination and consideration should be given to a patient's preference regarding the gender of the examining clinician and the presence of a chaperone. Skin colour should be taken into account when eliciting clinical signs such as jaundice. Differential diagnosis may need to be adjusted to consider racial or ethnic differences.

## General examination

### Examination sequence (Video 6)

- Note the patient's demeanour and general appearance. Are they in pain, cachectic, thin, well-nourished or obese? Record height, weight, waist circumference and body mass index (p. 32). Note whether obesity is truncal or generalised. Look for abdominal striae or loose skin folds.

- Inspect the patient's hands for clubbing, koilonychia (spoon-shaped nails) and signs of chronic liver disease (Fig. 6.9), including leuconychia (white nails) and palmar erythema.
- Inspect the mouth, throat and tongue.
- Ask the patient to look down and retract the upper eyelid to expose the sclera; look to see if it is yellow in natural light (see Fig. 6.8).
- Examine the cervical, axillary and inguinal lymph nodes (p. 34).

**6**

**Eyes**
- Jaundice

**Chest**
- Gynaecomastia (in men)
- Breast atrophy (in women)

A  Spider naevus

**Upper half of body (above umbilicus)**
- Spider naevi (A)

**Abdomen**
- Splenomegaly
- Hepatomegaly (but liver may be small)
- Dilated collateral vessels around umbilicus

B  Leuconychia

**Hands**
- Leuconychia (white nails) (B)
- Palmar erythema (C)
- Clubbing

**Genitalia**
- Testicular atrophy

**Legs**
- Oedema
- Hair loss

**General**
- Skin pigmentation
- Loss of body hair
- Bruising

C  Palmar erythema

**Fig. 6.9** Features of chronic liver disease.

Striae indicate rapid weight gain, previous pregnancy or, rarely, Cushing's syndrome. Loose skin folds signify recent weight loss.

Stigmata of iron deficiency include angular cheilitis (painful cracks at the corners of the mouth) and atrophic glossitis (pale, smooth tongue). The tongue has a beefy, raw appearance in folate and vitamin $B_{12}$ deficiency. Mouth and throat aphthous ulcers are common in coeliac and inflammatory bowel disease (see Fig. 6.3B).

Gastric and pancreatic cancer may spread to cause enlargement of the left supraclavicular lymph nodes (Troisier's sign). More widespread lymphadenopathy with hepatosplenomegaly suggests lymphoma.

## Liver disease

Do not confuse the diffuse yellow sclerae of jaundice with small, yellowish fat pads (pingueculae) sometimes seen at the periphery of the sclerae.

Certain signs (stigmata) suggest chronic liver disease (see Fig. 6.9):

- Palmar erythema and spider naevi are caused by excess oestrogen associated with the reduced hepatic breakdown of sex steroids. Spider naevi are isolated telangiectasias that characteristically fill from a central vessel and are found in the distribution of the superior vena cava (upper trunk, arms and face). Women may have up to five spider naevi in health; palmar erythema and numerous spider naevi are normal during pregnancy. In men, these signs suggest chronic liver disease.
- Gynaecomastia (breast enlargement in males), with loss of body hair and testicular atrophy, may occur due to reduced breakdown of oestrogens.
- Leuconychia, caused by hypoalbuminaemia, may also occur in protein-calorie malnutrition (kwashiorkor), malabsorption due to protein-losing enteropathy, as in coeliac disease, or heavy and prolonged proteinuria (nephrotic syndrome).
- Finger clubbing is found in liver cirrhosis, inflammatory bowel disease and malabsorption syndromes.

Other signs that may be associated with liver disease include:

- Dupuytren's contracture of the palmar fascia (see Fig. 3.5): linked with alcohol-related chronic liver disease
- bilateral parotid swelling due to sialoadenosis: may be a feature of chronic alcohol misuse.

Signs that suggest liver failure include:

- asterixis, a coarse flapping tremor when the arms are outstretched and hands dorsiflexed, which occurs with hepatic encephalopathy
- fetor hepaticus, a distinctive 'mousy' odour of dimethyl sulphide on the breath, which is evidence of portosystemic shunting (with or without encephalopathy)
- altered mental state, varying from drowsiness with the day/night pattern reversed, through confusion and disorientation, to unresponsive coma

- jaundice, yellowing of the skin may be less noticeable in patients with black or brown skin
- ascites
- late neurological features, which include spasticity, an extension of the arms and legs, and extensor plantar responses.

In a jaundiced patient, spider naevi, palmar erythema and ascites all strongly suggest chronic liver disease rather than obstructive jaundice.

## Abdominal examination

Examine the patient in good light and warm surroundings, positioned comfortably supine, arms by the side with the head resting on only one or two pillows to relax the abdominal wall muscles. Use extra pillows to support a patient with kyphosis or breathlessness.

## Inspection

### Examination sequence (Video 6A)

- Look at the teeth, tongue and buccal mucosa; check for mouth ulcers.
- Note any smells, including alcohol, fetor hepaticus, uraemia, melaena or ketones.
- Expose the abdomen from the xiphisternum to the symphysis pubis, leaving the chest and legs covered.

The normal abdomen is flat or slightly scaphoid and symmetrical. At rest, respiration is principally diaphragmatic; the abdominal wall moves out and the liver, spleen and kidneys move downwards during inspiration. The umbilicus is usually inverted.

### Skin

In older patients, seborrhoeic warts, ranging from pink to brown or black, and haemangiomas (Campbell de Morgan spots) are common and normal, but note any striae, bruising or scratch marks.

### Visible veins

Abnormally prominent veins on the abdominal wall suggest portal hypertension or vena cava obstruction. In portal hypertension, recanalisation of the umbilical vein along the falciform ligament produces distended veins that drain away from the umbilicus: the 'caput medusae'. The umbilicus may appear bluish and distended due to an umbilical varix. In contrast, an umbilical hernia is a distended and everted umbilicus that does not appear vascular and may have a palpable cough impulse. Dilated tortuous veins with blood flow superiorly are collateral veins caused by obstruction of the inferior vena cava. Rarely, superior vena cava obstruction gives rise to similarly distended abdominal veins, but these all flow inferiorly.

## Abdominal swelling

Diffuse abdominal swelling could be due to ascites or intestinal obstruction. If localised, it could be caused by urinary retention, a mass or an enlarged organ such as the liver. In obesity, the umbilicus is usually sunken; in ascites, it is flat or, more commonly, everted. Look tangentially across the abdomen and from the foot of the bed for any asymmetry suggesting a localised mass.

## Abdominal scars and stomas

Note any surgical scars or stomas and clarify what operations have been undertaken (Figs 6.10 and 6.11). A small infraumbilical incision usually indicates a previous laparoscopy. Puncture scars from laparoscopic surgical ports may be visible. An incisional hernia at the site of a scar is palpable as a defect in the abdominal wall musculature and becomes more obvious as the patient raises their head off the bed or coughs.

## | Palpation

### Examination sequence (Video 6B) ▶

- Ensure your hands are warm and clean.
- If the bed is low, kneel beside it but avoid touching the floor to prevent infection.
- Ask the patient to show you where any pain is and to report any tenderness during palpation.
- Ask the patient to place their arms by their sides to help relax the abdominal wall.
- Use your right hand, keeping it flat and in contact with the abdominal wall.

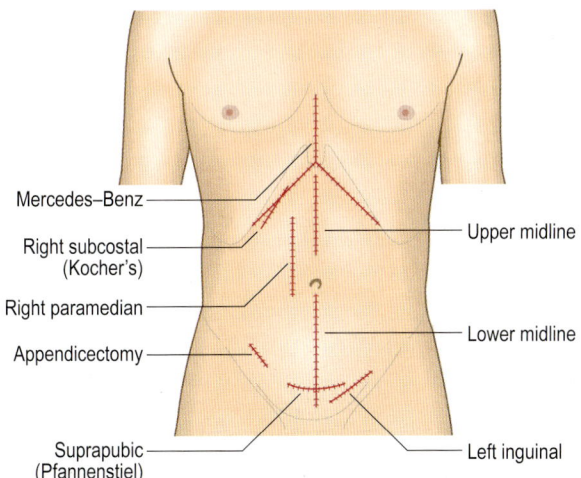

**Fig. 6.10 Some abdominal incisions.** The midline and oblique incisions avoid damage to innervation of the abdominal musculature and later development of incisional hernias. These incisions have been widely superseded by laparoscopic surgery, however.

Labels (top to bottom):
- Mercedes–Benz
- Right subcostal (Kocher's)
- Right paramedian
- Appendicectomy
- Suprapubic (Pfannenstiel)
- Upper midline
- Lower midline
- Left inguinal

**Fig. 6.11 Surgical stomas.** [A] An ileostomy is usually in the right iliac fossa and is formed as a spout. [B] A loop colostomy is created to defunction the distal bowel temporarily. It is usually in the transverse colon and has afferent and efferent limbs. [C] A colostomy may be terminal: that is, resected distal bowel. It is usually flush and in the left iliac fossa.

- Observe the patient's face throughout for any sign of discomfort.
- Begin with light superficial palpation away from any site of pain.
- Palpate each region in turn, and then repeat with deeper palpation.
- Test abdominal muscle tone using light, dipping finger movements.
- Describe any mass using the basic principles outlined in Chapter 3, p. 34. Describe its site, size, surface, shape and consistency, and note whether it moves on respiration. Is the mass fixed or mobile?
- To determine if a mass is superficial and in the abdominal wall rather than within the abdominal cavity, ask the patient to tense their abdominal muscles by lifting their head. An abdominal wall mass will still be palpable, whereas an intra-abdominal mass will not.
- Decide whether the mass is an enlarged abdominal organ or separate from the solid organs.

### Tenderness

Discomfort during palpation may vary and may be accompanied by resistance to palpation. Consider the patient's level of anxiety when assessing the severity of pain and degree of tenderness elicited. Tenderness in several areas on minimal pressure may be due to generalised peritonitis but is more often caused by anxiety. Severe superficial pain with no tenderness on deep palpation or pain that disappears if the patient is distracted also suggests anxiety. With these exceptions, tenderness usefully indicates underlying pathology.

Voluntary guarding is the voluntary contraction of the abdominal muscles when palpation provokes pain. Involuntary guarding is the reflex contraction of the abdominal muscles when there is inflammation of the parietal peritoneum. If the whole peritoneum is inflamed (generalised peritonitis) due to a

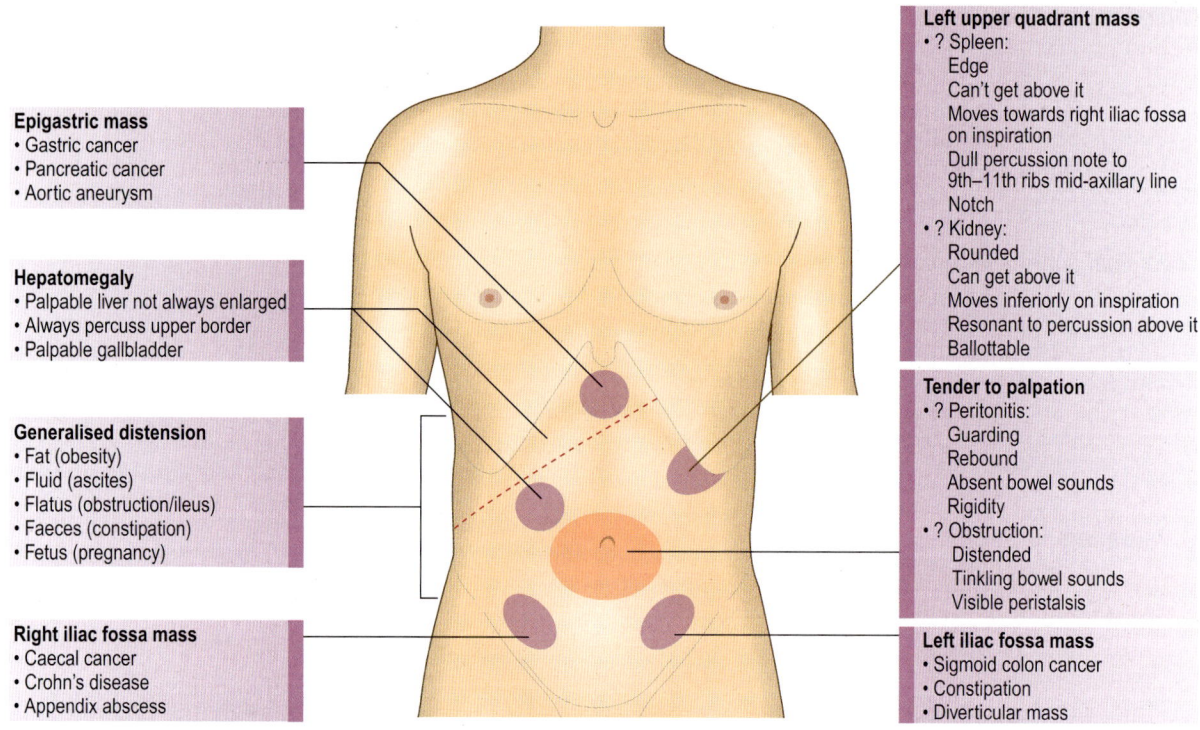

**Epigastric mass**
- Gastric cancer
- Pancreatic cancer
- Aortic aneurysm

**Hepatomegaly**
- Palpable liver not always enlarged
- Always percuss upper border
- Palpable gallbladder

**Generalised distension**
- Fat (obesity)
- Fluid (ascites)
- Flatus (obstruction/ileus)
- Faeces (constipation)
- Fetus (pregnancy)

**Right iliac fossa mass**
- Caecal cancer
- Crohn's disease
- Appendix abscess

**Left upper quadrant mass**
- ? Spleen:
  Edge
  Can't get above it
  Moves towards right iliac fossa on inspiration
  Dull percussion note to 9th–11th ribs mid-axillary line
  Notch
- ? Kidney:
  Rounded
  Can get above it
  Moves inferiorly on inspiration
  Resonant to percussion above it
  Ballottable

**Tender to palpation**
- ? Peritonitis:
  Guarding
  Rebound
  Absent bowel sounds
  Rigidity
- ? Obstruction:
  Distended
  Tinkling bowel sounds
  Visible peristalsis

**Left iliac fossa mass**
- Sigmoid colon cancer
- Constipation
- Diverticular mass

**Fig. 6.12** Palpable abnormalities in the abdomen.

### 6.10 Specific signs in the 'acute abdomen'

| Sign | Disease associations | Examination |
|---|---|---|
| Murphy's | Acute cholecystitis:<br>Sensitivity 50–97%<br>Specificity 50–80% | As the patient takes a deep breath in, gently palpate in the right upper quadrant of the abdomen; the acutely inflamed gallbladder contacts the examining fingers, evoking pain with the arrest of inspiration |
| Rovsing's | Acute appendicitis:<br>Sensitivity 20–70%<br>Specificity 40–96% | Palpation in the left iliac fossa produces pain in the right iliac fossa |
| Iliopsoas | Retroileal appendicitis, iliopsoas abscess, perinephric abscess | Ask the patient to flex their thigh against the resistance of your hand; a painful response indicates an inflammatory process involving the right psoas muscle |
| Grey Turner's and Cullen's | Haemorrhagic pancreatitis, aortic rupture and ruptured ectopic pregnancy (see Fig. 6.13) | Bleeding into the falciform ligament; bruising develops around the umbilicus (Cullen) or in the loins (Grey Turner) |

perforated viscus, the abdominal wall no longer moves with respiration; breathing becomes increasingly thoracic and the anterior abdominal wall muscles are held rigid (board-like rigidity).

The site of tenderness is important. Tenderness in the epigastrium suggests peptic ulcer; in the right hypochondrium, cholecystitis; in the left iliac fossa, diverticulitis; and in the right iliac fossa, appendicitis or Crohn's ileitis (Fig. 6.12). Ask the patient to cough or gently percuss the abdomen to elicit any pain or 'rebound tenderness'. This approach is preferable to rapidly removing your hand after deep palpation. Rebound tenderness is a sign of intra-abdominal disease but not necessarily of parietal peritoneal inflammation (peritonism). Specific abdominal signs are shown in Box 6.10; signs of Grey Turner's and Cullen's are shown in Fig. 6.13. Typical findings may be masked in patients taking glucocorticoids, immunosuppressants or anti-inflammatory drugs, in alcohol intoxication or altered states of consciousness.

### Palpable mass

A pulsatile mass palpable in the upper abdomen may be normal aortic pulsation in a thin person, a gastric or pancreatic tumour transmitting underlying aortic pulsation or an aortic aneurysm.

A                                                                    B

**Fig. 6.13 Acute pancreatitis.** A Bruising over the flanks (Grey Turner's sign). B Bruising around the umbilicus (Cullen's sign).

A pathological mass can usually be distinguished from normal palpable structures by site (Fig. 6.14), and from palpable faeces as these can be indented and may disappear following defecation. A hard subcutaneous nodule at the umbilicus may indicate metastatic cancer ('Sister Mary Joseph's nodule').

### Enlarged organs

Examine the liver, gallbladder, spleen and kidneys in turn during deep inspiration. Keep your examining hand still and wait for the organ to move with breathing. Do not start palpation too close to the costal margin, missing the edge of the liver or spleen.

### Hepatomegaly

### Examination sequence (Video 6C)

- Place your hand flat on the skin of the right iliac fossa.
- Point your fingers upwards and your index and middle fingers lateral to the rectus muscle, so that your fingertips lie parallel to the rectus sheath (Fig. 6.15). Keep your hand stationary.
- Ask the patient to breathe in deeply through the mouth.
- Feel for the liver edge as it descends on inspiration.
- Move your hand progressively up the abdomen, 1 cm at a time, between each breath the patient takes until you reach the costal margin or detect the liver edge.
- If you feel a liver edge, describe:
  - size
  - surface: smooth or irregular
  - edge: smooth or irregular; define the medial border
  - consistency: soft or hard
  - tenderness
  - pulsatility.
- To examine for gallbladder tenderness, ask the patient to breathe in deeply, then gently palpate the right upper quadrant in the mid-clavicular line.

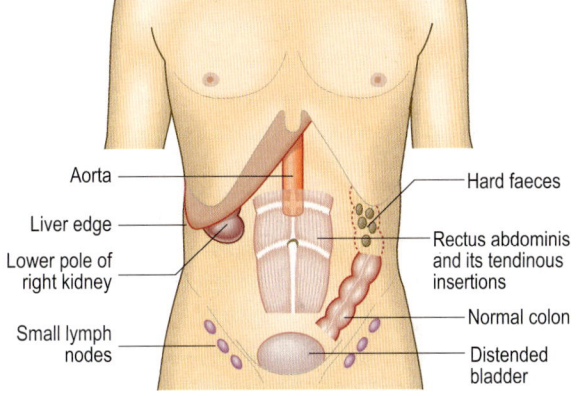

Aorta — Hard faeces

Liver edge —

Lower pole of right kidney — Rectus abdominis and its tendinous insertions

— Normal colon

Small lymph nodes — Distended bladder

**Fig. 6.14** Palpable masses that may be physiological rather than pathological.

**Fig. 6.15** Palpation of the liver.

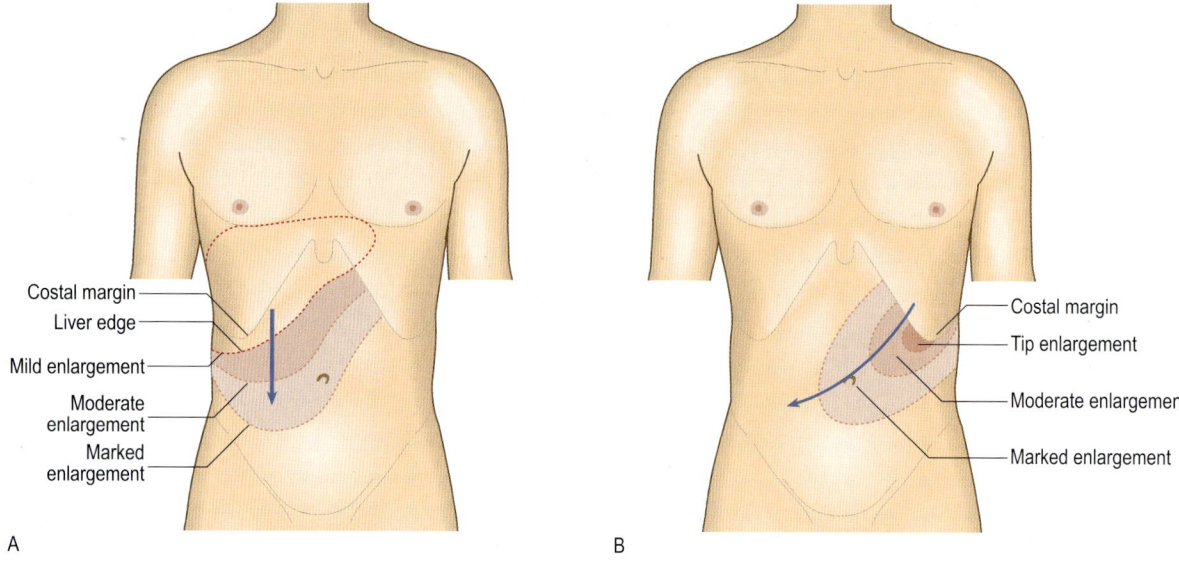

Costal margin
Liver edge
Mild enlargement
Moderate enlargement
Marked enlargement

Costal margin
Tip enlargement
Moderate enlargement
Marked enlargement

A

B

**Fig. 6.16 Patterns of progressive enlargement of the liver and spleen.** [A] Direction of enlargement of the liver. [B] Direction of enlargement of the spleen. The spleen moves downwards and medially during inspiration.

## Percussion

### Examination sequence

- Ask the patient to hold their breath in full expiration.
- Percuss downwards from the right fifth intercostal space in the mid-clavicular line, listening for dullness indicating the upper border of the liver.
- Measure the distance in centimetres below the costal margin in the mid-clavicular line or from the upper border of dullness to the palpable liver edge.

In the normal abdomen, you may feel:

- the liver edge below the right costal margin
- the aorta as a pulsatile swelling above the umbilicus
- the lower pole of the right kidney in the right flank
- faecal scybala (hardened masses of faeces) in the sigmoid colon in the left iliac fossa
- a full bladder arising out of the pelvis in the suprapubic region.

The normal liver is identified as an area of dullness to percussion over the right anterior chest between the fifth rib and the costal margin.

The liver may be enlarged (Fig. 6.16A) or displaced downwards by hyperinflated lungs.

Hepatic enlargement can result from chronic parenchymal liver disease from any cause (Box 6.11). The liver is enlarged in early cirrhosis but often shrunken in advanced cirrhosis. Fatty liver (hepatic steatosis) can cause marked hepatomegaly. Hepatic enlargement due to metastatic tumour is hard and irregular. An enlarged left lobe may be felt in the epigastrium or even

the left hypochondrium. In right heart failure, the congested liver is usually soft and tender; a pulsatile liver indicates tricuspid regurgitation. A bruit over the liver may be heard in acute alcoholic hepatitis, hepatocellular cancer, arteriovenous malformation and in patients with portal-systemic shunts. The most common reason for an audible bruit over the liver, however, is a transmitted heart murmur. Liver failure produces additional symptoms of encephalopathy, which can be graded (Box 6.12).

Resonance below the fifth intercostal space suggests hyperinflated lungs or occasionally the interposition of the transverse colon between the liver and the diaphragm (Chilaiditi's sign).

| 6.11 Causes of hepatomegaly | |
|---|---|
| **Chronic parenchymal liver disease** | |
| • Alcoholic liver disease | • Viral hepatitis |
| • Hepatic steatosis | • Primary biliary cirrhosis |
| • Autoimmune hepatitis | |
| **Malignancy** | |
| • Primary hepatocellular cancer | • Secondary metastatic cancer |
| **Right heart failure** | |
| **Haematological disorders** | |
| • Lymphoma | • Myelofibrosis |
| • Leukaemia | • Polycythaemia |
| **Rarities** | |
| • Amyloidosis | • Sarcoidosis |
| • Budd–Chiari syndrome | • Glycogen storage disorders |

## 6.12 Grading of hepatic encephalopathy (West Haven)

| Stage | State of consciousness |
|---|---|
| 0 | No change in personality or behaviour<br>No asterixis (flapping tremor) |
| 1 | Impaired concentration and attention span<br>Sleep disturbance, slurred speech<br>Euphoria or depression<br>Asterixis present |
| 2 | Lethargy, drowsiness, apathy or aggression<br>Disorientation, inappropriate behaviour, slurred speech |
| 3 | Confusion and disorientation, bizarre behaviour<br>Drowsiness or stupor<br>Asterixis usually absent |
| 4 | Comatose with no response to voice commands<br>Minimal or absent response to painful stimuli |

*Reproduced from Conn HO, Leevy CM, Vlahcevic ZR, et al. Comparison of lactulose and neomycin in the treatment of chronic portal-systemic encephalopathy. A double-blind controlled trial. Gastroenterology. 1977;72(4):573, with permission from Elsevier Inc.*

## 6.13 Differentiating a palpable spleen from the left kidney

| Distinguishing feature | Spleen | Kidney |
|---|---|---|
| Mass is smooth and regular in shape | More likely | Polycystic kidneys are bilateral irregular masses |
| Mass descends in inspiration | Yes, travels superficially and diagonally | Yes, moves deeply and vertically |
| Ability to feel deep into the mass | Yes | No |
| Palpable notch on the medial surface | Yes | No |
| Bilateral masses palpable | No | Sometimes (e.g. polycystic kidneys) |
| Percussion resonant over the mass | No | Sometimes |
| Mass extends beyond the midline | Sometimes | No (except with horseshoe kidney) |

In a patient with right upper quadrant pain, test for Murphy's sign (see Box 6.10); a positive test modestly increases the probability of acute cholecystitis. Palpable distension of the gallbladder is rare and has a characteristic globular shape. It results from either obstruction of the cystic duct, as in mucocoele or empyema of the gallbladder, or obstruction of the common bile duct with a patent cystic duct, as in pancreatic cancer. In a jaundiced patient, a palpable gallbladder is likely to be due to extrahepatic obstruction, such as from pancreatic cancer or, very rarely, gallstones (Courvoisier's sign). In gallstone disease, the gallbladder may be tender but impalpable because of fibrosis of the gallbladder wall.

### Splenomegaly

The spleen has to enlarge threefold before it becomes palpable, so a palpable spleen always indicates splenomegaly. It enlarges from under the left costal margin down and medially towards the umbilicus (Fig. 6.16B). A characteristic notch may be palpable midway along its leading edge, helping differentiate it from an enlarged left kidney (Box 6.13).

- If you cannot feel the splenic edge, palpate with your right hand, placing your left hand behind the patient's left lower ribs and pulling the ribcage forward (Fig. 6.17B), or ask the patient to roll towards you and on to their right side and repeat the above.
- Feel along the left costal margin and percuss over the lateral chest wall. The normal spleen causes dullness to percussion posterior to the left mid-axillary line beneath the 9th–11th ribs.

There are many causes of splenomegaly (Box 6.14). Massive enlargement in the developed world is usually due to myeloproliferative disease or haematological malignancy; worldwide, tropical splenomegaly syndrome due to malaria is a common cause.

Important causes of hepatosplenomegaly include lymphoma or myeloproliferative disorders, cirrhosis with portal hypertension, amyloidosis, sarcoidosis and glycogen storage disease.

### Ascites

Ascites is the accumulation of intraperitoneal fluid (see Fig. 6.6).

## Examination sequence (Video 6D)

- Place your hand over the patient's umbilicus. With your hand stationary, ask the patient to inhale deeply through the mouth.
- Feel for the splenic edge as it descends on inspiration.
- Move your hand diagonally upwards towards the left hypochondrium (Fig. 6.17A), 1 cm at a time between each breath the patient takes.
- Feel the costal margin along its length, as the position of the spleen tip is variable.

## Examination sequence (Video 6E)

### Shifting dullness

- With the patient supine, percuss from the midline out to the flanks (Fig. 6.18). Note any change from resonant to dull, along with areas of dullness and resonance.
- Keep your finger on the site of dullness in the flank and ask the patient to turn on to their opposite side.
- Pause for 10 seconds to allow any ascites to gravitate, then percuss again. If the area of dullness is now resonant, shifting dullness is present, indicating ascites.

A                                                                            B

**Fig. 6.17 Palpation of the spleen.** [A] Initial palpation for the splenic edge moving diagonally from the umbilicus to the left hypochondrium. [B] If the spleen is impalpable by the method shown in A, use your left hand to pull the ribcage forward and elevate the spleen, making it more likely to be palpable by your right hand.

| 6.14 Causes of splenomegaly | |
|---|---|
| **Haematological disorders** | |
| • Lymphoma and lymphatic leukaemias | • Haemolytic anaemia, congenital spherocytosis |
| • Myeloproliferative diseases, polycythaemia rubra vera and myelofibrosis | |
| **Portal hypertension** | |
| **Infections** | |
| • Glandular fever | • Brucellosis, tuberculosis, salmonellosis |
| • Malaria, kala-azar (leishmaniasis) | |
| • Bacterial endocarditis | |
| **Rheumatological conditions** | |
| • Rheumatoid arthritis (Felty's syndrome) | • Systemic lupus erythematosus |
| **Rarities** | |
| • Sarcoidosis | • Glycogen storage disorders |
| • Amyloidosis | |

## Fluid thrill

- If the abdomen is tensely distended and you are uncertain whether ascites is present, feel for a fluid thrill.
- Place the palm of your left hand flat against the left side of the patient's abdomen and flick a finger of your right hand against the right side of the abdomen.
- If you feel a ripple against your left hand, ask an assistant or the patient to place the edge of their hand on the midline of the abdomen (Fig. 6.19). This prevents transmission of the impulse via the skin rather than through the ascites. If you still feel a ripple against your left hand, a fluid thrill is present (detected only in gross ascites).

The causes of ascites are shown in Box 6.15.

## Auscultation

### Examination sequence (Video 6F)

- With the patient supine, place your stethoscope diaphragm to the right of the umbilicus and do not move it.

A                                    B                                    C

**Fig. 6.18 Percussing for ascites.** [A] and [B] Percuss towards the flank from resonant to dull. [C] Then ask the patient to roll onto their other side. In ascites the note then becomes resonant.

- Listen for up to 2 minutes before concluding that bowel sounds are absent.
- Listen above the umbilicus over the aorta for arterial bruits.
- Now listen 2–3 cm above and lateral to the umbilicus for bruits from renal artery stenosis.
- Listen over the liver for bruits.
- Test for a succussion splash; this sounds like a half-filled water bottle being shaken. Explain the procedure to the patient, then shake their abdomen by rocking their pelvis using both hands.

Normal bowel sounds are gurgling noises from the normal peristaltic activity of the gut. They normally occur every 5–10 seconds but the frequency varies.

The absence of bowel sounds implies paralytic ileus or peritonitis. In intestinal obstruction, bowel sounds occur with increased frequency and volume and have a high-pitched, tinkling quality. Bruits suggest an atheromatous or aneurysmal aorta or superior mesenteric artery stenosis. A friction rub, which sounds like rubbing your dry fingers together, may be heard over the liver (perihepatitis) or spleen (perisplenitis). An audible splash more than 4 hours after the patient has eaten or drunk anything indicates delayed gastric emptying, as in pyloric stenosis.

## Hernias

The inguinal canal extends from the pubic tubercle to the anterior superior iliac spine (Fig. 6.20). It has an internal ring at the mid-inguinal point (midway between the pubic symphysis and the anterior superior iliac spine) and an external ring at the pubic tubercle. The femoral canal lies below the inguinal ligament and lateral to the pubic tubercle.

Hernias are common and typically occur at openings of the abdominal wall, such as the inguinal, femoral and obturator canals, the umbilicus and the oesophageal hiatus. They may also occur at sites of the weakness of the abdominal wall, as in previous surgical incisions.

An external abdominal hernia is an abnormal protrusion of the bowel and/or omentum from the abdominal cavity. External hernias are more obvious when the pressure within the abdomen rises, such as when the patient is standing, coughing or straining at stool. Internal hernias occur through defects of the mesentery or into the retroperitoneal space and are not visible.

An impulse can often be felt in a hernia during coughing (cough impulse). Identify a hernia from its anatomical site and characteristics and attempt to differentiate between direct and indirect inguinal hernias.

### Examination sequence

- Examine the groin with the patient standing upright.

**Fig. 6.19** Eliciting a fluid thrill.

| 6.15 Causes of ascites | |
|---|---|
| **Diagnosis** | **Comment** |
| **Common**<br>Hepatic cirrhosis with portal hypertension | Transudate |
| Intra-abdominal malignancy with peritoneal spread | Exudate, cytology may be positive |
| **Uncommon**<br>Hepatic vein occlusion (Budd–Chiari syndrome) | Transudate in the acute phase |
| Constrictive pericarditis and right heart failure | Check jugular venous pressure and listen for pericardial rub |
| Hypoproteinaemia (nephrotic syndrome, protein-losing enteropathy) | Transudate |
| Tuberculous peritonitis | Low glucose content |
| Pancreatitis, pancreatic duct disruption | Very high amylase content |

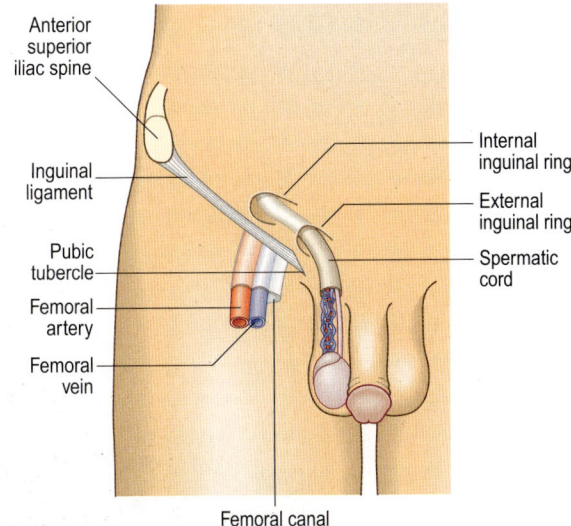

**Fig. 6.20** Anatomy of the inguinal canal and femoral sheath.

- Inspect the inguinal and femoral canals and the scrotum for any lumps or bulges.
- Ask the patient to cough; look for an impulse over the femoral or inguinal canal and scrotum.
- Identify the anatomical relationships between the bulge, the pubic tubercle and the inguinal ligament to distinguish a femoral from an inguinal hernia.
- Palpate the external inguinal ring and along the inguinal canal for possible muscle defects. Ask the patient to cough and feel for a cough impulse.
- Now ask the patient to lie down and establish whether the hernia reduces spontaneously.
- If so, press two fingers over the internal inguinal ring at the mid-inguinal point and ask the patient to cough or stand up while you maintain pressure over the internal inguinal ring. If the hernia reappears, it is a direct hernia. If it can be prevented from reappearing, it is an indirect inguinal hernia.
- Examine the opposite side to exclude the possibility of asymptomatic hernias.

An indirect inguinal hernia bulges through the internal ring and follows the course of the inguinal canal. It may extend beyond the external ring and enter the scrotum. Indirect hernias comprise 85% of all hernias and are more common in younger men.

A direct inguinal hernia forms at a site of muscle weakness in the posterior wall of the inguinal canal and rarely extends into the scrotum. It is more common in older men and women (Fig. 6.21).

A femoral hernia projects through the femoral ring and into the femoral canal. Inguinal hernias are palpable above and medial to the pubic tubercle. Femoral hernias are palpable below the inguinal ligament and lateral to the pubic tubercle.

In a reducible hernia, the contents can be returned to the abdominal cavity, spontaneously or by manipulation; if they cannot, the hernia is irreducible. An abdominal hernia has a covering sac of the peritoneum and the neck of the hernia is a common site of compression of the contents (Fig. 6.22). If the hernia contains bowel, obstruction may occur. If the blood supply to the contents of the hernia (bowel or omentum) is restricted, the hernia is strangulated. It is tense, tender and has no cough impulse, there may be bowel obstruction and, later,

signs of sepsis and shock. A strangulated hernia is a surgical emergency and, if left untreated, will lead to bowel infarction and peritonitis.

## Rectal examination

Digital examination of the rectum is important (Box 6.16). Do not avoid it because you or the patient find it disagreeable. The patient's verbal consent is needed, however, and the examination should be carried out in the presence of a chaperone.

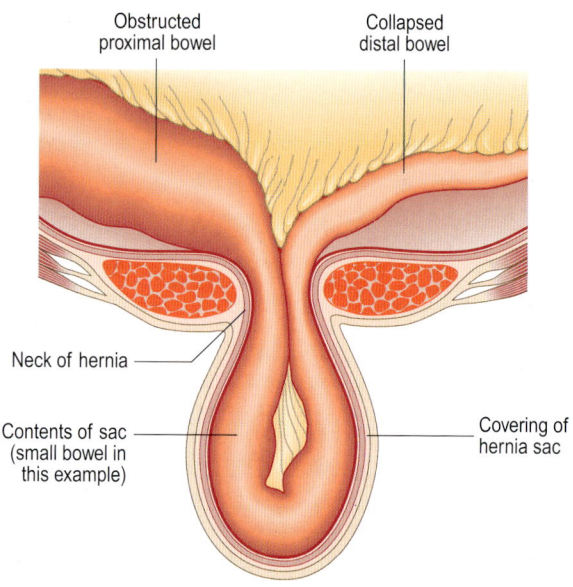

**Fig. 6.22** Hernia: anatomical structure.

| 6.16 Indications for rectal examination |
| --- |
| **Alimentary** |
| • Suspected appendicitis, pelvic abscess, peritonitis, lower abdominal pain |
| • Diarrhoea, constipation, tenesmus or anorectal pain |
| • Rectal bleeding or iron deficiency anaemia |
| • Unexplained weight loss |
| • Bimanual examination of lower abdominal mass for diagnosis or staging |
| • Malignancies of unknown origin |
| **Genitourinary** |
| • Assessment of prostate in prostatism or suspected prostatic cancer |
| • Dysuria, frequency, haematuria, epididymo-orchitis |
| • Replacement for vaginal examination when this would be inappropriate |
| **Miscellaneous** |
| • Unexplained bone pain, backache or lumbosacral nerve root pain |
| • Pyrexia of unknown origin |
| • Abdominal, pelvic or spinal trauma |

**Fig. 6.21** Right inguinal hernia.

The normal rectum is usually empty and smooth-walled, with the coccyx and sacrum lying posteriorly. In the male, anterior to the rectum from below upwards, lie the membranous urethra, the prostate and the base of the bladder. The normal prostate is smooth and firm, with lateral lobes and a median groove between them. In the female, the vagina and cervix lie anteriorly. The upper end of the anal canal is marked by the puborectalis muscle, which is readily palpable and contracts as a reflex action on coughing or conscious contraction by the patient. Beyond the anal canal, the rectum passes upwards and backwards along the curve of the sacrum.

Spasm of the external anal sphincter is common in anxious patients. When associated with local pain, it is probably due to an anal fissure (a mucosal tear). If you suspect an anal fissure, give the patient a local anaesthetic suppository 10 minutes before the examination to reduce the pain and spasm, and to aid examination.

## Examination sequence

- Explain what you are going to do and why it is necessary and ask for permission to proceed. Tell the patient that the examination may be uncomfortable but should not be painful.
- Offer a chaperone; record a refusal. Make a note of the name of the chaperone.
- Position the patient in the left lateral position with their buttocks at the edge of the couch, their knees drawn up to their chest and their heels clear of the perineum (Fig. 6.23).
- Put on gloves and examine the perianal skin, using an effective light source.
- Look for skin lesions, external haemorrhoids, fissures and fistulae.
- Lubricate your index finger with water-based gel.
- Place the pulp of your forefinger on the anal margin and apply steady pressure on the sphincter to push your finger gently through the anal canal into the rectum (Fig. 6.24).
- If an anal spasm occurs, ask the patient to breathe in deeply and relax. If necessary, use a local anaesthetic suppository or

**Fig. 6.24 Rectal examination.** The correct method for inserting your index finger in rectal examination.

gel before trying again. If pain persists, examination under general anaesthesia may be necessary.
- Ask the patient to squeeze your finger with their anal muscles and note any weakness of sphincter contraction.
- Palpate systematically around the entire rectum; note any abnormality and examine any mass (Fig. 6.25). Record the percentage of the rectal circumference involved by disease and its distance from the anus.
- Identify the uterine cervix in women and the prostate in men; assess the size, shape and consistency of the prostate and note any tenderness.
- If the rectum contains faeces and you are in doubt about palpable masses, repeat the examination after the patient has defecated.
- Slowly withdraw your finger. Examine it for stool colour and the presence of blood or mucus (Box 6.17).

Haemorrhoids ('piles', congested venous plexuses around the anal canal) are usually palpable if thrombosed. In patients with chronic constipation, the rectum is often loaded with faeces. Faecal masses are frequently palpable, should be movable and can be indented. In women, a retroverted uterus and the normal cervix are often palpable through the anterior rectal wall and a vaginal tampon may be confusing. Cancer of the lower rectum is palpable as a mucosal irregularity. Obstructing cancer of the upper rectum may produce ballooning of the empty rectal cavity below. Metastases or colonic tumours within the pelvis may be mistaken for faeces and vice versa. Lateralised tenderness suggests pelvic peritonitis. Gynaecological malignancy may cause a 'frozen pelvis' with a hard, rigid feel to the pelvic organs due to extensive peritoneal disease, such as post-radiotherapy or in metastatic cervical or ovarian cancer.

Benign prostatic hyperplasia often produces palpable symmetrical enlargement, but not if the hyperplasia is confined to the median lobe. A hard, irregular or asymmetrical gland with no palpable median groove suggests prostate cancer. Tenderness accompanied by a change in the consistency of the gland may

**Fig. 6.23 The correct position of the patient before a rectal examination.**

**Fig. 6.25 Examination of the rectum.** [A] and [B] Insert your finger, then rotate your hand. [C] The most prominent feature in the female is the cervix. [D] The most prominent feature in the male is the prostate.

### 6.17 Causes of abnormal stool appearance

| Stool appearance | Cause |
|---|---|
| Abnormally pale | Biliary obstruction |
| Pale and greasy | Steatorrhoea |
| Black and tarry (melaena) | Bleeding from the upper gastrointestinal tract |
| Grey/black | Oral iron or bismuth therapy |
| Silvery | Steatorrhoea plus upper gastrointestinal bleeding (e.g. pancreatic cancer) |
| Fresh blood in or in stool | Large bowel, rectal or anal bleeding |
| Stool mixed with pus | Infective colitis or inflammatory bowel disease |
| Rice-water stool (watery with mucus and cell debris) | Cholera |

be caused by prostatitis or prostatic abscess. The prostate is abnormally small in hypogonadism.

## Proctoscopy

Proctoscopy is the visual examination of the anal canal; it is an invasive procedure and should only be practised after appropriate training. Always undertake a digital rectal examination first. If examination of the rectal mucosa is required, perform flexible sigmoidoscopy rather than proctoscopy.

## Examination sequence

- Place the patient in the left lateral position, as for digital rectal examination.
- With gloved hands, separate the buttocks with the forefinger and thumb of one hand. With your other hand, gently insert a lubricated proctoscope with its obturator in place into the anal canal and rectum in the direction of the umbilicus.
- Remove the obturator and carefully examine the anal canal under good illumination, noting any abnormality. Check for fissures, particularly if the patient reports pain during the procedure.
- Ask the patient to strain down as you slowly withdraw the instrument to detect any degree of rectal prolapse and the presence and severity of any haemorrhoids.

Proctoscopic examination of the anus and lower rectum can confirm or exclude the presence of haemorrhoids, anal fissures and rectal prolapse. Rectal mucosa looks like buccal mucosa, apart from the presence of prominent submucosal veins. During straining, haemorrhoids distend with blood and may prolapse. If the degree of protrusion is more than 3–4 cm, a rectal prolapse may be present.

## Investigations

Selecting the relevant investigation depends on the clinical problem revealed on history and examination. Investigations are costly and many carry risks, so choose tests capable of distinguishing the likely diagnoses and prioritise the most decisive ones (Box 6.18 and Figs 6.26–6.30).

## 6.18 Investigations in gastrointestinal and hepatobiliary disease

| Investigation | Indication/comment |
|---|---|
| **Clinical samples** | |
| Stool: | |
|    Faecal occult blood by quantitative Faecal Immunochemical Test (qFIT) | Gastrointestinal haemorrhage; sensitive but not specific; used as a population screening tool for colorectal cancer |
| Faecal H pylori antigen test | Dyspepsia |
|    Faecal calprotectin | Inflammatory bowel disease—raised |
| Urine: dipstick or biochemistry | Jaundice (see Box 6.8) |
| | Acute abdominal pain |
| Ascitic fluid: diagnostic tap | Clear/straw-coloured—normal |
| | Uniformly blood-stained—malignancy |
| | Turbid—infection |
| | Chylous—lymphatic obstruction |
| | High protein (exudate)—inflammation or malignancy |
| | Low protein (transudate)—cirrhosis and portal hypertension |
| **Radiology** | |
| Chest X-ray | Suspected acute abdomen, suspected perforated viscus or subphrenic abscess |
| | Pneumonia, free air beneath diaphragm, pleural effusion, elevated diaphragm |
| Abdominal X-ray | Intestinal obstruction, perforation, renal colic |
| | Fluid levels, air above the liver, urinary tract stones |
| Barium swallow and meal | Only indicated when gastroscopy is not possible and there is suspicion of oesophageal dysmotility, or pharyngeal or gastric outlet obstruction on clinical symptoms (dysphagia or vomiting) |
| | Oesophageal obstruction (endoscopy preferable, especially if previous gastric surgery) |
| Small bowel follow-through | Subacute small bowel obstruction, duodenal diverticulosis |
| Small bowel magnetic resonance imaging or magnetic resonance enteroclysis (real-time imaging of liquid moving through the small bowel) | Crohn's disease, lymphoma, obscure gastrointestinal bleeding |
| CT colonography | Altered bowel habit, iron deficiency anaemia, rectal bleeding: alternative to colonoscopy in the frail, sick patient, if colonoscopy is unsuccessful or if not acceptable to the patient to diagnose colon cancer, inflammatory bowel disease or diverticular disease; useful in colon cancer screening |
| Abdominal ultrasound scan | Biliary colic, jaundice, pancreatitis, malignancy |
| | Gallstones, liver metastases, cholestasis, pancreatic calcification, subphrenic abscess |
| Abdominal CT | Acute abdomen, suspected pancreatic or renal mass, tumour staging, abdominal aortic aneurysm |
| | Confirms or excludes metastatic disease and leaking from the aortic aneurysm |
| MR cholangiopancreatography (MRCP) | Obstructive jaundice, acute and chronic pancreatitis |
| Pelvic ultrasound scan | Pelvic masses, inflammatory diseases, ectopic pregnancy, polycystic ovary syndrome |
| | Pelvic structures and abnormalities |
| | Ascitic fluid |
| **Invasive procedures** | |
| Upper gastrointestinal endoscopy | Dysphagia, dyspepsia, gastrointestinal bleeding, gastric ulcer, malabsorption |
| | Gastric and/or duodenal biopsies are useful |
| Lower gastrointestinal endoscopy (colonoscopy) | Rectal bleeding, obscure gastrointestinal bleeding, altered bowel habit, iron deficiency anaemia |
| | Able to biopsy lesions and remove polyps |
| Video capsule endoscopy | Obscure gastrointestinal bleeding with bidirectional negative endoscopies, suspected small bowel disease (vascular malformations, inflammatory bowel disease) |
| Endoscopic retrograde cholangiopancreatography (ERCP) | Obstructive jaundice, acute and chronic pancreatitis |
| | Mainly therapeutic role |
| | Stenting strictures and removing stones |
| Endoscopic ultrasound ± fine-needle aspiration (FNA) or Tru-Cut needle biopsy | Staging of upper gastrointestinal or pancreatobiliary cancer |
| | Gallstone detection in the biliary tree |
| | Drainage of pancreatic pseudocysts |
| Laparoscopy | Suspected appendicitis or perforated viscus, suspected ectopic pregnancy, chronic pelvic pain (e.g. due to endometriosis or pelvic inflammatory disease), suspected ovarian disease (e.g. ruptured ovarian cyst), peritoneal and liver disease |
| Ultrasound- or CT-guided aspiration cytology and biopsy | Liver metastases, intra-abdominal or retroperitoneal tumours |
| Liver biopsy | Parenchymal disease of the liver |
| | Tissue biopsy by percutaneous, transjugular or laparoscopic route |
| **Others** | |
| Pancreatic function tests | Faecal elastase, pancreolauryl test |

*CT*, computed tomography.

**Fig. 6.27** **Ultrasound scan of the gallbladder.** *A,* Thick-walled gallbladder containing gallstones. *B,* Posterior acoustic shadowing.

**Fig. 6.26** **Radiography in gastrointestinal disease.** [A] Air under the diaphragm on chest x-ray due to a perforated duodenal ulcer. [B] Dilated small bowel due to acute intestinal obstruction. [C] Dilated loop of large bowel due to sigmoid volvulus.

**Fig. 6.28** **Gastrointestinal endoscopy.** [A] Gastric ulcer. [B] Gastric varices.

**Fig. 6.29 Colonoscopy.** Colon cancer.

**Fig. 6.30 Computed tomogram of the pelvis.** *A,* Diverticular abscess.

6

---

## OSCE example 1: Abdominal pain and diarrhoea

Mr Reid, 29 years old, presents with a 6-month history of anorexia, 7 kg weight loss, abdominal pains and diarrhoea (liquid stool). He underwent appendicectomy 4 months ago following severe right iliac fossa pain.

### Please examine the gastrointestinal system

- Introduce yourself and clean your hands.
- Start with a general inspection: body habitus, signs of dehydration, fever and pallor.
- Inspect the hands: palmar erythema, finger clubbing, leuconychia, koilonychia, nicotine stains and swollen finger or wrist joints.
- Inspect the face: signs of anaemia (pallor, angular stomatitis), swollen lips and aphthous mouth ulcers.
- Inspect the skin: erythema nodosum or pyoderma gangrenosum.
- Inspect the abdomen: laparoscopy/laparotomy scars or skin fistulae.
- Palpate for right iliac fossa tenderness or the presence of a firm, non-tender mass.
- Offer to examine the perianal area for the presence of dusky blue discolouration, oedematous skin tags and the presence of fissures, fistulae or ulcerations.
- Thank the patient and clean your hands.

### Summarise your findings

This 29-year-old man with a history of weight loss and diarrhoea appears comfortable at rest but looks thin. He has a recently healed appendicectomy scar, mild periumbilical and left iliac fossa tenderness, and normal bowel sounds.

### Suggest a differential diagnosis

The differential diagnosis is Crohn's disease and irritable bowel syndrome.

### Suggest initial investigations

Full blood count, C-reactive protein, liver function tests, urea, creatinine and electrolytes, iron studies, vitamin $B_{12}$ and folate levels, ileocolonoscopy and small bowel magnetic resonance imaging, faecal calprotectin.

## OSCE example 2: Jaundice

Mr MacDonald, a 61-year-old retired salesman, presents with increasing tiredness and loss of appetite over 4 months. Two weeks ago, he noticed dark urine and pale stools, and his friends have remarked that his eyes have become yellow. He has drunk a litre of whisky a day for the last 5 years, although recently he has cut down to a bottle of whisky every 3 days.

### Please examine this patient's abdomen

- Introduce yourself and clean your hands.
- Unless prompted otherwise, proceed to peripheral examination prior to concentrating on the abdomen.
- Carry out a general inspection: body habitus, evidence of malnutrition, pallor or jaundice, scratch marks on the forearm and back, bruising.
- Examine the hands: palmar erythema, finger clubbing, leuconychia, Dupuytren's contractures.
- Check for a flapping tremor.
- Examine the face: telangiectasias, xanthelasmas, bilateral parotid enlargement and jaundice (yellow sclera of the eyes and skin).
- Smell for alcohol or fetor hepaticus.
- Inspect the neck and chest for spider naevi, gynaecomastia; look for axillary and chest hair loss.
- Inspect the abdomen for distension, everted umbilicus, caput medusae or scars of recent drain insertion.
- Palpate and percuss the abdomen for hepatomegaly and splenomegaly.
- Percuss for shifting dullness.
- Auscultate for hepatic bruits.
- Look for peripheral oedema.
- Thank the patient and your clean hands.

### Summarise your findings

This patient is jaundiced with multiple spider naevi on the chest and abdomen. He has generalised abdominal swelling with shifting dullness and a firm liver edge palpable 2 cm below the costal margin.

### Suggest a differential diagnosis

The differential diagnosis is alcoholic cirrhosis, chronic hepatitis and hepatoma.

### Suggested initial investigations

Liver function tests, ferritin, viral hepatitis screen, full blood count and prothrombin time, urea, creatinine and electrolytes, alpha-fetoprotein, abdominal ultrasound scan and upper digestive endoscopy (to check for oesophagogastric varices).

## Integrated examination sequence for the gastrointestinal system

- Position the patient: supine and comfortable on the examination couch. Expose the abdomen from the xiphisternum to the pubic symphysis.
- Inspection: start with general observation, then inspect the skin, face, neck and chest, and finally the abdomen.
- Palpation:
  - Begin with light, superficial palpation away from any site of pain, then repeat with deeper palpation.
  - Describe any mass and decide whether there is an enlarged abdominal organ.
- Palpation for hepatomegaly:
  - Ask the patient to breathe in deeply through the mouth and feel for the descent of the liver edge on inspiration.
  - Move your hand progressively up the abdomen, between each breath, until you reach the costal margin or detect the liver edge.
- Percussion to confirm hepatomegaly:
  - Ask the patient to hold their breath in full expiration.
  - Percuss for liver dullness and measure the distance in centimetres below the costal margin.
- Palpation and percussion for splenomegaly:
  - Start with your hand over the umbilicus, moving diagonally up and left to feel for the splenic edge as it descends and moves towards the midline on inspiration.
- Check for ascites (shifting dullness):
  - Percuss from the midline out to the flanks for dullness.
  - Keep your finger on the site of dullness in the flank; ask the patient to turn on to their opposite side and then percuss again. If the area of dullness is now resonant, shifting dullness is present.
- Check for a fluid thrill:
  - Place the palm of your left hand flat against the left side of the patient's abdomen and flick a finger of your right hand against the right side of the abdomen. If you still feel a ripple against your left hand, a fluid thrill is present.
- Auscultation:
  - Listen to the right of the umbilicus for bowel sounds, above the umbilicus over the aorta for arterial bruits, lateral to the umbilicus for bruits from renal artery stenosis, and over the liver for hepatic bruits.
- Check for peripheral oedema.
- Consider a rectal examination (always with a chaperone).

Richard Davenport
Hadi Manji

# 7

# The nervous system

Anatomy and physiology 134

The history 134
Common presenting symptoms 134
Past medical history 138
Drug history 138
Family history 138
Social history 138

The physical examination 139
Assessment of conscious level 139
Meningeal irritation 139
Speech 139
Dysphasia 140
Cortical function 140

Cranial nerves 142
Olfactory (I) nerve 142
Optic (II), oculomotor (III), trochlear (IV) and abducens (VI) nerves 144
Trigeminal (V) nerve 144
Facial (VII) nerve 145
The vestibulocochlear (VIII) nerve 148
Glossopharyngeal (IX) and vagus (X) nerves 148
Accessory (XI) nerve 148
Hypoglossal (XII) nerve 149

Motor system 150
Anatomy 150
Stance and gait 151

Inspection and palpation of the muscles 152
Tone 153
Power 154
Deep tendon reflexes 155
Primitive reflexes 158
Coordination 158

Sensory system 159
Anatomy 159
Common presenting symptoms 160
Sensory modalities 161

Peripheral nerves 162
Median nerve 162
Radial nerve 164
Ulnar nerve 164
Common peroneal nerve 164
Lateral cutaneous nerve of the thigh 164

Interpretation of the findings 164

Investigations 165
Initial investigations 165
Specific investigations 165

OSCE example 1: Headache history 167

OSCE example 2: Tremor 167

Integrated examination sequence for the nervous system 168

# Anatomy and physiology

The nervous system consists of the brain and spinal cord (central nervous system, CNS) and the peripheral nerves (peripheral nervous system, PNS). The PNS includes the autonomic nervous system, which is responsible for controlling involuntary functions.

The neuron is the functional unit of the nervous system. Each neuron has a cell body and axon terminating at a synapse, supported by astrocytes and microglial cells. Astrocytes provide the structural framework for the neurons, control their biochemical environment and form the blood-brain barrier. Microglial cells are blood-derived mononuclear macrophages with immune and scavenging functions. In the CNS, oligodendrocytes produce and maintain a myelin sheath around the axons. In the PNS, myelin is produced by Schwann cells.

The brain consists of two cerebral hemispheres, each with four lobes (frontal, parietal, temporal and occipital), the brainstem and the cerebellum. The brainstem comprises the midbrain, pons and medulla. The cerebellum lies in the posterior fossa, with two hemispheres and a central vermis attached to the brainstem by three pairs of cerebellar peduncles. Between the brain and the skull are three membranous layers called the meninges: dura mater next to the bone, arachnoid and pia mater next to the nervous tissue. The subarachnoid space between the arachnoid and pia is filled with cerebrospinal fluid (CSF) produced by the choroid plexuses. The total volume of CSF is between 140 and 270 mL, and there is a turnover of the entire volume three to four times a day; thus, CSF is produced at a rate of approximately 700 mL/day.

The spinal cord contains afferent and efferent fibres arranged in discrete bundles (pathways running to and from the brain), which are responsible for transmitting motor and sensory information. Peripheral nerves have myelinated and unmyelinated axons. The sensory cell bodies of peripheral nerves are situated in the dorsal root ganglia. The motor cell bodies are in the anterior horns of the spinal cord (Fig. 7.1).

# The history

For many common neurological symptoms such as headache, numbness, disturbance/loss of consciousness and memory loss, the history is the key to diagnosis, as the examination may be normal. Some symptoms, including loss of consciousness or amnesia, require an additional witness history; make every effort to contact such witnesses. Whilst histories can lend themselves to remote consulting, remote neurological examination is challenging if not impossible. People with communication difficulties (e.g. due to deafness, spoken language, cognitive impairment, or non-verbal such as autism) require particularly careful attention to overcome these barriers.

Remember the two key questions: where (in the nervous system) is the lesion and what is the lesion?

Neurological symptoms may be difficult for patients to describe, so clarify exactly what they mean. Words such as 'blackout', 'dizziness', 'weakness' and 'numbness' may have different meanings for different patients, so ensure you understand what the person is describing.

Ask patients what they think or fear might be wrong with them, as neurological symptoms cause much anxiety. Patients commonly research their symptoms on the internet; searches on common benign neurological symptoms, like numbness or weakness, usually list the most alarming (and unlikely) diagnoses such as multiple sclerosis, motor neuron disease or brain tumours first, and almost never mention more common conditions such as carpal tunnel syndrome or functional disorders.

## Time relationships

The onset, duration and pattern of symptoms over time often provide diagnostic clues: for example, in assessing headache (Box 7.1) or vertigo (see Box 9.3).

Ask:

- When did the symptoms start (or when was the patient last well)?
- Are they persistent or intermittent?
- If persistent, are they getting better, getting worse or staying the same?
- If intermittent, how long do they last, and how long does the patient remain symptom-free in between episodes?
- Was the onset sudden or gradual/evolving?

## Precipitating, exacerbating or relieving factors

- What was the patient doing when the symptoms occurred?
- Does anything make the symptoms better or worse, such as time of day, menstrual cycle, posture or medication?

## Associated symptoms

Associated symptoms can aid diagnosis. For example, headache may be associated with nausea, vomiting, photophobia (aversion to light) and/or phonophobia (aversion to sound) in migraine; headache with neck stiffness, fever and rash may be associated with meningitis (see Box 7.1).

## Common presenting symptoms

### Headache

Headache is the most common neurological symptom and may be either primary or secondary to other pathology. Primary (idiopathic) causes are the most common and include:

- migraine
- tension-type headache
- trigeminal autonomic cephalalgias (including cluster headache)
- primary stabbing, cough, exertional or sex headache
- primary thunderclap headache
- new daily persistent headache.

**A** Lateral surface of the brain.

Central sulcus

Precentral gyrus (motor area)

Postcentral gyrus (sensory area)

**Parietal lobe**

Sensory speech area (Wernicke's area)

**Occipital lobe**

**Frontal lobe**

Lateral sulcus (fissure)

Motor speech area (Broca's area)

**Temporal lobe**

Cerebellum

Pons

Medulla oblongata

**B** Spinal cord, nerve roots and meninges.

Posterior median septum

Dorsal intermediate septum

Dorsal root entry zone

Dorsal column

Central canal

Ventral grey horn

Dorsal grey horn

Lateral column

Ventral column

Spinal ganglion

**Rootlets**
Dorsal
Ventral

Pia mater

Arachnoid mater

Mixed spinal nerve

Dura mater

Dural root sleeve

Anterior median fissure

**C** Cross-section of the spinal cord.

Position sense
Vibration sense
1/2 touch

Fasciculus gracilis

Fasciculus cuneatus

Lateral (indirect) corticospinal tract

Posterior spino-cerebellar tract

Anterior spino-cerebellar tract

Lateral spino-thalamic tract

Areas of extrapyramidal tracts

Voluntary movement

Equilibrium

Pain
Temperature
1/2 touch

Voluntary movement

Anterior spino-thalamic tract

Anterior (direct) corticospinal tract

**D** Spinal motor neuron.

Presynaptic nerve fibres

Nucleus

Dendrites

Cell body

Axon

**Spinal motor neurone**

Myelin

Node of Ranvier

Nerve terminals

**Fig. 7.1 Anatomy of the central nervous system.** A Lateral surface of the brain. B Spinal cord, nerve roots and meninges. C Cross-section of the spinal cord. D Spinal motor neuron. The terminals of presynaptic neurons form synapses with the cell body and dendrites of the motor neurons.

## 7.1 Clinical characteristics of headache syndromes

| | Onset | Duration/periodicity | Pain location | Associated features |
|---|---|---|---|---|
| **Primary syndromes** | | | | |
| Migraine | Evolves over 30–120 min | Usually last <24 h, recurrent with weeks/months symptom-free | Classically unilateral but may be anywhere including face/neck | Aura (usually visual), nausea/vomiting, photophobia and phonophobia |
| Cluster headache | Rapid onset, often waking patient from sleep | 30–120 min, 1–4 attacks within 24 h, clusters usually last weeks to months, with months to years of remission | Orbital/retro-orbital; always same side during cluster, may switch sides between clusters | Autonomic features, including conjunctival injection, tearing, nasal stuffiness, ptosis, miosis, agitation |
| Stabbing headache | Abrupt, rarely from sleep | Very brief, seconds or less | Anywhere over head | Common in migraineurs |
| **Secondary syndromes** | | | | |
| Meningitis | Usually evolves over a day or two, can be abrupt | Depends on cause and treatment, usually days to weeks | Global, including neck stiffness | Fever, meningism, rash, false localising signs, signs of raised intracranial pressure |
| Subarachnoid haemorrhage | Abrupt, immediately maximal, rare from sleep | May be fatal at onset, usually days to weeks | Anywhere, poor localising value | 20% isolated headache only; nausea/vomiting, reduced consciousness, false localising signs, III nerve palsies |
| Temporal arteritis | Gradual onset of temple pain and scalp tenderness | Continuous | Temple and scalp | Usually in those >55 years; unwell, jaw pain on chewing, visual symptoms, tender temporal arteries, elevated erythrocyte sedimentation rate and C-reactive protein |

Secondary (or symptomatic) headaches include potentially life-threatening or disabling causes, such as subarachnoid haemorrhage or temporal arteritis. One of the key history aspects is rapidity of onset; isolated headache with a truly abrupt onset may represent a potentially serious cause, such as subarachnoid haemorrhage or cerebral vein thrombosis, whereas recurrent headache is much more likely to be migraine, particularly if associated with other migrainous features (see Box 7.1). Asking patients what they do when they have a headache can be instructive. For example, abandoning normal tasks and seeking a bed in a dark, quiet room suggest migraine, whereas pacing around the room in an agitated state, or even headbanging, suggests cluster headache.

## Transient loss of consciousness (TLOC)

Syncope is loss of consciousness due to inadequate cerebral perfusion and is the most common cause of transient loss of consciousness (TLOC). Vasovagal (or reflex) syncope (fainting) is the most common type and is precipitated by stimulation of the parasympathetic nervous system by factors such as pain or intercurrent illness. Exercise-related syncope, or syncope with no warning or trigger, suggests a possible cardiac cause. TLOC on standing is suggestive of orthostatic (postural) hypotension and may be caused by drugs (antihypertensives or levodopa) or associated with autonomic neuropathies, which may complicate conditions such as diabetes.

## Seizure

An epileptic seizure is caused by paroxysmal electrical discharges from either the whole brain (generalised seizure) or part of the brain (focal seizure). A tonic-clonic seizure (convulsion) is the most common form of generalised seizure and typically follows a stereotyped pattern with early loss of consciousness associated with body stiffening (tonic phase) succeeded by rhythmical jerking crescendoing and subsiding over 30 to 120 seconds (clonic phase); this is followed by a period of unresponsiveness (often with heavy breathing, the patient appearing to be deeply asleep) and finally confusion or amnesia as the patient reorientates (postictal phase). The history from the patient and witnesses can help distinguish syncope from epilepsy (Box 7.2). Focal seizures may or may not involve loss of awareness (complete loss of consciousness is less typical) and are characterised by whichever part of the brain is involved: for example, a focal motor seizure arising from the motor cortex, or temporal lobe seizures characterised by autonomic and/or psychic symptoms, often associated with automatisms such as lip smacking or swallowing. Functional dissociative attacks (also known as non-epileptic or psychogenic attacks, or pseudoseizures) are common and may be difficult to distinguish from epileptic seizures. These attacks are often more frequent than epilepsy, sometimes occurring multiple times in a day, and may last considerably longer, with symptoms waxing and waning. Other features may include asynchronous movements, pelvic

**7.2 Features that help discriminate vasovagal syncope from epileptic seizure**

| Feature | Vasovagal syncope | Seizure |
|---|---|---|
| Triggers | Typically, pain, illness, emotion | Often none (sleep deprivation, alcohol, drugs) |
| Prodrome | Feeling faint/lightheaded, nausea, tinnitus, vision dimming | Focal onset (not always present) |
| Duration of unconsciousness | <60 s | 1–2 min |
| Convulsion | May occur but usually brief myoclonic jerks | Usual, tonic-clonic 1–2 min |
| Colour | Pale/grey | Flushed/cyanosed, may be pale |
| Injuries | Uncommon, sometimes biting of tip of tongue | Lateral tongue biting, headache, generalised myalgia, back pain (sometimes vertebral compression fractures), shoulder fracture/dislocation (rare) |
| Recovery | Rapid, no confusion | Gradual, over 30 min; patient is often confused, sometimes agitated/aggressive, amnesic |

thrusts, side-to-side rather than flexion/extension movements and absence of postictal confusion. The widespread availability of smartphones allows witnesses to film such events, which may prove invaluable; the availability of secure platforms for families to upload such videos for viewing is an evolving area (e.g. https://www.vcreate.tv/).

## Focal neurological symptoms due to stroke or transient ischaemic attack

A stroke is a focal neurological deficit of rapid onset due to a vascular cause. A transient ischaemic attack (TIA) is the same, but symptoms resolve within 24 hours. TIAs are an important risk factor for impending stroke and demand urgent assessment and treatment. Hemiplegia following middle cerebral artery occlusion is a typical example, but symptoms are dictated by the vascular territory involved. Much of the cerebral hemispheres are supplied by anterior circulation (the anterior and middle cerebral arteries are derived from the internal carotid artery), while the occipital lobes and brainstem are supplied by posterior (vertebrobasilar) circulation (Fig. 7.2).

A useful and simple clinical system for classifying strokes is shown in Box 7.3.

Isolated vertigo, amnesia or TLOC are rarely, if ever, due to stroke. In the Western world about 80% of strokes are ischaemic, the remainder haemorrhagic. Haemorrhagic stroke is much more frequent in Asian populations. Factors in the history or examination that increase the likelihood of haemorrhage rather than ischaemia include the use of anticoagulation, headache, vomiting, seizures and early reduced consciousness, although brain imaging is necessary to be definitive. Spinal strokes are very rare; patients typically present with abrupt bilateral paralysis, depending on the level of spinal cord affected. Anterior spinal

Anterior cerebral artery
Anterior communicating artery
Internal carotid artery
Circle of Willis
Middle cerebral artery
Posterior communicating artery
Posterior cerebral artery
Basilar artery
Vertebral artery

**Fig. 7.2** The arterial blood supply of the brain (circle of Willis).

**7.3 Clinical classification of stroke**

**Total anterior circulation syndrome (TACS)**

- Hemiparesis, hemianopia and higher cortical deficit (e.g. dysphasia or visuospatial loss)

**Partial anterior circulation syndrome (PACS)**

- Two of the three components of a TACS
- OR isolated higher cortical deficit
- OR motor/sensory deficit more restricted than LACS (see below)

**Posterior circulation syndrome (POCS)**

- Ipsilateral cranial nerve palsy with contralateral motor and/or sensory deficit
- OR bilateral motor and/or sensory deficit
- OR disorder of conjugate eye movement
- OR cerebellar dysfunction without ipsilateral long-tract deficits
- OR isolated homonymous visual field defect

**Lacunar syndrome (LACS)**

- Pure motor >2 out of 3 of face, arm, leg
- OR pure sensory >2 out of 3 of face, arm, leg
- OR pure sensorimotor >2 out of 3 of face, arm, leg
- OR ataxic hemiparesis

artery syndrome is most common and causes loss of motor function and pain/temperature sensation, with relative sparing of joint position and vibration sensation below the level of the lesion.

## Dizziness and vertigo

Patients use 'dizziness' to describe many sensations. Recurrent 'dizzy spells' affect approximately 30% of those over 65 years and can be due to postural hypotension, cerebrovascular disease, cardiac arrhythmia or hyperventilation induced by anxiety and panic. Vertigo (the illusion of movement) specifically indicates a problem in the vestibular apparatus (peripheral) or, much less commonly, the brain (central) (see Box 9.3 and p. 201). Identifying a specific cause of dizziness is often challenging but may be rewarding in some cases, including benign paroxysmal positional vertigo (BPPV), which is eminently treatable. As a guide, recurrent episodes of vertigo lasting a few seconds are most likely to be due to BPPV; vertigo lasting hours may be caused by Ménière's disease (with associated symptoms including hearing loss, tinnitus, nausea and vomiting) or migrainous vertigo (with or without headache); brain stem or cerebellar stroke may also present with vertigo, often associated with ataxia, diplopia and other motor or sensory symptoms and is an important diagnosis not to miss.

## Functional neurological symptoms

Many neurological symptoms are not due to organic or structural disease. These symptoms are often called 'functional' but other (less useful and more pejorative) terms include psychogenic, hysterical, somatisation or conversion disorders. Presentations include blindness, tremor, weakness and collapsing attacks, and patients will often describe numerous other symptoms, with fatigue, lethargy, pain, anxiety and other mood disorders commonly associated. Diagnosing functional symptoms requires experience and patience (p. 424). Clues include symptoms not compatible with disease (such as retained awareness of convulsing, or being able to walk normally backwards but not forwards), considerable variability in symptoms (such as intermittent recovery of a hemiparesis), multiple symptoms (often with numerous previous assessments by other specialties, particularly gynaecology, gastroenterology, ear, nose and throat and cardiorespiratory) and multiple unremarkable investigations, leading to numerous different diagnoses. The size of a patient's case notes can sometimes be a clue in itself! Beware of labelling symptoms as functional simply because they appear odd or inexplicable, and remember that functional and organic disease may coexist. Like disease, most functional neurological disorders follow recognisable patterns, so be cautious when the pattern is atypical.

## Past medical history

Symptoms that the patient has forgotten about or overlooked may be important; for example, a history of previous visual loss (optic neuritis) in someone presenting with numbness suggests multiple sclerosis. Birth history and development may be significant, as in epilepsy. Contact parents or family doctors to obtain such information. If considering a vascular cause of neurological symptoms, ask about important risk factors, such as other vascular diseases, hypertension, family history and smoking.

## Drug history

Always enquire about drugs, including prescribed, over-the-counter, complementary and recreational/illegal ones, as they can give rise to many neurological symptoms (for example, phenytoin toxicity causing ataxia; excessive intake of analgesia causing medication overuse headache). Recent vaccinations may be relevant when faced with rapidly progressive weakness (Guillain-Barré syndrome) or cerebral venous thrombosis (COVID-19 vaccinations). The absence of vaccinations (e.g. polio or measles) may be overlooked initially but may provide crucial clues for diagnosis.

## Family history

Obtain a family history for at least first-degree relatives: parents, siblings and children. In some communities, parental consanguinity is common, increasing the risk of autosomal recessive conditions, so you may need to enquire sensitively about this. Some neurological disorders are caused by single-gene defects, such as myotonic dystrophy or Huntington's disease. Others have important polygenic influences, as in multiple sclerosis or migraine. Some conditions have a variety of inheritance patterns; for example, Charcot-Marie-Tooth disease may be autosomal dominant, autosomal recessive or X-linked. Mitochondria uniquely have their own DNA, and abnormalities in this DNA can cause a range of disorders (such as diabetes, short stature and deafness) that manifest in many different systems and may cause common neurological syndromes such as migraine or epilepsy. Some diseases, such as Parkinson's or motor neuron disease, may be either due to single-gene disorders or sporadic.

## Social history

Social circumstances are relevant. How are patients coping with their symptoms? Are they able to work and drive? What are their support circumstances, and are these adequate?

Alcohol is the most common neurological toxin and damages both the CNS (ataxia, seizures, dementia) and the PNS (neuropathy). Poor diet with vitamin deficiency may compound these problems and is relevant in areas affected by famine, alcoholism or dietary exclusion. Vegetarians may be susceptible to vitamin $B_{12}$ deficiency. Recreational drugs may affect the nervous system; for example, nitrous oxide inhalation causes subacute combined degeneration of the cord due to dysfunction of the vitamin $B_{12}$ pathway, cocaine can cause seizures and smoking contributes to vascular and malignant disease. Always consider sexually transmitted or blood-borne infection, such as human immunodeficiency virus (HIV) or syphilis, as both can cause a wide range of neurological symptoms and are treatable. A travel history may give clues to the underlying diagnosis, such as Lyme disease (facial palsy), neurocysticercosis (brain lesions and epilepsy) or malaria (coma). Post-viral syndromes, including post-COVID-19, may cause persistent and disabling symptoms in a minority.

### Occupational history

Occupational factors are relevant to several neurological disorders. For example, toxic peripheral neuropathy, due to exposure to heavy or organic metals like lead, causes motor neuropathy; manganese causes Parkinsonism. Some neurological diagnoses may adversely affect a patient's occupation, such as epilepsy in anyone who needs to drive or operate dangerous machinery. For patients with cognitive disorders, particularly dementias, it may be necessary to advise on whether to stop working.

## The physical examination

Although history-taking can be undertaken remotely, a neurological examination ideally requires direct patient contact. Neurological assessment begins with your first contact with the patient and continues during the history. Note facial expression, demeanour, dress, posture, gait and speech. Mental state examination (p. 368) and general examination (p. 385) are integral parts of the neurological examination.

### Assessment of conscious level

Consciousness has two main components:

- The state of consciousness depends largely on the integrity of the ascending reticular activating system, which extends from the brainstem to the thalamus.
- The content of consciousness refers to how aware the person is and depends on the cerebral cortex, the thalamus and their connections.

Do not use ill-defined terms such as stuporose or obtunded. Use the Glasgow Coma Scale (see Box 18.5), a reliable and reproducible tool, to record consciousness level.

### Meningeal irritation

Meningism (inflammation or irritation of the meninges) can lead to increased resistance to passive flexion of the neck (neck stiffness) or the extended leg (Kernig's sign). Patients may lie with flexed hips to ease their symptoms. Meningism suggests infection (meningitis) or blood within the subarachnoid space (subarachnoid haemorrhage) but can occur with non-neurological infections, such as a urinary tract infection or pneumonia. Conversely, the absence of meningism does not exclude pathology within the subarachnoid space. In meningitis, neck stiffness has relatively low sensitivity but higher specificity. The absence of all three signs of fever, neck stiffness and altered mental state virtually eliminates the diagnosis of meningitis in immunocompetent individuals.

**Fig. 7.3** Testing for meningeal irritation: Kernig's sign.

### Examination sequence (Video 7) ▶

- Position the patient supine with no pillow.
- Expose and fully extend both of the patient's legs.

#### Neck stiffness
- Place your hands on either side of the patient's head, supporting the occiput.
- Flex the patient's head gently until their chin touches their chest.
- Ask the patient to hold that position for 10 seconds. If neck stiffness is present, the neck cannot be passively flexed and you may feel a spasm in the neck muscles.
- Flexion of the hips and knees in response to neck flexion is Brudzinski's sign.

#### Kernig's sign
- Flex one of the patient's legs to 90 degrees at both the hip and the knee, with your left hand placed over the medial hamstrings (Fig. 7.3).
- Extend the knee while the hip is maintained in flexion. Look at the other leg for any reflex flexion. Kernig's sign is positive when extension is resisted by spasms in the hamstrings. Kernig's sign is absent with local causes of neck stiffness, such as cervical spine disease or raised intracranial pressure.

### Speech

Dysarthria refers to altered or abnormal speech caused by articulation problems due to a motor deficit. Dysphonia describes the loss of volume caused by laryngeal disorders. Both affect speech only, whereas dysphasia may affect other language functions (e.g. reading or writing).

## Examination sequence (Video 8)

- Listen to the patient's spontaneous speech, noting volume, rhythm and clarity.
- Ask the patient to repeat phrases such as 'yellow lorry' to test lingual (tongue) sounds and 'baby hippopotamus' for labial (lip) sounds, then a tongue twister such as 'The Leith police dismisseth us.'
- Ask the patient to count to 30 to assess fatigue.
- Ask the patient to cough and to say 'ah'; observe the soft palate rising bilaterally.

Disturbed articulation (dysarthria) may result from localised lesions of the tongue, lips or mouth, ill-fitting dentures or neurological dysfunction such as bulbar palsy or cerebellar disease.

Pseudobulbar versus bulbar palsies (see Box 7.5): bilateral upper motor neuron lesions of the corticobulbar tracts cause a pseudobulbar dysarthria, characterised by slow, harsh, strangulated speech with difficulty pronouncing consonants and may be accompanied by a brisk jaw jerk and emotional lability. The tongue is contracted and stiff. Bulbar palsy results from bilateral lower motor neuron lesions affecting the same group of cranial nerves (IX, X, XI, XII). The nature of the speech disturbance is determined by the specific nerves and muscles involved. Weakness of the tongue results in difficulty with lingual sounds, while palatal weakness gives a nasal quality to the speech. Other lower motor neuron signs such as a wasted, fibrillating tongue may be seen.

Cerebellar dysarthria is slow and slurred, similar to alcohol intoxication. Myasthenia gravis causes fatiguing speech that becomes increasingly nasal and may disappear altogether. Parkinsonism may cause dysarthria and dysphonia, with a low-volume, monotonous voice, words running into each other (festination of speech) and marked stuttering/hesitation.

Dysphonia usually results from either vocal cord pathology, as in laryngitis, or damage to the vagal (X) nerve supply to the vocal cords (recurrent laryngeal nerve). Inability to abduct one of the vocal cords leads to a 'bovine' (and ineffective) cough.

## Dysphasia

Dysphasia is a central disturbance of language resulting in abnormalities of speech production and/or understanding. It may involve other language symptoms, such as writing and/or reading problems, unlike dysarthria and dysphonia.

### Anatomy

The language areas are located in the dominant cerebral hemisphere, which is the left in almost all right-handed people and most left-handed people.

Broca's area (inferior frontal region) is concerned with word production and language expression.

Wernicke's area (superior posterior temporal lobe) is the principal area for comprehension of spoken language. Adjacent regions of the parietal lobe are involved in understanding written language and numbers.

The arcuate fasciculus connects Broca's and Wernicke's areas.

## Examination sequence

- During spontaneous speech, listen to the fluency and appropriateness of the content, particularly paraphasias (incorrect words) and neologisms (nonsense or meaningless new words).
- Show the patient a common object, such as a coin or pen, and ask them to name it.
- Give a simple three-stage command, such as 'Pick up this piece of paper, fold it in half and place it under the book.'
- Ask the patient to repeat a simple sentence, such as 'Today is Tuesday.'
- Ask the patient to read a passage from a newspaper.
- Ask the patient to write a sentence; examine the handwriting.

Expressive (motor) dysphasia results from damage to Broca's area. It is characterised by reduced verbal output with non-fluent speech and errors of grammar and syntax. Comprehension is intact.

Receptive (sensory) dysphasia occurs due to dysfunction in Wernicke's area. There is poor comprehension, and although speech is fluent, it may be meaningless and contain paraphasias and neologisms.

Global dysphasia is a combination of expressive and receptive difficulties caused by involvement of both areas.

Dysphasia (a focal sign) is frequently misdiagnosed as confusion (non-focal). Always consider dysphasia before assuming confusion, as this fundamentally alters the differential diagnosis and management.

Dominant parietal lobe lesions affecting the supramarginal gyrus may cause dyslexia (difficulty comprehending written language), dyscalculia (problems with simple addition and subtraction) and dysgraphia (impairment of writing). Gerstmann's syndrome is the combination of dysgraphia, dyscalculia, finger agnosia (inability to recognise the fingers) and inability to distinguish left from right. It localises to the left parietal lobe in the region of the angular gyrus.

## Cortical function

Thinking, emotions, language, behaviour, planning and initiation of movements and perception of sensory information are functions of the cerebral cortex and are central to awareness of, and interaction with, the environment. Certain cortical areas are associated with specific functions, so particular patterns of dysfunction can help localise the site of pathology (Fig. 7.4A). Assessment of higher cortical function can be difficult and time-consuming but is essential in patients with cognitive symptoms. There are various tools, primarily developed as screening and assessment tools for dementia. At the bedside, the Montreal Cognitive Assessment (MoCA; https://www.mocatest.org) may be used to detect mild cognitive impairment, while the 4AT

**2 Parietal lobe**

| Dominant side | | Non-dominant side | |
|---|---|---|---|
| FUNCTION<br>Calculation<br>Language<br>Planned movement<br>Appreciation of size,<br>shape, weight<br>and texture | LESIONS<br>Dyscalculia<br>Dysphasia<br>Dyslexia<br>Apraxia<br>Agnosia<br>Homonymous hemianopia | FUNCTION<br>Spatial orientation<br>Constructional skills | LESIONS<br>Neglect of non-dominant side<br>Spatial disorientation<br>Constructional apraxia<br>Dressing apraxia<br>Homonymous hemianopia |

**1 Frontal lobe**

FUNCTION
Personality
Emotional response
Social behaviour

LESIONS
Disinhibition
Lack of initiative
Antisocial behaviour
Impaired memory
Incontinence
Grasp reflexes
Anosmia

**3 Occipital lobe**

FUNCTION
Analysis of vision

LESIONS
Homonymous hemianopia
Hemianopic scotomas
Visual agnosia
Impaired face recognition
(prosopagnosia)
Visual hallucinations
(lights, lines and zigzags)

**4 Temporal lobe**

| Dominant side | | Non-dominant side | |
|---|---|---|---|
| FUNCTION<br>Auditory perception<br>Speech, language<br>Verbal memory<br>Smell | LESIONS<br>Dysphasia<br>Dyslexia<br>Poor memory<br>Complex hallucinations<br>(smell, sound, vision)<br>Homonymous hemianopia | FUNCTION<br>Auditory perception<br>Music, tone sequences<br>Non-verbal memory<br>(faces, shapes, music)<br>Smell | LESIONS<br>Poor non-verbal memory<br>Loss of musical skills<br>Complex hallucinations<br>Homonymous hemianopia |

A

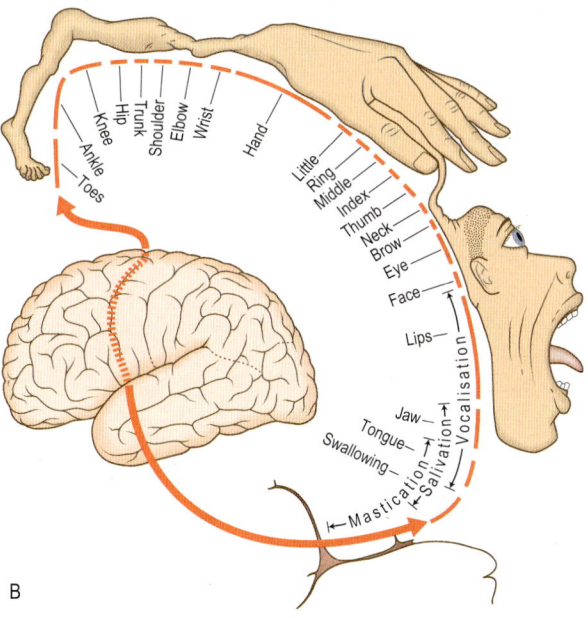

B

**Fig. 7.4 Cortical function.** [A] Features of localised cerebral lesions. [B] Somatotopic homunculus.

(the4AT.com) is a very useful rapid clinical test for delirium. None of these bedside tests is a substitute for detailed neuropsychological assessment. The assessment of cognitive function is covered in more detail on page 372.

## Frontal lobe

The posterior part of the frontal lobe is the motor strip (precentral gyrus), which controls voluntary movement. The motor strip is organised somatotopically (Fig. 7.4B). The area anterior to the precentral gyrus is concerned with personality, social behaviour, emotions, cognition and expressive language, and contains the frontal eye fields and cortical centre for micturition (Fig. 7.4A).

Frontal lobe damage may cause:

- personality and behaviour changes, such as apathy or disinhibition
- loss of emotional responsiveness, or emotional lability
- cognitive impairments, such as memory, attention and concentration
- dysphasia (dominant hemisphere)
- conjugate gaze deviation to the side of the lesion
- urinary incontinence
- primitive reflexes, such as grasp
- focal motor seizures (motor strip).

## Temporal lobe

The temporal lobe contains the primary auditory cortex, Wernicke's area and parts of the limbic system. The latter is crucially important in memory, emotion and smell appreciation. The temporal lobe also contains the lower fibres of the optic radiation and the area of auditory perception.

Temporal lobe dysfunction may cause:

- Memory impairment
- Focal seizures with psychic symptoms
- Contralateral upper quadrantanopia (see Fig. 8.5[4])
- Receptive dysphasia (dominant hemisphere).

## Parietal lobe

The postcentral gyrus (sensory strip) is the most anterior part of the parietal lobe and is the principal destination of conscious sensations. The upper fibres of the optic radiation pass through it. The dominant hemisphere contains aspects of language function, and the non-dominant lobe is concerned with spatial awareness.

Features of parietal lobe dysfunction include:

- cortical sensory impairments
- contralateral lower quadrantanopia (see Fig. 8.5[5])
- dyslexia, dyscalculia, dysgraphia
- apraxia (an inability to carry out complex tasks despite having an intact sensory and motor system)

- focal sensory seizures (postcentral gyrus)
- visuospatial disturbance (non-dominant parietal lobe).

## Occipital lobe

The occipital lobe blends with the temporal and parietal lobes and forms the posterior part of the cerebral cortex. Its main function is analysis of visual information.

Occipital lobe damage may cause:

- visual field defects: hemianopia (loss of part of a visual field) or scotoma (blind spot) (see Fig. 8.5[6])
- visual agnosia: the inability to recognise visual stimuli
- disturbances of visual perception, such as macropsia (seeing things larger) or micropsia (seeing things smaller)
- visual hallucinations.

# Cranial nerves

The 12 pairs of cranial nerves (with the exception of the olfactory [I] pair) arise from the brainstem (Fig. 7.5 and Box 7.4). Cranial nerves II, III, IV and VI relate to the eye (see Chapter 8) and the VIII nerve to hearing and balance (see Chapter 9).

## Olfactory (I) nerve

The olfactory nerve conveys the sense of smell.

## Anatomy

Bipolar cells in the olfactory bulb form olfactory filaments with small receptors projecting through the cribriform plate high in the nasal cavity. These cells synapse with second-order neurons, which project centrally via the olfactory tract to the medial temporal lobe and amygdala.

## Examination sequence

Bedside testing of smell is of limited clinical value and rarely performed, although objective 'scratch and sniff' test cards, such as the University of Pennsylvania Smell Identification Test (UPSIT), are available. You can ask patients if they think their sense of smell is normal, although self-reporting can be surprisingly inaccurate.

Hyposmia or anosmia (reduction or loss of the sense of smell) may result from upper respiratory infection (for example with the Sars-CoV-2 virus), sinus disease, damage to the olfactory filaments after head injury or infection, local compression (by olfactory groove meningioma, for example, see Fig. 7.29C) or invasion by basal skull tumours. Disturbance of smell may also occur very early in Parkinson's and Alzheimer's diseases. Patients often note hypogeusia/ageusia (altered taste) with anosmia too, as taste is crucially influenced by the sense of smell.

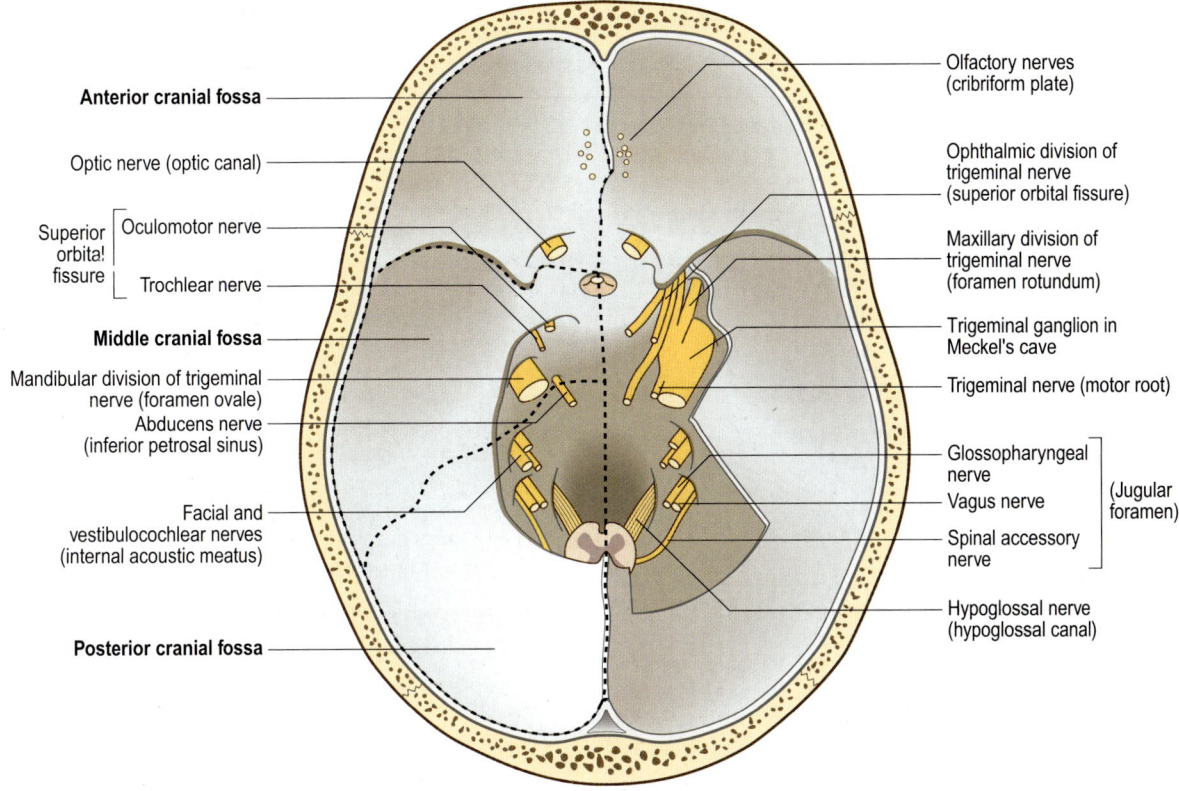

**7**

**Fig. 7.5 Base of the cranial cavity.** The dura mater, with the cranial nerves and their exits from the skull. On the right side, part of the tentorium cerebelli and the roof of the trigeminal cave have been removed.

## 7.4 Summary of the 12 cranial nerves

| Nerve | Examination | Abnormalities/symptoms |
|---|---|---|
| I | Sense of smell, each nostril | Anosmia/parosmia |
| II | Visual acuity | Partial sight/blindness |
| | Visual fields | Scotoma; hemianopia |
| | Pupil size and shape | Anisocoria |
| | Pupil light reflex | Impairment or loss |
| | Fundoscopy | Optic disc and retinal changes |
| III | Light and accommodation reflex | Impairment or loss |
| III, IV and VI | Eye position and movements | Strabismus, diplopia, nystagmus |
| V | Facial sensation | Impairment, distortion or loss |
| | Corneal reflex | Impairment or loss |
| | Muscles of mastication | Weakness of chewing movements |
| | Jaw jerk | Increase in upper motor neuron lesions |
| VII | Muscles of facial expression | Facial weakness |
| | Taste over anterior two-thirds of tongue | Ageusia (loss of taste) |
| VIII | Whisper and tuning fork tests | Impaired hearing/deafness |
| | Vestibular tests | Nystagmus and vertigo |
| IX | Pharyngeal sensation | Not routinely tested |
| X | Palate movements | Unilateral or bilateral impairment |
| XI | Trapezius and sternomastoid | Weakness of scapular and neck movement |
| XII | Tongue appearance and movement | Dysarthria and chewing/swallowing difficulties |

Parosmia is the perception of pleasant odours as unpleasant; it may occur with head trauma or sinus infection or be an adverse effect of drugs. Olfactory hallucinations may occur in Alzheimer's disease and focal epilepsies. Phantosmia, when patients describe a persistent smell, often cigarette smoke, is common and usually benign.

## Optic (II), oculomotor (III), trochlear (IV) and abducens (VI) nerves

See Chapter 8.

## Trigeminal (V) nerve

The V nerve conveys sensation from the face, mouth and part of the dura and provides motor supply to the muscles of mastication.

### ▌ Anatomy

The cell bodies of the sensory fibres are located in the trigeminal (Gasserian) ganglion, which lies in a cavity (Meckel's cave) in the petrous temporal dura (see Fig. 7.5). From the trigeminal ganglion, the V nerve passes to the pons. From here, pain and temperature pathways descend to the C2 segment of the spinal cord, so ipsilateral facial numbness may occur with cervical cord lesions.

There are three major branches of V (Fig. 7.6):

- ophthalmic ($V_1$): sensory
- maxillary ($V_2$): sensory
- mandibular ($V_3$): sensory and motor.

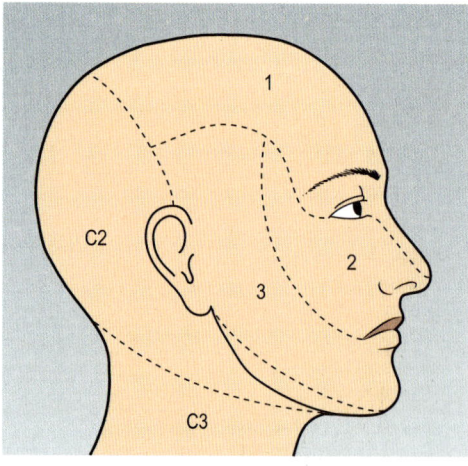

**Fig. 7.6** The sensory distribution of the three divisions of the trigeminal nerve. 1. Ophthalmic division. 2. Maxillary division. 3. Mandibular division.

The ophthalmic branch leaves the ganglion and passes forward to the superior orbital fissure via the wall of the cavernous sinus (see Fig. 8.3). In addition to the skin of the upper nose, upper eyelid, forehead and scalp, $V_1$ supplies sensation to the eye (cornea and conjunctiva) and the mucous membranes of the sphenoidal and ethmoid sinuses and upper nasal cavity.

The maxillary branch ($V_2$) passes from the ganglion via the cavernous sinus to leave the skull by the foramen rotundum. It contains sensory fibres from the mucous membranes of the upper mouth, roof of the pharynx, gums, teeth and palate of the upper jaw and the maxillary, sphenoidal and ethmoid sinuses.

The mandibular branch ($V_3$) exits the skull via the foramen ovale and supplies the floor of the mouth, sensation (but not taste) to the anterior two-thirds of the tongue, the gums and teeth of the lower jaw, mucosa of the cheek and the temporomandibular joint, in addition to the skin of the lower lips and jaw area, but not the angle of the jaw (see Fig. 7.6).

The motor fibres of V run in the mandibular branch ($V_3$) and innervate the muscles of mastication: temporalis, masseter and medial and lateral pterygoids.

## Examination sequence (Video 9)

Four aspects need to be assessed: sensory, motor and two reflexes.

### Sensory

- Ask the patient to close their eyes and say 'yes' each time they feel a light touch (you use a cotton-wool tip for this test). Do this in the areas of $V_1$, $V_2$ and $V_3$.
- Repeat using a fresh neurological pin, such as a Neurotip, to test superficial pain.
- Compare both sides. If you identify an area of reduced sensation, map it out. Does it conform to the distribution of the trigeminal nerve or branches? Remember the angle of the jaw is served by C2 and not the trigeminal nerve, but $V_1$ extends towards the vertex (see Fig. 7.6).
- 'Nasal tickle' test: use a wisp of cotton wool to 'tickle' the inside of each nostril and ask the patient to compare. The normal result is an unpleasant sensation easily appreciated by the patient.

### Motor (signs rare)

- Inspect for wasting of the muscles of mastication (most apparent in temporalis).
- Ask the patient to clench their teeth; feel the masseters, estimating their bulk.
- Ask the patient to open their jaw and note any deviation; the jaw may deviate to the paralysed side due to contraction of the intact contralateral pterygoid muscle.

### Corneal reflex

Routine testing of the corneal reflex is unnecessary but may be relevant when the history suggests a lesion localising to the brainstem or cranial nerves V, VII or VIII. The afferent limb is via the trigeminal nerve, the efferent limb via the facial nerve.

**Fig. 7.7 Testing the corneal reflex.** The cotton-wool wisp should touch the cornea overlying the iris, not the conjunctiva, and avoid visual stimulus.

## 7.5 Comparison of bulbar and pseudobulbar palsy

|  | Bulbar palsy | Pseudobulbar palsy |
|---|---|---|
| Level of motor Lesion | Lower motor neuron | Upper motor neuron |
| Speech | Dysarthria | Dysarthria and dysphonia |
| Swallowing | Dysphagia | Dysphagia |
| Tongue | Weak, wasted and fasciculating | Spastic, slow-moving |
| Jaw jerk | Absent | Present/brisk |
| Emotional lability | Absent | May be present |
| Causes | Motor neuron disease | Cerebrovascular disease, motor neuron disease, multiple sclerosis |

**7**

- Explain to the patient what you are going to do and ask them to remove their contact lenses, if relevant.
- Gently depress the lower eyelid while the patient looks up.
- Lightly touch the lateral edge of the cornea with a wisp of damp cotton wool (Fig. 7.7).
- Look for both direct and consensual blinking.

### Jaw jerk

- Ask the patient to let their mouth hang loosely open.
- Place your forefinger in the midline between lower lip and chin.
- Percuss your finger gently with the tendon hammer in a downward direction (Fig. 7.8), noting any reflex closing of the jaw.
- An absent, or just present, reflex is normal. A brisk jaw jerk occurs in pseudobulbar palsy (Box 7.5).

Sensory symptoms include facial numbness and pain. Unilateral loss of sensation in one or more branches of the V nerve may result from direct injury in association with facial fractures

(particularly $V_2$), local invasion by cancer or Sjögren's syndrome. Lesions in the cavernous sinus often cause loss of the corneal reflex and $V_1$ or $V_2$ cutaneous sensory loss. Cranial nerves III, IV and VI may also be involved (see Fig. 8.3). Trigeminal neuralgia causes severe, lancinating pain, typically in the distribution of $V_2$ or $V_3$. Reactivation of herpes varicella zoster virus (chickenpox) can affect any sensory nerve, but typically either $V_1$ or a thoracic dermatome (Fig. 7.9). In herpes zoster ophthalmicus (affecting $V_1$), there is a risk of sight-threatening complications. Hutchinson's sign, vesicles on the side or tip of the nose, may be present.

Clinically significant weakness of the muscles of mastication is unusual but may occur in myasthenia gravis, with fatigable chewing. Claudication (i.e. pain on chewing) of these muscles can occur in temporal arteritis.

## Facial (VII) nerve

The facial nerve supplies the muscles of facial expression (frontalis, orbicularis oculi, buccinators, orbicularis oris and platysma) and carries parasympathetic fibres to the lacrimal, submandibular and sublingual salivary glands (via nervus intermedius). It receives taste sensation from the anterior two-thirds of the tongue (via the chorda tympani; Fig. 7.10).

### Anatomy

From its motor nucleus in the lower pons, fibres of the VII nerve pass back to loop around the VI nerve nucleus before emerging from the lateral pontomedullary junction in close association with the VIII nerve (Fig. 7.11); together they enter the internal acoustic meatus (see Fig. 7.5). At the lateral end of the meatus, the VII nerve continues in the facial canal within the temporal bone, exiting the skull via the stylomastoid foramen. Passing through the parotid gland, it gives off its terminal branches. In its course in the facial canal, it gives off branches to the stapedius muscle and its parasympathetic fibres as well as being joined by the taste fibres of the chorda tympani (see Fig. 7.10).

**Fig. 7.8 Eliciting the jaw jerk.**

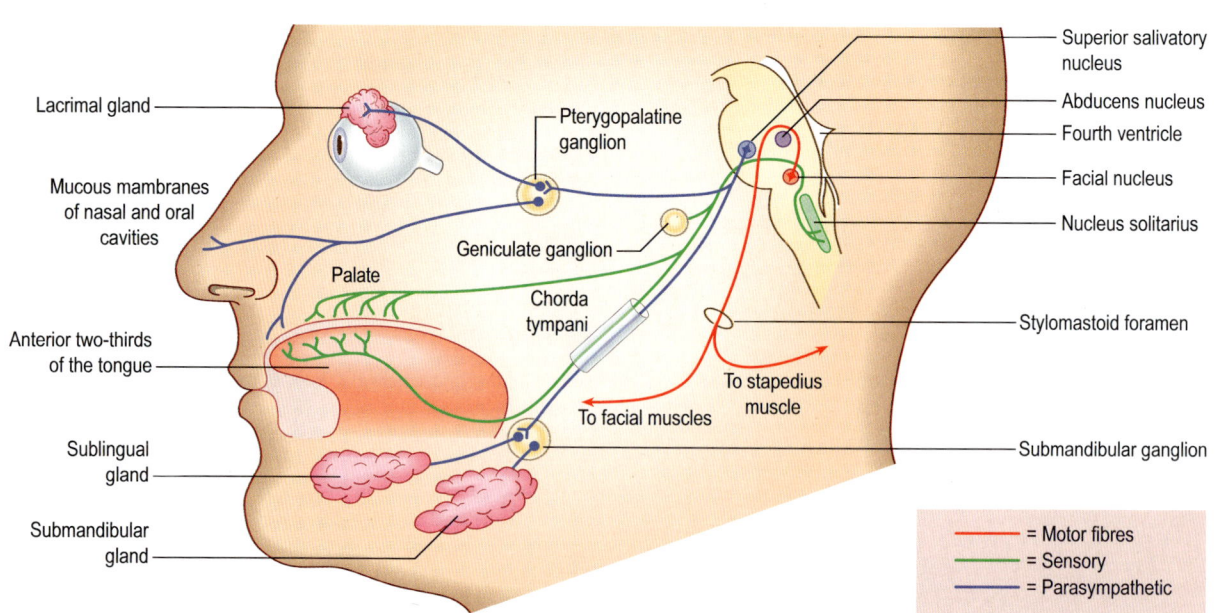

**Fig. 7.9 Herpes zoster.** [A] The ophthalmic division of the left trigeminal (V) nerve is involved. [B] The maxillary division of the left V nerve. [C] Cervical spinal root left C4. [D] Thoracic spinal root right T5.

Lacrimal gland

Mucous mambranes of nasal and oral cavities

Anterior two-thirds of the tongue

Sublingual gland

Submandibular gland

Pterygopalatine ganglion

Geniculate ganglion

Palate

Chorda tympani

To facial muscles

To stapedius muscle

Superior salivatory nucleus

Abducens nucleus

Fourth ventricle

Facial nucleus

Nucleus solitarius

Stylomastoid foramen

Submandibular ganglion

= Motor fibres
= Sensory
= Parasympathetic

**Fig. 7.10** Component fibres of the facial nerve and their peripheral distribution.

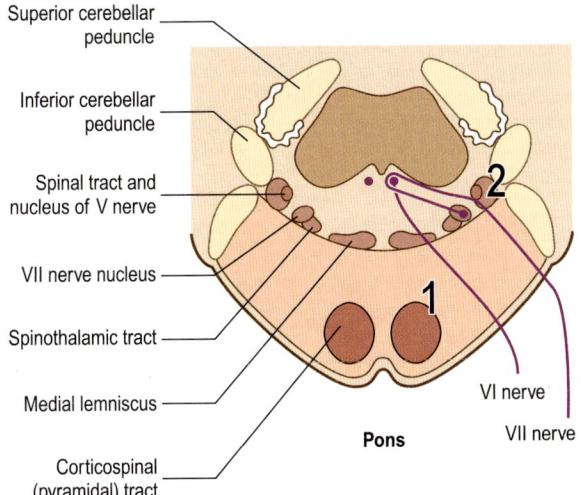

Superior cerebellar peduncle

Inferior cerebellar peduncle

Spinal tract and nucleus of V nerve

VII nerve nucleus

Spinothalamic tract

Medial lemniscus

Corticospinal (pyramidal) tract

**Pons**

VI nerve

VII nerve

**Fig. 7.11 Lesions of the pons.** Lesions at (1) may result in ipsilateral VI and VII nerve palsies and contralateral hemiplegia. At (2) ipsilateral cerebellar signs and impaired sensation on the ipsilateral side of the face and on the contralateral side of the body may occur.

## Examination sequence (Video 10) ▶

Examination is usually confined to motor function; taste is rarely tested.

### Motor function

- Inspect the face for asymmetry or differences in blinking or eye closure on one side. Note that minor facial asymmetry is common and rarely pathological.
- Watch for spontaneous or involuntary movement such as blepharospasm, hemifacial spasm or aberrant innervation after facial nerve palsy.
- For the following actions it is often easiest to demonstrate the actions yourself and ask the patient to copy you, observing for any asymmetry.

- Ask the patient to raise their eyebrows and observe for symmetrical wrinkling of the forehead (frontalis muscle).
- Ask the patient to screw their eyes tightly shut and resist you opening them (orbicularis oculi).
- Ask the patient to bare their teeth (orbicularis oris).
- Ask the patient to blow out their cheeks with their mouth closed (buccinators and orbicularis oris).

In a unilateral lower motor neuron VII nerve lesion, there is weakness of both upper and lower facial muscles. Bell's palsy is the term used to describe an idiopathic acute lower motor neuron VII nerve paralysis, often preceded by mastoid pain. It may be associated with impairment of taste and hyperacusis (high-pitched sounds appearing unpleasantly louder than normal). Bell's phenomenon occurs when a patient closes their eyes: as eye closure is incomplete, the globe can be seen to roll upwards to avoid corneal exposure (Fig. 7.12A). Ramsay Hunt syndrome occurs in herpes zoster infection of the geniculate (facial) ganglion. This produces a severe lower motor neuron facial palsy, ipsilateral loss of taste and buccal ulceration, and a painful vesicular eruption in the external auditory meatus. Other causes of a lower motor neuron VII lesion include cerebellopontine angle tumours (including acoustic neuroma), trauma and parotid tumours. Synkinesis (involuntary muscle contraction accompanying a voluntary movement: most commonly, twitching of the corner of the mouth with ipsilateral blinking) is a sign of aberrant reinnervation and may be seen in recovering lower motor neuron VII lesions.

In unilateral VII nerve upper motor neuron lesions, weakness is marked in the lower facial muscles with relative sparing of the upper face. This is because there is bilateral cortical innervation of the upper facial muscles. The nasolabial fold may be flattened and the corner of the mouth drooped, but eye closure is usually preserved (see Fig. 7.12B). Hemifacial spasm presents with synchronised twitching of the ipsilateral eye and mouth.

Bilateral facial palsies are less common but occasionally occur, as in Guillain–Barré syndrome, sarcoidosis or infection such as Lyme disease, HIV or leprosy. Facial weakness, especially with respect to eye closure, can also be found in some congenital myopathies (facioscapulohumeral or myotonic dystrophies).

**7**

Loss of frontal wrinkling

Bell's phenomenon

Loss of nasolabial fold

Mouth deviates to normal side

A

Preserved function in upper face

Loss of nasolabial fold

Mouth deviates to normal side

B

**Fig. 7.12 Types of facial weakness.** A Right-sided lower motor neuron lesion (within facial nerve or nucleus); Bell's phenomenon is also shown. B Right-sided upper motor neuron lesion.

Distinct from VII nerve palsies, Parkinson's disease can cause loss of spontaneous facial movements, including a slowed blink rate, and involuntary facial movements (levodopa-induced dyskinesias) may complicate advanced disease.

Involuntary emotional movements, such as spontaneous smiling, have different pathways and may be preserved in the presence of paresis.

## The vestibulocochlear (VIII) nerve

See page 194.

## Glossopharyngeal (IX) and vagus (X) nerves

The IX and X nerves have an intimate anatomical relationship. Both contain sensory, motor and autonomic components. The glossopharyngeal (IX) nerve mainly carries sensation from the pharynx and tonsils, and sensation and taste from the posterior one-third of the tongue. The IX nerve also supplies the carotid chemoreceptors. The vagus (X) nerve carries important sensory information but also innervates upper pharyngeal and laryngeal muscles. The main functions of IX and X that can be tested clinically are swallowing, phonation/articulation and sensation from the pharynx/larynx. In the thorax and abdomen, the vagus (X) nerve receives sensory fibres from the lungs and carries parasympathetic fibres to the lungs, heart and abdominal viscera.

### ▊ Anatomy

Both nerves arise as several roots from the lateral medulla and leave the skull together via the jugular foramen (see Fig. 7.5). The IX nerve passes down and forward to supply the stylopharyngeus muscle, the mucosa of the pharynx, the tonsils and the posterior one-third of the tongue, and sends parasympathetic fibres to the parotid gland. The X nerve courses down in the carotid sheath into the thorax, giving off several branches, including pharyngeal and recurrent laryngeal branches, which provide motor supply to the pharyngeal, soft palate and laryngeal muscles. The main nuclei of these nerves in the medulla are the nucleus ambiguus (motor), the dorsal motor vagal nucleus (parasympathetic) and the solitary nucleus (visceral sensation; Fig. 7.13).

### Examination sequence (Videos 11 and 11A) ▶

- Assess the patient's speech for dysarthria or dysphonia (p. 211).
- Ask them to say 'Ah'. Look at the movements of the palate and uvula using a torch. Normally, both sides of the palate elevate symmetrically and the uvula remains in the midline.
- Ask the patient to puff out their cheeks with their lips tightly closed. Listen for air escaping from the nose. For the cheeks to puff out, the palate must elevate and occlude the nasopharynx. If palatal movement is weak, air will escape audibly through the nose.
- Ask the patient to cough; assess the strength of the cough.

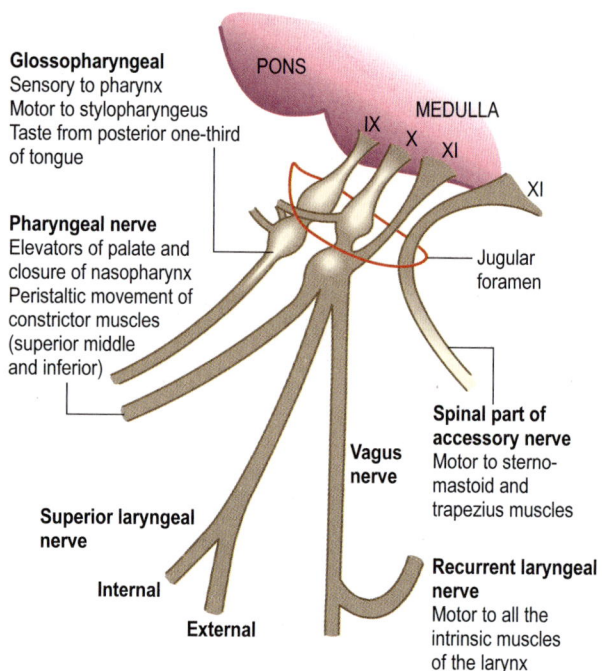

**Glossopharyngeal**
Sensory to pharynx
Motor to stylopharyngeus
Taste from posterior one-third of tongue

**Pharyngeal nerve**
Elevators of palate and closure of nasopharynx
Peristaltic movement of constrictor muscles (superior middle and inferior)

**Superior laryngeal nerve**

Internal

External

**Vagus nerve**

**Spinal part of accessory nerve**
Motor to sterno-mastoid and trapezius muscles

**Recurrent laryngeal nerve**
Motor to all the intrinsic muscles of the larynx

Jugular foramen

PONS

MEDULLA

IX X XI

XI

**Fig. 7.13** The lower cranial nerves: glossopharyngeal (IX), vagus (X) and accessory (XI).

- Testing pharyngeal sensation and the gag reflex is unpleasant and has poor predictive value for aspiration. Instead, and in fully conscious patients only, use the swallow test. Administer 3 teaspoons of water and observe for absent swallow, cough or delayed cough or change in voice quality after each teaspoon. If there are no problems, observe again while the patient swallows a glass of water.

Isolated unilateral IX nerve lesions are rare. Unilateral X nerve damage leads to ipsilateral reduced elevation of the soft palate, which may cause deviation of the uvula (away from the side of the lesion) when the patient says 'Ah'. Unilateral lesions of IX and X are most commonly caused by strokes, skull-base fractures or tumours. Damage to the recurrent laryngeal branch of the X nerve due to lung cancer, thyroid surgery, mediastinal tumours and aortic arch aneurysms causes dysphonia and a 'bovine' cough. Bilateral X nerve lesions cause dysphagia and dysarthria, and may be due to lesions at the upper (pseudobulbar palsy) or lower (bulbar palsy) motor neuron levels (see Box 7.5). Less severe cases can result in nasal regurgitation of fluids and nasal air escape when the cheeks are puffed out (dysarthria and nasal escape are often evident during history taking). Always consider myasthenia gravis in patients with symptoms of bulbar dysfunction, even if the examination seems normal.

## Accessory (XI) nerve

The accessory nerve has two components:
- a cranial part closely related to the vagus (X) nerve

- a spinal part that provides fibres to the upper trapezius muscles, responsible for elevating (shrugging) the shoulders and elevating the arm above the horizontal, and the sternomastoid muscles that control head turning and neck flexion.

The spinal component is discussed here.

## Anatomy

The spinal nuclei arise from the anterior horn cells of C1–5. Fibres emerge from the spinal cord, ascend through the foramen magnum and exit via the jugular foramen (see Fig. 7.5), passing posteriorly.

## Examination sequence (Video 11B)

- Face the patient and inspect the sternomastoid muscles for wasting or hypertrophy; palpate them to assess their bulk.
- Stand behind the patient to inspect the trapezius muscle for wasting or asymmetry.
- Ask the patient to shrug their shoulders, then apply downward pressure with your hands to assess the power.
- Test power in the left sternomastoid by asking the patient to turn their head to the right while you provide resistance with your hand placed on the right side of the patient's chin. Reverse the procedure to check the right sternomastoid.
- Test both sternocleidomastoid muscles simultaneously by asking the patient to flex their neck. Apply your palm to the forehead as resistance.

Isolated XI nerve lesions are uncommon, but the nerve may be damaged during surgery in the posterior triangle of the neck, penetrating injuries or tumour invasion. Wasting of the upper fibres of trapezius may be associated with displacement ('winging') of the upper vertebral border of the scapula away from the spine, while the lower border is displaced towards it. Wasting and weakness of the sternomastoids are characteristic of myotonic dystrophy. Weakness of neck flexion or extension, the latter causing head drop, may occur in myasthenia gravis, motor neuron disease, myotonic dystrophy and some myopathies. Dystonic head postures causing antecollis (neck flexed), retrocollis (neck extended) or torticollis (neck twisted to one side) are not associated with weakness.

## Hypoglossal (XII) nerve

The XII nerve innervates the tongue muscles; the nucleus lies in the dorsal medulla beneath the floor of the fourth ventricle.

## Anatomy

The nerve emerges anteriorly and exits the skull in the hypoglossal canal, passing to the root of the tongue (see Fig. 7.5).

## Examination sequence (Video 11C)

- Ask the patient to open their mouth. Look at the tongue at rest for wasting, fasciculation or involuntary movement.
- Ask the patient to put out their tongue. Look for deviation or involuntary movement.
- Ask the patient to move their tongue quickly from side to side.
- Test power by asking the patient to press their tongue against the inside of each cheek in turn while you press from the outside with your finger.
- Assess speech by asking the patient to say 'yellow lorry.'
- Assess swallowing with a water swallow test (p. 148).

Unilateral lower motor XII nerve lesions lead to tongue wasting on the affected side and deviation to that side on protrusion (Fig. 7.14). Bilateral lower motor neuron damage results in global wasting; the tongue appears thin and shrunken and fasciculation may be evident. Normal rippling or undulating movements may be mistaken for fasciculation, especially if the tongue is protruded; these usually settle when the tongue is at rest in the mouth. When associated with lesions of the IX, X and XI nerves, typically in motor neuron disease, these features are termed bulbar palsy (see Box 7.5).

Unilateral upper motor XII nerve lesions are uncommon; bilateral lesions lead to a tongue with increased tone (spastic), and the patient has difficulty flicking the tongue from side to side. Bilateral upper motor lesions of the IX–XII nerves are called pseudobulbar palsy (see Box 7.5). Tremor of the resting or protruded tongue may occur in Parkinson's disease, although jaw tremor is more common. Other orolingual dyskinesias (involuntary movements of the mouth and tongue) are often drug-induced and include tardive dyskinesias due to neuroleptics.

**Fig. 7.14 Left hypoglossal nerve lesion.** *From Epstein O, Perkin GD, de Bono DP, et al. Clinical Examination. 2nd ed. London: Mosby; 1997.*

7

# Motor system (Videos 12 and 13)

## Anatomy

The principal motor pathway has CNS (corticospinal or pyramidal tract: upper motor neuron) and PNS (anterior horn cell: lower motor neuron) components (Fig. 7.15). Other parts of the nervous system, such as the basal ganglia and cerebellum, have important modulating effects on movement. It is important to distinguish upper from lower motor neuron signs to help localise the lesion (Box 7.6).

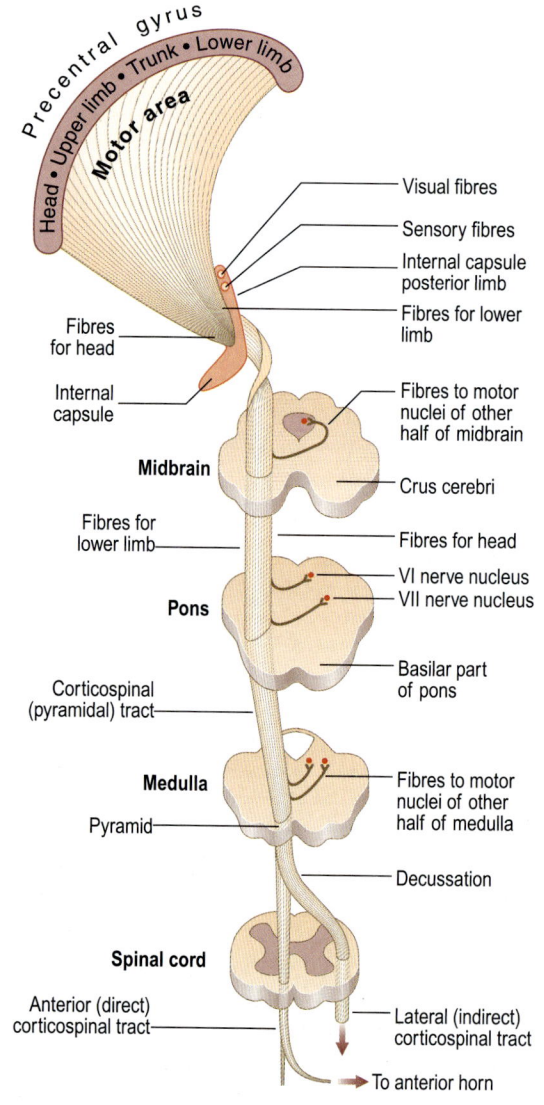

**Fig. 7.15** Principal motor pathways.

### 7.6 Features of motor neuron lesions

|  | Upper motor neuron lesion | Lower motor neuron lesion |
|---|---|---|
| Inspection | Usually normal (may be disuse wasting in longstanding lesions) | Muscle wasting, fasciculations |
| Tone | Increased with clonus | Normal or decreased, no clonus |
| Weakness | Preferentially affects extensors in arms, flexors in leg | Usually more focal, in distribution of nerve root or peripheral nerve |
| Deep tendon reflexes | Increased | Decreased/absent |
| Plantar response | Extensor (Babinski sign) | Flexor |

## Upper motor neuron lesions

If the lesion affects the CNS pathways, the lower motor neurons are under the uninhibited influence of the spinal reflex. The motor units then have an exaggerated response to stretch with increased tone (spasticity), clonus and brisk reflexes. There is weakness but not wasting (although atrophy may develop with longstanding lesions). Primitive reflexes, such as the plantar extensor response (Babinski sign), may be present.

## Lower motor neuron lesions

Motor fibres, together with input from other systems involved in the control of movement, including extrapyramidal, cerebellar, vestibular and proprioceptive afferents, converge on the cell bodies of lower motor neurons in the anterior horn of the grey matter in the spinal cord (see Fig. 7.15).

The group of muscle fibres innervated by a single anterior horn cell forms a 'motor unit.' A lower motor neuron lesion causes weakness and wasting in these muscle fibres, reduced tone (flaccidity), fasciculation and reduced or absent reflexes.

## Basal ganglia lesions

The basal ganglia are connected structures within the cerebral hemispheres and brainstem (Fig. 7.16). They include the caudate nucleus and putamen (collectively known as the striatum), globus pallidus, thalamus, subthalamic nucleus and substantia nigra (the latter in the brainstem). The basal ganglia receive much information from the cortex and are involved in regulating many activities, principally control of movement, but are also involved in eye movement, behaviour and executive function control. Disorders of the basal ganglia may cause reduced movement (typically Parkinsonism; p. 151) or, less commonly, excessive movement such as ballism or tics (p. 153).

Assess the motor system using the following method:

- assessing stance and gait
- inspecting and palpating muscles

A

- Caudate nucleus
- Putamen
- Thalamus
- Amygdala

B

- Thalamus
- Caudate nucleus — Striatum
- Putamen
- Globus pallidus externa (GPe)
- Globus pallidus interna (GPi)
- Subthalamic nucleus (STN)
- Substantia nigra (SN)

Fig. 7.16 **Basal ganglia.** **A** Anatomical location. **B** Coronal view.

- assessing tone
- testing movement and power
- examining reflexes
- testing coordination.

## Stance and gait

Stance and gait depend on intact visual, vestibular, sensory, corticospinal, extrapyramidal and cerebellar pathways, together with functioning lower motor neurons and spinal reflexes. Non-neurological gait disorders are discussed on page 152. Certain abnormal gait patterns are recognisable, suggesting diagnoses (Box 7.7 and Fig. 7.17).

## Examination sequence

### Stance

- Ask the patient to stand with their (preferably bare) feet together and eyes open.
- Swaying, lurching or an inability to stand with the feet together and eyes open suggests cerebellar ataxia.
- Ask the patient to close their eyes (Romberg's test) but be prepared to steady/catch them. Repeated falling is a positive result. Swaying is common and should not be misinterpreted.
- The 'pull test' assesses postural stability. Ask the patient to stand with their feet slightly apart. Inform them that you are

### 7.7 Common gait abnormalities

| Gait disturbance | Description | Causes |
|---|---|---|
| Parkinsonian | Stooped posture<br>Shuffling (reduced stride length)<br>Loss of arm swing<br>Postural instability<br>Freezing | Parkinson's disease and other Parkinsonian syndromes |
| Gait apraxia | Small, shuffling steps (*marche à petits pas*)<br>Difficulty in starting to walk/freezing<br>Better 'cycling' on bed than walking | Cerebrovascular disease<br>Hydrocephalus |
| Spastic | Stiff 'walking-through-mud' or scissors gait | Spinal cord lesions |
| Myopathic | Waddling (proximal weakness)<br>Bilateral Trendelenburg signs | Muscular dystrophies and acquired myopathies |
| Foot drop | Foot slapping | Neuropathies<br>Common peroneal nerve palsy<br>L5 radiculopathy |
| Central ataxia | Wide-based, 'drunken'<br>Tandem gait poor | Cerebellar disease |
| Sensory ataxia | Wide-based<br>Positive Romberg sign | Neuropathies<br>Spinal cord disorders |
| Functional | Variable, often bizarre, inconsistent<br>Knees flexed, buckling<br>Dragging immobile leg behind | Functional neurological disorders |

© Crown Copyright.

going to push them forwards or pull them backwards. They should maintain their position if possible. Standing behind the patient, deliver a brisk push forwards or pull backwards. You must be ready to catch them if they are unable to maintain their balance. If in doubt, have an assistant standing in front of the patient.

### Gait

- Look at the patient's shoes for abnormal wear patterns.
- Perform a timed get-up-and-go test (see Fig. 17.4)
- Note stride length, arm swing, steadiness (including turning), limping or other difficulties.
- Look for abnormal movements that may be accentuated by walking, such as tremor (in Parkinson's disease) or dystonic movements.
- Listen for the slapping sound of a foot-drop gait.
- Ask the patient to walk first on their tiptoes, then heels. Ankle dorsiflexion weakness (foot drop) is much more common than plantar flexion weakness and makes walking on the heels difficult or impossible.
- Ask the patient to walk heel to toe in a straight line (tandem gait). This emphasises gait ataxia and may be the only abnormal finding in midline cerebellar (vermis) lesions.

7

**A  Spastic hemiparesis**
One arm held immobile and
close to the side with elbow,
wrist and fingers flexed
Leg extended with plantar
flexion of the foot
On walking, the foot is
dragged, scraping the toe
in a circle (circumduction)
Caused by upper motor
neurone lesion, e.g. stroke

**B  Steppage gait**
Foot is dragged or lifted high
and slapped on to the floor
Unable to walk on the heels
Caused by foot drop owing to
lower motor neurone lesion

**C  Sensory or cerebellar ataxia**
Gait is unsteady and wide-
based. Feet are thrown forward
and outward and brought down
on the heels
In sensory ataxia, patients watch
the ground. With their eyes
closed, they cannot stand
steadily (positive Romberg sign)
In cerebellar ataxia, turns are
difficult and patients cannot
stand steadily with feet together
whether eyes are open or
closed
Caused by polyneuropathy or
posterior column damage, e.g.
syphilis

**D  Parkinsonian gait**
Posture is stooped with head
and neck forwards
Arms are flexed at elbows and
wrists. Little arm swing
Steps are short and shuffling
and patient is slow in getting
started (festinant gait)
Caused by lesions in the basal
ganglia

**Fig. 7.17** Abnormalities of gait.

Unsteadiness on standing with the eyes open is common in cerebellar disorders. Instability that only occurs, or is markedly worse, on eye closure (Romberg sign) indicates proprioceptive sensory loss (sensory ataxia) or bilateral vestibular failure. Cerebellar ataxia is not usually associated with a positive Romberg test.

Hemiplegic gait (unilateral upper motor neuron lesion) is characterised by extension at the hip, knee and ankle and circumduction at the hip such that the foot on the affected side is plantar flexed and describes a semicircle as the patient walks. The upper limb may be flexed (see Fig. 7.17A).

Bilateral upper motor neuron damage causes a scissor-like gait due to spasticity. Cerebellar dysfunction leads to a broad-based, unsteady (ataxic) gait, which usually makes walking heel to toe impossible. In Parkinsonism, initiation of walking may be delayed; the steps are short and shuffling with loss/reduction of arm swing (see Fig. 7.17D). A tremor may become more apparent. The stooped posture and impairment of postural reflexes can result in a festinant (rapid, short-stepped, hurrying) gait. As a doorway or other obstacle approaches, the patient may freeze. Turning involves many short steps, with the risk of falls. Postural instability on the pull test, especially backwards, occurs in Parkinsonian syndromes. Proximal muscle weakness

may lead to a waddling gait with bilateral Trendelenburg signs (see p. 296 and Fig. 13.38). Bizarre gaits, such as when patients drag a leg behind them, are often functional but some diseases, including Huntington's disease, produce unusual and chaotic gaits.

## Inspection and palpation of the muscles

### Examination sequence

- Completely expose the patient while maintaining their comfort and dignity.
- Look for asymmetry, inspecting both proximally and distally. Note deformities, such as flexion deformities or pes cavus (high foot arches).
- Inspect for wasting or hypertrophy, fasciculation and involuntary movement.

### Muscle bulk

Lower motor neuron lesions may cause muscle wasting. This is not seen in acute upper motor neuron lesions, although disuse atrophy may develop with longstanding lesions. A motor neuron lesion in childhood may impair growth (causing a smaller limb or hemiatrophy) or lead to limb deformity, such as pes cavus. Muscle disorders usually result in proximal wasting (the notable exception is myotonic dystrophy, in which it is distal, often with temporalis wasting). People in certain occupations, such as professional sports players, may have physiological muscle hypertrophy. Pseudohypertrophy may occur in muscular dystrophy, but the muscles are weak.

## Fasciculation

Fasciculations are visible irregular twitches of resting muscles caused by individual motor units firing spontaneously. This occurs in lower motor neuron disease, usually in wasted muscles. Fasciculation is seen, not felt, and you may need to observe carefully for several minutes to be sure that it is not present. Physiological (benign) fasciculation is common, especially in the calves, but is not associated with weakness or wasting. Myokymia – fine, involuntary fascicular contractions – involves rapid bursts of repetitive motor unit activity that often affects orbicularis oculi or the first dorsal interosseus and is rarely pathological.

## Abnormal movements

### Myoclonic jerks

These are sudden, shock-like contractions of one or more muscles that may be focal or diffuse and occur singly or repetitively. Healthy people commonly experience these when falling asleep (hypnic jerks). They may also occur pathologically in association with epilepsy, diffuse brain damage and some neurodegenerative disorders, such as prion diseases. Negative myoclonus (asterixis) is seen most commonly in liver disease (liver flap).

### Tremor

Tremor is an involuntary, oscillatory movement about a joint or a group of joints, resulting from alternating contraction and relaxation of muscles. Tremors are classified according to their frequency, amplitude, position (at rest, on posture or movement) and body part affected.

Physiological tremor is a fine (low-amplitude), fast (high-frequency, 3 to 30 Hz) postural tremor. A similar tremor occurs in hyperthyroidism and with excess alcohol or caffeine intake and is a common adverse effect of beta-agonist bronchodilators.

Essential tremor is the most common pathological cause of tremor; it is typically symmetrical in the upper limbs and may involve the head and voice. The tremor is noted on posture and with movement (kinetic). It may be improved by alcohol and often demonstrates an autosomal dominant pattern of inheritance.

Parkinson's disease causes a slow (3 to 7 Hz), coarse, 'pill-rolling' tremor, worse at rest but reduced with voluntary movement. It is more common in the upper limbs, is usually asymmetrical and does not affect the head, although it may involve the jaw/chin and sometimes the legs.

Isolated head tremor is usually dystonic and may be associated with abnormal neck postures such as torticollis, antecollis or retrocollis.

Intention tremor is absent at rest but maximal on movement and on approaching the target and is usually due to cerebellar damage. It is assessed with the finger-to-nose test (p. 158).

Other causes of tremor include hereditary or acquired demyelinating neuropathies (such as Charcot-Marie-Tooth disease) and are termed neuropathic tremors. Drugs commonly causing tremor include sodium valproate, glucocorticoids and lithium.

Movement disorders, including tremor, are common functional symptoms. They are often inconsistent and distractible with varying frequencies and amplitudes and may be associated with other functional signs.

### Other involuntary movements

These are classified according to their appearance.

Dystonia is caused by sustained muscle contractions, leading to twisting, repetitive movements and sometimes tremor. It may be focal (as in torticollis), segmental (affecting two or more adjacent body parts) or generalised.

Chorea describes brief, jerky, random, purposeless movements that may affect various body parts, commonly the arms.

Athetosis is a slower, writhing movement, more similar to dystonia than chorea.

Ballism refers to violent flinging movements sometimes affecting only one side of the body (hemiballismus).

Tics are repetitive, stereotyped movements that may be briefly suppressed by the patient.

## Tone

Tone is the resistance felt by the examiner when moving a joint passively.

### Examination sequence (Videos 12A and 13A)

- Ask the patient to lie supine on the examination couch and to relax and 'go floppy.' Enquire about any pain or limitations of movement before proceeding.
- Passively move each joint to be tested through as full a range as possible, both slowly and quickly in all anatomically possible directions. Be unpredictable with these movements, in both direction and speed, to prevent the patient actively moving with you; you want to assess passive tone. It may be helpful to distract the patient by asking them to count backwards from 20 while assessing tone.

### Upper limb

- Hold the patient's hand as if shaking hands, using your other hand to support their elbow. Assess tone at the wrist and elbow with supination/pronation and flexion/extension movements.
- Activation (or synkinesis) is a technique used to exaggerate subtle increase in tone and is particularly useful for assessing extrapyramidal tone increase. Ask the patient to describe circles in the air with the contralateral limb while you assess tone. A transient increase in tone with this manoeuvre (Froment's) is normal.

**7**

## Lower limb

- Roll the leg from side to side and then briskly flip the knee up into a flexed position, observing the movement of the foot. Typically, the heel moves up the bed, but increased tone may cause it to lift off the bed due to failure of relaxation.

## Ankle clonus

- Support the patient's leg, with both the knee and the ankle resting in 90-degree flexion.
- Briskly dorsiflex and partially evert the foot, sustaining the pressure. Clonus is felt as repeated beats of dorsiflexion/plantar flexion.

## Myotonia

- Ask the patient to make a fist and then to relax and open their hand; watch for the speed of relaxation.
- Using the tendon hammer, percuss the belly of the thenar eminence; this may induce contraction of the muscles, causing the thumb to adduct, and you may witness dimpling of the muscle belly.

### Hypotonia

Decreased tone may occur in lower motor neuron lesions and is usually associated with muscle wasting, weakness and hyporeflexia. It may also be a feature of cerebellar disease or signal the early phases of cerebral or spinal shock when the paralysed limbs are atonic prior to developing spasticity. Reduced tone can be difficult to elicit.

### Hypertonia

Increased tone may occur in two main forms: spasticity and rigidity.

Spasticity is velocity-dependent resistance to passive movement; it is detected with quick movements and is a feature of upper motor neuron lesions. It is usually accompanied by weakness, hyperreflexia, an extensor plantar response and sometimes clonus. In mild forms, it is detected as a 'catch' at the beginning or end of passive movement. In severe cases, it limits the range of movement and may be associated with contractures. In the upper limbs, it may be more obvious on attempted extension; in the legs, it is more evident on flexion.

Rigidity is a sustained resistance throughout the range of movement and is most easily detected when the limb is moved slowly. In Parkinsonism, this is classically described as 'lead pipe' rigidity. In the presence of a Parkinsonian tremor, there may be a regular interruption to the movement, giving it a jerky feel ('cog wheeling').

### Clonus

Clonus is a rhythmic series of contractions evoked by a sudden stretch of the muscle and tendon. Unsustained (<6 beats) clonus may be physiological. When sustained, it indicates upper motor neuron damage and is accompanied by spasticity. It is best elicited at the ankle; knee (patella) clonus is rare and not routinely tested.

| 7.8 Medical Research Council grading of muscle power | |
|---|---|
| Grade | Description |
| 0 | No muscle contraction visible |
| 1 | Flicker of contraction but no movement |
| 2 | Joint movement when effect of gravity eliminated |
| 3 | Movement against gravity but not against resistance |
| 4[a] | Movement against resistance but weaker than normal |
| 5 | Normal power |

[a]May be further classified as 4+ or 4−.

### Myotonia

Myotonia refers to the inability of muscles to relax normally and characterises a group of neuromuscular disorders, the most common of which is myotonic dystrophy. Patients may notice difficulty in letting go of things with their hands or a stiff gait.

## Power

Strength varies with age, occupation and fitness. Grade muscle power using the Medical Research Council (MRC) scale (Box 7.8). Record what patients can do in terms of daily activities; for example, whether they can stand, walk and raise both arms above their head. Lesions at different sites produce different clinical patterns of weakness; examination will help discriminate upper from lower motor neuron lesions.

## Examination sequence (Videos 12B and 13B)

- Do not test every muscle in most patients; the commonly tested muscles are listed in Box 7.9.
- Ask about pain that might interfere with testing.
- Observe the patient getting up from a chair and walking.
- Test upper limb power with the patient sitting on the edge of the couch. Test lower limb power with the patient reclining.
- Ask the patient to lift their arms above their head.
- Ask them to 'play the piano.' Check movements of the fingers; asymmetric loss of fine finger movement may be a very early sign of cortical or extrapyramidal disease.
- Observe the patient with their arms outstretched and supinated (palms up) and their eyes closed for 'pronator drift,' when one arm starts to pronate.
- Assess individual muscles depending on the history. Ask the patient to undertake a movement. First assess whether they can overcome gravity. For example, give the instruction 'Lift your right leg off the bed' to test hip flexion. Then apply resistance to this movement, testing across a single joint; for instance, apply resistance to the thigh in hip flexion, not the lower leg.
- To test truncal strength, ask the patient to sit up from a lying position.

Upper motor neuron lesions produce weakness of a relatively large group of muscles, such as a limb or more than one limb.

## 7.9 Nerve and muscle supplies of commonly tested movements

| Movement | Muscle | Nerve and root |
|---|---|---|
| Shoulder abduction | Deltoid | Axillary C5 |
| Elbow flexion | Biceps[a]<br>Brachioradialis (supinator reflex)[a] | Musculocutaneous C5[a]/6<br>Radial C6[a] |
| Elbow extension | Triceps[a] | Radial C7 |
| Wrist extension | Extensor carpi radialis longus | Radial (posterior interosseous branch) C6 |
| Finger extension | Extensor digitorum communis | Radial (posterior interosseous branch) C7 |
| Finger flexion | Flexor pollicis longus (thumb)<br>Flexor digitorum profundus (index and middle fingers)<br>Flexor digitorum profundus (ring and little fingers) | Median (anterior interosseous branch) C8<br><br>Ulnar C8 |
| Finger abduction | First dorsal interosseous | Ulnar T1 |
| Thumb abduction | Abductor pollicis brevis | Median T1 |
| Hip flexion | Iliopsoas | Iliofemoral nerve L1/2 |
| Hip extension | Gluteus maximus | Sciatic L5/S1 |
| Knee flexion | Hamstrings | Sciatic S1 |
| Knee extension | Quadriceps[a] | Femoral L3[a]/4 |
| Ankle dorsiflexion | Tibialis anterior | Common peroneal L4/5 |
| Ankle plantar flexion | Gastrocnemius and soleus[a] | Tibial S1[a]/2 |
| Great toe extension (dorsiflexion) | Extensor hallucis longus | Common peroneal L5 |
| Ankle eversion | Peronei | Common peroneal L5/S1 |
| Ankle inversion | Tibialis posterior | Tibial nerve L4/5 |

[a]Indicates nerve root innervation of commonly elicited deep tendon reflexes.

Lower motor neuron damage can cause paresis of an individual and specific muscle, so more detailed examination of individual muscles is required (see Chapter 13). Look for patterns of weakness that may suggest a diagnosis. In pyramidal weakness – after a stroke, for example – the extensors in the upper limbs are weaker than the flexors, and vice versa in the lower limbs. Myopathies tend to cause proximal weakness and neuropathies often give rise to more distal patterns, while mononeuropathies or radiculopathies lead to discrete focal weakness (such as a foot drop caused by a common peroneal nerve palsy or L5 radiculopathy).

Patients may find it difficult to sustain maximum power for reasons other than weakness, most commonly pain. You need only show that the patient can achieve maximum power briefly to be satisfied that the weakness is not neurological. Very few organic diseases cause power to fluctuate; the fatigable weakness of myasthenia is the chief exception. Wildly fluctuating or sudden 'give-way' weakness suggests a functional explanation. Hoover's sign (Fig. 7.18) refers to the improvement of apparently weak hip extension when it is tested at the same time as contralateral hip flexion (as hip flexion is associated with reflex contralateral hip extension) and is often present in functional leg weakness. This is helpful both diagnostically and therapeutically, as you can show patients that their leg is not actually weak using this sign.

## Deep tendon reflexes

### Anatomy

A tendon reflex is the involuntary contraction of a muscle in response to stretch. It is mediated by a reflex arc consisting of an afferent (sensory) and an efferent (motor) neuron with one synapse between (a monosynaptic reflex). Muscle stretch activates the muscle spindles, which send a burst of afferent signals that lead to direct efferent impulses, causing muscle contraction. These stretch reflex arcs are served by a particular spinal cord segment that is modified by descending upper motor neurons. The most important reflexes are the deep tendon and plantar responses, whereas others, such as abdominal and cremasteric reflexes, are rarely tested and of questionable value. Dermatomal involvement may further help localise a lesion; for example, pain going down one leg with an absent ankle jerk (S1) and sensory loss on the sole of the foot (S1 dermatome) localises to the S1 root, most commonly due to a prolapsed intervertebral disc (sciatica).

'Push down with your right heel'

Weak hip extension

'Lift your left leg'

Hip extension returns to normal

**Fig. 7.18** Hoover's sign.

## Examination sequence (Videos 13C and 13D) ▶

- Ask the patient to lie supine on the examination couch with the limbs exposed. They should be as relaxed and comfortable as possible, as anxiety and pain can cause an increased response.
- Extend your wrist and allow the weight of the tendon hammer head to determine the strength of the blow. Strike your finger that is palpating the biceps and supinator tendons (otherwise

it is painful for the patient) or the tendon itself for the triceps, knee and ankle jerks.
- Record the response as:
  - increased (+++)
  - normal (++)
  - decreased (+)
  - present only with reinforcement (+/-)
  - absent (0).

## Principal (deep tendon) reflexes

- Ensure that both limbs are positioned identically with the same amount of stretch. This is especially important for the ankle reflex, where the ankle is passively dorsiflexed before striking the tendon.
- Compare each reflex with the other side; check for symmetry of response (Figs 7.19 and 7.20).
- Use reinforcement whenever a reflex appears to be absent. For knee and ankle reflexes, ask the patient to interlock their fingers and pull one hand against the other on command ('Have a tug of war with yourself'), immediately before you strike the tendon (Jendrassik's manoeuvre).
- To reinforce upper limb reflexes, ask the patient to make a fist with the contralateral hand and squeeze tightly immediately before you strike the tendon.

## Hoffmann's reflex

- Place your right index finger under the distal interphalangeal joint of the patient's middle finger.
- Use your right thumb to flick the patient's finger downwards.
- Look for any reflex flexion of the patient's thumb.

## Finger jerk (C8)

- Place your middle and index fingers across the palmar surface of the patient's proximal phalanges.
- Tap your own fingers with the hammer.
- Watch for flexion of the patient's fingers.

## Plantar response (S1–2)

- Run a blunt object (orange stick) along the lateral border of the sole of the foot towards the little toe (Fig. 7.21).
- Watch both the first movement of the great toe and the other leg flexor muscles. The normal response is plantar flexion of the great toe (downward movement).

A

B

C

**Fig. 7.19** Testing the deep tendon reflexes of the upper limb. **A** Biceps jerk, C5. **B** Triceps jerk, C7. **C** Supinator jerk, C6.

A                B

**Fig. 7.20 Testing the deep tendon reflexes of the lower limb.** A Knee jerk (note that the patient's legs should not be in contact with each other), L3, L4. B Ankle jerk of the recumbent patient, S1.

**Fig. 7.21** Eliciting the plantar reflex.

- An extensor plantar response (Babinski sign), signifying an abnormal reflex due to an upper motor neuron lesion:
- involves activation of the extensor hallucis longus tendon (not movement of the entire foot, a common 'withdrawal' response to an unpleasant stimulus)
- coincides with contraction of other leg flexor muscles
- is reproducible.

## Abdominal reflexes (T8–12)

- The patient should be supine and relaxed.
- Use an orange stick and briskly but lightly stroke the upper and lower quadrants away from the midline of the relaxed abdomen, watching for a contraction.
- The normal response is contraction of the underlying muscle.

## Cremasteric reflex (L1–2): males only

- Explain what you are going to do and why it is necessary.
- Abduct and externally rotate the patient's thigh.

- Use an orange stick to stroke the upper medial aspect of the thigh.
- Normally the testis on the side stimulated will rise briskly.

Hyperreflexia (abnormally brisk reflexes) is a sign of upper motor neuron damage. Diminished or absent jerks are most commonly due to lower motor neuron lesions. In healthy older people, the ankle jerks may be reduced or lost, and in Holmes-Adie syndrome, myotonic pupils (p. 180) are associated with loss of some reflexes. Isolated loss of a reflex suggests a mono-neuropathy or radiculopathy, such as loss of ankle jerk with L5/S1 lumbosacral disc prolapse compressing the S1 nerve root. Reflex patterns are helpful in localising neurological lesions, and you should know the nerve roots that serve the commonly tested reflexes (see Box 7.9). There are several reflex grading systems, but interobserver agreement is poor; record reflexes as present (and, if so, whether normal, increased or decreased) or absent. Never conclude that a reflex is absent until you have used reinforcement.

An 'inverted' biceps reflex is caused by combined spinal cord and root pathology localising to a specific spinal level. It is most common at the C5/6 level. When elicited, the biceps reflex is absent or reduced but finger flexion occurs. This is because the lesion at the C5/6 level affects the efferent arc of the biceps jerk (C5 nerve root), causing it to be reduced or lost, and also the spinal cord, increasing reflexes below this level (including the finger jerks, C8). It is most commonly seen in cervical spondylotic myeloradiculopathy.

A Hoffmann's reflex and increased finger jerks suggest hypertonia; they may occur in healthy individuals but can be informative if asymmetric. In cerebellar disease, the reflexes may be pendular and muscle contraction and relaxation tend to be slow, but these are neither sensitive nor specific signs.

An extensor plantar response is a sign of upper motor neuron damage and is usually associated with other upper motor neuron signs, such as spasticity, clonus and hyperreflexia. Fanning of the toes is normal and not pathological.

Superficial abdominal reflexes (T8–12) are lost in upper motor neuron lesions but are also affected by lower motor neuron damage affecting thoracic roots T8–12. They are usually absent in the obese and the elderly or after abdominal surgery and are not part of the routine examination.

The cremasteric reflex in males (L1, 2) may be absent on the side of spinal cord or root lesions, but this is of little clinical significance.

## Primitive reflexes

These are present in normal neonates and young infants but disappear as the nervous system matures (p. 350). People with congenital or hereditary cerebral lesions and a few healthy individuals retain these reflexes, but their return after early childhood is often associated with brain damage or degeneration. Although often referred to as frontal, the primitive reflexes (snout, grasp, palmomental and glabellar tap) have little localising value and in isolation are of little significance, but in combination suggest diffuse or frontal cerebral damage (Box 7.10). Unilateral grasp and palmomental reflexes may occur with contralateral frontal lobe pathology. The glabellar tap is an unreliable sign of Parkinson's disease.

## Coordination

Performing complex movements smoothly and efficiently depends on intact sensory and motor function and an intact cerebellum.

### Anatomy

The cerebellum lies in the posterior fossa and consists of two hemispheres with a central vermis. Afferent and efferent pathways convey information to and from the cerebral motor cortex, basal ganglia, thalamus, vestibular and other brainstem nuclei and the spinal cord. In general, midline structures, such as the vermis, influence body equilibrium, while each hemisphere controls ipsilateral coordination.

---

| 7.10 **Primitive reflexes** |
|---|
| **Snout reflex** |
| • Lightly tap the lips. Lip pouting is an abnormal response. |
| **Grasp reflex** |
| • Firmly stroke the palm from the radial side. In an abnormal response, your finger is gripped by the patient's hand. |
| **Palmomental reflex** |
| • Apply firm pressure to the palm next to the thenar eminence with a tongue depressor. An abnormal response is ipsilateral puckering of the chin. |
| **Glabellar tap** |
| • Stand behind the patient and tap repeatedly between their eyebrows with the tip of your index finger. Normally, the blink response stops after three or four taps. |

---

### Examination sequence (Videos 12C and 13E)

Test cerebellar function by assessing stance and gait (p. 151), including tandem gait (walking in a straight line, heel to toe), eye movements (looking for nystagmus; p. 196), speech (dysarthria; p. 139) and limb coordination.

#### Finger-to-nose test

- Ask the patient to touch their nose with the tip of their index finger and then touch your fingertip. Hold your finger at the extreme of the patient's reach (you should make the patient stretch).
- Ask them to repeat the movement between nose and target finger as quickly as possible.
- Make the test more sensitive by changing the position of your target finger. Timing is crucial; move your finger just as the patient's finger is about to leave their nose, otherwise you will induce a false-positive finger-to-nose ataxia.
- Some patients are so ataxic that they may injure their eye/face with this test. If so, use your two hands as the targets or ask the patient to touch their chin rather than nose (Fig. 7.22).

A                                                                     B

**Fig. 7.22 Finger-to-nose test.** **A** Ask the patient to touch the tip of their nose (**1**) and then your finger (**2**). **B** Move your finger from one position to another, towards and away from the patient (**1**), as well as from side to side (**2**).

## Rapid alternating movements

- Demonstrate repeatedly patting the palm of your hand with the palm and then the back of your opposite hand as quickly and regularly as possible.
- Ask the patient to copy your actions.
- Repeat with the opposite hand.
- Alternatively, ask the patient to tap a steady rhythm rapidly with one hand on the other hand or table and 'listen to the cerebellum'; ataxia makes this task difficult, producing a slower, more irregular rhythm than normal.

## Heel-to-shin test

- With the patient lying supine, ask them to lift the heel into the air and to place it on their opposite knee, then slide their heel up and down their shin between knee and ankle (Fig. 7.23).

The finger-to-nose test may reveal a tendency to fall short of or overshoot the examiner's finger (dysmetria or past-pointing). In more severe cases, there may be a tremor (or an increase in amplitude of tremor) of the finger as it approaches the target finger and the patient's own nose (intention or hunting tremor). The movement may be slow, disjointed and clumsy (dyssynergia). The heel-to-shin test is the equivalent test for the legs. It is abnormal if the heel wavers away from the line of the shin. Weakness may produce false-positive finger-to-nose or heel-to-shin tests, so demonstrate that power is normal first.

Dysdiadochokinesis (impairment of rapid alternating movements) is evident as slowness, disorganisation and irregularity of movement. Dysarthria and nystagmus also occur with cerebellar disease. Much less reliable signs of cerebellar disease include the rebound phenomenon (when the displaced outstretched arm may fly up past the original position), pendular reflexes and hypotonia.

In disorders predominantly affecting midline cerebellar structures, such as tumours of the vermis and alcoholic cerebellar damage, the tests described may be normal and truncal ataxia (that is, ataxic gait) may be the only finding. In the most severe cases, this may mean that the patient cannot sit unsupported.

**Fig. 7.23** Performing the heel-to-shin test with the right leg.

Cerebellar dysfunction occurs in many conditions, and the differential diagnosis varies with age and speed of presentation.

## Apraxia

Apraxia, or dyspraxia, is difficulty or inability to perform a task, despite no sensory or motor abnormalities. It is a sign of higher cortical dysfunction, usually localising to the non-dominant frontal or parietal lobes.

### Examination sequence (Video 12D)

- Ask the patient to perform an imaginary act, such as drinking a cup of tea, combing their hair, or folding a letter and placing it in an envelope.
- Ask the patient to copy movements you make with your fingers, such as pointing or making a V sign.
- Ask the patient to copy a geometric figure (interlocking pentagons or cube).
- Ask the patient to put on a pyjama top or dressing gown, one sleeve of which has been pulled inside out.
- Ask the patient to lie on the couch and perform cycling movements with their legs.

The patient may be unable to initiate a task or may perform it in an odd or bizarre fashion. Constructional apraxia (difficulty drawing a figure) is a feature of parietal disturbance. Dressing apraxia, often associated with spatial disorientation and neglect, is usually due to parietal lesions of the non-dominant hemisphere. Patients with gait apraxia have difficulty walking but are able to perform cycling movements on the bed surprisingly well.

## Sensory system

The sensory system comprises the simple sensations of light touch, pain, temperature and vibration, together with joint position sense (proprioception) and higher cortical sensations, which include two-point discrimination, stereognosis (tactile recognition), graphaesthesia (identification of letters or numbers traced on the skin) and localisation.

Detailed examination of sensation is time-consuming and unnecessary unless the patient volunteers sensory symptoms or you suspect a specific pathology, such as spinal cord compression or mononeuropathy. In patients without sensory symptoms, assessing light touch only of all four limbs as a screening process may suffice. It is useful to have a working knowledge of the dermatomal distribution (a dermatome is an area of skin innervated by a single nerve root) and sensory distribution of the more commonly entrapped peripheral nerves (see Figs 7.26 and 7.27 later).

### Anatomy

Proprioception and vibration are conveyed in large, myelinated fast-conducting fibres in the peripheral nerves and in the posterior (dorsal) columns of the spinal cord. Pain and temperature sensation are carried by small, slow-conducting fibres of the peripheral nerves and the spinothalamic tract of the spinal cord. The posterior column remains ipsilateral from the point of entry up to the medulla, but most pain and temperature fibres cross to the contralateral spinothalamic tract within one or two segments of entry to the spinal cord. All sensory fibres relay in the thalamus before sending information to the sensory cortex in the parietal lobe (Fig. 7.24).

## Common presenting symptoms

Sensory symptoms are common, and it is important to discern what the patient is describing. Clarify that, by 'numbness', the patient means lack of sensation rather than weakness or clumsiness. Neuropathic pain (pain due to disease or dysfunction of the PNS or CNS) is often severe and refractory to simple analgesia. Reduced ability to feel pain may be accompanied by scars from injuries or burns (trophic injuries). Sensory symptoms are defined as follows:

- paraesthesia: tingling, or pins and needles
- dysaesthesia: unpleasant paraesthesia
- hypoaesthesia: reduced sensation to a normal stimulus
- analgesia: numbness or loss of sensation
- hyperaesthesia: increased sensitivity to a stimulus
- allodynia: painful sensation resulting from a non-painful stimulus
- hyperalgesia: increased sensitivity to a painful stimulus.

## Examination sequence (Videos 14 and 15)

The aim here is to focus the examination. Look for a sensory level if the history and examination suggest spinal cord pathology; a glove and stocking pattern usually starting distally, caused by a peripheral neuropathy; or sensory disturbance in a specific nerve territory or dermatome. Be guided by the history and the examination findings from the motor system and reflexes. It is useful to ask the patient to map out their area(s) of sensory disturbance if they can.

### Light touch
- While the patient looks away or closes their eyes, use a wisp of cotton wool (or lightly apply your finger) and ask the patient to say 'yes' to each touch.
- Time the stimuli irregularly and make a dabbing rather than a stroking or tickling stimulus.
- Start distally in the feet and hands; work proximally for a neuropathy or focus on a specific nerve distribution or dermatome.

### Superficial pain
- Use a fresh neurological pin, such as a Neurotip, not a hypodermic needle. Dispose of the pin after each patient.
- Explain and demonstrate (on an area of skin not affected by the lesion, such as the sternum) that the ability to feel a sharp pinprick is being tested.
- Map out the boundaries of any area of reduced, absent or increased sensation. Move from reduced to higher sensibility

**Fig. 7.24 The sensory system.** A Main sensory pathways. B Spinothalamic tract: layering of the spinothalamic tract in the cervical region. C represents fibres from cervical segments, which lie centrally; fibres from thoracic, lumbar and sacral segments (labelled T, L and S, respectively) lie progressively more laterally.

– that is, from hypoaesthesia to normal, or normal to hyperaesthesia.

### Temperature
- Touch the patient with a cold metallic object, such as a tuning fork, and ask if it feels cold. More sensitive assessment requires tubes of hot and cold water at controlled temperatures, but this is seldom performed.

## Vibration

Note that ankle oedema may affect perception. Strike the tuning fork on your own palm; an average healthy person should be able to detect the vibration this causes for over 10 seconds.

- Place a vibrating 128-Hz tuning fork over the patient's sternum.
- Ask the patient, 'Do you feel it buzzing?'
- Place the fork on the patient's big toe. If vibration is not felt, then move it proximally to the medial malleolus; if this is not perceived, move to the patella, then the anterior iliac spine, lower chest wall or clavicle. Repeat on the other side. Record the level at which the patient detects vibration.
- Repeat the process in the upper limb. Start at the distal interphalangeal joint of the forefinger; if sensation is impaired, proceed proximally to the metacarpophalangeal joints, wrist, elbow, shoulder and finally clavicle.
- If in doubt as to the accuracy of the response, ask the patient to close their eyes and to report when you stop the fork vibrating with your fingers.

## Joint position sense (proprioception)

- With the patient's eyes open, demonstrate the procedure.
- Lightly hold the distal phalanx of the patient's great toe at the sides. Tell the patient you are going to move their toe up or down, demonstrating as you do so.
- Ask the patient to close their eyes and to identify the direction of small movements in random order.
- If perception is impaired, move to more proximal joints – ankle, knees and hips. Repeat for the other side.
- Repeat for the upper limbs. Start with movements at the distal interphalangeal joint of the index finger; if the movements are not accurately felt, move to the first metacarpophalangeal joint, wrist, elbow and finally shoulder.

## Stereognosis and graphaesthesia

- Ask the patient to close their eyes.
- Place a familiar object, such as a coin or key, in their hand and ask them to identify it (stereognosis).
- Use the blunt end of a pencil or orange stick and trace letters or digits on the patient's palm. Ask the patient to identify the figure (graphaesthesia).

## Sensory inattention

- Only test if sensory pathways are otherwise intact.
- Ask the patient to close their eyes.
- Touch their arms/legs in turn and ask which side has been touched.
- Now touch both sides simultaneously and ask whether the left side, right side or both sides were touched.

## Sensory modalities

In addition to the modalities conveyed in the principal ascending pathways (touch, pain, temperature, vibration and joint position sense), sensory examination includes tests of discriminative aspects of sensation, which may be impaired by lesions of the sensory cortex. Assess these cortical sensory functions only if the main pathway sensations are intact. Consider abnormalities on sensory testing according to whether the lesion (or lesions) is in the peripheral nerve(s), dorsal root(s) or spinal cord, or is intracranial.

## Peripheral nerve and dorsal root

Many diseases affect peripheral nerves, generally resulting in peripheral neuropathies or polyneuropathies. Peripheral neuropathies tend to affect the lower limbs, first starting in the toes. In these length-dependent neuropathies, the upper limbs may become involved once the symptoms extend above the knees. Symptoms first affecting the upper limbs suggest a demyelinating rather than axonal neuropathy or a disease process in the nerve roots or spinal cord. In many cases, touch and pinprick sensation are lost in a 'stocking-and-glove' distribution (Fig. 7.25A). There may also be autonomic involvement, causing symptoms affecting sweating, sphincter control and the cardiovascular system (such as orthostatic hypotension). In mononeuritis multiplex, different nerves in the upper and lower limbs can be affected in a stepwise fashion.

In 'large-fibre' neuropathies, such as Guillain-Barré syndrome, vibration and joint position sense may be disproportionately affected (reduced vibration sense at the ankle may be normal in people over 60 years). Patients may report staggering when they close their eyes during hair washing or in the dark (Romberg sign, p. 152). When joint position sense is affected in the arms, pseudoathetosis may be demonstrated by asking the patient to close their eyes and hold their hands outstretched; the fingers/arms will make involuntary, slow, wandering movements, mimicking athetosis. Reflexes will be absent or depressed. Interpretation of sensory signs requires knowledge of the relevant anatomy of sensory nerves and dermatomes (Figs 7.26 and 7.27). In 'small-fibre' neuropathies, in which pain and temperature sensation are mainly affected, the only finding may be reduced pinprick and temperature sensation; there may also be autonomic involvement. The most common causes worldwide are diabetes mellitus and HIV infection.

## Spinal cord

Traumatic and compressive spinal cord lesions cause loss or impairment of sensation in a dermatomal distribution below the level of the lesion. A zone of hyperaesthesia may be found in the dermatomes immediately above the level of sensory loss. Syringomyelia (a fluid-filled cavity within the spinal cord) can result in a dissociated pattern of altered spinothalamic (pain and temperature) sensation and motor function, with sparing of dorsal column (touch and vibration) sensation.

When one-half of the spinal cord is damaged, Brown–Séquard syndrome may occur. This is characterised by ipsilateral upper motor neuron weakness and loss of touch, vibration and joint position sense, with contralateral loss of pain and temperature (see Fig. 7.25B).

## Intracranial lesions

Brainstem lesions are often vascular, and you must understand the relevant anatomy to determine the site of the lesion. Lower

Light touch causes
exquisite pain
(hyperpathia)

Distribution
of sensory
impairment

Impaired pain and
temperature sense

Impaired light touch
and vibration sense

Pyramidal weakness
Increased tendon reflexes in left
leg and extensor plantar response

A                                                                B

**Fig. 7.25 Patterns of sensory loss.** **A** Length-dependent peripheral neuropathy. **B** Brown-Séquard syndrome. Note the distribution of corticospinal, posterior column and lateral spinothalamic tract signs. The cord lesion is in the left half of the cord.

brainstem lesions may cause ipsilateral numbness on one side of the face (V nerve nucleus) and contralateral body numbness (spinothalamic tract).

Thalamic lesions may cause patchy sensory impairment on the opposite side with unpleasant, poorly localised pain, often of a burning quality.

Cortical parietal lobe lesions typically cause sensory inattention but may also affect joint position sense, two-point discrimination, stereognosis (tactile recognition) and localisation of point touch. Two-point discrimination and touch localisation are not helpful signs, and tests are not performed routinely.

# Peripheral nerves (Video 16)

Peripheral nerves may be damaged individually (mono-neuropathy) or multiply (peripheral neuropathy or mononeuritis multiplex). Certain nerves (median nerve at the wrist, common peroneal nerve at the knee) are particularly prone to compression.

## Median nerve

The medial nerve may be compressed as it passes between the flexor retinaculum and the carpal bones at the wrist (carpal tunnel syndrome). This is the most common entrapment

neuropathy and initially produces sensory symptoms and pain in the hands, occasionally radiating up the arm, typically at night. Carpal tunnel syndrome occurs commonly during pregnancy (Box 7.11).

# Examination sequence (Video 16A)

- Look for wasting of the thenar eminence.
- Test thumb abduction with the patient's hand held palm up on a flat surface. Ask the patient to move their thumb verti-cally against your resistance (abductor pollicis brevis).
- Test opposition by asking the patient to touch their thumb and ring finger together while you attempt to pull them apart (opponens pollicis).
- Test for altered sensation over the hand involving the thumb, index and middle fingers and the lateral half of the ring finger, splitting the ring finger (see Fig. 7.27A). Weakness of distal flexion of the thumb and the index finger indicates the lesion is proximal due to involvement of the anterior interosseus branch of the median nerve.
- Tinel's sign is elicited by tapping the distal wrist crease with the tendon hammer, which may produce tingling in the me-dian nerve territory. Although often used, it has poor sensi-tivity and specificity.
- Phalen's test is forced flexion of the wrist for up to 60 sec-onds to induce symptoms; it also has limited sensitivity and specificity.

7

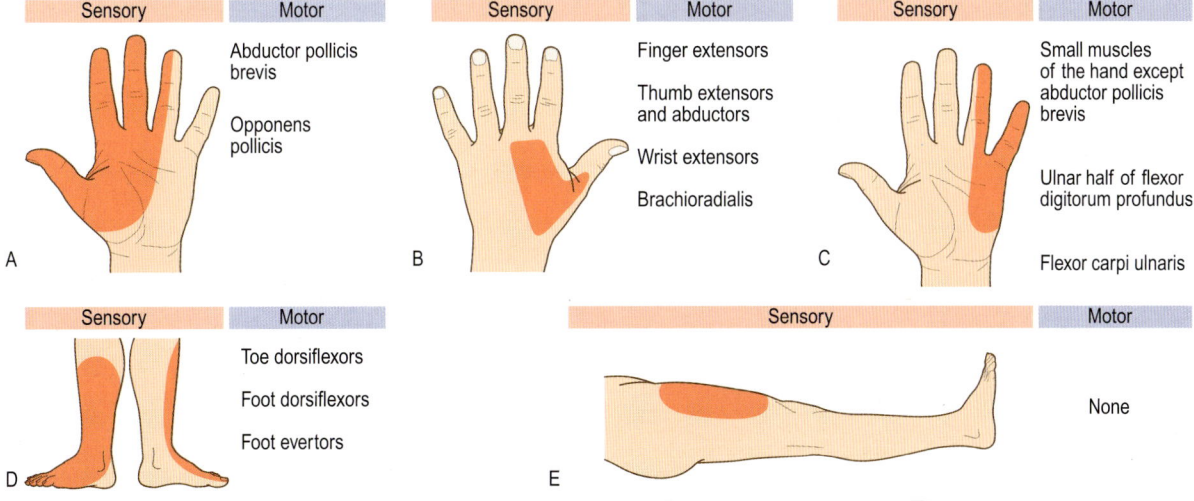

**Fig. 7.26 Dermatomal and sensory peripheral map innervation.** Points (shown in blue) for testing cutaneous sensation of the limbs. By applying stimuli at the points marked, both the dermatomal and main peripheral nerve distributions are tested simultaneously. **A** Anterior view. **B** Posterior view.

**Fig. 7.27 Sensory and motor deficits in nerve lesions.** **A** Median. **B** Radial. **C** Ulnar. **D** Common peroneal. **E** Lateral cutaneous of the thigh.

## 7.11 Common features of carpal tunnel syndrome

- It is more common in women.
- There is unpleasant tingling in the hand.
- It may not observe anatomical boundaries, radiating up the arm to the shoulder.
- Weakness is uncommon; if it does occur, it affects thumb abduction.
- Symptoms are frequently present at night, waking the patient from sleep.
- The patient may hang the hand and arm out of the bed for relief.
- There is thenar muscle wasting (in longstanding cases).
- It is commonly associated with pregnancy, diabetes and hypothyroidism.

## Radial nerve

This may be compressed as it runs through the axilla, in the spiral groove of the humerus (Saturday night palsy) or may be injured in fractures of the humerus. It typically causes wrist drop.

### Examination sequence (Video 16B)

- Test for weakness of brachioradialis (elbow flexor) and the extensors of the arm (triceps). There will also be weakness of wrist and finger extension.
- Look for sensory loss over the dorsum of the hand (see Fig. 7.27B) and loss of triceps tendon jerk.

## Ulnar nerve

The ulnar nerve is most often affected at the elbow by external compression as the nerve is superficial in some individuals and vulnerable to pressure, or by injury, as in elbow dislocation/fracture. Compression usually occurs as the nerve passes through the condylar groove behind the medial epicondyle of the humerus or as it passes through the cubital tunnel.

### Examination sequence (Video 16C)

- Examine the medial elbow, palpating the nerve in the ulnar groove (the most common place of entrapment). Note any scars or other signs of trauma.
- Look for wasting of the interossei (dorsal guttering).
- Test for weakness of finger abduction with the patient's fingers on a flat surface, and ask them to spread the fingers against resistance from your fingers.
- Test adduction by asking them to grip a card placed between their fingers and pulling it out using your own fingers.
- Assess for sensory loss on the ulnar side of the hand, splitting the ring finger (see Fig. 7.27C).

## Common peroneal nerve

The nerve may be damaged by fractures as it winds around the fibular head, or it may be compressed, particularly in thin, immobile patients or as a result of repetitive kneeling, squatting or sitting with the legs crossed at the knees. It typically causes a foot drop.

### Examination sequence

- Test for weakness of ankle dorsiflexion and eversion; test for extension of the big toe (extensor hallucis longus). Inversion and the ankle reflex will be preserved.
- Test for sensory loss over the dorsum of the foot (see Fig. 7.27D).

## Lateral cutaneous nerve of the thigh

This purely sensory nerve may be compressed as it passes under the inguinal ligament, producing paraesthesiae in the lateral thigh (meralgia paraesthetica, 'burning numbness') (see Fig. 7.27E).

### Examination sequence

- Ask the patient to map out the area of disturbance.
- Test for disturbed sensation over the lateral aspect of the thigh. Palpate the abdomen and groin for masses or inguinal lymph nodes.

## Interpretation of the findings

Having completed the history and examination, first decide whether the symptoms are due to neurological disease, a functional neurological disorder or non-neurological causes, remembering that many neurological symptoms (e.g. fasciculation, intermittent sensory disturbance, hypnic jerks) occur in normal people. Try to localise the lesion to a single area of the nervous system if possible (Is the lesion in the CNS or PNS?) and then localise in more detail (e.g. if the lesion is in the PNS, is it in the root, nerves or neuromuscular junction muscle?). Some conditions, like multiple sclerosis, may give rise to multiple symptoms and signs because they involve several lesions; others, like migraine or functional disorders, do not follow strict neurological and anatomical rules.

Having localised the lesion, consider the likely underlying pathology (What is the lesion?). This will depend on the history (e.g. syncope versus seizure; see Box 7.2), and also epidemiology (sudden-onset leg weakness in a 72-year-old man with diabetes and previous angina is unlikely to have the same explanation as a new foot drop in a 20-year-old carpet fitter). Draw up a differential diagnosis and then consider which (if any) investigations are pertinent. Sometimes during the summarising process, it may become clear that there are aspects of the history that have not been adequately addressed. Go back and resolve these areas. Time spent reviewing the history is never wasted; undertaking unnecessary tests, on the other hand, is more than just a waste of time.

Do not place undue emphasis on an isolated sign that fails to fit with the history, such as an apparently isolated extensor plantar response in a patient with typical migraine. It is more likely that this is a false-positive sign due to an inept examination/interpretation of a ticklish patient rather than an indication of underlying pathology.

## Investigations

### Initial investigations

Not all patients require investigation. Most patients with headache, for example, need no tests, but some do (such as a 75-year-old man with new-onset headache and temporal tenderness on examination, who should have urgent measurement of the erythrocyte sedimentation rate and C-reactive protein and a temporal artery biopsy). Unfortunately, the increasing availability of tests means that many patients are investigated unnecessarily, which creates new problems (such as what to do with the incidental finding of an unruptured intracranial aneurysm identified in a patient with migraine). Avoid doing tests because you can or because you do not know what else to do; further investigations should be guided by the history and physical examination. Magnetic resonance imaging (MRI) of the brain may unearth incidental findings of no clinical relevance in up to 20%, depending on age, and there is an irony – usually lost on your patient – in attempting reassurance with a scan only to identify an incidental 'abnormality.' Sometimes a single carefully chosen test is all that is necessary to confirm a diagnosis. For example, a patient with chorea whose father died of Huntington's disease will almost certainly have the diagnosis confirmed with genetic testing without the need for imaging or other tests.

Consider your diagnosis and start with any necessary simple blood tests (such as exclusion of metabolic disturbance, including diabetes); then work upwards. If imaging is required, decide what to image using which modality (computed tomography, MRI, ultrasound or functional imaging) and whether any special sequences or techniques are necessary (like intravenous contrast; Figs 7.28–7.30). Discuss the case with the radiologists if you are unsure. For some PNS disorders, nerve conduction studies and electromyography may be helpful. Electroencephalography is perhaps the most misused test in neurology. Think carefully about whether it will add anything to what you already know; it should not be used to *diagnose* epilepsy. The more invasive tests (lumbar puncture, nerve/muscle/brain biopsy) all require careful consideration and should be guided by specialists. Lastly, knowledge of antibody-mediated and genetic diseases is evolving rapidly, so you may need to have a discussion with the relevant experts about which specialised test might be most appropriate.

### Specific investigations

#### Lumbar puncture

Lumbar puncture is a key investigation in a number of acute and chronic neurological conditions. Always measure the CSF opening pressure (in a lying position, not sitting), using an atraumatic (blunt) needle. CSF is routinely examined for cells, protein content and glucose (compared to simultaneously taken blood glucose); it is also stained and cultured for bacteria. Other specific tests may be carried out, such as analysis for oligoclonal bands, meningococcal and pneumococcal antigens, polymerase chain reaction (PCR) for certain viruses or cytology for malignant cells.

A                        B                        C

**Fig. 7.28 Imaging of the head.** [A] DaTscan showing uptake of tracer (dopamine receptors) in the basal ganglia on cross-section of the brain. [B] Magnetic resonance scan showing ischaemic stroke. T2 imaging demonstrates bilateral occipital infarction and bilateral hemisphere lacunar infarction. [C] Unenhanced computed tomogram showing subarachnoid blood in both Sylvian fissures *(white arrows)* and early hydrocephalus. The temporal horns of the lateral ventricles are visible *(black arrows)*.

A        B        C

**Fig. 7.29** **Imaging of the head.** [A] Computed tomogram (CT) showing a cerebral abscess. [B] Magnetic resonance scan showing multiple sclerosis with white demyelinating plaques. [C] CT scan showing a large meningioma arising from the olfactory groove.

A                B

**Fig. 7.30** T2 magnetic resonance images showing a large left paracentral L4–5 disc protrusion *(arrowed)* compressing the L5 nerve root. [A] Sagittal section. [B] Axial section.

## Neurophysiological tests

Electroencephalography (EEG) records spontaneous electrical activity of the brain, using scalp electrodes. It is employed in the investigation of epilepsy, encephalopathies or dementia. Modifications to standard EEG improve sensitivity and include sleep-deprived studies, prolonged videotelemetry and invasive EEG monitoring.

Electromyography (EMG) involves needle electrodes inserted into muscle. Electrical activity is displayed on an oscilloscope and an audio monitor, allowing the neurophysiologist to see and hear the pattern of activity. Neurogenic and myopathic pathology causes characteristic EMG abnormalities.

Nerve conduction studies involve applying electrical stimuli to nerves and measuring the speed of impulse conduction. They are used for both motor and sensory nerves, and are helpful in diagnosing peripheral nerve disorders, such as nerve compressions or polyneuropathies. They are also helpful is distinguishing between axonal and demyelinating neuropathies, the underlying causes and management of which are very different.

## OSCE example 1: Headache history

Miss Das, 32 years old, presents acutely with a severe global headache, associated with vomiting and feeling dreadful.

### Please take a history from this patient

Confirm:
- Onset – gradual or sudden
- Site – lateralised or global
- Severity
- Aggravating and relieving factors, such as bright light
- Associated symptoms, such as vomiting, photophobia, neck pain or visual disturbance
- Relevant family history.

### Summarise your findings

This 32-year-old woman's headache began gradually last night and is worse today; she has been in bed in a darkened room trying to sleep. She has vomited the analgesic she took. She often has headaches at the time of her period, but this is the worst headache she has ever experienced. She recalls having one or two migraines as a child, and her mother had migraines. She is otherwise well and takes no medication other than the oral contraceptive. The examination is normal, although she looks tired and distressed.

### Suggest a differential diagnosis

The most likely diagnosis is migraine; the headache evolved and worsened over a few hours, with no 'red flags,' on a background of a predisposition to migraine. The differential includes more sinister causes such as meningitis, cerebral venous sinus thrombosis or intracranial haemorrhage, but there are no features to support these. The headache is likely to resolve in the next day or two.

### Suggest initial investigations

She does not need any tests, as there are no features to suggest she needs brain imaging or lumbar puncture to exclude a subarachnoid haemorrhage or meningitis.

## OSCE example 2: Tremor

Mr Anderson, 76 years old, presents with a tremor of his arm.

### Please examine his arms

- Introduce yourself and clean your hands.
- Observe the patient sitting at rest; note any tremor, abnormal postures, facial expression, jaw/chin tremor or drooling.
- Listen to his speech.
- Ask him to raise both arms above his head, then to stretch them out in front of him; observe any tremor on posture.
- Ask him to perform piano-playing movements; look carefully for asymmetry and reduced fine finger movements.
- Assess tone, looking specifically for asymmetry, and cog wheeling or lead pipe rigidity in the affected right arm.
- Test power in shoulder abduction, elbow flexion/extension and finger extension.
- Test upper limb deep tendon reflexes (biceps, supinator and triceps).
- Omit sensory testing, as this is unlikely to add anything.
- Test finger-to-nose movements.
- Ask him to walk, observing what happens to the tremor and right arm swing.
- Thank the patient and clean your hands.

### Summarise your findings

The patient has an asymmetric pill-rolling rest tremor of the right arm, which briefly disappears on movement but quickly returns (re-emergent tremor). He also has a tremor affecting the jaw/chin. There is a lack of facial expression; drooling; monotonous, hypophonic speech; bradykinesia (reduced fine finger movements, difficulty with repetitive movements); increased tone with cog wheeling; and loss of right arm swing and increased tremor when walking, with short stride length.

### Suggest a diagnosis

These findings are typical of Parkinson's disease.

### Suggest initial investigations

A diagnosis of Parkinson's disease is usually based on the clinical features, and investigation is unnecessary. In selected cases, structural imaging (MR or CT) to rule out the rare mimics of Parkinson's disease or functional imaging (DaTscan) may be appropriate. Blood tests are rarely helpful, but a strong family history may precipitate consideration of genetic testing.

## Integrated examination sequence for the nervous system

A complete neurological examination is demanding for both doctor and patient and in many cases will not be necessary. The history will dictate a more targeted examination, and time spent on the history is always more productive than an amateur neurological examination.

### Cranial nerve examination

- Ask about sense of smell and taste (I).
- Assess visual acuity (using a Snellen chart) and visual fields (by confrontation) (II).
- Observe pupils and test pupillary reactions bilaterally: direct and consensual (II).
- Observe both eyes in the neutral position. Are they orthotropic (both pointing in the same direction)? Test eye movements, observing for completeness of movement in pursuit and looking for nystagmus (III, IV, VI).
- Test facial sensation (V) and corneal reflex (V and VII).
- Observe for facial asymmetry and test facial muscles of the upper and lower parts of the face (VII).
- Perform a bedside test of hearing (VIII).
- Assess speech, swallow and palatal movement (IX, X, XI).
- Inspect the tongue and assess movement (XII).

### Neurological examination of the upper limbs

- Expose the upper limbs, ensuring maintenance of dignity and privacy; request a chaperone if appropriate.
- Inspect for wasting, fasciculations, abnormal movements and contractures/other deformities.
- As a screening test, ask the patient to hold their arms out (palms up) and close their eyes. Watch for pronator drift.
- Assess tone.
- Test muscle power: shoulder abduction (axillary nerve C5), elbow flexion (musculocutaneous nerve, C5, C6) and extension (radial nerve, C7), finger extension (posterior interosseus nerve, C7), index finger abduction (ulnar nerve, T1), little finger abduction (ulnar nerve, T1) and thumb abduction (median nerve, T1).
- Assess reflexes at biceps (C5), triceps (C7) and supinator (brachioradialis, C6).
- Test coordination with finger-to-nose test and look for dysdiadokinesia.
- Test sensory modalities: pinprick, temperature, vibration sense, joint position sense.

### Neurological examination of the lower limb

- Undress the patient to expose both lower limbs fully, ensuring maintenance of dignity and privacy; request a chaperone if appropriate.
- Carry out a general inspection, noting walking aids and other associated neurological signs, such as facial droop or ipsilateral arm flexion.
- If the patient is able to do so, ask them to stand and walk so that you can assess stance and gait. Assess tandem gait.
- Inspect both legs, noting any scars, muscle wasting or fasciculations, abnormal postures or movements.
- Assess tone at the hip, knee and ankle. Test for ankle clonus.
- Test muscle power. As a simple screen, assess hip flexion (iliofemoral nerve, L1, 2) and extension (sciatic, L5/S1), knee flexion (sciatic, S1) and extension (femoral, L3, 4), and ankle plantar flexion (tibial, S1, 2) and dorsiflexion (deep peroneal, L4, 5).
- Assess reflexes at the knee (L3) and ankle (S1), comparing sides. Test the plantar response.
- Test coordination via heel-to-shin tests.
- Test sensory modalities: pinprick, temperature, vibration and joint position sense. Map out any symptomatic areas of disturbed sensation.

Shyamanga Borooah
Naing Latt Tint

# The visual system

**Anatomy and physiology 170**
Eye 170
Extraocular muscles 170
Refractive elements of the eye 171
Visual pathway 172
Pupillary pathways 172

**Patient history 173**
Common presenting symptoms 173
Past ocular history 178
Past medical history 178
Drug and allergy history 178
Family history 178
Social history 178

**The physical examination  179**

General examination 179
Visual acuity 179
Orbit and periorbital examination 180
Pupils   180
Visual fields 182
Ocular alignment and eye movements 183
Ophthalmoscopy 184
Retinopathies 186

**Investigations 188**

**Ophthalmic examination and COVID-19 189**

**OSCE example 1: Gradual visual loss 191**

**OSCE example 2: Double vision 191**

**Integrated examination sequence for ophthalmology 192**

## Anatomy and physiology

The eye lies in the bony orbit of the skull and is covered by the eyelid, which protects it from foreign bodies and keeps the anterior surface moist by maintaining the tear film. The upper lid is elevated by two muscles: the levator palpebrae superioris, innervated by cranial nerve III; and Müller's muscle, innervated by sympathetic nerves. The orbicularis oculi muscle closes both upper and lower eyelids and is innervated by cranial nerve VII.

The orbit also contains the six extraocular muscles responsible for eye movement; the lacrimal gland; blood vessels; autonomic nerve fibres; and cranial nerves II, III, IV and VI, cushioned by orbital fat (Fig. 8.1).

The conjunctiva is a thin mucous membrane lining the inner aspects of the eyelids and the anterior surface of the eyeball. It is reflected at the superior and inferior fornices. The conjunctiva is coated in a tear film that protects and nourishes the ocular surface.

### Eye

The eyeball is normally approximately 25 mm in diameter and comprises three layers (see Fig. 8.1). These are:

- Outer fibrous layer: this includes the white sclera and the clear cornea anteriorly.
- Middle vascular layer (uveal tract): anteriorly, this consists of the ciliary body and the iris, and posteriorly, the choroid.

- Inner neurosensory layer (retina): the retina is a thin layered structure responsible for transducing light to neurological signals. There are two main types of photoreceptors: cones function maximally under photopic (light) conditions and enable colour vision while rods are primarily used in scotopic (dark) conditions. Cones are concentrated at the centre of the retina and are most highly concentrated at the centre of the macula (the fovea). Photoreceptors transduce light into neuronal signals that pass via bipolar cells and ganglion cells to the nerve fibre layer of the inner retina before entering the optic nerve.

### Extraocular muscles

Six extraocular muscles are responsible for eye movement: (1) the superior rectus, (2) medial rectus, (3) lateral rectus, (4) inferior rectus, (5) superior oblique and (6) inferior oblique. Each muscle is responsible for a specific vector of eye movement (Fig. 8.2). They work together to move the eye in other directions.

Cranial nerve III innervates the superior rectus, medial rectus, inferior oblique and inferior rectus muscles. Cranial nerve IV innervates the superior oblique muscle, and cranial nerve VI innervates the lateral rectus muscle. The cranial nerves originate in the midbrain and pons and pass through the cavernous sinus (Fig. 8.3). Examining for eye movement deficits reveals cranial nerve deficits. For instance, a complete loss of cranial nerve III results in a loss of function of the superior rectus,

**Fig. 8.1** Cross-section of the eye and orbit (sagittal view).

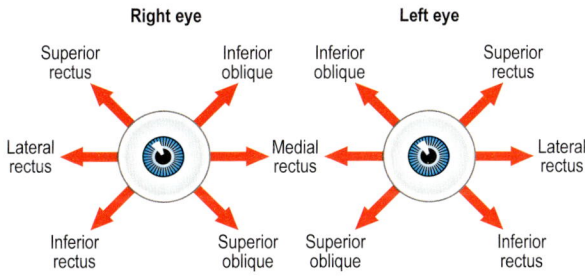

**Fig. 8.2 Control of eye movements.** The direction of displacement of the pupil by normal contraction of a particular muscle can be used to work out which eye muscle is paretic.

inferior oblique, medial rectus and inferior rectus. If cranial nerves IV and VI are intact, the lateral rectus and the superior rectus continue to pull the eye inferiorly and laterally. This gives the classical 'down and out' resting position of an eye with cranial nerve III palsy.

## Refractive elements of the eye

The major refractive elements of the eye are the tear film, cornea and crystalline lens. The cornea accounts for approximately two-thirds of the refractive power of the eye while the lens provides additional controllable refraction, allowing light to focus onto the retina at varying focal lengths. When light is precisely focused at the retina, the eye is called emmetropic (Fig. 8.4A). When the focus point falls behind the retina, the result is hypermetropia (see Fig. 8.4B, long-sightedness). When the focal point is in front of the retina, the result is myopia (see Fig. 8.4C, short-sightedness). These refractive errors can be corrected with lenses or partially corrected with a pinhole (see Fig. 8.4D).

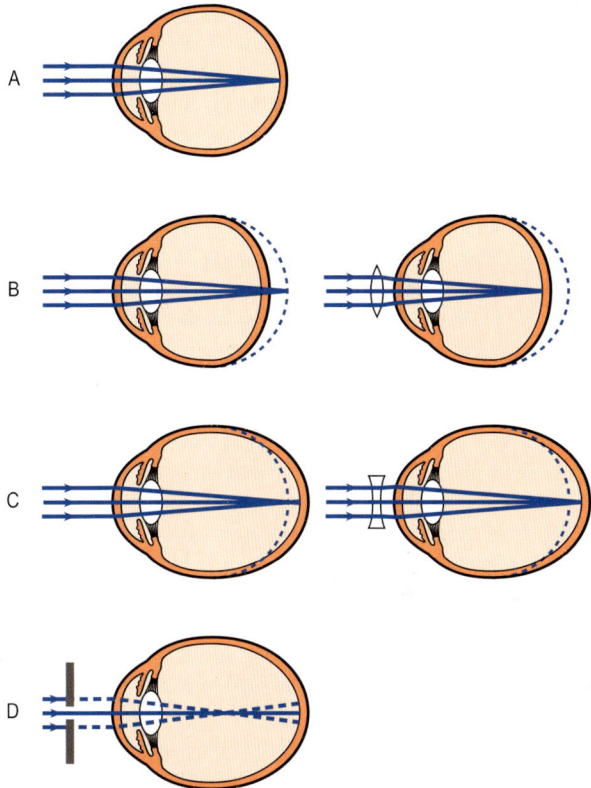

**Fig. 8.4 Normal and abnormal refraction by the cornea and lens.** [A] Emmetropia (normal refraction). Cornea and lens focus light on the retina. [B] Hypermetropia (long-sightedness). The eye is too short and the image focuses behind the retina. A convex (plus) lens focuses the image on the retina. [C] Myopia (short-sightedness). The eye is too long and the image focuses in front of the retina. A concave (minus) lens focuses the image on the retina. [D] Myopia corrected using a pinhole, which allows only rays not requiring refraction to pass to the retina.

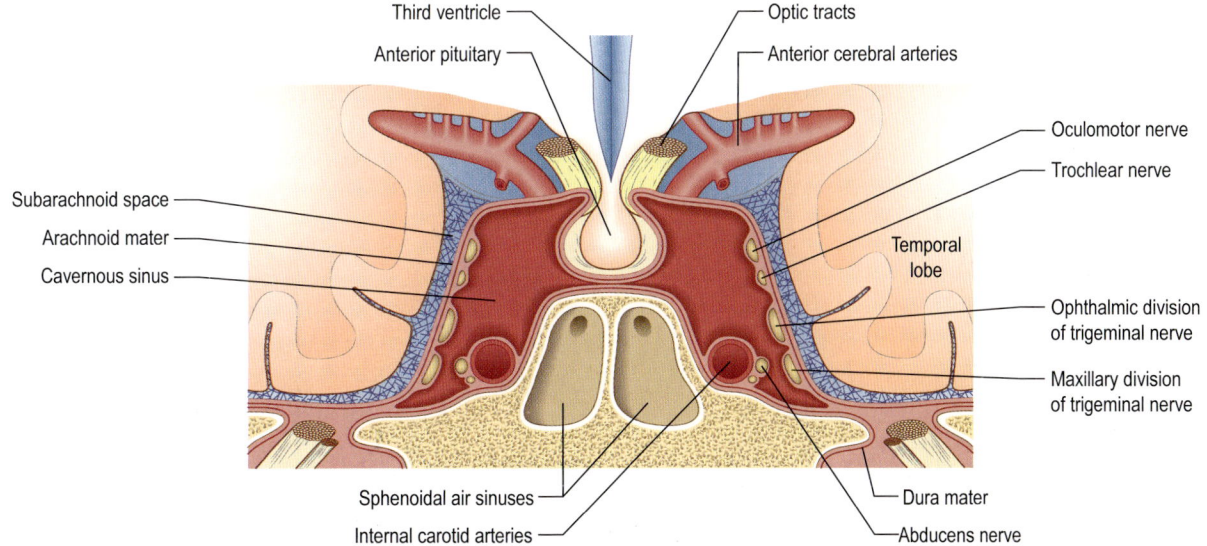

**Fig. 8.3 Cavernous sinus (coronal view).** Neuroanatomy of cranial nerves III, IV and VI.

## Visual pathway

The visual pathway connects the eye to the brain and consists of the retina, optic nerve, optic chiasm, optic tracts, lateral geniculate bodies, optic radiations and visual cortex. Deficits in the visual pathway lead to specific field defects (Fig. 8.5).

## Pupillary pathways

The pupil controls the amount of light entering the eye. The intensity of light determines the pupillary aperture through autonomic reflexes. The parasympathetic pathway controlling pupillary constriction is shown in Fig. 8.6A; the sympathetic pathway controlling pupillary dilatation is shown in Fig. 8.6B.

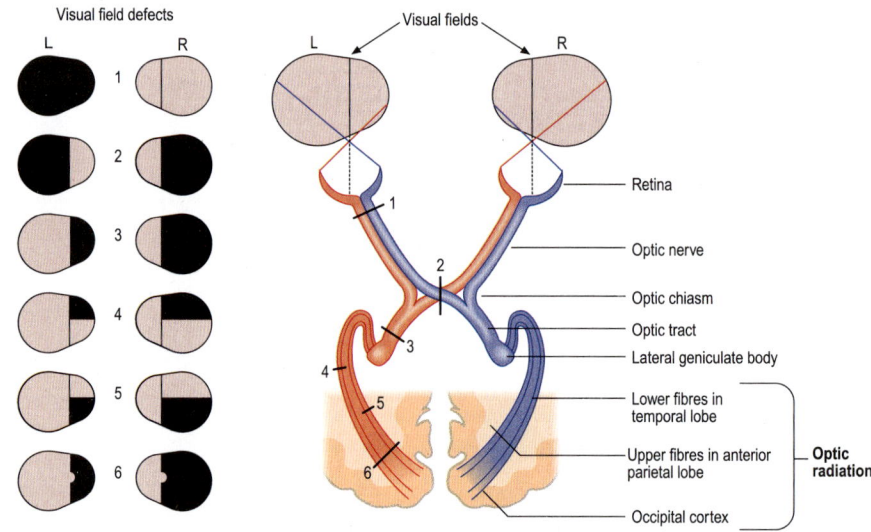

**Fig. 8.5 Visual field defects.** 1, Total loss of vision in one eye because of a lesion of the optic nerve. 2, Bitemporal hemianopia due to compression of the optic chiasm. 3, Right homonymous hemianopia from a lesion of the optic tract. 4, Upper right quadrantanopia from a lesion of the lower fibres of the optic radiation in the temporal lobe. 5, Lower quadrantanopia from a lesion of the upper fibres of the optic radiation in the anterior part of the parietal lobe. 6, Right homonymous hemianopia with sparing of the macula due to a lesion of the optic radiation in the occipital lobe.

**Fig. 8.6 Pupillary innervation.** A Parasympathetic pathway. B Sympathetic pathway.

# Patient history

To guide your ophthalmic history, remember the anatomy of the eye. This will enable you to work from 'front to back' to include or exclude differential diagnoses.

## Common presenting symptoms

Start the ophthalmic history with open questions so the patient can describe their symptoms in their own words. Use the patient's description to inform more directed questions later.

Specific visual symptoms prompt specific sets of directed questions. The most common symptoms are described below.

### Change in vision

Loss or reduced vision is the most common change. Patients often describe blurred vision. Ocular disease is the most common cause of a change in vision. Any intraocular condition that prevents light from activating retinal photoreceptors or the signal from photoreceptors reaching the optic nerve can cause altered vision. Rarely, damage to the extraocular visual pathway may cause altered vision (see Fig. 8.5).

When patients present with a change in vision, ask:

- *Was the onset of visual change sudden or gradual?* Sudden or gradual visual loss leads to specific differential diagnoses (Box 8.1 and Fig. 8.7; Box 8.2 and Fig. 8.8). If sudden, then enquire about possible causes (e.g. trauma, foreign body, chemical injury).

- *Does the vision change affect one or both eyes?* Sudden onset of bilateral change in vision suggests a post chiasmal cause.
- *Is the change in vision associated with any additional features (e.g. haloes, flashing lights, floaters, distortion, discharge, red eye, pain)?* Haloes are bright or rainbow-coloured rings seen surrounding a light source. They occur when there is corneal oedema and are most commonly associated with angle-closure glaucoma. Flashes and floaters result from a disturbance of the vitreous–retinal interface, most commonly due to a posterior vitreous detachment. This usually occurs with age as the vitreous degenerates, liquefies and peels away from the retina, resulting in floaters. Detachment sometimes causes retinal traction, resulting in flashing lights. More rarely, posterior vitreous detachment causes a retinal tear (releasing cells seen as floaters), which may progress to retinal detachment with visual field loss. Distortion is most commonly seen in diseases of the macula, such as age-related macular degeneration, epiretinal membrane, vitreous traction on the retina or central serous retinopathy.
- *Does the change in vison affect part or whole of the visual field?* If part, which part? Specific types of visual field loss may point to retinal disease, such as macular degeneration, optic nerve disease such as glaucoma or visual pathway defects (see Fig. 8.5).

### Pain

Ask:

- *Can you describe the nature of the pain?*
- *How severe is it?*
- *Did anything cause the pain?*

**Fig. 8.7 Common causes of an acute change in vision.** **A** Central retinal vein occlusion. **B** Retinal detachment. Elevation of the retina around the 'attached' optic disc; the retina may even be visible on viewing the red reflex. **C** Central retinal arterial occlusion. **D** Herpes simplex virus keratitis. **E** Wet age-related macular degeneration. **F** Swollen optic nerve head in acute optic neuritis.

## 8.1 Common causes of an acute change in vision

| Cause | Clinical features | Cause | Clinical features |
|-------|-------------------|-------|-------------------|
| **Unilateral** | | | |
| Giant cell arteritis | • Painless loss of vision<br>• Age >50 years<br>• Weight loss<br>• Loss of appetite, fatigue<br>• Jaw or tongue claudication<br>• Temporal headache<br>• Pale or swollen optic disc<br>• RAPD | Vitreous haemorrhage | • Painless loss of vision<br>• Risk in proliferative diabetic retinopathy<br>• History of flashing lights or floaters may precede haemorrhage in posterior vitreous detachment<br>• Poor fundus view on examination<br>• Reduction or loss of the red reflex<br>• Usually no RAPD if retina is intact |
| Central retinal vein occlusion | • Acute, painless loss of vision<br>• May have RAPD if severe<br>• Greater risk if hypertensive<br>• Haemorrhages, exudates and tortuous retinal veins (Fig. 8.7A) | Wet age-related macular degeneration | • Sudden painless loss of central vision<br>• Age >55 years<br>• Increased risk in smokers<br>• Haemorrhage at the macula (Fig. 8.7E) |
| Retinal detachment | • Painless loss of vision<br>• Association with flashing lights or floaters<br>• History of a curtain coming across vision<br>• Myopic patients at greater risk<br>• RAPD if macula is involved<br>• Pale raised retina usually with a retinal tear (Fig. 8.7B) | Anterior ischaemic optic neuropathy | • Painless loss of upper or lower visual field<br>• Increased risk in vasculopaths<br>• Examination may reveal optic disc swelling |
| Central retinal arterial occlusion | • Acute, painless loss of vision<br>• Carotid bruit may be heard<br>• RAPD<br>• Increased risk in vasculopaths<br>• Examination: pale retina with a cherry red spot at the fovea (Fig. 8.7C) | Optic neuritis/retrobulbar neuritis | • Visual reduction over hours<br>• Usually aged 20–50<br>• Pain exacerbated by eye movement<br>• RAPD<br>• Reduced colour sensitivity<br>• Swollen optic disc in optic neuritis (Fig. 8.7F) or normal appearances in retrobulbar neuritis |
| Corneal disease | • Usually painful<br>• Foreign body sensation<br>• Corneal opacity may be visible (e.g. Fig. 8.7D) | Amaurosis fugax | • Painless loss of vision for minutes<br>• History of cardiovascular disease<br>• May have associated atrial fibrillation or carotid bruit<br>• Normal ocular examination |
| **Bilateral** | | | |
| Giant cell arteritis | • Painless loss of vision<br>• Age >50 years<br>• Weight loss<br>• Loss of appetite, Fatigue<br>• Jaw or tongue, claudication<br>• Temporal headache<br>• Pale or swollen optic disc | Cerebral infarct | • May have associated headache and/or neurological signs<br>• Usually specific field defects dependent on how the visual pathway is affected (Fig. 8.5)<br>• Normal fundus examination<br>• If post chiasmal visual pathway affected, bilateral visual field abnormalities |
| Raised intracranial pressure | • Headache<br>• Often asymmetric<br>• Pulsatile tinnitus<br>• Swollen optic discs | Migraine | • Gradually evolving usually bilateral visual loss<br>• Vision loss is usually preceded by visual aura<br>• Normal ocular examination<br>• Ocular examination: normal<br>• Vision usually returns to normal after hours |

*RAPD*, Relative afferent pupillary defect (p. 182).

• *Is pain exacerbated or relieved by anything?*
• *Any other associated features (e.g. change in vision, red eye, discharge, photophobia, watering eye)?*

The most common cause of a painful eye is corneal irritation from a foreign body or infection. The cornea is one of the most highly innervated parts of the body. When the corneal nerves are activated, a patient experiences foreign body sensation, pain, reflex watering and photophobia. There are, however, many other causes of a painful eye. Box 8.3 summarises the history and examination findings associated with a painful eye.

**Fig. 8.8 Common causes of a gradual loss of vision.** $\boxed{A}$ Cataract. $\boxed{B}$ Altered red reflex in cataract. $\boxed{C}$ Dry age-related macular degeneration. $\boxed{D}$ Compressive optic neuropathy. Optic nerve sheath meningioma causing optic disc pallor and increased disc cupping with sparing of the outer optic nerve rim. $\boxed{E}$ Retinitis pigmentosa: a triad of optic atrophy, attenuated retinal vessels and pigmentary changes. The latter typically start peripherally with an associated ring scotoma and symptoms of night blindness.

### 8.2 Common causes of a gradual loss of vision

| Cause | Clinical features |
|---|---|
| Refractive error | • No associated symptoms<br>• Normal ocular examination<br>• Vision can be improved by pinhole (Fig. 8.4D) |
| Glaucoma | • Usually bilateral but asymmetric loss of visual field<br>• Cupped optic discs on examination |
| Cataract | • Gradual clouding of vision<br>• May be associated with glare<br>• Usually seen in the elderly<br>• Examination: clouding of the pupil and altered red reflex (Fig. 8.8A and B) |
| Diabetic maculopathy | • History of diabetes<br>• Central vision reduced or distorted<br>• Haemorrhages and exudates at the macula on examination (Fig. 8.17A) |
| Compressive optic neuropathy | • Gradual unilateral loss of vision<br>• Pale optic disc on examination (Fig. 8.8D) |
| Retinitis pigmentosa | • Gradual bilateral symmetric loss of peripheral visual field<br>• Nyctalopia (poor vision in dim light)<br>• Family history<br>• Examination: bone spicule fundus, attenuated blood vessels and waxy optic disc (Fig. 8.8E) |
| Dry age-related macular degeneration | • Gradual loss of central vision<br>• Usually bilateral<br>• Examination: drusen, atrophy and pigmentation at the macula (Fig. 8.8C) |

## Red eye

The eye is covered in a network of vessels in the conjunctiva, episclera and sclera. Ciliary vessels are also found around the cornea. Dilatation or haemorrhage of any of these vessels can lead to a red eye. Additionally, in uveitis, acute angle-closure glaucoma and corneal irritation, the ciliary vessels around the cornea become more prominent ('ciliary flush'). The appearance is distinct from conjunctivitis, in which there is classically a relative blanching of vessels around the cornea.

Ask:

• *Is there any pain or photophobia?*
• *Is vision affected? If so, how?*
• *Has there has been any recent trauma or foreign body?*
• *Is the eye itchy?*
• *Is there any discharge? If so, what kind (e.g. watery, sticky, clear, yellow)?*
• *Has there been any recent contact lens use?*

Box 8.4 summarises the features of the common causes of a red eye on history and examination.

## Double vision (diplopia)

Ask:

• *Does the double vision occur with one eye open or only with both eyes open?* Binocular double vision is caused by an

### 8.3 Causes and distinguishing features of a painful eye

| Cause | History | Examination |
|---|---|---|
| Blocked gland on lid | • Pain on lid | • Tenderness to touch<br>• Redness and swelling of lid |
| Corneal foreign body | • Foreign body sensation<br>• Watery eye<br>• Photophobia | • Foreign body visible or found under the eyelid |
| Corneal infection | • Foreign body sensation<br>• Photophobia | • Red eye<br>• Corneal ulcer, (highlighted with fluorescein stain (Fig. 8.7D)<br>• White infiltrates may be visible |
| Scleritis | • Severe pain disturbing sleep<br>• Association with recent infection, surgery or rheumatic disease | • Eye is sore to touch<br>• Scleral injection |
| Angle-closure glaucoma | • Constant pain around eye<br>• Acute reduction in vision<br>• Haloes seen around lights<br>• Associated nausea and vomiting | • Fixed mid-dilated pupil, hazy cornea and usually a cataract |
| Conjunctivitis | • Clear or purulent discharge<br>• Vision usually unaffected | • Red eye |
| Uveitis | • Floaters<br>• Blurry vision<br>• Photophobia | • Ciliary flush |
| Optic neuritis | • Reduction in vision<br>• Reduction in colour sensitivity<br>• Constant pain, worsened by eye movement | • Swollen disc in optic neuritis (Fig. 8.7F), normal disc in retrobulbar neuritis |
| Orbital cellulitis | • Constant ache around eyes<br>• Reduced vision<br>• Double vision<br>• Associated with recent infection/sinus blockage | • Conjunctival chemosis and injection<br>• Restricted eye movements<br>• Severe cases: visual reduction with RAPD |
| Thyroid eye disease | • Symptoms of hyperthyroidism (p. 222)<br>• Sore, gritty eyes<br>• Double vision | • Lid retraction<br>• Proptosis<br>• Restricted eye movements<br>• Conjunctival injection or chemosis (Fig. 10.2B) |

*RAPD,* Relative afferent pupillary defect (p. 182).

imbalance in eye movement between the eyes. Monocular diplopia results from intraocular disease in one eye.

- *What is the character of the double vision* (e.g. are images seen side by side, one above the other or at an angle)?
- *Has there been any recent trauma?*

In binocular diplopia, test the eye movements (Fig. 8.9) and use your knowledge of the function of the extraocular muscles (see Fig. 8.2) to work out which cranial nerve is affected.

The causes of double vision are summarised in Box 8.5 and Figs. 8.10 and 8.11.

### Discharge

Ocular discharge results from either an increase in production or a decrease in drainage from the ocular surface. Irritation of corneal nerves activates cranial nerve V(I), resulting in a reflex tearing response.

Tears normally drain from the ocular surface through the puncta, small openings to the medial end of the upper and lower eyelid, into the nasolacrimal duct, which opens below the inferior turbinate in the nasal cavity. Consequently, blockage of tear drainage or an abnormal lid position can also result in excessive discharge.

Ask:

- *Is the discharge clear or opaque? If opaque, what colour?*
- *Is the discharge watery or sticky?*
- *Is the discharge associated with any other features (e.g. pain, foreign body sensation, red eye or itchiness)?*

The clinical features of different types of eye discharge are summarised in Box 8.6.

## 8.4 Common causes and distinguishing features of a red eye

| Causes | History | Examination |
|---|---|---|
| Allergic conjunctivitis | • Itchy eyes<br>• Clear discharge<br>• May be seasonal | • Conjunctival injection |
| Viral conjunctivitis | • Watery discharge<br>• Possible itch<br>• Usually bilateral | • Swollen conjunctiva<br>• Gland swelling and follicles under lid |
| Bacterial conjunctivitis | • Purulent discharge<br>• Pain | • Purulent discharge |
| Trauma | • History of trauma | • May reveal subconjunctival haemorrhage or injection |
| Acute angle-closure glaucoma | • Acute reduction in vision<br>• Pain<br>• Blurring of vision<br>• Haloes seen around lights<br>• Nausea | • Fixed, mid-dilated pupil with a hazy cornea |
| Acute anterior uveitis | • Gradual onset of pain<br>• Photophobia<br>• Floaters | • Ciliary flush |
| Episcleritis | • Red eye without pain<br>• Vision not affected | • Focal or diffuse injection<br>• Possible association with a nodule |
| Scleritis | • Focal or diffuse injection<br>• Vision may be affected<br>• Association with recent infection, surgery or rheumatic disease<br>• Severe pain disturbing sleep | • Eye painful to touch |
| Dry eyes | • Gritty or burning sensation<br>• Watery eyes | • Corneal fluorescein staining |
| Subconjunctival haemorrhage | • No pain<br>• Vision unaffected | • Mildly raised conjunctiva with a bleed |
| Corneal ulcer/abrasion | • Vision usually reduced<br>• Foreign body sensation<br>• Photophobia<br>• Watering | • Ulcer seen on fluorescein staining (Fig. 8.7D)<br>• May be associated with a white corneal infiltrate |
| Orbital cellulitis | • Usually affects young children<br>• Recent intercurrent viral illness<br>• Vision may be affected<br>• Possible double vision | • Reduced vision and colour vision<br>• Proptosis<br>• Eye movement restriction<br>• In severe cases, RAPD |
| Thyroid eye disease | • Chronic red eyes<br>• Sore, gritty sensation<br>• Foreign body sensation<br>• Double vision | • Lid retraction<br>• Proptosis<br>• Conjunctival injection and chemosis (see Fig. 10.2B) |

*RAPD,* Relative afferent pupillary defect (p. 182).

## Swollen eyes

The orbit is enclosed by bone on all sides, except anteriorly. As a result, orbital swelling can lead to the anterior displacement of the globe and proptosis.

Ask if the swelling is:

• *Unilateral or bilateral?*
• *Acute or gradual in onset?*
• *Associated with pain?*
• *Associated with itch or irritation?*
• *Associated with double vision?*

Box 8.7 summarises the common causes of swollen eyes.

| 8.5 Causes of double vision |
|---|
| **Monocular** |
| • High astigmatism |
| • Corneal opacity |
| • Abnormal lens |
| • Iris defect |
| **Binocular** |
| • Myasthenia gravis (p. 190) |
| • VI nerve palsy (Fig. 8.10) |
| • IV nerve palsy |
| • III nerve palsy (Fig. 8.11) |
| • Internuclear ophthalmoplegia |
| • Thyroid eye disease (see Fig. 10.2A,B) |
| • Complex or combined palsy |
| • Severe orbital cellulitis or orbital inflammation |

## Past ocular history

Ask the patient whether they have any known ophthalmic conditions. Enquire specifically about amblyopia (a reduction in vision in one eye from childhood), as this may limit best-corrected visual acuity. Check whether the patient normally wears glasses or contact lenses, and ask about the last time they had their eyes checked for refractive correction. Also ask about any previous eye surgery, as this may also limit vision.

## Past medical history

Focus on systemic diseases that can affect the eyes. In particular:

- a history of diabetes or hypertension, especially in the context of visual loss
- thyroid disease in the context of red, swollen eyes or double vision.

## Drug and allergy history

The eyes may, rarely, be affected by medication prescribed for other medical conditions. For example, oral glucocorticoids can cause glaucoma and cataract. Additionally, medication prescribed to treat eye conditions (such as beta-blocker eye drops) can aggravate systemic conditions like asthma.

Ask about a history of allergies, including hay fever, if the patient has itchy or red eyes.

## Family history

Several eye diseases can be inherited. Ask specifically about a history of glaucoma in first-order relatives. The most common

| 8.6 Common causes of increased discharge from the eyes | |
|---|---|
| **Causes** | **Clinical features** |
| Bacterial conjunctivitis | • Red eye<br>• Yellow or green sticky discharge<br>• Vision usually unaffected |
| Viral conjunctivitis | • Red eye<br>• Clear, watery discharge<br>• Occasionally itchy eyes<br>• Vision usually unaffected<br>• Ocular examination: conjunctival chemosis and injection |
| Blocked tear duct | • White eye<br>• Clear, colourless tearing<br>• Possible occluded punctum<br>• Possible malposition of the lid |
| Trichiasis/ foreign body | • Foreign body sensation<br>• Clear discharge<br>• Positive fluorescein staining |
| Allergic conjunctivitis | • Red eyes<br>• Itchy eyes<br>• Clear discharge<br>• Possible history of hay fever or atopy, or recent start of eye medication |
| Blepharitis | • Mild injection of lids<br>• Deposits on lashes |
| Poor tear film/ dry eyes | • Constant tearing<br>• Watering increased in the wind<br>• Improvement with tear supplements<br>• Ocular examination: early break-up time ($<3$ seconds) with fluorescein staining of tear film |

Mendelian inherited eye disease is retinitis pigmentosa (see Fig. 8.8E).

## Social history

Visual impairment can affect activities of daily living. If vision is reduced, ask about:

- Daily activities requiring vision, such as reading, television, sport, hobbies and driving.
- Effects on occupation. Certain professions are required to meet specific visual standards, including drivers of heavy goods vehicles and pilots.
- Smoking and alcohol. These may affect retinal vascular disease and optic nerve function.

## 8.7 Common causes of periorbital swelling and proptosis

| Category | Causes | Clinical features |
|---|---|---|
| Infective | • Orbital cellulitis | • Rapid onset unilateral swelling and erythema<br>• Pyrexia and signs of sepsis<br>• Restricted ocular movements<br>• Optic nerve compression in severe cases |
| Inflammatory | • Granulomatous polyangiitis<br>• Idiopathic orbital inflammatory disease<br>• Vasculitis | • Proptosis with conjunctival redness and swelling is seen.<br>• Restricted eye movements<br>• In severe cases optic nerve compression |
| Neoplastic | • Orbital tumours<br>• Lymphoma<br>• Metastases | • Gradual onset unilateral periocular swelling.<br>• Not inflamed and rarely any erythema<br>• Restricted eye movements |
| Systemic | • Thyroid eye disease | • Bilateral asymmetric periocular swelling<br>• Associated proptosis and reduced ocular movements.<br>• Most cases are not associated with inflammation |
| Vascular | • Caroticocavernous fistula<br><br>• Orbital varices | • Unilateral proptosis with conjunctival swelling<br>• Reduced ocular movements<br>• Patient aware of a bruit<br>• Intermittent unilateral swelling and proptosis associated with Valsalva manoeuvre<br>• Occasional pain |
| Pseudoproptosis | • Ptosis<br>• Severe viral conjunctivitis<br>• Myopia<br><br>• Lid retraction | • Asymmetric palpebrae aperture<br>• Bilateral conjunctival injection and oedema associated with serous discharge<br>• Significant difference in prescription between the two eyes<br>• The eye with the more minus prescription will look more prominent<br>• Difference in height of palpebral aperture between the two eyes |

## The physical examination (Video 17)

### General examination

Carefully and systematically examine:

- posture and gait
- head position
- facial asymmetry and dysmorphic features
- eyelid position and periocular skin
- position and symmetry of gaze (any squint/strabismus?).

### Visual acuity

The assessment of visual acuity is mandatory in all ophthalmic patients. Each eye must be tested separately. The most commonly used method of testing distance visual acuity uses a Snellen chart, which displays a random selection of letters in diminishing font sizes in successive lines. Ask patients to wear their distance spectacles if they usually require them. Near/reading spectacles should be worn only when testing reading vision.

## Examination sequence (Video 17A)

- Use a backlit Snellen chart positioned at 6 metres and dim the room's lighting.
- Cover one eye and ask the patient to read the chart from the top down until they cannot read any further. Repeat for the other eye.
- If the patient cannot see the largest font, reduce the test distance to 3 metres, then to 1 metre if necessary.
- If they still cannot see the largest font, document instead whether they can count fingers, see hand movement or just perceive the difference between light and dark.
- On the Snellen chart, lines of decreasing font size are numbered according to the distance in metres that a person with normal vision could read them. Express visual acuity as the distance at which text is read (usually 6 metres) over the number of the smallest font line read correctly on the chart. For example, 6/60 means that the patient sees at 6 metres the font size that is seen at 60 metres by a person with normal vision.
- If the patient cannot read down to line 6 (6/6), place a pinhole directly in front of the eye (with the patient keeping their usual spectacles on, if used) to correct any residual refractive error (see Fig. 8.4D).
- If visual acuity is not improved with a pinhole, this indicates the presence of eye disease not related to the refractive apparatus alone, such as amblyopia, or retinal or optic nerve pathology.

- Assess near vision with a similar test using text of reducing font size held at a comfortable reading distance. It is important to consider the need for reading spectacles in patients over the age of 40 years because of presbyopia (age-related deterioration in near vision).

**Fig. 8.9** **Testing the six positions of gaze.** Sit facing the patient, 1 metre away. Perform the test with both eyes open. Hold a pen torch or target in front of the patient and move it to the six positions of gaze *(blue arrows)*. Ask if they see the target as double.

## Orbit and periorbital examination

### Examination sequence (Video 17B)

- Observe the face and orbit for asymmetry and any obvious abnormalities, including swelling or erythema.
- Look for abnormalities in the position of the lids, such as ptosis (Box 8.8).
- Look for asymmetry in the position of the eyeballs. Eyeball protrusion (proptosis) is best detected by examining the head from above.
- Palpate around the orbital rim and orbit and look for any masses.
- Check eye movements (see Fig. 8.9).
- Use an ophthalmoscope (Fig. 8.12) to look for optic disc swelling from compression.

### Pupils (Video 17C)

Inspect first for squint and ptosis, which may reveal the cause of abnormal pupils. Examine pupil shape and symmetry. Physiological anisocoria (unequal pupil size) is seen in 20% of the population.

### Anisocoria

Assess which is the abnormal pupil.

**Fig. 8.10** **L sided sixth nerve palsy causing weakness of the lateral rectus.** The patient is attempting to look left.

A

B

**Fig. 8.11** **Third nerve palsy.** A Complete ptosis in R third nerve palsy. B The same patient looking down and left. The affected R eye is unable to adduct or depress and remains slightly abducted due to unopposed action of the lateral rectus. *From Forbes CD, Jackson WF. Color Atlas of Clinical Medicine. 3rd ed, Edinburgh: Mosby; 2003.*

### Examination sequence

- With the patient fixating at a point in the distance, increase and decrease the illumination and look for any change in the degree of anisocoria.

If the degree of anisocoria is greater in brighter lighting, then it is the larger pupil that is abnormal; if it is more pronounced in dim lighting, the smaller pupil is the abnormal one. An equal degree of anisocoria in all levels of lighting indicates physiological anisocoria.

### Direct and consensual light reflex

### Examination sequence

- With the patient fixating on a point in the distance and in ambient lighting, shine a bright light from the temporal side into one eye and look for constriction of the ipsilateral pupil.

### 8.8 Causes of eyelid ptosis

| Cause | Diagnosis | Associated distinguishing features |
|---|---|---|
| Neurogenic | Horner's syndrome | Ptosis, miosis, eye movement spared (Fig. 5.10, p. 96) |
| | Cranial nerve III palsy | Dilated pupil, eye movements affected (Fig. 8.11) |
| Myogenic | Myotonic dystrophy | Frontal balding, sustained handgrip |
| | Chronic progressive external ophthalmoplegia | Bilateral ptosis and impairment of eye movements, often without diplopia, sparing of pupil reflexes |
| | Oculopharyngeal dystrophy | History of swallowing abnormalities |
| Neuromuscular junction | Myasthenia gravis | History of variable muscular fatigue |
| Mechanical | Eyelid tumour | Evident on inspection |
| | Eyelid inflammation/infection | Evident on inspection |
| | Trauma | Scarring/history of trauma |
| Degenerative | Levator aponeurosis degeneration | Often unilateral, eye movement normal |
| | Long-term contact lens wear | History of contact lens use |

- To test the consensual reflex, assess the pupil response in the contralateral pupil when light is directed towards the ipsilateral pupil. Repeat for the other pupil.

## Relative afferent pupillary defect

Relative afferent pupillary defect (RAPD) is an important clinical sign that occurs when disease of the retina or optic nerve reduces the response of the eye to a light stimulus. Testing for RAPD is an extension of the direct and consensual light responses.

## Examination sequence

- Use a bright light source.
- Maintain the light on each eye for a minimum of 3 seconds, then move it between the eyes briskly.

In normal patients, the RAPD test results in symmetrical constriction of both pupils. If an RAPD is present, the pupil will dilate when the light is shone in the affected eye.

### 8.9 Causes of anisocoria

| Dilated pupil | Clinical features |
|---|---|
| • Physiological | • Normal pupillary reactions<br>• Seen in 20% of population |
| • Cranial nerve III palsy | • Pupil dilated and unresponsive to light<br>• Partial or complete ptosis<br>• Eye deviated down and out |
| • Trauma | • History of significant ocular trauma<br>• Rupture of pupillary sphincter muscle sometimes seen on slit lamp examination |
| • Adie's tonic pupil | • Slow to react to light<br>• Vermiform movement of the iris seen on slit lamp examination.<br>• Constricts with dilute pilocarpine (0.125%) |
| • Pharmacological treatment with a dilating agent (e.g. tropicamide or atropine) | • Unreactive dilated pupil, resolves with time<br>• History of pharmacological administration |
| **Constricted pupil** | |
| • Physiological | • Normal pupil reactions<br>• Seen in 20% of population |
| • Horner's syndrome | • Partial ptosis<br>• Ipsilateral anhidrosis<br>• Anisocoria more pronounced in dim light |
| • Mechanical (e.g. secondary to posterior synechiae in iritis or trauma) | • History of trauma or iritis<br>• Pupil margin may be irregular |
| • Late-stage Adie's tonic pupil | • Small slowly reactive pupil<br>• History of the pupil being the larger one in the past |
| • Pharmacological treatment with a constricting agent (e.g. pilocarpine) | • Unreactive constricted pupil that will dilate with time<br>• History of pharmacological administration |

## Accommodation

## Examination sequence

- Ask the patient to look at a distant target and then to quickly focus on a close fixation target (do not use a light source).
- The pupils will constrict on near gaze.
- Failure to constrict to light but constriction on near gaze is referred to as light-near dissociation.

There are many causes of a dilated or constricted pupil (Box 8.9).

## Horner's syndrome

Horner's syndrome results from a dysfunction of the sympathetic supply to the eye. The sympathetic innervation of the eye originates in the hypothalamus and emerges in the root of the neck before innervating the pupil (see Fig. 8.6B). Damage at any point along this pathway will result in Horner's syndrome. On examination, the pupil will be constricted (loss of sympathetic dilator tone) and have a partial ptosis resulting from denervation of Müller's muscle in the upper eyelid (see Fig. 5.10, p. 96). There may also be anhidrosis (loss of sweating) on the affected side.

The diagnosis of Horner's syndrome can be confirmed by administering drops of the alpha-2 adrenergic agonist apraclonidine to both eyes. This causes reversal of pupil constriction in the affected eye and no change in the unaffected eye. This results in a reduction of anisocoria (difference in pupil size between the eyes). Causes of Horner's syndrome include demyelination, neck trauma/surgery, apical lung tumour (Pancoast tumour) and carotid artery dissection.

## Adie's pupil

Adie's pupil is a dilated pupil that responds poorly to both light and accommodation. With time, however, the affected pupil can become constricted. Adie's pupil is thought to result from parasympathetic pathway dysfunction in the orbit leading to a lack of pupil constriction. It typically affects young women and is benign. When associated with diminished Achilles tendon reflexes, it is referred to as Holmes-Adie syndrome.

## Argyll Robertson pupil

Argyll Robertson pupils are bilaterally small and irregular and react to near accommodation but not to light ('light-near dissociation'). These pupils are classically the result of neurosyphilis; however, they can also occur in diabetes mellitus, severe optic nerve disease and midbrain lesions.

## Visual fields

The normal visual field extends 160 degrees horizontally and 130 degrees vertically. The physiological blind spot is located approximately 15 degrees temporal to the point of visual fixation and represents the entry of the optic nerve head into the eye.

The aim of the visual field examination is to test the patient's visual fields against your own (assuming that you have normal visual fields). The visual field can be tested using the fingers for gross examination. Finer examination is performed using a hatpin.

 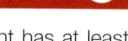
- Check visual acuity and ensure that the patient has at least enough vision to count fingers.
- Sit about 1 metre away directly facing the patient and at the same height.
- With your eyes and the patient's eyes open, ask the patient to look at your face and comment on whether they have any difficulty seeing parts of your face.
- Ask the patient to keep looking straight at your face. Test each eye separately. Ask the patient to close or cover one eye and look directly at your opposite eye; you should similarly close your contralateral eye.
- Bring an extended finger in from the periphery towards the centre of the visual field. For an accurate assessment of the patient's fields, it is vital that the testing finger is always kept in a plane exactly halfway between yourself and the patient. Wiggle your fingertip and ask the patient to say when they first see it (Fig. 8.12). If the patient fails to notice your finger when it is clearly visible to you, their field is reduced in that area.
- Test all four quadrants separately, testing each eye separately.
- More subtle visual field defects can be elicited using a small white hatpin or a white Neurotip. With the patient looking directly at your eye, bring the white target in from the periphery to the centre (always in the plane halfway between you and the patient). Ask the patient to say when they first see the target.

**Fig. 8.12 Confrontation visual field testing.** Sit facing the patient, 1 metre away. To compare your visual field (assumed normal) with the patient's, present a white target or your fingers at a point equidistant between yourself and the patient in the periphery. Bring the target inwards in the direction of the blue arrows, asking the patient to alert you when they first see it. Test each eye separately.

**Fig. 8.13 Testing the central visual field.** Sit facing the patient, 1 metre away. Present a red target at a point equidistant between yourself and the patient in the periphery, starting when you can first see the target as red. Bring the target inwards in the direction of the blue arrows, asking the patient to alert you when they first see the target as red. Test each eye separately.

- Check all four quadrants, testing each eye separately.
- To assess very early visual field loss, repeat the same test using a red hatpin or a red Neurotip (Fig. 8.13).
- It is important to show the patient the red target and ask them to report what colour they see. A dull or pale red suggests colour desaturation, which may indicate optic nerve dysfunction.
- When testing each quadrant with a red target, be sure to explain to the patient that they should say when they first see that the target is red and not when they first see it. The target may be visualised before they appreciate the red colour.
- To test the blind spot, place a red-tipped target equidistant between the patient and yourself at the visual fixation point.
- Move the target temporally from central fixation until it disappears.
- Once you have identified the blind spot, move the target slowly up and down and side to side until it reappears. This allows you to compare the patient's blind spot with yours.

## Ocular alignment and eye movements

The eyes normally move in the same direction (conjugate motion) in all positions of gaze except during convergence. Any misalignment is referred to as a squint (strabismus). Squints are described as manifest (tropia) if present with both eyes open or latent (phoria) if revealed only by covering one eye. In addition, they can be concomitant (where the angle of squint remains the same in all positions of gaze) or incomitant (where the angle of squint deviation is greatest in a single position of gaze). The latter is commonly the result of extraocular muscle paralysis.

## Detection of a squint

### Examination sequence

- Sit directly facing the patient, approximately 1 metre away and at a similar height.
- Check visual acuity as part of the examination.
- Look for any abnormal head posture, such as head tilts (seen in cranial nerve IV palsy) or head turns (cranial nerve VI palsy). These signs may be subtle.
- Hold a pen torch directly in front of the patient and instruct them to look at the light. Observe the reflection of the light on the cornea in relation to the pupil. The reflections should be symmetrical between the two eyes. Ask the patient if they see a single or double light. If they see double, this may indicate the presence of a squint, but not seeing double does not exclude a squint. If the reflection is on the nasal aspect of the pupil in one eye, this suggests that the eye is deviated outwards and is described as an exotropia.
- To confirm the presence of a squint, perform the cover/uncover test:
  - Ask the patient to look at the pen torch at all times and then cover one eye.
  - Look at the uncovered eye for any movement. It may be helpful to repeat this several times.
  - Inward movement of the uncovered eye suggests that it was positioned abnormally outwards and is described as an exotropia (divergent manifest squint).
  - Conversely, if the eye moves outwards when the contralateral eye is covered, this suggests that it was abnormally positioned inwards and is described as an esotropia (convergent manifest squint).
  - Repeat the cover/uncover test for the other eye.
- Failure of an eye to move despite an obvious corneal light reflex may indicate that the eye has such poor vision that it cannot take up fixation or else it is restricted from moving.
- The alternating cover test involves covering the eyes alternately and quickly while the patient is fixated on the pen torch. Leave the cover on each eye for about 2 seconds but move between the eyes in less than 1 second. The movement is repeated multiple times. This test will help to elicit latent squint.

8

## Ocular movements

### Examination sequence (Video 17E)

- In the same seating position, ask the patient to look at a target or pen-torch light about 50 cm away.
- Ask them to say if and when they experience diplopia.
- Starting from the primary position, move the target in the six positions of gaze (see Fig. 8.9) and up and down.
- If diplopia is present, ask whether this is horizontal, vertical or a combination of the two, and determine where the image separation is most pronounced.
- Look for nystagmus and determine whether the eye movement is smooth.

Interpretation of any limitation of excursion is made by reference to the functions of the extraocular muscles (see Fig. 8.2).

## Oculocephalic (doll's-eye) reflex

- This reflex is the ability of the eyes to remain fixated while the head is turned in the horizontal plane (Fig. 8.14). An impaired reflex indicates a brainstem abnormality. This test can also be performed on an unconscious patient to check for brainstem function.

### Examination sequence

- With the patient supine, ask them to look at your face. Gently turn their head from side to side, noting the eye movements.

## Nystagmus

Nystagmus is continuous, uncontrolled movement of the eyes. Biphasic or jerk nystagmus is the most common type. It is characterised by slow drift in one direction, followed by fast correction/recovery in the opposite direction. The direction of the fast phase designates the direction of the nystagmus. If there are equal oscillations in both directions, it is called pendular nystagmus.

Nystagmus commonly indicates vestibular disease, and the examination sequence and differential diagnosis are covered on page 197.

### Ophthalmoscopy

The direct ophthalmoscope is a useful tool for assessing both the anterior and the posterior segments of the eye. Pharmacological pupil dilatation is essential for a thorough fundus examination, though the optic disc can be examined sufficiently without dilatation.

**Fig. 8.14 Oculocephalic reflex.** Move the head in the horizontal plane. Note that the eyes move in the opposite direction to head movement.

## Examination sequence (Video 17F) ▶

- Ask the patient to look at a distant target.
- When using the direct ophthalmoscope to examine the patient's right eye, hold the ophthalmoscope in your right hand and use your right eye to examine. Hold it in your left hand and use your left eye to examine the patient's left eye.
- Place your free hand on the patient's forehead and brow, as this will steady the head and improve your proprioception when moving closer to the patient with the ophthalmoscope.
- Rotate the ophthalmoscope lens to +10. This will allow a magnified view of the anterior segment. Examine the eyelid margins, conjunctiva, cornea and iris. If epithelial defects are suspected, fluorescein can be administered and a cobalt blue filter used to highlight the epithelial defect.
- To examine the fundus, dial the lens back to 0.
- With your hand on the forehead and the brow, use the ophthalmoscope to see the red reflex (red light reflected off the retina) at a distance of about 10 cm. When the red reflex is in focus, look for opacities and determine whether they are static or mobile. Static opacities are usually due to cataract, while mobile opacities indicate vitreous opacities.
- Slowly move the ophthalmoscope closer to the patient almost to the point that your forehead touches your thumb, which is resting on the patient's forehead and brow (see Fig. 8.15).
- Turn the lens dial until the optic disc comes into focus; if it does not, focus on a blood vessel.

- The optic disc can usually be located easily; if not, follow a blood vessel centrally (in the direction opposite to its branches) to locate it.
- Examine the optic disc, paying particular attention to its shape, colour, edges and cup size.
- Follow each blood-vessel arcade and examine each of the retinal quadrants.
- To examine the macula, ask the patient to look directly at the light.

The normal retina looks different in Asian and Caucasian patients (Fig. 8.16).

**Fig. 8.15 Ophthalmoscopy.** Ask the patient to focus on a distant target. To examine the left eye, use your left eye to look through the ophthalmoscope and left hand to hold it, index finger on the wheel. Hold the patient's head with your free hand. Gradually move in to visualise the optic disc. Rotate the wheel to obtain a clear, focused image.

A

B

**Fig. 8.16 The normal fundus.** A Caucasian. B Asian.

## 8.10 Causes of optic disc swelling

| Unilateral | Clinical features |
|---|---|
| Optic neuritis | • Onset over 1–2 weeks days, recovery starts after 1–3 months<br>• Reduced colour vision<br>• Orbital pain<br>• Relative afferent pupillary defect<br>• Associated with multiple sclerosis |
| Arteritic anterior ischaemic optic neuropathy | • Sudden onset visual loss<br>• Associated features of giant cell arteritis (scalp tenderness, jaw claudication, fever)<br>• Optic disc rapidly becomes chalky white |
| Non-arteritic anterior ischemic optic neuropathy | • Age usually >50<br>• Usually causes loss of superior or inferior hemi-field<br>• Painless<br>• Associated cardiovascular risk factors (hypertension, diabetes, poor lipid profile) |
| Lyme disease | • Recent tick bite<br>• Erythema chronicum migrans<br>• Associated uveitis, cardiovascular or neurological deficits |
| *Bartonella* infection | • Recent history of cat scratch<br>• Pustules at site of cat contact<br>• New lymphadenopathy<br>• May show neuroretinitis with subretinal fluid and a macular star |
| Other neuroretinitis (syphilis, tuberculosis, toxocara, sarcoid) | • May present with unilateral optic disc swelling and macular star without systemic features of disease |
| Optic nerve glioma | • History of neurofibromatosis type 1<br>• May be associated with proptosis |
| Optic nerve head metastases | • History of malignancy |
| **Bilateral** | **Clinical features** |
| Papilloedema | • Headache<br>• Nausea/vomiting<br>• Pulsatile tinnitus<br>• Transient visual obscurations<br>• Enlarged blind spot on testing |
| Optic disc drusen | • Usually asymptomatic<br>• Yellow or white bodies at the optic disc head<br>• Confirmed by autofluorescence imaging or ocular ultrasound |
| Diabetic papillitis | • History of diabetes<br>• Vision relatively spared compared to optic disc examination<br>• Diabetic retinopathy (microaneurysms, exudates, blot haemorrhages and neovascularisation) |
| Pseudopapilloedema in hypermetropes | • Positive refraction<br>• Short axial length confirmed by ocular ultrasound |
| Hypertensive papillopathy | • History of hypertension<br>• Headaches<br>• Blurred vision<br>• Hypertensive retinopathy (cotton wools spots, hard exudates and flame shaped haemorrhages) |

Swelling of the optic disc is a very important clinical sign. Causes of unilateral and bilateral optic disc swelling, and their distinguishing features, are summarised in Box 8.10.

A variety of diseases that can damage the optic nerve cause an abnormally pale optic disc (see Fig. 8.8D). The differential diagnosis of optic disc pallor is summarised in Box 8.11.

## Retinopathies

Diabetes mellitus leads to a wide range of important abnormalities in the retina, which are summarised in Fig. 8.17.

Hypertension also results in retinal changes (Fig. 8.18). The retinal arteries are effectively arterioles. Chronic arteriosclerosis

## 8.11 Differential diagnosis of optic disc pallor

| Type | Clinical features |
|---|---|
| **Inherited** – Congenital optic atrophy | • Present from birth or young age<br>• May have family history |
| **End-stage glaucoma** | • Progressive loss of visual fields with reduced acuity<br>• Optic disc cupped in addition to pallor |
| **Trauma** | • History of trauma resulting in decreased vision |
| **Compressive**<br>Orbital cellulitis | • Acute proptosis with periocular inflammation and swelling<br>• Pyrexia and signs of sepsis<br>• Reduced ocular movements<br>• Unilateral proptosis<br>• Reduced vision in late stages |
| Orbital neoplasm | • Progressive proptosis with gradual loss of vision<br>• May have reduced ocular movements<br>• History of malignancy (e.g. breast, prostate, lymphoma) |
| Thyroid eye disease | • Unilateral or bilateral proptosis<br>• Lid retraction, unable to close eye<br>• Conjunctival chemosis and hyperaemia (acute disease)<br>• Reduced eye movements<br>• Reduced vision (late) |
| **Neurological**<br>End-stage papilloedema | • Bilateral optic disc swelling with pallor.<br>• Headache and nausea<br>• Visual obscuration not uncommon<br>• Occasionally pulsatile tinnitus.<br>• Enlarged blind spot |
| **Metabolic**<br>Diabetes mellitus<br>Nutritional deficiency<br>Toxic amblyopia<br>Ethambutol<br>Sulphonamide | • Metabolic and nutritional causes are bilateral<br>• Associated with gradual decline in vision<br>• Detailed history and examination essential |
| **Vascular**<br>Central retinal artery occlusion (CRAO) | • History of sudden painless loss of vision<br>• Associated cardiovascular disease, including atrial fibrillation or carotid bruit<br>• Occasionally results from giant cell arteritis |
| Anterior ischaemic optic neuropathy (AION) | • Sudden painless loss of vision.<br>• May show altitudinal loss of visual field (either top or bottom half of visual field reduced) |
| **Inflammatory**<br>Meningitis | • History of headache<br>• Photophobia<br>• Severely ill with signs of sepsis |
| Retrobulbar neuritis | • Retrobulbar pain worsened by eye movement<br>• Slight or profound visual loss – usually recovers over weeks<br>• Optic nerve changes not immediate; take time to develop |

**8**

leads to vessel-wall thickening and hyalinisation that appears as widening of the arterioles, arteriovenous nicking where arterioles cross venules and a 'silver and copper wiring' light reflex.

More acute changes can also be seen in malignant hypertension. Various grading systems have been created to try to link retinal findings to end-organ damage. The retinal appearances in hypertension are classified using the Modified Scheie classification:

• Grade 0: no changes

• Grade 1: barely detectable arteriolar narrowing
• Grade 2: obvious retinal arteriolar narrowing with focal irregularities
• Grade 3: grade 2 plus retinal haemorrhages, exudates, cotton-wool spots or retinal oedema
• Grade 4: grade 3 plus optic disc swelling.

Inherited retinopathies result from a wide range of genetic mutations. The most common inherited retinopathy is retinitis

**Fig. 8.17 Retinal abnormalities in diabetes mellitus.** [A] Diabetic maculopathy with yellowish hard exudates near the fovea and macular blot haemorrhages. [B] Background diabetic retinopathy: dot and blot haemorrhages and a cotton wool spot in the macula. [C] Severe non-proliferative diabetic retinopathy: dot and blot haemorrhages in all quadrants, intraretinal microvascular abnormalities superotemporally and scattered cotton wool spots. [D] Proliferative diabetic retinopathy with extensive neovascularisation at the disc. [E] Proliferative diabetic retinopathy: vitreous haemorrhage and circinate hard exudates in the macula. [F] Treated proliferative diabetic retinopathy: pigmented scars from panretinal laser photocoagulation and persistent haemorrhage in a regressed neovascular complex inferotemporally.

pigmentosa, which causes symptoms of nyctalopia (difficulty seeing in dim light) and tunnel vision. Examination reveals a pale optic disc, attenuated arterioles and bone-spicule retinal pigmentation (see Fig. 8.8E).

## Investigations

Appropriate initial tests for a variety of common presenting eye problems are summarised in Box 8.12.

**Fig. 8.18 Hypertensive retinopathy.** **A** Increased reflectance, giving a silver wiring appearance to the arteriole *(arrow)*. **B** Focal arteriolar narrowing *(double arrows)* seen in grade 2 disease. **C** Exudates and flame haemorrhages in grade 3 retinopathy. **D** Signs of malignant hypertension in grade 4 disease with a swollen optic disc and macular exudate.

## Ophthalmic examination and COVID-19

Ophthalmic examination requires close proximity, infectious patients may be asymptomatic and infection can occur through not only the oral and nasal mucosa but also the ocular surface. Ophthalmic examination, therefore, poses a relatively high risk of transmission of COVID-19 to both patient and examiner. To minimise risk, every patient should be treated as potentially COVID-19 positive and staff should be tested for infection regularly.

Precise advice on personal protective equipment will depend on local prevalence and policy, but the following is a reasonable minimum:

- Wash hands with soap and water or 70% alcohol before and after seeing patients.
- Wipe down equipment before and after each encounter.
- Patients should wear three-ply surgical face masks covering their mouth and nose. Patients known to be infected should wear N95 masks or equivalent to prevent aerosolised spread.
- Clinical examiners should wear a three-ply surgical face mask covering their mouth and nose and goggles or face shields to prevent ocular surface transmission.
- Minimise the time spent in proximity to patients.

## 8.12 Investigations

| Investigation | Indication |
|---|---|
| **Clinic tests** | |
| Refraction | Refractive error, cataract and corneal disorders |
| Fluorescein staining | Corneal epithelial disease |
| Schirmer's test | Dry eyes, Sjögren's syndrome |
| Nasolacrimal duct washout | Watery eyes |
| Blood pressure | Hypertensive retinopathy, retinal vein occlusion |
| Bacterial culture and sensitivity | Bacterial conjunctivitis |
| Viral swab | Viral conjunctivitis |
| **Blood tests** | |
| Erythrocyte sedimentation rate, C-reactive protein | Vasculitis, including giant cell arteritis |
| Antinuclear antibody | Systemic lupus erythematosus |
| Rheumatoid factor | Scleritis |
| Fasting glucose | Diabetic retinopathy |
| Anti-acetylcholinesterase receptor antibody | Myasthenia gravis |
| Quantiferon | Uveitis |
| Serum angiotensin-converting enzyme | Uveitis |
| Human immunodeficiency virus serology | Vasculitis, uveitis |
| Syphilis serology | Unexplained pathology and uveitis/vasculitis |
| Thyroid function tests | Thyroid eye disease |
| **Radiology** | |
| Chest x-ray | Sarcoidosis/tuberculosis |
| Orbital ultrasound | Incomplete fundal view |
| Optical coherence tomography | Macular disease, glaucoma |
| Fundus fluorescein angiography | Diabetic retinopathy, retinal vein occlusion |
| Computed tomography of brain and sinuses | Orbital cellulitis, thyroid eye disease, intracranial tumours, orbital compressive disease |
| Magnetic resonance imaging of brain and orbits | Pituitary tumour, compressive lesion |
| Carotid Doppler ultrasound | Carotid artery stenosis in ocular ischaemic syndrome or retinal artery occlusion |
| **Invasive tests** | |
| Lumbar puncture | Idiopathic intracranial hypertension, inflammatory orbital neuropathies |
| Temporal artery biopsy | Giant cell arteritis |

## OSCE example 1: Gradual visual loss

Mrs. Rahman, 55 years old, presents with a gradual reduction of vision over the last 6 months in both eyes. She says that she also has distortion in her vision when she is looking at straight lines. In addition, she feels constantly thirsty and is passing urine frequently.

### Please examine this patient's eyes

- Introduce yourself and clean your hands.
- Perform a general inspection, looking for any signs of squint. Check the bedside for any clues that the patient wears glasses.
- Assess visual acuity using a Snellen chart at the appropriate distance.
- Examine the eyes, looking for any conjunctival injection, chemosis or swelling.
- Dim the room lights.
- Test the pupillary light reflexes.
- Ideally, dilate the pupils at this stage.
- Test the red reflex in each eye.
- Dial the fundoscope to +10 and examine the anterior portion of the eye, including the lens.
- Dial the fundoscope back to 0 and examine the fundus, looking at the disc and superior, nasal, inferior and temporal fundus.
- Finally, inspect the macula.
- Thank the patient and clean your hands.

### Summarise your findings

Visual acuity is reduced to 6/18 in both eyes, and fundoscopy reveals multiple retinal haemorrhages and exudates which include changes at the macula.

### Suggest a diagnosis

The most likely diagnosis is diabetic retinopathy with diabetic maculopathy.

### Suggest initial investigations

Urine dipstick, fasting blood glucose, and blood pressure.

### Advanced level comments

Diabetic macular oedema is the most common cause of reduced vision in diabetic patients. It may result in distortion, making straight lines appear bent.

## OSCE example 2: Double vision

Mr. Penrose, 75 years old, presents with double vision that has increased rapidly over the last week. He says that not only do objects appear side by side but also that the two images are separated vertically. He feels that his eyelid is drooping on his left side. He constantly has to lift his eyelid to see out of his left eye.

### Please examine the patient's eye movements

- Introduce yourself and clean your hands.
- Perform a general inspection: look for ptosis and squint, and examine the bedside for any spectacles that may contain a prism.
- Inspect visual acuity in each eye.
- Dim the room lights.
- Test pupillary light reflexes.
- Test all eye movements for ophthalmoplegia.
- Examine the optic nerve using an ophthalmoscope.
- Examine cranial nerves I, V, VI, VII, VIII, IX, X, XI and XII.
- Thank the patient and clean your hands.

### Summarise your findings

The patient has a partial ptosis on the left with a dilated pupil. Eye movements are diminished with impaired adduction and elevation of the eyeball. Double vision is confirmed on testing of eye movements.

### Suggest a diagnosis

The most likely diagnosis is left incomplete III nerve palsy (complete palsy would cause total ptosis with relief of double vision).

### Suggested investigations

Fasting glucose and cholesterol, blood pressure, erythrocyte sedimentation rate and a magnetic resonance angiogram to check for an underlying cerebral artery aneurysm.

### Advanced level comments

Palsies of the III nerve result in ptosis and diplopia. Microvascular damage to the III nerve usually spares the pupil. Compressive lesions, such as an aneurysm, cause a dilated pupil (as pupillary fibres are located on the outside of cranial nerve III), which responds poorly or is completely unresponsive to light.

## Integrated examination sequence for ophthalmology

- Introduce yourself and clean your hands.
- Explain what you will be doing.
- Observe the patient as they walk into the room, looking for:
  - Facial asymmetry
  - Proptosis
  - Gait (may indicate a possible cerebrovascular accident).
- Check visual acuity in each eye for distance and near vision.
- Undertake an assessment of the visual fields:
  - Look for homonymous hemianopia, bitemporal hemianopia or any other obvious visual field defect.
- Check the pupils:
  - Assess direct and consensual reflex.
  - Test for a relative afferent pupillary defect. Note that the pupils should be checked only after visual acuity and visual field assessments have been undertaken, as the lights used to examine the pupils may dazzle the patient and interfere with accurate visual field and acuity assessment.
- Dilate both pupils using tropicamide 1% eye drops.
- Examine each eye using the direct ophthalmoscope:
  - Assess the ocular surface.
  - Look at the red reflex (opacity may indicate either a cataract or vitreous opacities such as debris or haemorrhage).
  - Focus on the optic disc: look at colour, shape and cupping, as well as swelling.
  - Examine the blood vessel arcades in each quadrant.
  - Examine the macula.
  - Ask patient to look up, down, right and left so you can examine the peripheral retina.
- Examine extraocular movements if the patient presents with diplopia or if it is clinically indicated.

Iain Hathorn

# 9

# The ear, nose and throat

**Ear 194**

**Anatomy and physiology 194**
External ear 194
Middle ear 194
Inner ear 194

**The history 195**
Common presenting symptoms 195
Past medical history 196
Drug history 196
Family history 196
Social history 196

**The physical examination 197**
Testing hearing 198
Testing vestibular function 201

**Investigations 203**

**Nose and sinuses 203**

**Anatomy and physiology 203**

**The history 204**
Common presenting symptoms 204
Past medical history 205
Drug history 206
Family history 206

Social history 206

**The physical examination 206**

**Investigations 207**

**Mouth, throat and neck 208**

**Anatomy and physiology 208**
Mouth 208
Throat 208
Teeth 208
Neck 209

**The history 209**
Common presenting symptoms 209
Past medical history 211
Drug history 212
Social and family history 212

**The physical examination 213**
Mouth and throat 213
Neck 214

**Investigations 214**

**OSCE Example 1: Hoarseness 215**

**OSCE Example 2: Neck lump 216**

**Integrated examination sequence for ear, nose and throat disease 217**

# EAR

## Anatomy and physiology

The ear is the specialised sensory organ of hearing and balance; it is divided anatomically into the external, middle and inner ear.

### External ear

The external ear consists of the cartilaginous pinna, the external auditory canal (cartilage in the lateral one-third, bone in the medial two-thirds), and the lateral surface of the tympanic membrane (Fig. 9.1). Sound is collected and channelled by the pinna and transmitted via the external auditory canal to the tympanic membrane. The external auditory canal has an elongated S-shaped curve; hence it is important to retract the pinna when examining the ear to see the tympanic membrane clearly. The outer portion of the canal has hair and glands that produce ear wax, which forms a protective barrier.

### Middle ear

The middle ear is an air-filled space that contains the three bony, articulated ossicles: the malleus, incus and stapes. The eustachian tube opens into the middle ear inferiorly and allows equalisation of pressure and ventilation. Vibrations of the tympanic membrane are transmitted and amplified through the ossicular chain and focus on to the smaller oval window on which the stapes sits (see Fig. 9.1B). The malleus is attached to the tympanic membrane and can be seen clearly on otoscopy (Fig. 9.2). The long process of the incus can also be visible occasionally. The tympanic membrane has a flaccid upper part (pars flaccida), and it is important to look carefully in this area as this is where a cholesteatoma (an invasive collection of keratinising squamous epithelium) can form. The chorda tympani nerve runs through the middle ear carrying taste fibres from the anterior two-thirds of the tongue; these 'hitch a ride' with the facial nerve, which runs through the mastoid bone in the wall of the middle ear.

### Inner ear

The inner ear contains the organs of hearing (cochlea) and balance (vestibular system). The vibration of the stapes footplate stimulates fluid within the cochlea, resulting in the movement of hair cells in the cochlea which are converted to electrical impulses along the vestibulocochlear nerve (VIII).

The vestibular system helps maintain balance, along with visual input and proprioception. The vestibular part of the inner ear contains:

- The lateral, superior and posterior semicircular canals: these lie at right angles to detect rotational motion of their fluid (endolymph) in three planes.
- The utricle and the saccule: their hair cells are embedded in a gel layer containing small crystals (otoliths), which are subject to gravity and enable detection of head tilt and linear acceleration.

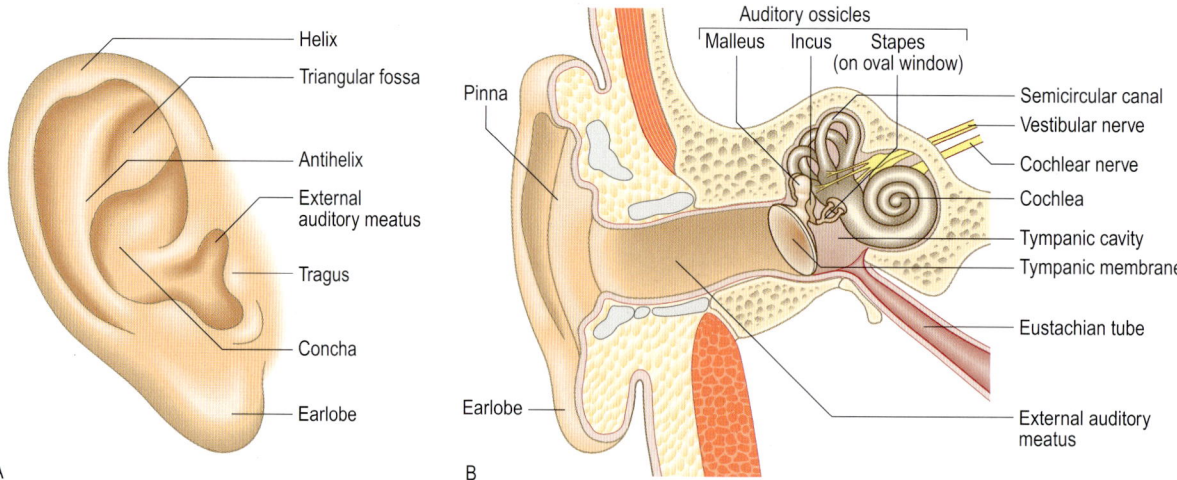

**Fig. 9.1 The ear.** **A** The pinna. **B** Cross-section of the outer, middle and inner ear.

**Fig. 9.2** Structures seen on otoscopic examination of the right ear. [A] Main structures. [B] Normal tympanic membrane.

## The history

### Common presenting symptoms

#### Pain and itching

Ask about:

- quality of the pain
- preceding trauma, upper respiratory tract infection (URTI)
- associated symptoms: dysphagia/voice change (suggesting possible referred pain from a throat lesion).

Otalgia (ear pain) associated with pruritus (itching) is often due to otitis externa. Acute otitis media is common in children and otalgia often follows an URTI. Other causes of otalgia are described in Box 9.1.

#### Ear discharge

Ask about:

- purulent, mucoid or blood-stained discharge (otorrhoea)
- associated pain.

A purulent discharge can be caused by otitis externa or acute otitis media with a perforation. A chronic offensive discharge may be a sign of cholesteatoma.

Blood-stained discharge may suggest the presence of granulation tissue from infection or can be a result of trauma, with or without an associated cerebrospinal fluid (CSF) leak.

#### Hearing loss

Ask about:

- sudden or gradual onset

### 9.1 Causes and features of earache (otalgia)

| Cause | Clinical features |
|---|---|
| **Otological** | |
| Acute otitis externa | Pain worsens on touching outer ear, tragus Swelling of ear canal Purulent discharge and itching |
| Acute otitis media | Severe pain, red, bulging tympanic membrane, purulent discharge if tympanic membrane perforation present |
| Perichondritis | Erythematous, swollen pinna |
| Trauma | Pinna haematoma, pinna laceration, haemotympanum (blood behind tympanic membrane); cerebrospinal fluid leak or facial nerve palsy may be present |
| Herpes zoster (Ramsay Hunt syndrome) | Vesicles in ear canal, facial nerve palsy may be present; vertigo is common |
| Malignancy | Mass in ear canal or on pinna |
| **Non-otological** | |
| Tonsillitis | Sore throat, tonsil inflammation |
| Peritonsillar abscess | Trismus, soft-palate swelling in peritonsillar abscess |
| Temporomandibular joint dysfunction | Tenderness, clicking of joint on jaw opening |
| Dental disease | Toothache, e.g. due to dental abscess |
| Cervical spine disease | Neck pain/tenderness |
| Cancer of the pharynx or larynx | Associated sore throat, hoarseness, dysphagia, weight loss, neck lump |

- precipitating factors: trauma, URTI, noise exposure, antibiotics
- impact of the hearing loss on the patient's function.

Hearing loss can be a result of disruption in the conduction mechanism or may have sensorineural causes such as failure of the VIII nerve or cochlea (Box 9.2). Profound loss before speech acquisition affects speech development and quality.

## Tinnitus

Tinnitus is an awareness of a noise in the absence of an external stimulus.

Ask about:

- quality of tinnitus: high-pitched, ringing, pulsatile
- intermittent or constant nature
- whether it is unilateral or bilateral
- associated hearing loss or other ear symptoms.

Tinnitus is usually associated with hearing loss. An acoustic neuroma (a tumour of the vestibulocochlear nerve, cranial nerve VIII) needs to be considered in unilateral tinnitus or tinnitus with an asymmetrical sensorineural hearing loss.

## Vertigo

Vertigo is a sensation of movement relative to one's surroundings. Rotational movements are most common, and patients often have associated nausea, vomiting, and postural or gait instability. Vertigo can originate peripherally or, less often, centrally (brainstem, cerebellum). Patients will often say they are 'dizzy' when describing the illusion of movement that is vertigo. It is very important to clarify exactly what they mean by this. Lightheadedness is not a vestibular symptom, but unsteadiness may be.

Ask about:

- duration and frequency of episodes
- aggravating or provoking factors (position, head movement)

### 9.2 Causes of hearing loss

**Conductive[a]**

- Wax
- Otitis externa
- Middle ear effusion
- Trauma to the tympanic membrane/ossicles
- Otosclerosis
- Chronic middle ear infection
- Tumours of the middle ear

**Sensorineural[b]**

- Genetic, e.g. Alport's syndrome
- Prenatal infection, e.g. rubella
- Birth injury
- Infection:
  - Meningitis
  - Measles
  - Mumps
- Trauma
- Ménière's disease
- Degenerative (presbyacusis)
- Occupation- or other noise-induced
- Acoustic neuroma
- Idiopathic

[a]Disruption to the mechanical transfer of sound in the outer ear, eardrum or ossicles.
[b]Cochlear or central damage.

- associated 'fullness in the ear' during the episode (Ménière's disease)
- associated focal neurology (cerebrovascular event)
- fluctuating hearing loss or tinnitus
- associated headaches, nausea or aura (migraine)
- previous significant head injury; previous URTI.
- The most common causes of vertigo include benign paroxysmal positional vertigo (attributed to debris within the posterior semicircular canal), vestibular neuritis (also known as vestibular neuronitis, a viral or postviral inflammatory disorder) and Ménière's disease (caused by excess endolymphatic fluid pressure). Other causes include migraine, cerebral ischaemia, drugs and head trauma. Discriminating features are described in Box 9.3.

## Nystagmus

Nystagmus is an involuntary rhythmic oscillation of the eyes, which can be horizontal, vertical, rotatory or multidirectional. It may be continuous, paroxysmal, or evoked by manoeuvres such as gaze or head position. The most common form, 'jerk nystagmus', consists of alternating phases of a slow drift in one direction with a corrective saccadic 'jerk' in the opposite direction. The direction of the fast jerk is used to define the direction of nystagmus (Box 9.4). Pendular nystagmus, in which there is a sinusoidal oscillation without a fast phase, is less common. Nystagmus may be caused by disorders of the vestibular, visual or cerebellar pathway.

## Past medical history

Ask about:

- previous ear surgery, trauma
- recurrent ear infections
- systemic conditions associated with hearing loss (such as granulomatosis with polyangiitis)
- any significant previous illnesses, such as meningitis, which can result in sensorineural hearing loss.

## Drug history

The aminoglycoside antibiotics (such as gentamicin), aspirin, furosemide and some chemotherapy agents (cisplatin) are ototoxic.

## Family history

Some causes of sensorineural hearing loss and otosclerosis are congenital. Otosclerosis causes a conductive hearing loss due to fixation of the stapes footplate.

## Social history

The patient's occupation should be noted, as well as any significant previous exposure to loud noise.

## 9.3 Diagnosing vertigo

| | Benign paroxysmal positional vertigo | Vestibular neuritis | Ménière's disease | Central vertigo (migraine, MS, brainstem ischaemia, drugs) |
|---|---|---|---|---|
| Duration | Seconds | Days | Hours | Hours–migraine<br>Days and weeks – MS |
| Hearing loss | – | – | ++ | – |
| Tinnitus | – | – | ++ | – |
| Aural fullness | – | – | ++ | – |
| Episodic | Yes | Rarely | Recurrent vertigo; persistent tinnitus and progressive sensorineural deafness | Migraine–recurs<br>Central nervous system damage–usually some recovery but often persistent |
| Triggers | Lying on affected ear | Possible presence of upper respiratory symptoms | None | Drugs (e.g., aminoglycosides) cardiovascular disease |

*MS*, Multiple sclerosis.

## 9.4 Characteristics of nystagmus

| Nystagmus type | Clinical pathology | Characteristics | |
|---|---|---|---|
| | | Fast phase | Maximal on looking |
| Jerk: | | | |
|   Peripheral | Semicircular canal, vestibular nerve | Unidirectional<br>Not suppressed by optic fixation<br>Patient too dizzy to walk<br>Dix–Hallpike fatigues on repetition | Away from affected side |
|   Central | Brainstem, cerebellum | Bidirectional (changes with direction of gaze)<br>Suppressed by optic fixation<br>Patient can walk (even with nystagmus)<br>Dix–Hallpike persists | To either side |
|   Dysconjugate (ataxic) | Interconnections of III, IV and VI nerves (medial longitudinal bundle) | Typically affects the abducting eye | To either side |
| Pendular | Eyes, e.g., congenital blindness | No fast phase | Straight ahead |

## The physical examination

### Examination sequence (Video 18)

#### Inspection
- Pinna skin, shape, size, position, scars from previous surgery/trauma, deformity

#### Palpation
- Gently pull on the pinna and push on the tragus to check for pain.
- Gently palpate over the mastoid bone behind the ear to assess for pain or swelling.

### Otoscopy
- Use the largest otoscope speculum that will comfortably fit the meatus.
- Explain to the patient what you are going to do.
- Hold the otoscope in your right hand for examining the right ear (left hand to examine left ear). Rest the ulnar border of your hand against the patient's cheek to enable better control and to avoid trauma if the patient moves (Fig. 9.3).
- Gently pull the pinna upwards and backwards to straighten the cartilaginous external auditory canal. Use the left hand to retract the right pinna (see Fig. 9.3).
- Inspect the external auditory canal through the speculum, noting wax, foreign bodies or discharge. You should identify

9

**Fig. 9.3** Examination of the ear using an otoscope.

the tympanic membrane and the light reflex anteroinferiorly (see Fig. 9.2).

Congenital deformities of the pinna, like microtia (Fig. 9.4A) or low-set ears, can be associated with other conditions such as hearing loss and Down's syndrome. Children can also have protruding ears that occasionally require corrective surgery (pinnaplasty). Trauma can result in a pinna haematoma (see Fig. 9.4B) and subsequent 'cauliflower ear' due to cartilage necrosis if untreated. Trauma may also cause mastoid bruising ('Battle's sign'), suggesting a possible skull-base fracture. Lesions on the pinna are relatively common and can be related to sun exposure; they include actinic keratosis, and basal cell and squamous cell cancers (see Fig. 9.4C).

If discharge is noted on otoscopy and the tympanic membrane is intact, otitis externa is the likely cause (Fig. 9.5A). The canal can reveal exostoses, abnormal bone growth due to cold water exposure, often seen in surfers (see Fig. 9.5B).

Scarring on the tympanic membrane (tympanosclerosis) can be caused by previous grommet insertion or infections.

Tympanic membrane perforations can be central or marginal, and the position and size of the perforation should be noted as a percentage (Fig. 9.6A). A severe retraction pocket of the pars tensa can mimic a perforation (see Fig. 9.6B). A retraction of the pars flaccida can contain a cholesteatoma, which may cause an offensive discharge and erode the bony ossicles, resulting in a conductive hearing loss (see Fig. 9.5C). Fluid behind the tympanic membrane is called otitis media with effusion (OME, or 'glue ear', Fig. 9.7A), and a fluid level may be seen (see Fig. 9.7B). This commonly affects children and can be treated surgically with insertion of a ventilation tube or grommet (see Fig. 9.6C). If persistent OME is seen in adults, the postnasal space needs to be examined by a specialist to exclude a lesion in that site. Acute otitis media presents with pain; the tympanic membrane can become inflamed (see Fig. 9.7C), and may bulge and eventually perforate.

## Testing hearing (Video 19)

### Whispered voice test

## Examination sequence (Video 19A)

- Stand behind the patient.
- Start testing with your mouth about 15 cm from the ear you are assessing.
- Mask hearing in the patient's other ear by rubbing the tragus ('masking').
- Ask the patient to repeat a combination of numbers and letters (e.g. 3-B-7). Start with a normal speaking voice to confirm that the patient understands the test. Then, lower your voice to a clear whisper.
- Repeat the test but this time at arm's length from the patient's ear. People with normal hearing can repeat the sequence correctly when whispered at 60 cm.
- If the patient responds incorrectly, the test is repeated using a different number/letter combination.
- If 50% or more of the items in the two triplets are incorrect, the test is abnormal.

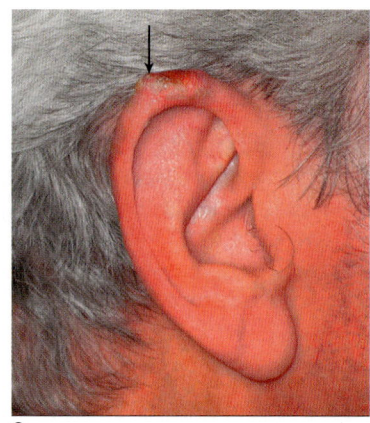

A          B          C

**Fig. 9.4** The pinna. **A** Microtia. **B** Haematoma. **C** Squamous cancer *(arrow)*.

**Fig. 9.5 Auditory canal abnormalities.** [A] Otitis externa. [B] Exostosis of the external auditory meatus. [C] Cholesteatoma.

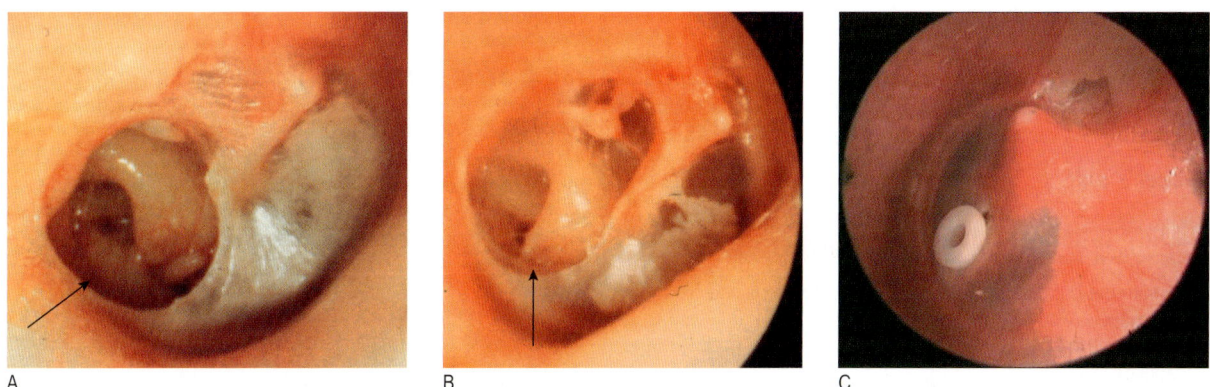

**Fig. 9.6 Tympanic membrane abnormalities.** [A] Tympanic membrane perforation *(arrow)*. [B] Retraction pocket of the pars tensa *(arrow)*. [C] Grommet in situ.

**Fig. 9.7 Otitis media.** [A] With effusion. [B] Fluid level behind the tympanic membrane *(arrow)*. [C] Acute otitis media.

**Fig. 9.8** Weber's test.

## Tuning fork tests

A 512-Hz tuning fork can be used to help differentiate between conductive and sensorineural hearing loss.

### Weber's test

**Examination sequence (Video 19B)**

- Strike the prongs of the tuning fork against a padded surface to make it vibrate.
- Place the base of the vibrating tuning fork in the middle of the patient's forehead (Fig. 9.8).
- Ask the patient, 'Where do you hear the sound?'
- Record which side Weber's test lateralises to if not central.

In a patient with normal hearing, the sound would be expected to be heard in the middle, or equally in both ears; however, up to 40% of people with normal hearing will lateralise on Weber's test.

Therefore, Weber's test should only be interpreted in patients with hearing loss.

In conductive hearing loss, the sound is heard louder in the affected ear. In unilateral sensorineural hearing loss, it is heard louder in the unaffected ear. If there is symmetrical hearing loss, it will be heard in the middle.

### Rinne's test

**Examination sequence (Video 19C)**

- Strike the prongs of the tuning fork against a padded surface to make it vibrate.
- Place the vibrating tuning fork on the mastoid process (Fig. 9.9A) and ask, 'Can you hear this?' Then ask the patient to 'tell me when you hear it stop'.
- Now place the tuning fork at the external auditory meatus and ask, 'Can you still hear it' (see Fig. 9.9B). In a patient with normal hearing, they will still hear it.

To maximise the sound for the patient, the "U" of the tuning fork should face forward.

### Alternative technique: loudness comparison

- Strike the prongs of the tuning fork against a padded surface to make it vibrate.
- Place the vibrating tuning fork on the mastoid process for about 2 seconds.
- Now place the still-vibrating tuning fork at the external auditory meatus and ask, 'Is it louder in front of your ear or behind?'

With normal hearing, sound is heard louder or longer when the tuning fork is at the external auditory meatus. That is, air conduction (AC) is better than bone conduction (BC), recorded as AC>BC. This normal result is recorded as 'Rinne-positive'.

In conductive hearing loss, bone conduction is better than air conduction (BC>AC); thus, sound is heard louder when the tuning fork is on the mastoid process ('Rinne-negative'). This finding is associated with a high likelihood that the patient has a

A                                                        B

**Fig. 9.9** Rinne's test. **A** Testing bone conduction. **B** Testing air conduction.

conductive hearing loss of at least 20 dB. A false-negative Rinne's test may occur if there is profound hearing loss on one side. This is due to sound being conducted through the bone of the skull to the other 'good' ear. Weber's test can detect a hearing loss of just 5 dB; therefore, the tuning fork will lateralise to the affected ear in conductive hearing loss before Rinne's test becomes abnormal (negative). In sensorineural hearing loss, Rinne's test will be positive, as air conduction is better than bone conduction.

Tuning fork test findings are summarised in Box 9.5.

## Testing vestibular function

### Testing for nystagmus

- Patients should be tested with spectacles or contact lenses for best corrected vision.

| 9.5 Tuning fork tests | Weber's test | Rinne's test |
|---|---|---|
| Bilateral normal hearing | Central | AC>BC, bilateral |
| Bilateral symmetrical sensorineural loss | Central | AC>BC, bilateral |
| Unilateral or asymmetrical sensorineural loss LEFT | Louder right | AC>BC, bilateral[a] |
| Unilateral conductive loss LEFT | Louder left | BC>AC, left<br>AC>BC, right |
| Bilateral conductive loss (worse on LEFT) | Louder left | BC>AC, bilateral |

[a]Patients with a severe sensorineural loss may have BC > AC due to BC crossing to the other better-hearing cochlea that is not being tested (false-negative Rinne's test).
*AC*, Air conduction; *BC*, bone conduction.

- With the patient seated, ask them to fixate on a stationary target in a neutral gaze position and observe for spontaneous nystagmus.
- Hold your finger an arm's length away, level with the patient's eye, and ask the patient to focus on and follow the tip of your finger. Slowly move your finger from side to side and up and down and observe the eyes for any oscillations, avoiding extremes of gaze where physiological nystagmus may occur. This assesses for gaze nystagmus and smooth pursuit.
- If any oscillations are present, note:
- whether they are horizontal, vertical or rotatory
- which direction of gaze causes the most marked nystagmus
- in which direction the fast phase of jerk nystagmus occurs

Discriminating characteristics of nystagmus are detailed in Box 9.4.

**9**

### Dix–Hallpike positional test

- Ask the patient to sit upright, close to the end of the couch.
- Turn the patient's head 45 degrees to one side (Fig. 9.10A).
- Rapidly lower the patient backward so that their head is now 30 degrees below the horizontal. Keep supporting the head and ask the patient to keep their eyes open, even if they feel dizzy (see Fig. 9.10B).
- Observe the eyes for nystagmus. If it is present, note latency (time to onset), direction, duration and fatigue (decrease on repeated manoeuvres).
- Repeat the test, turning the patient's head to the other side (see Fig. 9.10C).

Normal patients have no nystagmus or symptoms of vertigo. A positive Dix–Hallpike manoeuvre is diagnostic for benign paroxysmal positional vertigo. There is a delay of 5–20 seconds before the patient experiences vertigo and before rotatory jerk nystagmus toward the lower ear (geotropic) occurs; this lasts for

A          B          C

**Fig. 9.10 Dix–Hallpike position test.** The examiner looks for nystagmus (usually accompanied by vertigo). Both nystagmus and vertigo typically decrease (fatigue) on repeat testing. See text for details.

## 9.6 Investigations in ear disease

| Investigation | Indication/comment |
| --- | --- |
| Swab from external auditory meatus | Otorrhoea, such as in otitis externa or otitis media with a tympanic membrane perforation; microscopy and culture can help guide treatment |
| Magnetic resonance imaging | Acoustic neuroma (see Fig. 9.11)<br>Asymmetrical sensorineural hearing loss or unilateral tinnitus |
| Audiometry | Hearing loss<br>A single-frequency tone at different noise levels is presented to each ear in turn through headphones in a soundproof booth. The intensity of sound is reduced in 10-decibel steps until patients can no longer hear it. The hearing threshold is the quietest sound they can hear. Audiograms display air and bone conduction thresholds, and conductive and sensorineural hearing loss can therefore be differentiated (see Fig. 9.12) |
| Impedance audiometry (tympanometry) | Conductive hearing loss (e.g., otitis media with effusion, ossicular discontinuity, otosclerosis)<br>Eustachian tube dysfunction<br>The compliance of the tympanic membrane is measured during changes in pressure in the ear canal; compliance should be maximal at atmospheric pressure |
| Vestibular testing<br>    Caloric tests<br><br>    Posturography | Unilateral vestibular hypofunction<br>Water at 30°C and then 44°C is irrigated into the external ear canal. Electronystagmography records nystagmus. The response is reduced in vestibular hypofunction<br>Reveals whether patients rely on vision or proprioception more than usual<br>Usually reserved for specialist balance clinics |

**Fig. 9.11** Magnetic resonance image showing a right acoustic neuroma *(arrow).*

less than 30 seconds. The response fatigues on repeated testing due to adaptation. Immediate nystagmus without adaptation, and not necessarily with associated vertigo, can be caused by central pathology.

### Head impulse test (or head thrust test)

## Examination sequence

- Sit opposite the patient and ask them to focus on a target (usually your nose).
- Hold the patient's head, placing a hand on each side of it.

- Rapidly turn the patient's head to one side in the horizontal plane (roughly 15 degrees) and watch for any corrective movement of the eyes. Repeat, turning the head towards the other side. The eyes remain fixed on the examiner's nose in a normal test. When the head is turned towards the affected side, the eyes move with the head, and there is then a corrective saccade.

This is a test of the vestibulo-ocular reflex. The presence of a corrective saccade is a positive test and indicates a deficiency in the vestibulo-ocular reflex. It is useful to identify unilateral peripheral vestibular hypofunction. You must be careful when performing this test in patients with neck problems because of the rapid movements of the head.

### Unterberger's test

## Examination sequence

- Ask the patient to march on the spot with their eyes closed and their arms outstretched in front of them. The patient will rotate to the side of the damaged labyrinth.

### Fistula test

## Examination sequence

- Compress the tragus repeatedly against the external auditory meatus to occlude it.

**A**

**B**

**C**

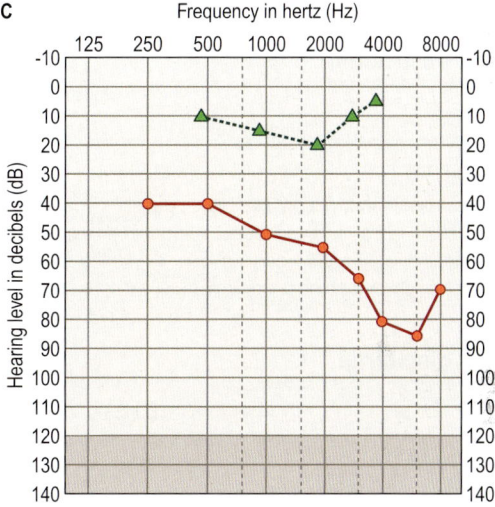

**Fig. 9.12 Hearing test (audiogram). [A]** Normal-hearing right and left ears. **[B]** Right sensorineural loss. **[C]** Right conductive hearing loss. (● Right air conduction, ✕ Left air conduction, ▲ Bone conduction)

If imbalance or vertigo with nystagmus is induced, it suggests an abnormal communication between the middle ear and vestibular system (such as erosion due to cholesteatoma).

## Investigations

Initial investigations in ear disease are summarised in Box 9.6 and Figs 9.11 and 9.12.

# NOSE AND SINUSES

## Anatomy and physiology

The external nose consists of two nasal bones that provide support and stability to the nose. The nasal bones articulate with each other and the bones of the face: the frontal bone, the ethmoid bone and the maxilla. The nasal bones also attach to the nasal septum and paired upper lateral cartilages of the nose. There are two further paired cartilages, the lower lateral cartilages, which form the nasal tip. Internally the nasal septum, which is bone posteriorly and cartilage anteriorly, separates the nose into two nasal cavities that join posteriorly in the postnasal space. There are three turbinates on each side of the nose, superior, middle and inferior, which warm and moisten nasal airflow (Figs 9.13 and 9.14A).

One important function of the nose is olfaction. The olfactory receptors are situated high in the nose in the olfactory cleft. Olfactory fibres from the nasal mucosa pass through the cribriform plate to the olfactory bulb in the anterior cranial fossa.

The paranasal sinuses are air-filled spaces in the skull. There are paired frontal, sphenoid, maxillary, and anterior and posterior ethmoid sinuses. The anterior nasal sinuses (frontal, maxillary and anterior ethmoid) drain into the middle meatus (between the middle turbinate and lateral wall of the nose). The posterior ethmoid and sphenoid sinuses drain into the sphenoethmoidal recess (between the superior turbinate and nasal septum).

# The history

## Common presenting symptoms

### Nasal obstruction

Ask about:

- unilateral or bilateral obstruction
- associated symptoms (bleeding, swelling, pain).

Unilateral nasal obstruction may be caused by anatomical blockage, such as a deviated septum possibly secondary to trauma. Bilateral obstruction can be due to rhinitis (allergic or non-allergic) or chronic rhinosinusitis with or without polyps.

### Nasal discharge

Ask about:

- unilateral or bilateral discharge (rhinorrhoea)
- purulent or clear nature
- anterior discharge or postnasal drip.

Clear, bilateral watery discharge suggests allergic or non-allergic rhinitis. Purulent discharge can point to acute bacterial rhinosinusitis or chronic rhinosinusitis. A unilateral, purulent discharge in a child raises the possibility of a foreign body in the nose. Following a head injury, unilateral clear rhinorrhoea suggests a possible CSF leak secondary to an anterior skull-base fracture.

### Epistaxis (bleeding from inside the nose)

Ask about:

- unilateral or bilateral bleeding
- frequency and duration of episodes

- provoking factors such as trauma, sneezing, or blowing or picking nose
- bleeding from the front or back of the nose.

The nasal septum has a very rich blood supply, particularly in Little's area (anterior septum), which is a common site for bleeding. If bleeding is unilateral and associated with nasal obstruction and pain, the possibility of sinonasal malignancy should be considered. In adolescent males with unilateral nasal obstruction and epistaxis, the rare diagnosis of juvenile angiofibroma should be excluded on nasendoscopy by an ear, nose and throat specialist.

### Sneezing

Ask about:

- associated itchy, red eyes
- whether symptoms occur all year round, only during certain seasons, or during contact with allergens.

Sneezing is a protective sudden expulsive effort triggered by local irritants in the nose and is most commonly due to allergy or viral URTIs.

### Disturbance of smell

Ask about:

- complete loss of smell (anosmia)
- reduced sense of smell (hyposmia)
- unpleasant smells (cacosmia)
- associated nasal symptoms such as obstruction and rhinorrhoea, which may suggest rhinitis or nasal polyps
- recent head injury
- recent URTI.

A sudden onset of anosmia can occur following a significant head injury or viral URTI due to damage to the olfactory epithelium. Inflammation and swelling in the nasal mucosa as a result of rhinitis, chronic rhinosinusitis or nasal polyps usually cause hyposmia. Cacosmia is usually caused by infection in the nose or sinuses, or occasionally by a foreign body in the nose. Phantosmia describes olfactory hallucinations, which may occur in temporal lobe epilepsy.

### Nasal and facial pain

Nasal pain is rare, except following trauma. Facial pain can be caused by a number of problems but is often incorrectly attributed to sinusitis. The key to identifying the cause of facial pain is an accurate history.

Ask about:

- quality of pain: for example, throbbing, aching, sharp, stabbing, tight-band

- location of pain: unilateral or bilateral
- duration and frequency of pain
- associated nasal symptoms
- associated nausea, photophobia or aura (migraine)
- relieving and exacerbating factors.

The differential diagnosis of facial pain includes temporomandibular joint dysfunction, migraine, dental disease, chronic rhinosinusitis, trigeminal neuralgia (severe, sharp pain in a trigeminal distribution), tension headache (band-like, tight pain) and cluster headaches (unilateral nasal discharge, eye watering).

## Nasal deformity

The most common cause of nasal deformity is trauma, resulting in swelling, bruising and deviation of the nose. The swelling following trauma will settle over a couple of weeks, but residual deviation may remain if the nasal bones were fractured and displaced. It is important to establish the impact of the nasal injury on function (nasal breathing, sense of smell) and cosmetic appearance.

Nasal septal destruction or perforation can result in 'saddle deformity' of the nasal bridge. Causes include granulomatosis with polyangiitis, trauma, cocaine abuse, congenital syphilis and iatrogenic factors (septal surgery, Fig. 9.14B).

The nose can appear widened in acromegaly or with advanced nasal polyposis (see Fig. 9.14C). Rhinophyma can also result from chronic acne rosacea of the nasal skin (Fig. 9.15).

## Past medical history

Ask about:

- history of atopy
- asthma (around one-third of patients with allergic rhinitis have asthma)
- prior nasal trauma or surgery
- history of bronchial infection (cystic fibrosis or ciliary disorders may affect the nose and lower airways).

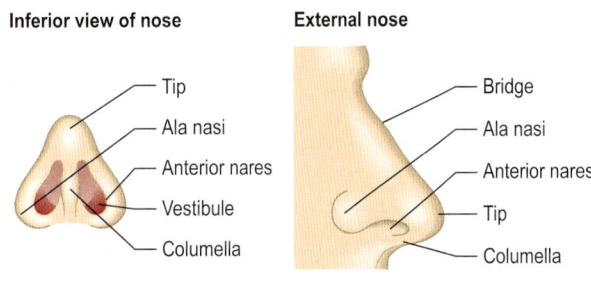

**Inferior view of nose**
- Tip
- Ala nasi
- Anterior nares
- Vestibule
- Columella

**External nose**
- Bridge
- Ala nasi
- Anterior nares
- Tip
- Columella

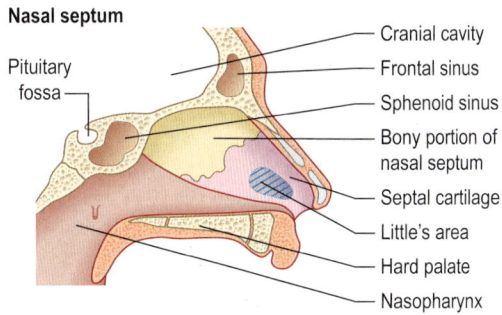

**Nasal septum**
- Pituitary fossa
- Cranial cavity
- Frontal sinus
- Sphenoid sinus
- Bony portion of nasal septum
- Septal cartilage
- Little's area
- Hard palate
- Nasopharynx

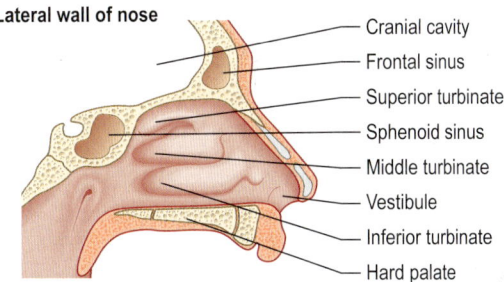

**Lateral wall of nose**
- Cranial cavity
- Frontal sinus
- Superior turbinate
- Sphenoid sinus
- Middle turbinate
- Vestibule
- Inferior turbinate
- Hard palate

**Fig. 9.13** The nose and paranasal sinuses.

A

B

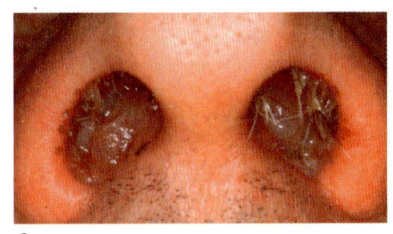

C

**Fig. 9.14 Nasal abnormalities.** **A** Turbinate hypertrophy. **B** Nasal septum perforation post-surgery. **C** Nasal polyps.

9

**Fig. 9.15** Rhinophyma as a complication of rosacea.

For patients with epistaxis, it is important to identify any history of bleeding diathesis or hypertension.

## Drug history

Ask about:

- use of anticoagulants, including warfarin, apixaban or rivaroxaban
- use of antiplatelet drugs (aspirin, clopidogrel).

Intranasal cocaine use can cause septal perforation, epistaxis, crusting and whistling.

## Family history

A family history of atopy is relevant in rhinitis. In patients with epistaxis, it is important to establish a family history of hereditary haemorrhagic telangiectasia or inherited bleeding disorders.

## Social history

Occupation is relevant because exposure to inhaled allergens, occupational dusts and chemicals may exacerbate rhinitis. Exposure to hardwood dust is associated with an increased risk of sinonasal cancers. Atopic patients should be asked about pets.

Heavy alcohol intake, leading to liver disease, can affect coagulation and is relevant for epistaxis. Smoking impedes mucociliary clearance and can contribute to nasal problems.

# The physical examination

## Examination sequence

- Assess the external appearance of the nose, noting swelling, bruising, skin changes and deformity.
- Stand above the seated patient to assess any external deviation.
- Ask the patient to look straight ahead. Elevate the tip of their nose using your non-dominant thumb to align the nostrils with the rest of the nasal cavity.
- Look into each nostril and assess the anterior nasal septum (Fig. 9.16); note the mucosal covering, visible vessels in Little's area, crusting, ulceration and septal perforation. In trauma, a septal haematoma should be excluded.
- Using an otoscope with a large speculum in an adult, assess the inferior turbinates. Note any hypertrophy and swelling of the turbinate mucosa.
- You may see large polyps on anterior rhinoscopy. To distinguish between hypertrophied inferior turbinates and nasal polyps, you can lightly touch the swelling with a cotton bud (polyps lack sensation).
- Palpate the nasal bones to assess for bony or cartilaginous deformity.
- In trauma, palpate the infraorbital ridges to exclude a step deformity and to check infraorbital sensation. Eye movements should be assessed to rule out restriction of movement related to 'orbital blowout'.

**Fig. 9.16** **Nasal examination.** [A] Elevation of the tip of the nose to give a clear view of the anterior nares. [B] Anterior rhinoscopy using an otoscope with a large speculum.

- Place a metal spatula under the nostrils and look for condensation marks to assess airway patency.
- Palpate for cervical lymphadenopathy (p. 36).
- Note that rigid nasendoscopy and tests of olfaction are confined to specialist clinics.

The mucosa of the inferior turbinate on anterior rhinoscopy is pale, moist and hypertrophied in allergic rhinitis (see Fig. 9.14A). In chronic rhinitis, the mucosa is swollen and red. Large polyps may be seen on anterior rhinoscopy as pale yellow/grey swellings (see Fig. 9.14C).

A septal haematoma will appear as a soft, red, fluctuant swelling of the anterior septum. The septal cartilage receives its blood supply from the overlying perichondrium; a septal haematoma interrupts this supply and can result in cartilage necrosis, septal perforation and 'saddle deformity'. It must therefore be identified and referred for early drainage.

Facial swelling is not usually seen in chronic sinusitis but can occur with dental abscesses and cancer of the maxillary antrum.

## Investigations

Initial investigations are summarised in Box 9.7 and Fig. 9.17.

### 9.7 Investigations in nasal disease

| Investigation | Indication/comment |
|---|---|
| Plain X-ray | Not indicated for nasal bone fracture<br>Only required if associated facial fracture is suspected |
| Nasal endoscopy | Inflammatory sinus disease, malignancy |
| Allergy tests | Skin-prick tests for common inhaled allergens, specific immunoglobulin E blood test (RAST) |
| Computed tomography | Inflammatory sinus disease, trauma and malignancy<br>Demonstrates extent of sinus disease, provides evidence of invasion into local structures and shows detailed bony anatomy, enabling planning of endoscopic surgical procedures (see Fig. 9.17) |
| Tests of olfaction | Used in specialist clinics only<br>Include the UPSIT smell test and Sniffin' Sticks |

*RAST,* Radioallergosorbent test; *UPSIT,* University of Pennsylvania smell identification test.

A　　　　　　　　　　　　　B

**Fig. 9.17 Computed tomograms of the paranasal sinuses.** A Normal scan. B Right-sided chronic sinusitis.

# MOUTH, THROAT AND NECK

## Anatomy and physiology

### Mouth

The mouth extends from the lips anteriorly to the anterior tonsillar pillar posteriorly and is divided into the vestibule; between the buccal (cheek), mucosa and the teeth; and the oral cavity internal to the teeth. The oral cavity contains the anterior two-thirds of the tongue, the floor of the mouth, the hard palate and the inner surfaces of the gums and teeth (Fig. 9.18). The tongue anteriorly has filiform papillae containing taste buds, giving the tongue its velvety texture. The circumvallate papillae are groups of taste buds marking the boundary between the anterior two-thirds and posterior third of the tongue.

Saliva is secreted into the mouth from the parotid, submandibular and sublingual salivary glands (Fig. 9.19). The parotid gland is situated anterior to the ear and has a superficial and deep lobe relative to the facial nerve that runs through it. The parotid duct opens into the buccal mucosa opposite the second upper molar. The submandibular gland lies anterior and medial to the angle of the mandible and its duct opens into the floor of the mouth next to the frenulum of the tongue (see Fig. 9.18).

### Throat

The pharynx is a shared upper aerodigestive channel that runs from the anterior tonsillar pillar to the laryngeal inlet. The larynx ('voice box') is responsible for phonation and has a protective function to prevent aspiration. It consists of two external cartilages, the thyroid cartilage (Adam's apple) and the cricoid cartilage (prominence at the top of the trachea; see Fig. 10.1A). The membrane between the two is called the cricothyroid membrane; a cricothyroidotomy may be performed by an experienced clinician at this site as an emergency procedure to

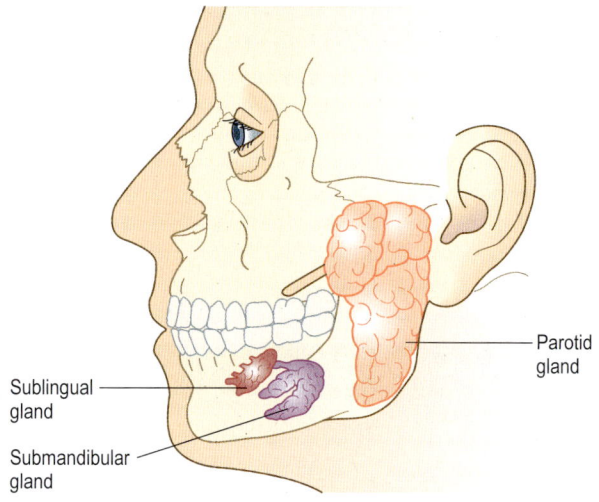

Fig. 9.19 The position of the major salivary glands.

obtain an airway. The sensory supply to the larynx is via the superior and recurrent laryngeal branches of cranial nerve X (vagus). The motor supply is mainly from the recurrent laryngeal nerve, which loops round the aortic arch on the left side and the subclavian artery on the right. Due to its longer pathway, the left recurrent laryngeal nerve is exposed to greater risk of damage during surgery to the neck or thorax, or from an upper lobe lung lesion.

### Teeth

In children the 20 deciduous teeth erupt by 3 years. There are 32 secondary teeth, erupting from ages 6 to 16 or later (Fig. 9.20).

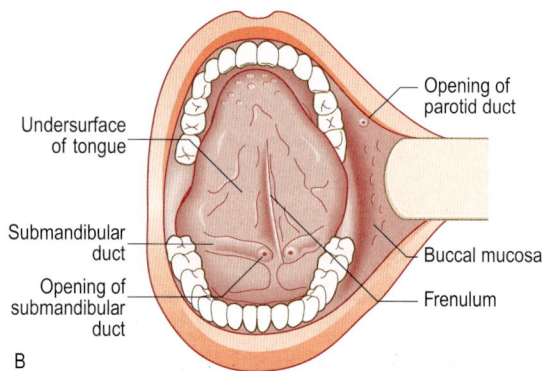

A             B

Fig. 9.18 Anatomy of the mouth and throat. [A] Examination with the mouth open. [B] Examination with the tongue touching the roof of the mouth.

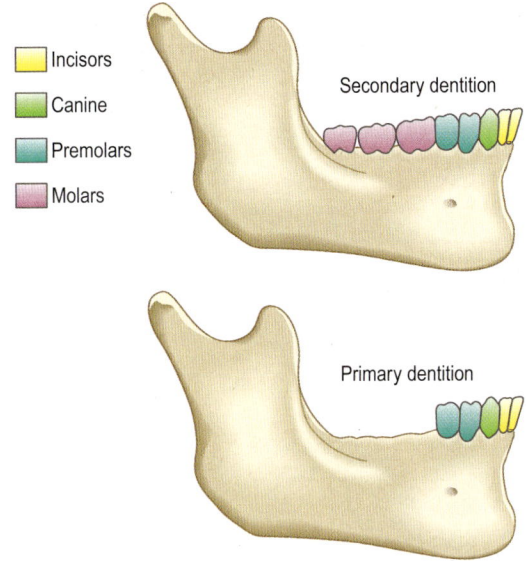

- Incisors
- Canine
- Premolars
- Molars

Secondary dentition

Primary dentition

**Fig. 9.20** Primary and secondary dentition.

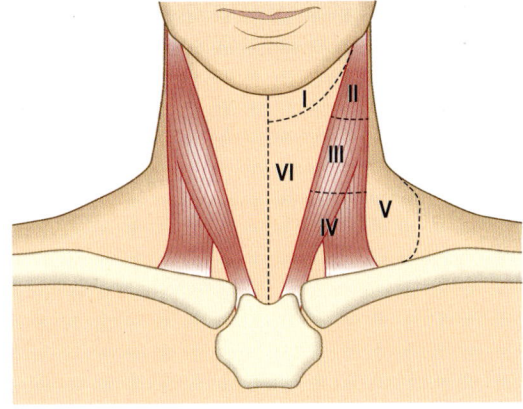

I   Submental and submandibular nodes
II  Upper third sternocleidomastoid (SCM) muscle
III Middle third SCM (between hyoid and cricoid)
IV  Lower third SCM (between cricoid and clavicle)
V   Posterior to SCM (posterior triangle)
VI  Midline from hyoid to manubrium

**Fig. 9.22** Cervical lymph node levels.

9

## Neck

Anatomically, the neck is divided into anterior and posterior triangles (Fig. 9.21). The anterior triangle is bounded by the midline, the anterior border of the sternocleidomastoid muscle and the body of the mandible. The posterior triangle of the neck is bounded by the posterior border of sternocleidomastoid, the trapezius muscle, and the clavicle. The cervical lymph nodes drain the head and neck (see Fig. 3.26). Examination of these nodes is described on page 37 and shown in Fig. 3.27. Palpable lymphadenopathy is most commonly due to URTI but may be caused by atypical infection, inflammation, lymphoma or metastatic malignancy. The neck can also be subdivided further into different levels that are used to describe the location of enlarged lymph nodes in the neck (Fig. 9.22).

## The history

## Common presenting symptoms

### Sore mouth

Ask about:

- how long pain has been present and any progression
- trauma to the mouth
- mouth ulcers
- problems with teeth or gums
- associated bleeding.

Aphthous ulcers are small, painful, superficial ulcers on the tongue, palate or buccal mucosa. They are common and usually heal spontaneously within a few days. Oral ulcers can be caused by trauma, vitamin or mineral deficiency, cancer, lichen planus or inflammatory bowel disease.

A sore mouth can also be due to conditions of the gums, including inflammation (gingivitis) or systemic conditions (Box 9.8).

Infections, including candidiasis (caused by *Candida albicans*), herpes simplex and herpes zoster, as well as dental sepsis, can cause a painful mouth. Candidiasis may be secondary to poorly fitted dentures, the use of inhaled glucocorticoids or immuno-deficiency. Herpes zoster of the maxillary division of the

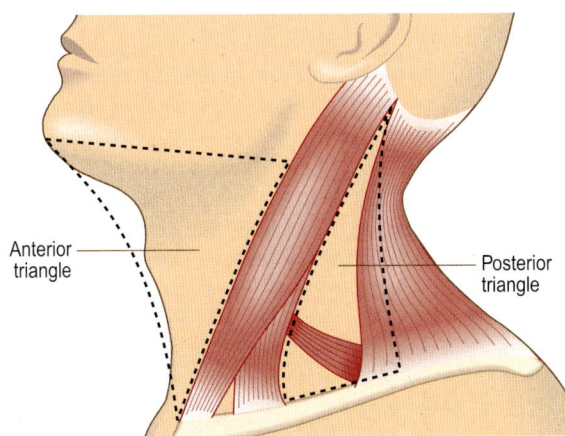

Anterior triangle

Posterior triangle

**Fig. 9.21** Sites of swellings in the neck.

| 9.8 The gums in systemic conditions | |
|---|---|
| Condition | Description |
| Phenytoin treatment | Firm and hypertrophied |
| Scurvy | Soft and haemorrhagic |
| Acute leukaemia | Hypertrophied and haemorrhagic |
| Cyanotic congenital heart disease | Spongy and haemorrhagic |

trigeminal nerve (see Fig. 7.9B) can cause unilateral painful vesicles on the palate.

## Sore throat

Ask about:

- unilateral or bilateral pain
- otalgia (earache)
- difficulty opening the mouth (trismus, due to spasm of the jaw muscles)
- associated fever, malaise, anorexia, neck swelling
- associated red flag symptoms (dysphagia, odynophagia, hoarseness, weight loss).

Throat pain can radiate to the ear because of the dual innervation of the pharynx and external auditory meatus via the vagus nerve (referred pain). The most common cause of sore throat is pharyngitis (inflammation of the pharynx) and is usually viral. Acute tonsillitis may be viral or caused by streptococcal bacterial infection (Fig. 9.23A) and cannot be distinguished clinically.

Infectious mononucleosis caused by Epstein–Barr virus (EBV) (glandular fever) results in tonsil erythema and swelling, a white pseudomembrane covering the tonsil, palatal petechiae (see Fig. 9.23B), cervical lymphadenopathy and sometimes hepatosplenomegaly. A peritonsillar abscess (quinsy) can lead to unilateral throat pain, trismus, drooling of saliva, soft-palate swelling, deviation of the uvula to the opposite side (see Fig. 9.23C) and 'hot-potato voice' (as though you were trying to speak with a hot potato in your mouth).

It is important to establish whether there are any 'red flag' symptoms associated with sore throat. Progressive dysphagia or hoarseness associated with weight loss should raise suspicion of malignancy. A mass or ulcer on the tonsil associated with throat pain may be a tonsil squamous cancer. Human papillomavirus-related oropharyngeal cancer is now the most common primary head and neck malignancy in young, sexually active non-smokers.

Globus pharyngeus is a sensation of something in the throat in the context of a normal clinical examination. Patients classically describe the feeling of a lump in the throat, usually in the midline, which fluctuates from day to day and eases when swallowing. Anxiety, habitual throat clearing and acid reflux are thought to be contributory factors.

A

B

C

**Fig. 9.23 Sore throat.** A Acute tonsillitis. The presence of pus strongly suggests a bacterial (streptococcal) aetiology. B Glandular fever showing palatal petechiae. C A left peritonsillar abscess. (A) From Bull TR. Color Atlas of ENT Diagnosis. 3rd edn. London: Mosby–Wolfe; 1995.

## Stridor

Stridor is a high-pitched noise produced by turbulent airflow through a narrowed, partially obstructed upper airway and can indicate laryngeal or tracheobronchial (p. 88) obstruction. It most commonly occurs on inspiration but may also be expiratory or biphasic. The level of obstruction determines the type of stridor. Inspiratory stridor suggests narrowing at the level of the vocal cords, biphasic stridor suggests subglottic/tracheal obstruction, and stridor on expiration suggests tracheobronchial obstruction. Common causes of stridor include infection/inflammation, trauma, foreign bodies (particularly in children) and tumours. Stridor should always be urgently evaluated.

Ask about:

- sudden or gradual onset
- associated fever
- associated hoarseness.

Stertor differs from stridor. It is a low-pitched snoring or gasping sound audible during inspiration and is due to obstruction at the level of the nasopharynx or oropharynx. This can result from enlarged inflamed tonsils, peritonsillar abscess or tongue swelling (trauma, anaphylaxis).

## Dysphonia

Ask about:

- how long dysphonia (hoarseness) has been present
- whether it is persistent or intermittent
- progression
- voice quality (croaky, breathy, weak)
- associated stridor, dysphagia, otalgia or weight loss.

If hoarseness has been present continuously for more than 3 weeks, urgent laryngoscopy is indicated to exclude laryngeal cancer. If voice quality is breathy and associated with a weak (bovine) cough (p. 87), a recurrent laryngeal nerve palsy due to lung or oesophageal cancer should be considered. Recurrent laryngeal nerve palsy may also be iatrogenic (thyroid surgery) or secondary to trauma or neurological conditions (Box 9.9).

## Dysphagia

The approach to dysphagia is described on page 110.

## Neck lump

Neck lumps are common; they may be reported by patients or found incidentally on physical examination. While many lumps are benign, there may be a more serious underlying diagnosis (Box 9.10).

Ask about:

- sudden or gradual onset
- progression
- associated pain
- associated hoarseness or dysphagia
- fever or other systemic symptoms (weight loss, night sweats).

Sudden, painful, unilateral salivary gland swelling (sialadenopathy) is due to a stone obstructing the duct (sialolithiasis). Other causes of enlarged salivary glands are mumps (usually bilateral), sarcoidosis, human immunodeficiency virus-related cysts, bacterial infection (suppurative parotitis; Fig. 9.24) and cancer. The clinical features of important neck lumps are summarised in Box 9.10.

### 9.9 Causes and features of dysphonia

| Causes | Features |
|---|---|
| **Neonate** | |
| Congenital abnormality | Laryngomalacia most frequent cause |
| | More common in preterm neonates |
| | Associated stridor due to immature larynx folding in on inspiration |
| Neurological disorder | Examples include vocal cord palsy |
| | Unilateral causing weak, breathy cry |
| | Bilateral may cause stridor and airway obstruction |
| **Child** | |
| Infection: | |
| Croup (laryngotracheobronchitis) | Barking cough, stridor, hoarse voice |
| Laryngitis | Bacterial or viral |
| Voice abuse (screamer's nodules) | History of voice abuse |
| **Adult** | |
| Infection: | |
| Upper respiratory tract infection | Associated features of upper respiratory tract infection |
| Laryngitis | |
| Trauma | Mechanical or chemical injuryCigarette smoking |
| | Gastro-oesophageal reflux disease (reflux laryngitis) |
| Lung cancer | Vocal cord paralysis, breathy voice |
| Vocal cord nodules (singer's nodules) | Prolonged vocal strainRough voice |
| | Reduced vocal range |
| | Vocal fatigue |
| Neurological disorder | Weak, wet or dysarthric voice |
| Cancer of the larynx | Rough voice, constant, progressive, often affects smokersAssociated with dysphagia, odynophagia, otalgia |
| Functional cause | |

## Past medical history

It is important to establish whether there are any previous dental problems or systemic disease – particularly those affecting the gastrointestinal tract – as the mouth is part of this. Neurological conditions may affect swallowing and cause drooling or dry mouth with secondary infection. Previous head and neck surgery and trauma should be noted.

Any prior intubations or admissions to intensive care should be recorded, as repeated or prolonged intubation can result in subglottic stenosis and stridor.

## 9.10 Causes and features of neck lumps

| Location in neck | Diagnosis | Clinical features |
|---|---|---|
| Midline | Thyroglossal cyst | Smooth, round, cystic lump that moves when patient sticks out tongue |
| | Submental lymph nodes | Associated infection of lower lip, floor of mouth, tip of tongue or cheek skin |
| | Thyroid isthmus swelling | Lump moves on swallowing |
| | Dermoid cyst | Small, non-tender, mobile subcutaneous lump |
| Lateral<br>Anterior triangle | Thyroid lobe swellings:<br>  Simple, physiological goitre<br>  Multinodular goitre<br>  Solitary nodule<br>  Thyroid tumours: benign (adenoma) and malignant (papillary, follicular, medullary, anaplastic) | Lump moves with swallowing but not on tongue protrusion |
| | Submandibular gland swelling:<br>  Infection, stones, autoimmune disease<br>  Benign or malignant tumours | Swelling below the angle of the mandible. Can be felt bimanually. Involvement of more than one gland suggests a systemic condition. A lump within the gland suggests a tumour. Uniform enlargement with pain suggests infection or stones |
| | Parotid gland swelling:<br>  Mumps, parotitis, stones, autoimmune disease | Swelling in the preauricular area or just below the ear |
| | Parotid gland mass:<br>  Benign<br>  Malignant tumours | Hard, fixed mass with facial nerve weakness suggests a malignant tumour of the parotid gland |
| | Branchial cyst | Smooth, non-tender, fluctuant mass. Not translucent. Slowly enlarging, may increase after upper respiratory tract infection |
| | Lymph nodes:<br>  Malignant: lymphoma, metastatic cancer<br>  Infection: bacterial infection of head and neck, viral infection (e.g., infectious mononucleosis), human immunodeficiency virus, tuberculosis | Large, hard, fixed, matted, painless mass suggests malignancy<br>Lymph nodes can be reactive to infection and are usually smooth, firm, mobile and tender |
| Posterior triangle | Lymph nodes:<br>  Malignant<br>  Benign | See p. 34 |
| | Carotid body tumour | Firm, rubbery, pulsatile neck mass fixed vertically due to attachment to bifurcation of common carotid. A bruit may be present |
| | Carotid artery aneurysm | Rare, present as pulsatile neck mass |
| | Cystic hygroma | Soft, fluctuant, compressible and transilluminable mass, usually seen in children |
| | Cervical rib | Hard, bony mass |
| Supraclavicular fossa | Supraclavicular lymphadenopathy | Left supraclavicular (Virchow's) node may suggest gastric malignancy |

## Drug history

Many drugs, including tricyclic antidepressants and anticholinergics, cause a dry mouth. Multiple repeated courses of antibiotics increase the risk of oral candidiasis, as do any prolonged illness.

## Social and family history

Risk factors for head and neck squamous cancer include alcohol and smoking. Oral cancer is more common in those who experience orogenital contact and in those who chew tobacco or betel nuts. Any history of head and neck cancer in the family should be established.

Fig. 9.24 Pus discharging from the parotid duct.

Fig. 9.25 **Torus palatinus.** This benign asymptomatic central palatal bony mass is more common in Asian populations. From Scully C. Oral and Maxillofacial Medicine. 2nd edn. Edinburgh: Churchill Livingstone; 2008.

**9**

## The physical examination

### Mouth and throat

### Examination sequence

- Listen to the patient's voice (rough, breathy, wet, muffled, nasal escape).
- Use a head light to leave both of your hands free to use instruments.

#### Inspection

- Ask the patient to remove any dentures.
- Look at their lips. Ask them to half-open their mouth and inspect the mucosa of the vestibule, buccal surfaces and buccogingival sulci for discoloration, inflammation or ulceration, then at bite closure. Inspect the parotid duct opening opposite the second upper molar for any pus or inflammation.
- Ask the patient to open their mouth fully and put the tip of their tongue behind their upper teeth. Check the mucosa of the floor of the mouth and the submandibular duct openings.
- Ask them to stick their tongue straight out, noting any deviation to either side (XII nerve dysfunction), mucosal change, ulceration, masses or fasciculation.
- Ask them to deviate their tongue to one side. Retract the opposite buccal mucosa with a tongue depressor to view the lateral border of the tongue. Repeat on the other side.
- Inspect the hard palate (Fig. 9.25) and note any cleft, abnormal arched palate or telangiectasia.
- Inspect the oropharynx. Ask the patient to say 'Aaah' and use a tongue depressor to improve visualisation.
- Assess the soft palate for any cleft, bifid uvula, swelling or lesions.
- Inspect the tonsils, noting size, symmetry, colour and any pus or membrane.
- Touch the posterior pharyngeal wall gently with the tongue depressor to stimulate the gag reflex. Check for symmetrical movement of the soft palate.

#### Palpation

- If any lesion is seen in the mouth or salivary glands, palpate it (wearing gloves) with one hand outside on the patient's cheek or jaw and a finger of your other hand inside the mouth (bimanual palpation).
- Feel the lesion and identify its characteristics (p. 36).
- If the base of the tongue or the tonsils are asymmetrical, palpate it using a gloved finger.
- If the parotid gland is enlarged or abnormal on inspection, examine the facial nerve and check if the deep lobe (tonsil area) is displaced medially.
- Palpate the parotid and submandibular duct, feeling for stones.
- Palpate the cervical lymph nodes (p. 36).

Cracking of the lips can be the result of cold exposure ('chapped lips'), riboflavin deficiency, chronic atrophic candidiasis or iron deficiency (Fig. 9.26). Squamous and basal cell cancers occur on the lips and are associated with smoking and sun exposure.

The normal tongue appearance includes areas of smooth mucosa ('geographic tongue') or, conversely, excessive furring. A smooth red tongue with diffuse papillary atrophy occurs in iron or vitamin $B_{12}$ deficiency. Tongue protrusion may be limited by neurological disease, painful mouth or a tight frenulum.

Fig. 9.26 **Angular stomatitis.**

**Fig. 9.27 Disorders of the tongue and teeth.** [A] Oral thrush. [B] Leukoplakia. [C] Aphthous stomatitis causing a deep ulcer in a patient with inflammatory bowel disease. [D] Dental caries. (B) From Bull TR. Color Atlas of ENT Diagnosis. 3rd edn. London: Mosby–Wolfe; 1995.

Macroglossia (enlarged tongue) occurs in Down's syndrome, acromegaly (see Fig. 10.9), hypothyroidism and amyloidosis. Wasting and fasciculation of the tongue are features of motor neuron disease.

White plaques of candidiasis on the tongue or mucosa (Fig. 9.27A) come away easily when scraped but leukoplakia (a keratotic precancerous condition) does not and requires excision biopsy (see Fig. 9.27B). Cancers (usually squamous) may occur at any site in the mouth. Any painless persistent mass in the mouth should be assumed to be oral cancer and referred urgently for biopsy. Similarly, any mouth ulcer persisting for over 3 weeks requires biopsy to exclude cancer (see Fig. 9.27C).

A stone may be felt in the submandibular (or, rarely, the parotid) duct. Rotten teeth (dental caries) are common in patients with poor oral hygiene (see Fig. 9.27D).

## Neck

The neck must be examined in all patients with mouth or throat symptoms, or a neck mass.

### Examination sequence (Video 20) ▶

- With the patient sitting down and their neck fully exposed (ties and scarves removed and shirt unbuttoned), look at their neck from in front. Inspect for scars, masses or pulsation.
- From behind, palpate the neck. Work systematically around the neck. Start in the midline and gently palpate the submental, submandibular and preauricular areas, assessing for the presence of any masses or swelling. Then palpate down the anterior border of the sternocleidomastoid muscle to the midline inferiorly.
- Palpate the midline structures of the neck from inferior to superior up to the submental area, noting any masses.
- If a midline mass is present, ask the patient to swallow (offer a glass of water if needed) and then instruct them to stick out their tongue while you palpate the mass. Movement superiorly on swallowing suggests a thyroid swelling (p. 224), while movement on tongue protrusion suggests a thyroglossal cyst (Fig. 9.28).
- Palpate the posterior triangle of the neck, including the posterior border of sternocleidomastoid and anterior border of trapezius. Palpate for occipital lymph nodes posteriorly.
- For any mass, note the size, site, consistency, edge, fixation to deeper structures, tethering to the skin, warmth, fluctuance, pulsatility and transillumination (p. 35).

## Investigations

Initial investigations are summarised in Box 9.11.

Fig. 9.28 Thyroglossal cyst.

9

### 9.11 Mouth, throat and neck investigations

| Investigation | Indication/comment |
|---|---|
| Full blood count | Infective causes of mouth, throat or neck symptoms |
| Monospot | Infectious mononucleosis<br>Hepatosplenomegaly can occur in infectious mononucleosis so liver function tests can be useful |
| Throat swab | Acute tonsillitis and pharyngitis<br>Patients may carry *Streptococcus pyogenes* and have a viral infection (detected by PCR), so swab does not always help direct management<br>PCR may help identify viral causes |
| Endoscopy and biopsy | Cancer of larynx and pharynx, changes in vocal cords<br>Under general anaesthetic |
| Ultrasound ± fine-needle aspiration | Neck lumps, swellings |
| Computed tomography | Cancer and metastases<br>Useful in staging |

*PCR,* Polymerase chain reaction.

### OSCE Example 1: Hoarseness

Mr Smith, 65 years old, presents with hoarseness.

#### Please take a history from the patient

- Introduce yourself and clean your hands.
- Invite the patient to describe the presenting symptoms, using open questioning.
- Take a detailed history of the presenting symptoms, asking specifically about onset, progression, fluctuation or constancy, provoking factors (work, singing, shouting) and weak or croaky voice. Enquire about associated cough, shortness of breath, throat pain, ear pain, dysphagia or weight loss.
- Ask about relevant history, including previous neck surgery, neck trauma, prolonged intubation, reflux disease and significant systemic conditions, including neurological problems.
- Enquire about drug history: specifically, recent courses of antibiotics (laryngeal candidiasis), anticholinergics (causing dry throat) or angiotensin-converting enzyme inhibitors (causing chronic dry cough).
- Ask about social history, including profession (singer, teacher), smoking and alcohol consumption.
- Address any patient concerns.
- Thank the patient and clean your hands.

#### Summarise your findings

The patient is a heavy smoker and reports slowly progressive hoarseness associated with breathlessness and a dry cough.

#### Suggest a diagnosis

This history suggests recurrent laryngeal nerve damage from a bronchial carcinoma. The differential diagnosis would include laryngeal carcinoma.

#### Suggest initial investigations

Full ear, nose and throat examination, including oral cavity, throat and neck, with a chest x-ray to exclude a bronchial carcinoma at the left hilum causing recurrent laryngeal nerve palsy. Persistent hoarseness (>3 weeks) requires referral for laryngoscopy to exclude laryngeal malignancy.

## OSCE Example 2: Neck lump

Mrs. Lee, 55 years old, presents with a lump just under her left ear at the angle of her jaw.

### Please examine her neck lump

- Introduce yourself and clean your hands.
- Inspect the neck for scars or swelling. If a neck lump is visible, describe its size, shape and site, as well as any skin changes. If it is in the midline, ask the patient to swallow and stick out their tongue.
- Ask if the lump is painful and if the patient minds you examining it.
- Palpate the lump to assess consistency, edge, fixation to deeper structures, tethering to the skin, warmth, fluctuance, pulsatility and transillumination.
- Palpate the anterior and posterior triangles of the neck, and the parotid region.
- Examine the oral cavity, throat, nose and ears (as potential primary sites of infection or malignancy that might be causing the neck mass).
- Assess facial nerve function if you suspect a parotid mass.
- Thank the patient and clean your hands.

### Summarise your findings

Examination confirms a firm, non-tender, mobile lump about 1 cm in diameter behind the angle of the jaw on the left.

### Suggest a diagnosis

The most likely diagnosis is a pleomorphic salivary adenoma in the tail of the parotid.

### Suggest investigations

Ultrasound scan with or without fine-needle aspiration.

## Integrated examination sequence for ear, nose and throat disease

- Position the patient: on an examination couch with the upper body at 45 degrees and neck fully exposed.
- Examine the ears:
  - Inspect: pinna skin, shape, size, position, deformity, scars.
  - Palpate: pinna, tragus, mastoid.
  - Otoscopy: external auditory canal (swelling, discharge), tympanic membrane (red, perforated).
  - If there is hearing loss: whispered voice test and tuning fork tests.
  - If there are balance symptoms: vestibular examination, including Dix–Hallpike.
- Examine the nose:
  - Inspect:
    - External nose (swelling, bruising, skin changes, deformity).
    - Anterior nasal septum (swelling, visible vessels, crusting ulceration, septal perforation). Exclude septal haematoma in nasal trauma.
    - Inferior turbinates (hypertrophy, swelling, polyps).
  - Palpate:
    - Nasal bones (bony or cartilaginous deformity).
    - Airway patency using metal spatula.
- Examine the mouth and throat:
  - Listen to the voice (rough, breathy, wet, muffled, nasal escape).
  - Remove any dentures.
  - Inspect:
    - Oral cavity, oropharynx.
    - Mucosal discoloration, inflammation, ulceration, masses, opening of parotid and submandibular ducts.
    - Hard palate for cleft, abnormal arched palate, telangiectasia.
    - Soft palate for cleft, bifid uvula, swelling or lesions.
    - Tonsils, noting size, symmetry, colour, pus or membrane.
  - Palpate:
    - Any lesion, identifying characteristics.
    - Base of tongue or tonsils if asymmetrical.
    - Parotid and submandibular ducts, feeling for stones.
- Examine the neck:
  - Inspect:
    - Scars, skin changes.
    - If there is midline swelling, ask the patient to swallow and stick out their tongue.
  - Palpate:
    - Anterior and posterior triangles of the neck and parotid region.
    - If there is a neck lump, note size, site, shape, consistency, edges, attachments, tenderness, warmth, pulsatility, transillumination.
    - If there is a parotid lump, assess the facial nerve.

**9**

Anna R Dover
Nicola Zammitt

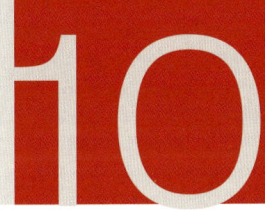

# The endocrine system

**The thyroid 220**

Anatomy and physiology 220

The history 222

Common presenting symptoms 222
Past medical, drug, family and social history 222

The physical examination 222

General examination 222
Thyroid gland 224
Eyes 225

**The parathyroids 225**

Anatomy and physiology 225

The history 225

Common presenting symptoms 225
Past medical, drug, family and social history 226

The physical examination 226

**The pituitary 226**

Anatomy and physiology 226

The history 226

Common presenting symptoms 226
Family history 227

The physical examination 227

**The adrenals 228**

Anatomy and physiology 228

The history 228

Common presenting symptoms 228
Past medical and drug history 231

The physical examination 231

**The gonads 231**

Anatomy and physiology 231

Common presenting symptoms and signs 231

**Diabetes 232**

Anatomy and physiology 232

The history 233

Common presenting symptoms 233
Past medical, drug, family and social history 234

The physical examination 234

OSCE example 1: Neck swelling 238

OSCE example 2: The diabetic foot 238

Endocrine glands synthesise hormones that are released into the circulation and act at distant sites. Diseases may result from excessive or inadequate hormone production, target organ hypersensitivity or resistance to the hormone. The main endocrine glands are the pituitary, thyroid, adrenals, gonads (testes and ovaries), parathyroids and the endocrine pancreas. With the notable exception of the pancreatic islet cells (which release insulin) and the parathyroids, most endocrine glands are themselves controlled by hormones released from the pituitary.

Since hormones circulate throughout the body, symptoms and signs of endocrine disease are frequently non-specific, affecting many body systems (Box 10.1). Often, endocrine disease is picked up incidentally during biochemical testing or radiological imaging. Careful history taking and examination are required to recognise characteristic patterns of disease. Thyroid disease and diabetes mellitus are common and frequently familial; establishing a detailed family history is therefore important. Some less common endocrine disorders (such as multiple endocrine neoplasia) show an autosomal dominant pattern of inheritance.

# THE THYROID

## Anatomy and physiology

The thyroid is a butterfly-shaped gland that lies inferior to the cricoid cartilage, approximately 4 cm below the superior notch of the thyroid cartilage (Fig. 10.1A). The normal thyroid has a volume of less than 20 mL and is palpable in about 50% of women and 25% of men. It features a central isthmus approximately 1.5 cm wide, overlying the second to fourth tracheal rings, and two lateral lobes that are usually no larger than the distal phalanx of the patient's thumb. The thyroid may extend into the superior mediastinum and can be partly or entirely retrosternal. Rarely, it is located along the line of the thyroglossal duct, along which the embryological thyroid descends from the base of the tongue to its final position. Thyroglossal cysts can also arise from the thyroglossal duct, often at the level of the hyoid bone (Fig. 10.1A); these characteristically move upwards on tongue protrusion. The thyroid is attached to the pretracheal fascia and thus moves superiorly on swallowing or neck extension.

Thyrotoxicosis is a clinical state of increased metabolism caused by elevated circulating levels of thyroid hormones. Graves' disease is the most common cause (Fig. 10.2 and Box 10.2). It is an autoimmune condition with a familial component and is 5–10 times more common in women, usually presenting between 30 and 60 years of age. Other causes include toxic multinodular goitre, solitary toxic nodule, thyroiditis and excessive thyroid hormone ingestion.

Hypothyroidism is caused by reduced levels of thyroid hormones, usually due to autoimmune Hashimoto's thyroiditis, and

### 10.1 Common clinical features in endocrine disease

| Symptom, sign or problem | Differential diagnoses |
|---|---|
| Tiredness | Hypothyroidism, hyperthyroidism, diabetes mellitus, hypopituitarism |
| Weight gain | Hypothyroidism, PCOS, Cushing's syndrome |
| Weight loss | Hyperthyroidism, diabetes mellitus, adrenal insufficiency |
| Diarrhoea | Hyperthyroidism, gastrin-producing tumour, carcinoid |
| Diffuse neck swelling | Simple goitre, Graves' disease, Hashimoto's thyroiditis |
| Polyuria and excessive thirst | Diabetes mellitus, diabetes insipidus, hyperparathyroidism, Conn's syndrome |
| Hirsutism | Idiopathic, PCOS, congenital adrenal hyperplasia, Cushing's syndrome |
| 'Funny turns' | Hypoglycaemia, phaeochromocytoma, neuroendocrine tumour |
| Sweating | Hyperthyroidism, hypogonadism, acromegaly, phaeochromocytoma |
| Flushing | Hypogonadism (especially menopause), carcinoid syndrome |
| Resistant hypertension | Conn's syndrome, Cushing's syndrome, phaeochromocytoma, acromegaly |
| Amenorrhoea/oligomenorrhoea | PCOS, hyperprolactinaemia, thyroid dysfunction |
| Erectile dysfunction | Primary or secondary hypogonadism, diabetes mellitus, non-endocrine systemic disease, medication-induced (e.g. beta-blockers, opiates) |
| Muscle weakness | Cushing's syndrome, hyperthyroidism, hyperparathyroidism, osteomalacia |
| Bone fragility and fractures | Hypogonadism, hyperthyroidism, Cushing's syndrome, primary hyperparathyroidism |

*PCOS,* Polycystic ovary syndrome.

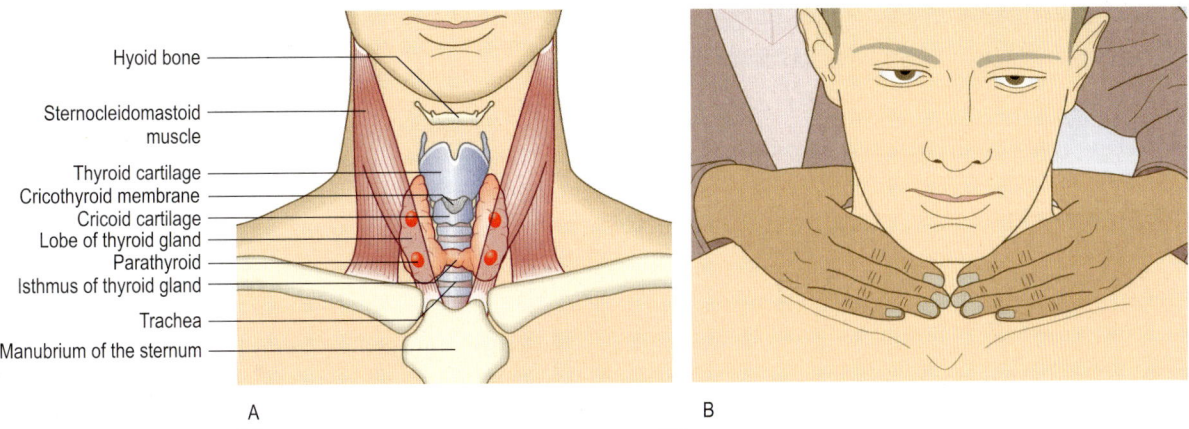

Hyoid bone
Sternocleidomastoid muscle
Thyroid cartilage
Cricothyroid membrane
Cricoid cartilage
Lobe of thyroid gland
Parathyroid
Isthmus of thyroid gland
Trachea
Manubrium of the sternum

A

B

**Fig. 10.1** **The thyroid gland.** A Anatomy of the gland and surrounding structures. B Palpating the thyroid gland from behind.

**10**

**Fig. 10.2** **Graves' hyperthyroidism.** A Typical facies. B Severe inflammatory thyroid eye disease. C Thyroid acropachy. D Pretibial myxoedema. *(A) From Strachan MWJ, Newell Price JDC. Endocrinology. In Ralston S, Penman I, Strachan MWJ, et al. (eds). Davidson's Principles and Practice of Medicine. 23rd ed. Philadelphia: Elsevier; 2018.*

---

**10.2 Features suggestive of Graves' hyperthyroidism**

**History**

- Female sex
- Family history of thyroid or other autoimmune disease
- Ocular symptoms ('grittiness', redness, pain, periorbital swelling)

**Physical examination**

- Vitiligo
- Thyroid acropachy
- Diffuse thyroid enlargement (can be nodular)
- Thyroid bruit
- Pretibial myxoedema
- Signs of Graves' ophthalmopathy (proptosis, redness, oedema)

---

affects women approximately six times more commonly than men. Most other causes are iatrogenic and include previous radioiodine therapy or surgery for Graves' disease.

# The history

## Common presenting symptoms

### Neck swelling

Goitre is an enlargement of the thyroid gland (Fig. 10.3). It is not necessarily associated with thyroid dysfunction; indeed, most patients with goitre are euthyroid. Large, or retrosternal, goitres may compress adjacent structures, causing stridor, breathlessness or dysphagia.

Thyroid enlargement can be due to diffuse goitre, multinodular goitre or a solitary nodule (Box 10.3). Thyroid nodules may be solitary (see Fig. 10.3C) or may be present as a dominant nodule within a multinodular gland. Palpable nodules (usually >2 cm in diameter) occur in up to 5% of women and less commonly in men, although up to 50% of patients have occult nodules; thus many are found incidentally on neck or chest imaging.

### Neck pain

Neck pain is uncommon in thyroid disease and, if sudden in onset and associated with thyroid enlargement, may represent bleeding into an existing thyroid nodule. Pain can also occur in viral subacute (de Quervain's) thyroiditis.

### History suggesting hyperthyroidism

Ask about:

- fatigue, poor sleep
- tremor, heat intolerance, excessive sweating (hyperhidrosis)
- pruritus (itch), onycholysis (loosening of the nails from the nail bed), hair loss
- irritability, anxiety, emotional lability

- dyspnoea, palpitations, ankle swelling
- weight loss, hyperphagia, faecal frequency, diarrhoea
- proximal muscle weakness (difficulty rising from sitting or bathing)
- oligomenorrhoea or amenorrhoea (infrequent or ceased menses, respectively)
- eye symptoms: 'grittiness', excessive tearing, retroorbital pain, eyelid swelling or erythema, blurred vision or diplopia (these symptoms of ophthalmopathy occur in the setting of autoimmune thyroid disease)

### History suggesting hypothyroidism

Ask about:

- fatigue, mental slowing, depression
- cold intolerance
- weight gain, constipation
- symptoms of carpal tunnel syndrome
- dry skin or hair

### Past medical, drug, family and social history

Ask about:

- prior neck irradiation (risk factor for thyroid malignancy)
- recent pregnancy (postpartum thyroiditis usually occurs in the first 12 months)
- drug therapy: antithyroid drugs or radioiodine therapy; amiodarone and lithium can cause thyroid dysfunction
- family history of thyroid or other autoimmune disease
- residence in an area of iodine deficiency, such as the Andes, Himalayas, Central Africa: can cause goitre and, rarely, hypothyroidism
- smoking (increases the risk of Graves' ophthalmopathy).

# The physical examination

## General examination

Look for signs of weight loss or gain (calculate the body mass index), and assess the patient's behaviour for signs of agitation, restlessness, apathy or slowed movements. Patients may have abnormal speech (pressure of speech suggests hyperthyroidism, while speech is often slow and deep in hypothyroidism). Hoarseness suggests vocal cord paralysis and should raise suspicion of thyroid malignancy.

Features of hyperthyroidism and hypothyroidism on examination are summarised in Fig. 10.4. A patient with hyperthyroidism may have warm, moist skin, proximal muscle weakness (due to a catabolic energy state), tremor and brisk deep tendon reflexes. Hyperthyroidism may also be associated with tachycardia or atrial fibrillation, and a midsystolic cardiac flow murmur due to increased cardiac output.

Dermopathy is an uncommon autoimmune extrathyroidal manifestation of Graves' disease. It occurs most commonly as

**10**

**Fig. 10.3 Thyroid enlargement.** A 99mTechnetium radionuclide scan demonstrating diffuse goitre due to Graves' disease. B Diffuse goitre due to Graves' disease. C Solitary toxic nodule. D 99mTechnetium radionuclide scan confirming multinodular goitre. *(A and D) Courtesy Dr Dilip Patel.*

## 10.3 Causes of thyroid enlargement

| Type of enlargement | Associated clinical features |
|---|---|
| *Diffuse goitre* | |
| Simple/physiological (puberty, pregnancy) | Soft, symmetrical, non-tender |
| Graves' disease | Hyperthyroidism, ophthalmopathy, pretibial myxoedema |
| Thyroiditis (Hashimoto's, subacute) | Hypothyroidism with Hashimoto's, tender goitre with hypo- or hyperthyroidism in subacute |
| Drugs (lithium, amiodarone, iodine) | Relevant drug history |
| Iodine deficiency (endemic goitre) | Particularly in mountainous regions |
| Infiltrative (amyloidosis, sarcoidosis, tuberculosis) | May be tender, other features of systemic disease |
| Dyshormonogenesis (e.g. Pendred's syndrome) | Congenital hypothyroidism, sensorineural deafness (Pendred's) |
| *Multinodular goitre* | Multiple nodules palpable or on scan |
| *Solitary nodule* | |
| Dominant nodule in a multinodular goitre | Distinguishing these may require ultrasound and/or fine needle aspiration |
| Colloid cyst | |
| Hyperplastic nodule | |
| Follicular adenoma | |
| Thyroid carcinoma (papillary, follicular, medullary, anaplastic) | May be fixed, with vocal cord involvement and/or lymph nodes |
| Lymphoma | Lymphadenopathy |
| Metastasis | Other clinical evidence of malignancy |

**Hyperthyroidism**

**Hypothyroidism**

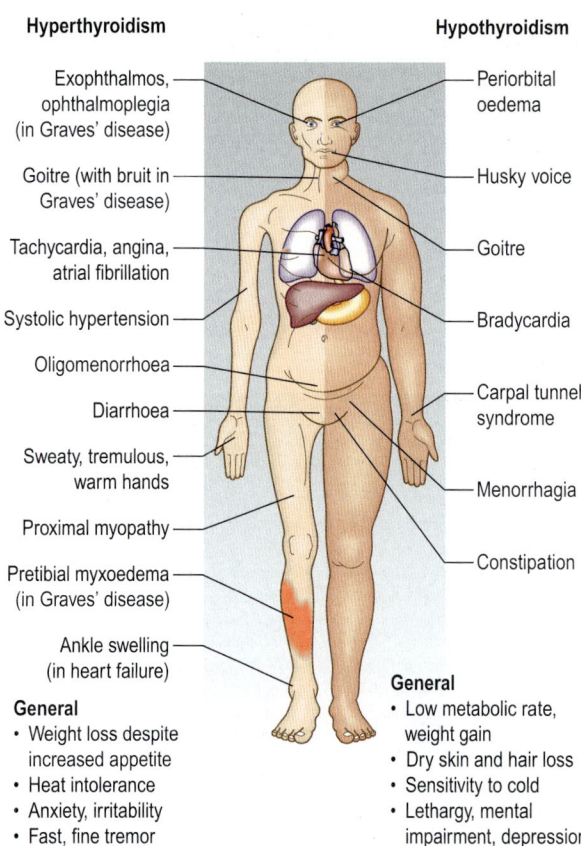

Exophthalmos, ophthalmoplegia (in Graves' disease)

Periorbital oedema

Goitre (with bruit in Graves' disease)

Husky voice

Tachycardia, angina, atrial fibrillation

Goitre

Systolic hypertension

Bradycardia

Oligomenorrhoea

Diarrhoea

Carpal tunnel syndrome

Sweaty, tremulous, warm hands

Menorrhagia

Proximal myopathy

Pretibial myxoedema (in Graves' disease)

Constipation

Ankle swelling (in heart failure)

**General**
• Weight loss despite increased appetite
• Heat intolerance
• Anxiety, irritability
• Fast, fine tremor

**General**
• Low metabolic rate, weight gain
• Dry skin and hair loss
• Sensitivity to cold
• Lethargy, mental impairment, depression

**Fig. 10.4** Features of hyper- and hypothyroidism.

pretibial myxoedema: a raised, discoloured (usually pink or brown), indurated appearance over the anterior shins; despite its name, it is specifically associated with Graves' disease and not hypothyroidism (see Fig. 10.2D). A less common extrathyroidal manifestation of Graves' disease is thyroid acropachy, a soft tissue swelling and periosteal hypertrophy of the distal phalanges which mimics finger clubbing (see Fig. 10.2C). It is almost always associated with dermopathy and ophthalmopathy.

Many clinical features of hypothyroidism are produced by myxoedema (non-pitting oedema caused by tissue infiltration by mucopolysaccharides, chondroitin and hyaluronic acid; Figs. 10.4 and 10.5). Other common findings in hypothyroidism include goitre, cool, dry or coarse skin, bradycardia, delayed ankle reflexes and a slowing of movement.

## Examination sequence

• Observe the facial appearance, noting dry or coarse hair and periorbital puffiness (see Fig. 10.5).
• Inspect the hands for vitiligo, thyroid acropachy (see Fig. 10.2C), onycholysis and palmar erythema.
• Assess the pulse (tachycardia, atrial fibrillation, bradycardia) and blood pressure.

**Fig. 10.5** Typical facies in hypothyroidism.

• Ask the patient to extend their arms. Inspect for a fine tremor due to sympathetic overactivity; laying a sheet of paper over the patient's fingers may improve detection.
• Auscultate the heart for a midsystolic flow murmur (hyperthyroidism).
• Inspect the limbs for coarse, dry skin or pretibial myxoedema (see Fig. 10.2D).
• Assess proximal muscle power and deep tendon (ankle) reflexes (p. 155).

## Thyroid gland

## Examination sequence (Video 21)

• Inspect the neck from the front, noting any asymmetry or scars. Inspect the thyroid from the side with the patient's neck slightly extended. Extending the neck will cause the thyroid (and trachea) to rise by a few centimetres and may make the gland more apparent. Give the patient a glass of water and ask them to take a sip and then swallow. The thyroid rises with the trachea on swallowing.
• Palpate the thyroid by placing your hands gently on the front of the neck with your index fingers just touching, while standing behind the patient (see Fig. 10.1B). The patient's neck should be slightly flexed to relax the sternocleidomastoid muscles. Ask the patient to swallow again and feel the gland as it moves upwards.
• Note the size, shape and consistency of any goitre and feel for any thrill.

- Palpate for cervical lymphadenopathy (Fig. 3.27, the neck examination sequence on p. 214, and the new neck video).
- Percuss the manubrium to assess for dullness due to retrosternal extension of goitre.
- Auscultate with your stethoscope for a thyroid bruit. A thyroid bruit (sometimes associated with a palpable thrill) indicates abnormally high blood flow and is most commonly associated with Graves' disease. It may be confused with other sounds, but carotid bruits or murmurs transmitted from the aorta are louder over the carotid artery.

Early simple goitres are relatively symmetrical but may become nodular with time. In Graves' disease, the surface of the thyroid is usually smooth and the gland diffusely enlarged; in uninodular or multinodular goitre, it is irregular (see Fig. 10.3). Diffuse tenderness is typical of viral thyroiditis. Localised tenderness may follow bleeding into a thyroid cyst. Fixation of the thyroid to surrounding structures (such that it does not move on swallowing) and associated cervical lymphadenopathy increase the likelihood of thyroid malignancy. Further investigation of thyroid disorders is summarised in Box 10.4.

## Eyes

### Examination sequence

- Look for periorbital puffiness or oedema and lid retraction (this is present if the white sclera is visible above the iris in the primary position of gaze; Fig. 10.2A).
- Examine for features of Graves' ophthalmopathy, including exophthalmos (look down from above and behind the patient), lid swelling or erythema and conjunctival redness or swelling (chemosis; Fig. 10.2B).
- Assess for lid lag: ask the patient to follow your index finger as you move it from the upper to the lower part of the visual field. Lid lag means delay between downward movement of the eyeball and descent of the upper eyelid, exposing the sclera above the iris.
- Assess eye movements (Fig. 8.9, p. 189). Graves' ophthalmopathy is characteristically associated with restriction of upgaze.

| 10.4 Investigations in thyroid disease | |
|---|---|
| **Investigation** | **Indication/comment** |
| **Biochemistry** | |
| Thyroid function tests | To assess thyroid status |
| **Immunology** | |
| Antithyroid peroxidase (TPO) antibodies | Non-specific, high in autoimmune thyroid disease |
| Antithyroid stimulating hormone receptor antibodies (TRAbs) | Specific for Graves' disease |
| **Imaging** | |
| Ultrasound | Goitre, nodule |
| Thyroid scintigraphy ($^{123}$I, $^{99m}$Tc) | To assess areas of hyper-/hypoactivity |
| Computed tomography | To assess goitre size and aid surgical planning |
| **Invasive/other** | |
| Fine-needle aspiration cytology | Thyroid nodule |
| Respiratory flow-volume loops | To assess tracheal compression from a large goitre |

Lid retraction (a staring appearance due to widening of the palpebral fissure) and lid lag (see above) are common eye signs associated with hyperthyroidism. Both are thought to be due to contraction of the levator palpebrae muscles as a result of sympathetic hyperactivity. Periorbital puffiness (myxoedema) is sometimes seen in hypothyroidism.

Graves' ophthalmopathy is an inflammatory infiltration of the soft tissues and extraocular muscles which affects around 20% of patients with Graves' disease (see Fig. 10.2A and B). Features suggestive of active inflammation include spontaneous or gaze-evoked eye pain, and redness or swelling of the lids or conjunctiva. Proptosis (protrusion of the globe from the orbit) may occur in both active and inactive Graves' ophthalmopathy and is often called exophthalmos. Inflammation of the orbital soft tissues may lead to other more severe features, including corneal ulceration, diplopia, ophthalmoplegia and compressive optic neuropathy (Fig. 8.8D).

10

# THE PARATHYROIDS

## Anatomy and physiology

There are usually four parathyroid glands situated posterior to the thyroid (see Fig. 10.1A). Each is about the size of a pea and produces parathyroid hormone, a peptide that increases circulating calcium levels.

## The history

### Common presenting symptoms

Parathyroid disease is commonly asymptomatic. In hyperparathyroidism, the most common symptoms relate to hypercalcaemia: polyuria, polydipsia, renal stones, peptic ulceration, tender areas of bone fracture or deformity ('Brown tumours') and delirium or psychiatric symptoms. In hypoparathyroidism, hypocalcaemia may cause hyper-reflexia or tetany (involuntary muscle contraction), most commonly in the hands or feet. Paraesthesiae of the hands and feet, or around the mouth, may occur. Hypoparathyroidism is most often caused by inadvertent damage to the glands during thyroid surgery but may also be caused by autoimmune disease. Patients with the rare autosomal dominant condition pseudohypoparathyroidism have end-organ resistance to parathyroid hormone and typically have short stature, a round face and shortening of the fourth and fifth metacarpal bones.

Ask about:

- Symptoms of hypercalcaemia:
  - polyuria, polydipsia
  - abdominal pain or constipation
  - confusion or psychiatric symptoms
  - bone pain
- Symptoms of hypocalcaemia:
  - muscle cramps, perioral or peripheral paraesthesia.

## Past medical, drug, family and social history

Ask about:

- recent neck surgery or irradiation
- past history of bone fractures
- past history of renal stones
- family history of hyperparathyroidism (which can be part of the autosomal dominant multiple endocrine neoplasia syndrome) or other endocrine disease (Addison's disease and type 1 diabetes can occur with hypoparathyroidism in the autosomal recessive type 1 autoimmune polyglandular syndrome).

**Fig. 10.6** Trousseau's sign.

## The physical examination

### Examination sequence

- Hands: ask the patient to make a fist and assess the length of the metacarpals (4th and 5th are shortened in pseudohypoparathyroidism).
- Examine the neck for scars. Parathyroid tumours are rarely palpable.
- Measure blood pressure and assess hydration (p. 279). Inflating the blood pressure cuff in a patient with hypocalcaemia may precipitate a typical pattern of muscle contraction, with the thumb adducted, the proximal interphalangeal and distal interphalangeal joints extended and the metacarpophalangeal joints flexed ('*main d'accoucheur*' (hand of the obstetrician), or Trousseau's sign; Fig. 10.6).
- Test for muscle weakness and hyper-reflexia (p. 254).
- Look for evidence of recent fractures or bone deformity/tenderness.
- Perform urinalysis (renal stones may cause haematuria).

# THE PITUITARY

## Anatomy and physiology

The pituitary gland is enclosed in the sella turcica at the base of the skull beneath the hypothalamus. It is bridged over by a fold of dura mater (diaphragma sellae) with the sphenoidal sinus below and the optic chiasm above. Lateral to the pituitary fossa are the cavernous sinuses, containing cranial nerves III, IV and VI and the internal carotid arteries (Fig. 8.3, p. 171). The gland comprises anterior and posterior lobes. The anterior lobe secretes adrenocorticotrophic hormone (ACTH), prolactin, growth hormone (GH), thyroid-stimulating hormone (TSH) and gonadotrophins (luteinising hormone (LH) and follicle-stimulating hormone (FSH)). The posterior lobe is an extension of the hypothalamus and secretes vasopressin (antidiuretic hormone) and oxytocin.

## The history

### Common presenting symptoms

Pituitary tumours are common and are found incidentally in around 10% of patients undergoing head computed tomography (CT) or magnetic resonance imaging (MRI). Hypopituitarism can result from a space-occupying lesion or from a destructive or infiltrative

**Fig. 10.7 Pituitary macroadenoma.** The tumour extends into the suprasellar cistern and is compressing the optic chiasm. *Courtesy Dr Dilip Patel.*

process such as trauma, radiotherapy, sarcoidosis, tuberculosis or metastatic disease. Pituitary infarction or haemorrhage can result in acute hypopituitarism (pituitary apoplexy) and is a medical emergency; it is often associated with headache, vomiting, visual impairment and altered consciousness. Secondary adrenal insufficiency due to pituitary apoplexy may be life-threatening and must be identified and treated urgently (see p. 231).

Non-functioning pituitary adenomas may be asymptomatic or may present with local effects such as compression of the optic chiasm causing visual loss (typically bitemporal upper quadrantanopia or hemianopia; Fig. 10.7 and Fig. 8.5) or headache due to expansion of the sella. Adenomas may produce hormones such as prolactin, GH or ACTH; the resulting symptoms and signs will depend on the excess hormone present.

## Prolactinoma

Ask about:

- galactorrhoea (breast milk secretion)
- oligomenorrhoea, amenorrhoea or infertility (in women)
- reduced libido, erectile dysfunction and reduced shaving frequency (in men)

## Acromegaly

GH excess prior to puberty presents as gigantism; after puberty, it causes acromegaly.

Ask about:

- headache
- excessive sweating
- changes in facial features (ask to see old photographs)
- an increase in shoe, ring or glove size
- associated medical conditions: arthropathy, carpal tunnel syndrome, hypertension, diabetes, colonic malignancy, sleep apnoea.

## Hypopituitarism

Apart from headache due to stretching of the diaphragma sellae and visual abnormalities, clinical presentation depends on the deficiency of the specific anterior pituitary hormones involved. Individual or multiple hormones may be involved, so questioning in relation to deficiencies of the thyroid, adrenocortical and reproductive hormones is needed.

## Family history

**10**

Enquire about family history since pituitary disease can occur as part of inherited multiple endocrine neoplasia or familial pituitary syndromes.

## The physical examination

### Acromegaly

#### Examination sequence

- Look at the face for coarsening of features, thick, greasy skin, prominent supraorbital ridges, enlargement of the nose, prognathism (protrusion of the mandible) and separation of the lower teeth (Fig. 10.8A and B).
- Examine the hands and feet for soft-tissue enlargement and tight-fitting rings or shoes, carpal tunnel syndrome and arthropathy (see Fig. 10.8C and D).
- Assess the visual fields (p. 183).
- Check the blood pressure and perform a urinalysis. Hypertension and diabetes mellitus are common associations.

### Hypopituitarism

#### Examination sequence

Look for:
- extreme skin pallor (a combination of mild anaemia and melanocyte-stimulating hormone deficiency)
- absent axillary hair
- reduced/absent secondary sexual hair and testicular atrophy (caused by gonadotrophin deficiency)
- visual field defects (most often bitemporal hemianopia), optic atrophy or cranial nerve defects (III, IV and VI), caused by a tumour compressing the optic chiasm, optic nerve or cavernous sinus.

**Fig. 10.8 Acromegaly.** A Typical facies. B Prognathism and separation of the lower teeth. C Large, fleshy hands. D Widening of the feet.

# THE ADRENALS

## Anatomy and physiology

The adrenals are small, pyramidal organs lying immediately above the kidneys on their posteromedial surface. The adrenal medulla is part of the sympathetic nervous system and secretes catecholamines. The adrenal cortex secretes cortisol (a gluco-corticoid), mineralocorticoids and androgens.

## The history

### Common presenting symptoms

Adrenal insufficiency is due to inadequate secretion of cortisol and can be due to intrinsic disease of the adrenal gland (primary) or due to failure, or suppression, of ACTH signalling (secondary).

**Fig. 10.9 Addison's disease.** [A] Hyperpigmentation in a patient with coexistent vitiligo. [B] Buccal pigmentation.

Primary adrenal insufficiency (Addison's disease; Fig. 10.9) is usually secondary to autoimmune destruction of the adrenal cortex but can also be due to infections (tuberculosis, HIV, fungal etc.), infarction, metastatic disease, or drugs (e.g. etomidate, ketoconazole, phenytoin). Secondary adrenal insufficiency is most often due to long-term exogenous glucocorticoid use but can also be due to pituitary disease. Symptoms are often non-specific.

Asymptomatic, non-functioning adenomas may be detected incidentally on abdominal CT or MRI scans. Functioning adrenal adenomas may present with refractory hypertension (Box 10.5) or features of androgen excess (p. 231).

Cushing's syndrome is caused by excess exogenous or endogenous glucocorticoid exposure. Most cases are iatrogenic and caused by side effects of glucocorticoid therapy. 'Endogenous' Cushing's usually results from an ACTH-secreting pituitary microadenoma, but other causes include a primary adrenal adenoma or 'ectopic' ACTH secretion by a non-pituitary tumour. The catabolic effects of glucocorticoids cause widespread tissue breakdown (leading to proximal myopathy, fragility fractures, spontaneous bruising and skin thinning) and a central accumulation of body fat (Fig. 10.10). Patients may develop hypertension or diabetes and are susceptible to infection.

| 10.5 Adrenal causes of endocrine hypertension | | |
|---|---|---|
| **Condition** | **Hormone produced in excess** | **Associated features** |
| Conn's syndrome | Aldosterone | Hypokalaemia |
| Cushing's syndrome | Cortisol | Central obesity, proximal myopathy, fragility fractures, spontaneous bruising, skin thinning, violaceous striae, hypokalaemia |
| Phaeochromocytoma | Noradrenaline (norepinephrine), adrenaline (epinephrine) | Paroxysmal symptoms, including hypertension, palpitations, sweating |

- nausea, vomiting, diarrhoea, constipation, abdominal pain and weight loss
- muscle cramps
- altered skin pigmentation (vitiligo or hyperpigmentation).

## Adrenal insufficiency

Ask about:

- weakness
- postural light-headedness

## Cushing's syndrome

Ask about:

- increase in weight, particularly if the weight is centrally distributed

**Fig. 10.10 Cushing's syndrome.** [A] Cushingoid facies. [B] After curative pituitary surgery. [C] Typical features: facial rounding and plethora, central obesity, proximal muscle wasting and violaceous skin striae. [D] Skin thinning: purpura caused by wristwatch pressure.

- bruising, violaceous striae and skin thinning
- difficulty rising from a chair/bath (may indicate proximal myopathy).

## Past medical and drug history

Enquire about recent or past exogenous glucocorticoid usage (route, dose, duration) as this may contribute to either iatrogenic Cushing's syndrome or suppression of the hypothalamic–pituitary–adrenal axis and resultant glucocorticoid insufficiency.

## The physical examination

### Adrenal insufficiency

#### Examination sequence

- Look for signs of weight loss.
- Examine the skin for abnormal or excessive pigmentation. This is most prominent in sun-exposed areas, or epithelia, subject to trauma or pressure: skin creases, buccal mucosa (see Fig. 10.9B) and recent scars. In primary adrenal insufficiency, the pituitary increases ACTH secretion in response to low cortisol levels. High levels of ACTH increase melanocyte-stimulating hormone, leading to increased skin pigmentation (most striking in Caucasians). Vitiligo (depigmentation of areas of skin) occurs in 10–20% of autoimmune Addison's disease cases (see Fig. 10.9A).

- Measure the blood pressure and test for postural hypotension (p. 48), resulting from salt and water loss due to inadequate mineralocorticoid.
- Patients on long-term glucocorticoids may have features of Cushing's syndrome (see below). Patients with an existing diagnosis of primary or secondary adrenal insufficiency may be carrying a steroid emergency alert card (Fig. 10.11).

### Cushing's syndrome

#### Examination sequence

- Look at the face and general appearance for central obesity; there may be a round, plethoric 'moon' face (see Fig. 10.10A) or dorsocervical fat pad ('buffalo hump').
- Examine the skin for thinning and bruising (see Fig. 10.10D), striae (especially abdominal; Fig. 10.10C), acne, hirsutism, signs of infection or poor wound healing.
- Measure the blood pressure.
- Perform ophthalmoscopy for cataracts and hypertensive retinal changes (Fig. 8.18, p. 189), and assess the visual fields (p. 162).
- Examine the spine for kyphosis and/or tenderness due to vertebral compression fractures (p. 297).
- Examine the legs for proximal muscle weakness and oedema.
- Perform urinalysis for glycosuria.

**10**

# THE GONADS

## Anatomy and physiology

The gonads (testes and ovaries) secrete sex hormones (testosterone and oestrogen) in response to gonadotrophin (FSH and LH) release by the pituitary. The reproductive system is covered in Chapter 11.

## Common presenting symptoms and signs

Most commonly, men present with androgen deficiency, whereas women present with hyperandrogenism.

Hypogonadism can be primary (failure of the gonad itself) or secondary (where reduced gonadotrophin levels cause gonadal failure). Klinefelter's syndrome (47XXY) is the most common cause of primary hypogonadism in men (1:600 live male births).

Secondary hypogonadism may be caused by pituitary disease, extremes of weight, or drugs that suppress hypothalamic gonadotrophin releasing hormone release (such as anabolic steroids or opiates). Presenting symptoms in men include loss of libido, erectile dysfunction, loss of secondary sexual hair, reduction in testicular size and gynaecomastia.

Hyperandrogenism in women usually presents with hirsutism (excessive male-pattern hair growth), acne and/or oligomenorrhoea and is commonly due to polycystic ovary syndrome (PCOS; usually also associated with obesity). Other less common causes, such as congenital adrenal hyperplasia, should also be considered. Virilisation is suggested by malepattern baldness, deepening of the voice, increased muscle bulk and clitoromegaly; if present in women with a short history of severe hirsutism, consider a testosterone-secreting tumour.

### Steroid Emergency Card (Adult)

**IMPORTANT MEDICAL INFORMATION FOR HEALTHCARE STAFF**
**THIS PATIENT IS PHYSICALLY DEPENDENT ON DAILY STEROID THERAPY** as a critical medicine. It must be given/taken as prescribed and never omitted or discontinued. Missed doses, illness or surgery can cause adrenal crisis requiring emergency treatment

**Patients not on daily steroid therapy or with a history of steroid usage may also require emergency treatment.**

Name .............................................................................................

Date of Birth ............................... NHS Number ...................................

Why steroid prescribed ...........................................................

Emergency Contact ...........................................................

---

When calling 999 or 111, emphasise this is a likely adrenal insufficiency/Addison's/Addisonian crisis or emergency AND describe symptoms (vomiting, diarrhoea, dehydration, injury/shock).

**Emergency treatment of adrenal crisis**

1) **Immediate 100mg** Hydrocortisone i.v. or i.m. injection.
   **Followed by** 24 hr continuous i.v. infusion of 200mg Hydrocortisone in Glucose 5% **OR** 50mg Hydrocortisone i.v. or i.m. qds (100mg if severely obese).

2) Rapid rehydration with Sodium Chloride 0.9%.

3) Liaise with endocrinology team.

 Scan here for further information or search
https://www.endocrinology.org/adrenal-crisis

**Fig. 10.11** Example of a steroid emergency alert card. *Courtesy Society for Endocrinology.*

## DIABETES

### Anatomy and physiology

The pancreas lies behind the stomach on the posterior abdominal wall. Its endocrine functions include production of insulin (from beta cells), glucagon, gastrin and somatostatin. Its exocrine function is to produce alkaline secretions containing digestive enzymes.

Diabetes mellitus is characterised by hyperglycaemia caused by absolute or relative insulin deficiency.

Diabetes can be classified into the following categories:

- Type 1: severe insulin deficiency due to autoimmune destruction of the pancreatic islets. These patients are susceptible to acute decompensation due to ketoacidosis or insulin-induced hypoglycaemia, both of which require prompt treatment.
- Type 2: commonly affects people who are obese and insulin-resistant, although impaired beta-cell function is also important. These patients may decompensate by developing a hyperosmolar hyperglycaemic state.
- Gestational diabetes: diabetes first diagnosed in the second or third trimester of pregnancy that is not clearly pre-existing type 1 or type 2 diabetes.
- Specific types of diabetes due to other causes. Examples with associated history and examination features are described in Box 10.6.

## 10.6 Causes of secondary diabetes[a]

| Cause of diabetes | Examples | Clinical features |
|---|---|---|
| Pancreatic disease | Pancreatitis<br>Trauma/pancreatectomy<br>Neoplasia<br>Cystic fibrosis<br>Haemochromatosis | Abdominal pain<br>Surgical scar<br>Weight loss<br>Chronic cough, purulent sputum<br>Skin pigmentation ('bronze diabetes') |
| Endocrinopathies | Acromegaly, Cushing's syndrome | p. 226 |
| Drugs | Glucocorticoids (e.g. prednisolone)<br>Antipsychotics (e.g. olanzapine)<br>Immunosuppressants (e.g. ciclosporin, tacrolimus) | Features of Cushing's syndrome (see Fig. 10.10)<br><br>Gum hypertrophy may be seen with ciclosporin use |
| Pregnancy | Gestational diabetes may develop in the third trimester | Gravid uterus |
| Monogenic defects in beta-cell function | Glucokinase deficiency | Glucokinase deficiency is present from birth with stable mild hyperglycaemia |
| Genetic syndromes associated with diabetes | Down's syndrome<br>Turner's syndrome | p. 39<br>p. 39 |

[a]Based on classification by the American Diabetes Association.

**10**

# The history

Diabetes is a long-term condition where self-management is key, and the language we use when speaking with people living with diabetes matters. Always use non-judgemental, respectful and empathic language, and avoid labelling people as 'diabetic'; most people prefer to be described as a 'person with diabetes'.

## Common presenting symptoms

### Newly diagnosed diabetes mellitus

Diabetes mellitus commonly presents with a classical triad of symptoms:

- polyuria (and nocturia): due to osmotic diuresis caused by glycosuria
- thirst: due to the resulting loss of fluid
- weight loss: due to fluid depletion and breakdown of fat and muscle, secondary to insulin deficiency.

Other common symptoms are tiredness, mood changes and blurred vision (due to glucose-induced changes in lens refraction). Bacterial and fungal skin infections are common because of the combination of hyperglycaemia, impaired immune resistance and tissue ischaemia. Itching of the genitalia (pruritus vulvae in women, balanitis in men) suggests *Candida* yeast infection (thrush).

### Diabetic ketoacidosis

Diabetic ketoacidosis (DKA) is an acute complication of insulin deficiency resulting in the production of ketone bodies and a consequent metabolic acidosis and osmotic diuresis. It may occur as the first presentation of diabetes or can develop in people with existing diabetes. It commonly presents with symptoms of hyperglycaemia (polyuria, thirst) alongside abdominal pain, vomiting and shortness of breath resulting from the underlying metabolic acidosis. Many people with type 1 diabetes have capillary blood glucose meters, which can also check capillary blood ketones. A blood ketone level of $\geq 3$ mmol/L suggests DKA. The history should cover possible triggers, such as omission of insulin or symptoms of intercurrent illness or infection.

### Hypoglycaemia

Hypoglycaemia may result from treatment with insulin or sulfonylureas. Symptoms of hypoglycaemia can be categorised as follows:

- Autonomic: e.g. hunger, sweating, tremor, palpitations
- Neuroglycopenic: e.g. confusion, irritability
- General malaise: e.g. tiredness, nausea

The history should include questions about possible precipitants, including missed meals, recent alcohol intake, insulin doses, exercise and the presence of lumpy insulin injection sites (lipohypertrophy). If the patient is unconscious or too confused to give a history, they should be assessed and treated using the ABCDE approach (Chapter 18, p. 395). Any episode requiring assistance from a third party is defined as severe and has implications for the person's ability to hold a driving licence (in the UK, this is governed by DVLA regulations https://www.gov.uk/guidance/assessing-fitness-to-drive-a-guide-for-medical-professionals). After the acute episode has been treated, the history should be completed by enquiring about the person's occupation and driving status.

## Past medical, drug, family and social history

Ask about:

- Other autoimmune conditions such as thyroid disease (increased incidence of type 1 diabetes).
- Previous glucose intolerance or gestational diabetes, which are risk factors for developing type 2 diabetes.
- Drug therapy: glucocorticoids can cause steroid-induced diabetes.
- Family history of diabetes or autoimmune disease. Monogenic diabetes is usually inherited in an autosomal dominant manner. Patients are often slim (unlike those with type 2 diabetes) but do not require insulin at diagnosis (unlike those with type 1 diabetes). Monogenic diabetes should be considered in people presenting with diabetes under the age of 30 who have an affected parent or a family history of early-onset diabetes in around 50% of first-degree relatives.
- Smoking: combines with diabetes to increase the risk of vascular complications.
- Alcohol: raises the possibility of pancreatic diabetes.

In established diabetes, key aspects of the history (Box 10.7) and examination should be reviewed at least annually. The history should cover any issues with daily glucose variability. Clinicians have historically focused on HbA1c as a measure of overall glycaemic control, as lower values reduce the long-term risk of complications of diabetes. However, for people living with diabetes, the daily variability in glucose levels is often of much greater immediate importance. For example, hypoglycaemia can affect the ability to exercise, drive or work. Recent advances in wearable technology which measure interstitial fluid glucose (continuous glucose monitors or flash glucose monitors; Fig. 10.12A) make it easier for the clinician and the person with diabetes to have meaningful conversations about glycaemic control as they provide more detailed information than intermittent or infrequent capillary blood glucose testing. Many patients link their data with their diabetes clinic, which supports virtual consultations. Clinicians should routinely ask what the individual uses to measure their

| **10.7 Routine history taking as part of the annual review in diabetes** |
|---|

**Glycaemic control**

- Frequency of blood or interstitial glucose checking
- Frequency and awareness of symptoms of hypoglycaemia
- When relevant, give guidance on driving and/or pre-pregnancy preparation

**Injection sites**

- Enquire about any lumpiness (lipohypertrophy), bruising or discomfort

**Symptoms of macrovascular disease**

- Enquire if any angina, myocardial infarction, claudication, stroke or transient ischaemic attack since the last clinic review

**Symptoms of microvascular disease**

- Ask if there has been any change in vision or any numbness or altered sensation in the feet

**Feet**

- Ask about neuropathy and peripheral vascular symptoms as above
- Enquire about any breaks in the skin, infections or ulcers

**Autonomic neuropathy**

- Enquire about erectile dysfunction in men
- Ask about postural hypotension, sweating, diarrhoea and vomiting in all patients

glucose levels, how often they check these, and whether they have identified any particular problems that they wish to discuss.

## The physical examination

The physical examination will differ, depending on whether this is a new presentation of diabetes or a person with established diabetes attending for annual review.

### Assessment of a person with newly diagnosed diabetes

#### Examination sequence

- Look for evidence of weight loss and dehydration. Unintentional weight loss is suggestive of insulin deficiency.
- Check for clinical features of acromegaly (see Fig. 10.8) or Cushing's syndrome (see Fig. 10.10).
- Assess for Kussmaul respiration (Box 18.4; hyperventilation with a deep, sighing respiratory pattern) or the sweet smell of

A                                                                              B

**Fig. 10.12** **A** Sensor measuring interstitial glucose and **B** Continuous subcutaneous insulin infusion pump. *(A) FreeStyle Libre is a trademark of Abbott or its related companies. Reproduced with permission of Abbott, © 2021. All rights reserved. (B) Courtesy Tandem Diabetes Care, Inc.*

acetone (a ketone), both of which suggest insulin deficiency and diabetic ketoacidosis.

- Skin: look for signs of infection such as cellulitis, boils, abscesses and fungal infections, paying particular attention to the feet (see later). Look for signs of insulin resistance such as acanthosis nigricans (Fig. 10.13A). Necrobiosis lipoidica, a yellow, indurated or ulcerated area surrounded by a red margin indicating collagen degeneration (see Fig. 10.13B), may occur on the shins in type 1 diabetes and often causes chronic ulceration.
- Look for xanthelasmata and xanthomata (Fig. 4.6, p. 52); these are suggestive of dyslipidaemia, which may occur in type 2 diabetes.
- Measure the pulse and blood pressure, and examine the cardiovascular and peripheral vascular systems with a particular emphasis on arterial pulses in the feet (p. 76).
- Examine the peripheral nervous system, with a particular focus on sensation in the lower limbs (p. 144).
- Test visual acuity and perform fundoscopy (p. 183 and Fig. 8.17, p. 188).
- Perform near-patient screening tests, such as capillary blood samples and urinalysis, both of which can be used to check for raised glucose or ketones. Diagnostic investigations are covered in Box 10.8.

Microvascular, neuropathic and macrovascular complications of hyperglycaemia can occur in patients with any type of diabetes mellitus, and may be present at diagnosis in patients with slow-onset type 2 disease.

Glycosuria is suggestive of diabetes; the presence of urinary (or blood) ketones suggests insulin deficiency and the possibility of diabetic ketoacidosis. Other investigations to consider are summarised in Box 10.8.

## Routine review of a person with diabetes

### Examination sequence

- Weight: an increase in weight in type 2 diabetes is likely to be associated with worsening insulin resistance, while weight loss in type 1 diabetes often suggests poor glycaemic control and inadequate insulin dosage.
- For patients using insulin, examine insulin injection sites or pump sites (see Fig. 10.12B) for evidence of lipohypertrophy (which may cause unpredictable insulin release; Fig. 10.13C), lipoatrophy (rare) or signs of infection (very rare).
- Measure the pulse and blood pressure.
- Test visual acuity and perform fundoscopy (p. 183 and Fig. 8.17, p. 188).
- Examine the feet (see the next section).
- Perform routine biochemical screening (see Box 10.8).

## The diabetic foot

Up to 40% of people with diabetes have peripheral neuropathy and 40% have peripheral vascular disease, both of which contribute to

**Fig. 10.13 Diabetes and the skin.** [A] Acanthosis nigricans. [B] Necrobiosis lipoidica. [C] Lipohypertrophy at insulin injection sites. *(A) Courtesy Istanbul Medeniyet University, Department of Dermatology; published in Uzuncakmak TK, Akdeniz N, Karadag AS. Cutaneous manifestations of obesity and the metabolic syndrome. Clin Dermatol. 2018;36(1):81–8. (C) From James WD, Elston DM, McMahon PJ. Diseases of subcutaneous fat. Andrews' Diseases of the Skin: Clinical Atlas. 1st ed. London: Elsevier; 2018.*

a 15% lifetime risk of foot ulcers (Fig. 10.14). Early recognition of the 'at-risk' foot is essential. There are two main presentations:

- Neuropathic: neuropathy predominates but the major arterial supply is intact.
- Neuroischaemic: reduced arterial supply produces ischaemia and exacerbates neuropathy.

Infection may complicate both presentations.

## Examination sequence (Video 5)

- Look for hair loss and nail dystrophy.
- Examine the skin (including the interdigital clefts) for excessive callus, skin breaks, infections and ulcers. Distal pallor can suggest early ischaemia, while purple/black discoloration suggests gangrene.

### 10.8 Investigations in diabetes

| Investigation | Indication/comment |
|---|---|
| **Diagnostic investigations** | |
| Fasting glucose, random glucose, oral glucose tolerance test | To make a diagnosis of diabetes. Patients also monitor capillary blood glucose to adjust their treatment |
| HbA1c | Can be used for diagnosis of type 2 diabetes and to assess glycaemic burden |
| Urine or blood ketone measurement | Ketones suggest insulin deficiency, which occurs in type 1 diabetes and in diabetes due to pancreatic pathology |
| Pancreatic antibodies (anti-GAD, anti-IA-2 and anti-ZnT8) | To confirm a diagnosis of autoimmune diabetes |
| C peptide | Used in established diabetes to distinguish between insulin-deficiency (low C peptide) and insulin-resistance (high C peptide) |
| **Annual review investigations** | |
| HbA1c | A measure of glycaemic control over the preceding 3 months; predicts risk of complications |
| Urea and electrolytes | To assess for diabetic nephropathy |
| Lipid profile | To aid estimation of cardiovascular risk and guide treatment with lipid-lowering therapy |
| Thyroid function tests | To screen for the commonly associated hypothyroidism |
| Urine albumin: creatinine ratio | To assess for early diabetic nephropathy (microalbuminuria) |
| Digital retinal photography or fundoscopy | To screen for diabetic retinopathy and/or maculopathy |

*GAD, glutamic acid decarboxylase, IA-2, insulinoma antigen 2, ZnT8, zinc transporter 8.*

- Ask the person to stand so that you can assess the foot arch; look for deformation of the joints of the feet.
- Feel the temperature of the feet.
- Examine the dorsalis pedis and posterior tibial pulses. If absent, arrange for Doppler studies and evaluate the ankle: brachial pressure index (p. 76).
- Test for peripheral neuropathy: use a 10-g monofilament to apply a standard, reproducible stimulus. The technique and the best sites to test are shown in Fig. 10.15. Avoid areas of untreated callus. Sensory loss typically occurs in a stocking distribution.
- Assess dorsal column function by testing vibration and proprioception.
- Undertake a foot risk assessment to guide management (Box 10.9).

When a consultation is being performed remotely and the clinician cannot examine the feet, they can direct the individual to the Diabetes UK website, which has videos demonstrating the self-administered 'Touch the Toes' test (www.diabetes.org.uk/guide-to-diabetes/complications/feet/touch-the-toes).

A

B

C

**Fig. 10.14 Diabetic foot complications.** **A** Infected foot ulcer with cellulitis and ascending lymphangitis. **B** Ischaemic foot: digital gangrene. **C** Charcot arthropathy with plantar ulcer.

A                                    B

**Fig. 10.15 Monofilament sensory testing of the diabetic foot.** **A** Apply sufficient force to allow the filament to bend. **B** Sites at highest risk (toes and metatarsal heads).

**10**

| 10.9 Risk assessment of the diabetic foot | | |
|---|---|---|
| **Level of risk** | **Definition** | **Action required** |
| Low | No sensory loss, peripheral vascular disease or other risk factors | Annual foot screening can be undertaken by any trained healthcare professional |
| Moderate | One risk factor present, e.g., absent pulses or reduced sensation | Annual foot screening should be undertaken by a podiatrist |
| High | Previous ulceration or amputation, or more than one risk factor present | Annual screening should be undertaken by a specialist podiatrist |
| Active foot disease | Ulceration, spreading infection, critical ischaemia or an unexplained red, hot, swollen foot | Prompt referral to a multidisciplinary diabetic foot team is required |

Hair loss and nail dystrophy occur with ischaemia. Feet are warm in neuropathy and cold in ischaemia. Ischaemic ulcers are typically found distally, at the tips of toes (see Fig. 10.14B), for example. There may be skin fissures or tinea infection ('athlete's foot'). Loss of sensation to vibration (p. 161) and proprioception (p. 161) are early signs of diabetic peripheral neuropathy. Sensory neuropathy is present if the person cannot feel the monofilament on the sites shown in Fig. 10.15. This suggests loss of protective pain sensation and is a good predictor of future ulceration.

With significant neuropathy, the foot arch may be excessive or collapsed (rocker-bottom sole). Both conditions cause abnormal pressures and increase the risk of plantar ulceration (see Fig. 10.14C), particularly in the forefoot. Charcot's arthropathy is disorganised foot architecture, acute inflammation, fracture and bone thinning in a person with neuropathy. It presents acutely as a hot, red, swollen foot and is often difficult to distinguish clinically from infection.

## OSCE example 1: Neck swelling

Miss Tan, 27 years old, presents with a 6-month history of palpitations, weight loss and neck swelling.

### Please examine her thyroid status

- Introduce yourself and clean your hands.
- Carry out a general inspection, observing dress, body habitus, agitation, restlessness, diaphoresis, anxiety, exophthalmos, goitre and neck scars.
- Inspect the hands for vitiligo, palmar erythema, thyroid acropachy and fine tremor (hands outstretched with paper over the dorsum).
- Palpate the pulse for bounding pulse, tachycardia and atrial fibrillation.
- Inspect the eyes for lid retraction (scleral show) and exophthalmos (look down from above and behind the patient).
- Test eye movements for ophthalmoplegia and lid lag.
- Examine the neck for scars, goitre, lymphadenopathy. Ask the patient to swallow to see the thyroid gland rise on swallowing.
- Palpate the thyroid (again on swallowing) and cervical lymph nodes; percuss manubrium for retrosternal goitre.
- Auscultate any goitre for bruit.
- Assess the patient for proximal myopathy (ask them to stand from sitting, with their arms crossed).
- Examine the shins for pretibial myxoedema and test for hyper-reflexia.
- Thank the patient and clean your hands.

### Summarise your findings

The patient is thin, with a fine tremor, tachycardia, exophthalmos and lid lag. In the neck there is a smooth, non-tender goitre.

### Suggest a diagnosis

These findings suggest autoimmune thyrotoxicosis (Graves' disease).

### Suggest investigations

Thyroid function tests, thyroid receptor autoantibodies and thyroid scintigraphy.

### Advanced level comments

Thyrotoxicosis may cause elevated alkaline phosphatase and hypercalcaemia due to increased bone turnover and normochromic normocytic anaemia.

## OSCE example 2: The diabetic foot

Mr Birnam, 67 years old, has type 2 diabetes and presents with pain in his lower limbs.

### Please examine his feet

- Introduce yourself and clean your hands.
- Carry out a general inspection of the lower limbs, looking for hair loss, nail dystrophy or discoloration.
- Inspect the skin for excessive callus, skin breaks, infections and ulcers.
- Inspect the joints. Ask the patient to stand so that you can assess the foot arch and look for deformation of the joints of the feet.
- Palpate the feet to assess the temperature of the skin.
- Palpate the dorsalis pedis and posterior tibial pulses.
- Test for peripheral neuropathy using a 10-g monofilament and tuning fork.
- Thank the patient and clean your hands.

### Summarise your findings

The patient has pale, cool feet with absent dorsalis pedis pulses bilaterally. The skin is intact but there is loss of sensation in stocking distribution in both feet.

### Suggest a diagnosis

The most likely diagnosis is peripheral vascular disease and peripheral neuropathy secondary to diabetes.

### Suggest investigations

Doppler studies to evaluate the ankle: brachial pressure index. Review of diabetes control.

### Advanced-level comments

With peripheral neuropathy, also take an alcohol history and check vitamin $B_{12}$ levels to take other common causes of peripheral sensory loss into account. Peripheral neuropathy can be confirmed in nerve conduction studies. Offer an examination for other microvascular complications, such as retinopathy (fundoscopy) and nephropathy (test urine for microalbuminuria).

# The reproductive system

Christina Yip
Colin Duncan
Kirsty Dundas
Alexander Laird

**11**

| | |
|---|---|
| **Breast 240** | Social history 255 |
| **Anatomy and physiology 240** | **Investigations 256** |
| **The history 240** | **Routine antenatal check in later pregnancy 257** |
| Common presenting symptoms 241 | **The history 257** |
| **The physical examination 242** | Common presenting symptoms 258 |
| **Examination sequence 242** | **The physical examination 258** |
| **Investigations 244** | **Investigations 260** |
| **Female reproductive system 245** | **Male reproductive system 262** |
| **Anatomy and physiology 245** | **Anatomy and physiology 262** |
| **The history 246** | **The history 263** |
| Common presenting symptoms 247 | Common presenting symptoms 263 |
| Drug history 249 | Past medical history 265 |
| Family and social history 249 | Drug history 265 |
| Sexual history 249 | Social history 265 |
| **The physical examination 249** | **The physical examination 265** |
| Passing a speculum 249 | Skin 265 |
| Taking a cervical smear 251 | Penis 266 |
| Bimanual examination 252 | Scrotum 266 |
| **Investigations 253** | Prostate 268 |
| **Obstetric history and examination: the booking visit 254** | **Investigations 268** |
| **The history 254** | **OSCE example 1: Breast examination 268** |
| Past medical history 254 | **OSCE example 2: Scrotal pain history 269** |
| Drug history 254 | **OSCE example 3: Gynaecological examination 269** |
| Family history 254 | |

# BREAST

## Anatomy and physiology

The adult breast lies over the pectoralis major and serratus anterior muscles; it extends from the lateral border of the sternum into the lower axilla as the tail of Spence. The centre of the breast is the nipple, which is composed mostly of smooth muscle fibres. The areola is the pigmented skin around the nipple that contains numerous Montgomery glands. The breast is divided into four quadrants by two invisible lines running horizontally and vertically through the nipple (Fig. 11.1). Accessory breast tissue (Fig. 11.2) is usually found in the axilla, whilst accessory nipples are most commonly seen just inferior to a normal breast or above the groins.

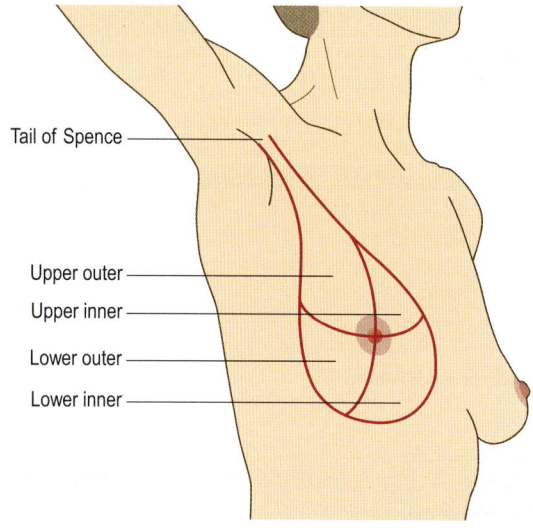

**Fig. 11.1** Adult right breast.

**Fig. 11.2** Accessory breast tissue in the axilla.

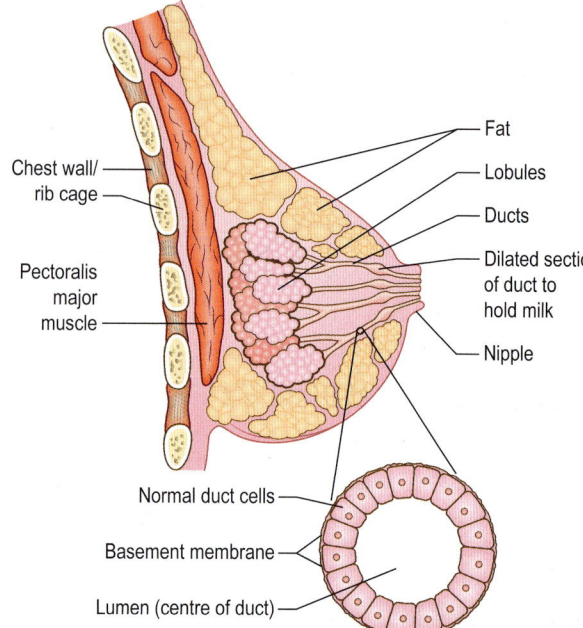

**Fig. 11.3** Cross-section of the female breast.

The breast is composed of mammary glands, which are modified sweat glands surrounded by connective tissue stroma (Fig. 11.3). The mammary glands consist of 15–20 duct and lobular units that open individually onto the nipple-areolar complex. The connective tissue stroma has a fibrous and a fatty component. The fibrous bands, called the suspensory ligaments of Cooper, anchor the breast tissue to the dermis and underlying pectoral fascia and separate the secretory lobules of the breast. The fibrous stroma maintains the shape of the breast, while the fatty component contributes to the breast volume. Advancing age, body weight fluctuations and hormonal changes during puberty, menstruation, pregnancy and lactation can alter the consistency and density of the breast, resulting in changes to breast shape and volume.

Four groups of lymph nodes drain each breast: supraclavicular, infraclavicular, internal mammary and axillary. More than 75% of the lymphatic drainage of the breast is to the ipsilateral axillary lymph nodes.

## The history

Breast symptoms affect all ages. Most patients present with a single breast complaint, but it is not uncommon for patients to have multiple breast concerns. The most common presenting symptoms are breast lumps, breast pain and changes to the skin and nipples. Malignancy is more common as patients get older.

An older patient who presents with a painless breast lump with skin dimpling and nipple inversion would raise suspicion of malignancy. On the other hand, a red, painful, swollen breast lump in a patient who is breastfeeding would suggest lactational mastitis.

For each presenting symptom, it is important to establish the duration and progression of the symptom and any association with the menstrual cycle.

In addition, ask about previous breast investigations, breast surgeries, breast cancer diagnoses and treatments. Document any exposure to exogenous oestrogen, especially the use of hormonal replacement therapy. Previous mantle field radiation for the treatment of lymphoma is also relevant.

Family history of cancer, especially breast and ovarian cancer, should be established. Be specific about the degree of relatives affected and their age at diagnosis.

## Common presenting symptoms

### Breast pain (mastalgia)

Ask if the pain varies during the menstrual cycle (if relevant) and establish the site, duration, severity and characteristics of the pain.

Breast pain associated with the menstrual cycle (cyclical mastalgia) is commonest among young women. Non-cyclical mastalgia may suggest a non-breast origin, for example, the chest wall. Ask about the association of pain with arm movements and the presence of underlying shoulder pathologies to distinguish a non-breast cause.

### Breast lump

A breast lump is the commonest reason for referral to a breast clinic. Many patients describe lumpiness or nodularity rather than a discrete mass. Patients may also present with an axillary lump. The general approach to history taking is the same for all these scenarios.

Ask:

- Is it a single lump or multiple lumps?
- When was it first noticed?
- Has it changed in size?
- Is there any relation to the menstrual cycle?

Establish:

- Any association with other symptoms, such as skin dimpling or nipple retraction?
- Any recent trauma to the breast?

In addition, for an axillary lump, establish:

- Any recent systemic illness?
- Any previous history of skin malignancy?

The commonest causes of an axillary lump are lymph nodes, skin lesions such as cysts, and accessory breast tissue.

### Breast volume and shape changes

Patients may report a change in the size or shape of their breasts. To quantify breast volume changes, it is best to ask the

**Fig. 11.4** Breast volume and shape changes to right breast following lumpectomy (scar at upper outer quadrant) and radiotherapy (tattoo indicated by *arrow*). Radiotherapy has also resulted in right breast skin thickening and hyperpigmentation

patient if they have recently changed their bra size. In addition, ask if the changes are:

- unilateral or bilateral,
- recent or longstanding

Breast cancer surgery or treatment, especially radiotherapy, are likely to cause scarring that results in breast skin colour, texture, shape and volume changes (Fig. 11.4).

Breast implant surgery is increasingly common, and changes to breast volume and shape may be a consequence of implant changes, such as capsular contracture or implant rupture.

### Skin changes

- Ask about skin colour and textural changes and their site, duration and progression. Common descriptions of skin changes used by patients include rash, dimpling, puckering and thickening. It is essential to understand what they are referring to and establish any association with other symptoms.
  - Rash can be a sign of infection. It is important to establish if the patient has been treated with antibiotics and if the rash has responded to them. If not, further investigation is necessary, as it may be a sign of inflammatory breast cancer (Fig. 11.5).
  - 'Orange peel appearance' or 'peau d'orange' describes thickened and dimpled breast skin (Fig. 11.6). It is a sign of breast lymphoedema and may be a consequence of infection or malignancy.

### Nipple changes

Patients may report changes to the nipple, or these may be noted on examination. Common nipple complaints are: pain, discharge, inversion and nipple and/or areola skin changes.

- Nipple pain: establish the duration, severity and characteristics of the pain.

11

**Fig. 11.5** Inflammatory breast cancer: patchy erythema, flattened nipple, peau d'orange of right breast.

**Fig. 11.6** *Peau d'orange* of the breast.

- Nipple discharge: establish if unilateral or bilateral and if spontaneous or provoked by massage. Ascertain the frequency, quantity (from single or multiple ducts) and the colour (white, yellow, green or blood-stained) of the discharge. Nipple discharge can be part of the ageing process (e.g. duct ectasia). Galactorrhoea, which is bilateral milky discharge not associated with pregnancy or breastfeeding, can be drug-induced or secondary to hyperprolactinaemia. A persistent, blood-stained (Fig.11.7), spontaneous, single duct nipple discharge should be investigated in order to exclude malignancy.
- Nipple and areola skin changes: may be skin colour changes, irritation or ulceration. Dermatitis of the nipple-areola complex can be part of a generalised skin condition; however, if it fails to respond to conservative treatments, Paget's disease of the nipple and skin malignancy should be excluded.
- Nipple inversion: retraction of the nipple is common. Establish its duration, whether it is correctible or not, and any associated

**Fig. 11.7** Single duct, blood-stained nipple discharge.

symptoms. Malignant nipple retraction is unlikely to be correctable and often presents with other signs of malignancy.

## Gynaecomastia

Gynaecomastia is the enlargement of the male breast and is usually, but not always, bilateral. It can be due to physiological, pharmacological or pathological causes, often when there is relative oestrogen excess or testosterone insufficiency (Box 11.1).

| 11.1 Causes of gynaecomastia | |
|---|---|
| Physiological | • Neonatal, puberty and old age |
| Pharmacological | • Prescription: cimetidine, digoxin, diazepam, spironolactone, Angiotension Converting Enzyme (ACE) inhibitor<br>• Recreational: cannabis, marijuana, alcohol, anabolic steroids |
| Pathological | • Cirrhosis, thyrotoxicosis, hypogonadism, Klinefelter's syndrome, testicular and adrenal tumours |

## The physical examination

Breast examination should be conducted in a well-illuminated room, on an examination bed, in the presence of a chaperone, whose name should be recorded. Ask your patient to undress to the waist and explain that you will be examining them sitting up as well as lying down.

## Examination sequence

- Ask the patient to sit with hands relaxed by their side (Fig.11.8A).
- Look for:
  - breast asymmetry: shape/contour and volume differences

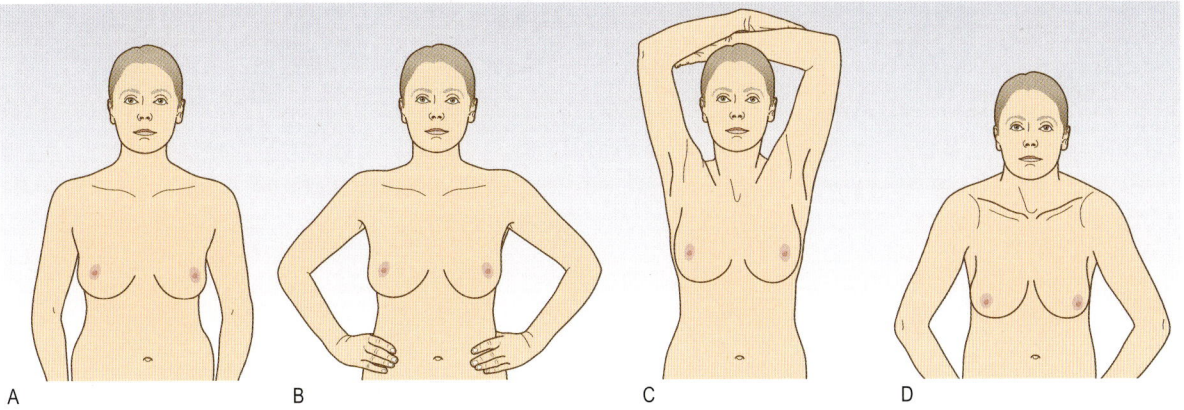

**Fig. 11.8 Positions for inspecting the breasts.** ⒶHands resting on the thighs. ⒷHands pressed on to the hips. ⒸArms above the head. ⒹLeaning forward with the breasts pendulous.

11

- breast skin colour and textural variation
- nipple-areola complex changes: spontaneous discharge, skin ulceration, nipple retraction.
- Operative scars and tattoos from previous chest wall radiotherapy
- chest asymmetry (see Chapter 5)
- Ask the patient to press their hands firmly on their hips to contract the pectoral muscles (see Fig. 11.8B), raise their arms above their head (see Fig. 11.8C) and then lean forward (see Fig. 11.8D).
- Look for any breast abnormality that becomes more visible with arm movements and note its association with the overlying skin, adjacent nipple-areola complex and underlying pectoral muscles.
- Ask the patient to lie supine, head on one pillow with their hand under their head on the side to be examined (Fig.11.9).
- Use both hands to palpate the breast and feel for abnormality under your fingertips. Avoid pressing too firmly as breasts can be very tender.
- Examine each quadrant of the breast from the outside towards the nipple, including under the nipple (Fig. 11.10).
- Examine the axillary tail between your finger and thumb.
- Gently squeeze the nipple between your index finger and thumb to determine if a discharge is present, either from a single or multiple ducts, and whether blood is present (either frankly or on urine dipstick testing).
- Palpate any breast abnormality. Assess its site, size, contour, texture and any fixation to the overlying skin, nipple-areolar complex or underlying muscle (Fig 11.11). Compare examination findings between the two breasts (Box 11.2).

**Fig. 11.9 Position for palpation of the right breast.**

A                        B                        C

**Fig. 11.10** **Clinical examination of the breast.** Examine each quadrant of the breast systematically, from the outside towards the nipple, including under the nipple.

**Fig. 11.11** Malignancy in the upper outer quadrant of left breast: painless, solid, irregular mass, fixed to the overlying skin.

### 11.2 Summary of examination findings in commonly presented breast conditions

| Conditions | Examination findings | Commonly affect |
|---|---|---|
| Fibroadenoma | • Extremely mobile, discrete, rubbery lump<br>• Solitary or multiples in one or both breasts | • Young women <35 years |
| Breast cyst | • Firm, discrete, smooth lump<br>• Solitary or in clusters | • Perimeno-pausal women |
| Lactational mastitis | • Pain, localised erythema and swollen breast<br>• Usually a history of cracked nipple | • Breastfeeding women |
| Non-lactational mastitis | • Peri-areolar infection: peri-areolar erythema and a mass or abscess<br>• Peri-areolar fistula | • Young female smokers |
| Malignancy | • Painless, solid, irregular mass, which can be fixed to surrounding tissues, leading to other skin and nipple changes (see Fig. 11.11) | • Women >50 years |

• Palpate the regional lymph nodes. The axilla and supra-clavicular fossa are best examined with the patient in a sitting position.
  • Support the full weight of the patient's arm at the wrist with your ipsilateral arm, place your contralateral hand high into the axilla and move it upwards over the chest to the apex. Compress the contents of the axilla against the chest wall. Define the characteristics of any mass (see Box 3.8 in the 14th edition).
  • Palpate the neck for the supraclavicular lymph nodes from behind (see Chapter 9).

## Investigations

Any breast abnormality, especially a breast lump, should be assessed by triple assessment: a combination of clinical, radio-logical and pathological examination.

Radiological examination options include mammography (Fig. 11.12) and ultrasonography (Fig. 11.13). Digital breast tomosynthesis (Fig.11.14) is sometimes used as an adjunct to standard mammography. Mammography is offered to women aged 40 or over, often in conjunction with ultrasonography, to detect malignancy. For women under 40, ultrasound is often the only imaging required. High breast density in younger women decreases the sensitivity of mammography for the detection of cancer. However, if there is a strong clinical and ultrasonographic suspicion of malignancy, then mammography is performed. Digital breast tomosynthesis increases cancer detection by increasing visibility between overlapped dense breast tissue. Breast MRI is the most sensitive technique for the detection of breast cancer; in selected cases, it can be used to evaluate the extent of cancer and for screening. It is also useful in assessing breast implant integrity.

The pathological examination involves a biopsy (Box 11.3). Image-guided biopsy improves diagnostic accuracy.

**Fig. 11.12 Digital mammogram.** A spiculate opacity characteristic of a cancer *(arrow)*.

**Fig. 11.13 Ultrasound of a breast cyst.** A characteristic smooth-walled, hypoechoic lesion *(arrow)*.

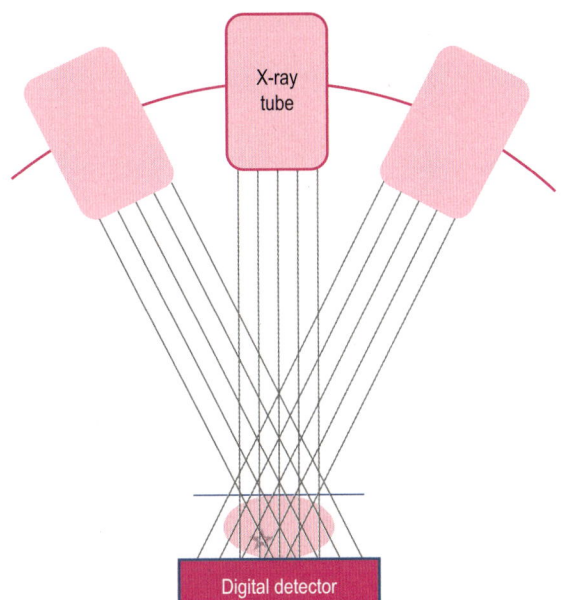

**Fig. 11.14 Digital breast tomosynthesis.** The x-ray tube moves along an acquisition angle obtaining projectional images (slices) of the compressed breast. These stacked images are then reconstructed to create three-dimensional images of the breast.

| 11.3 Fine-needle aspiration vs core biopsy | | |
|---|---|---|
| | Fine-needle aspiration | Core biopsy |
| Material examined | Cells | Tissue |
| Indications | Aspiration of cysts Lymph node assessment Sampling an area where core biopsy is technically not possible | Breast lump assessment Lymph node assessment |
| Advantages and disadvantages | Unable to distinguish between non-invasive and invasive cancer Molecular markers difficult to obtain | Can differentiate between non-invasive and invasive cancer Enables tumour grade and molecular markers assessment |

# FEMALE REPRODUCTIVE SYSTEM

## Anatomy and physiology

The female reproductive organs are situated within the bony pelvis (Fig. 11.15). They cannot normally be felt on abdominal palpation. A vaginal examination is required for their routine assessment.

The vulva (Fig. 11.16) consists of fat pads, called labia majora, covered with hair. The labia minora are hairless skin flaps at each side of the vulval vestibule, which contains the urethral opening and the vaginal orifice. The clitoris is situated anteriorly where the labia minora meet and is usually obscured by the prepuce. Posteriorly the labia meet at the fourchette, and the perineum is the fibromuscular region posteriorly that separates it from the anus.

The vagina is a rugged tube 10–15 cm in length. There is an irregular mucosal ring two centimetres into the vagina that represents the remnants of the hymen (see Fig. 11.16). Bulging into the top of the vagina is the grape-sized fibrous uterine cervix,

Fig. 11.15 Pelvis and pelvic organs.

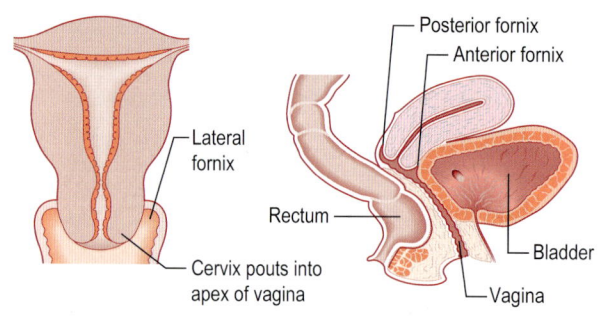

Fig. 11.18 Sagittal and coronal sections of the uterus. The vaginal fornices are shown.

Fig. 11.16 External female genitalia.

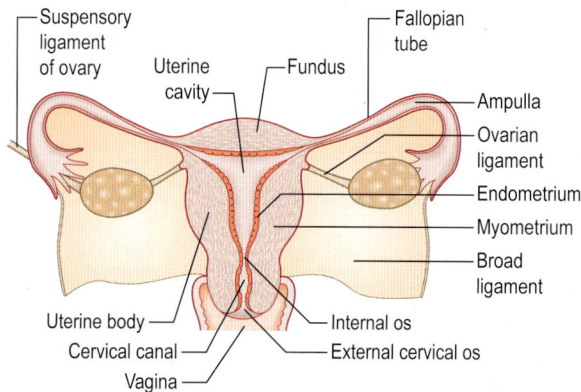

Fig. 11.17 Section through the pear-shaped, muscular uterus. The cervix, uterine body (corpus), fundus and Fallopian tubes, with the ligamentous attachments of the ovary. The uterine mucosa is the endometrium. The cervical canal has an internal and an external os.

with the external cervical os on its surface (Fig. 11.17). The fornices are the areas of the top of the vagina next to the cervix (Fig. 11.18).

The uterus is a muscular pear-shaped structure, about the size of a large plum, situated in the midline and usually tilted anteriorly over the bladder (Fig. 11.19). Its internal cavity is lined by endometrium that proliferates, secretes and breaks down during the menstrual cycle. The Fallopian tubes run laterally from the uterine fundus towards the ovaries (see Fig. 11.17). Their distal finger-like fimbriae collect the oocyte after ovulation.

The ovaries are about the size of a walnut and sit behind and above the uterus close to the pelvic sidewall. At mid-cycle, one ovary will have developed a fluid-filled preovulatory follicle measuring around 2 cm in diameter. The female reproductive tract is in close proximity to the bladder, ureter and lower gastrointestinal tract (see Fig. 11.19).

## The history

Identify the patient's main symptoms, how these developed, their day-to-day impact, how they cope and their ideas, concerns and expectations of the encounter. Document any previous investigations and management. Check the history, even if an asymptomatic patient has come for a routine cervical smear.

**Fig. 11.19 Lateral view of the female internal genitalia.** The relationship to the rectum and bladder.

Take a gynaecological history by asking about:

- (in pre- or perimenopausal patients) last menstrual period (LMP) and whether it was normal; always consider that these patients might be pregnant
- past and present contraceptive use
- plans for fertility
- previous cervical smears, when taken, and any treatment required for abnormalities
- prior abdominal surgery, pelvic infection or sexually transmitted disease
- prior pregnancies and their outcomes
- current or previous hormone replacement therapy
- other medication with potential gynaecological effects (see later).

## Common presenting symptoms

### Abnormal vaginal bleeding

If patients present with heavy periods, ask about:

- flooding: whether menstrual blood soaks through protection, increased requirements for sanitary protection
- passing of blood clots.

Menstruation normally occurs monthly from the menarche (average age 12) until the menopause (average age 51). Menstrual bleeding for 3–6 days normally occurs every 22–35 days (average 28). A menstrual cycle with bleeding for 4–5 days every 25–29 days is recorded as 4–5/25–29. Heavy menstrual bleeding (HMB, previously called menorrhagia) affects 20% of menstruating patients over 35 and is defined as >80 mL blood loss during a period (average 35 mL). As this is not quantified in routine practice, HMB is subjective. Anaemia implies heavy bleeding.

Unexpected bleeding suggests endometrial or cervical pathology. Ask when the bleeding occurs:

- between periods (intermenstrual bleeding, IMB)
- after intercourse (postcoital, PCB)
- more than 1 year after menopause (postmenopausal bleeding, PMB).

Approximately 4% of postmenopausal patients experience bleeding, which must be investigated as 10% have endometrial cancer.

Lack of periods (amenorrhoea) in the absence of pregnancy implies ovarian dysfunction and affects 5–7% of females in their reproductive years. Distinguish between:

- Primary amenorrhoea: periods have not started by age 16. Both ovarian function and the structure of the reproductive tract should be investigated.
- Secondary amenorrhoea: there have been no periods for ≥6 months, but there was previous menstruation.
- Oligomenorrhoea: the menstrual cycle is longer than 35 days.

Thirty percent of patients experience vaginal bleeding in early pregnancy. Establish if this is associated with lower abdominal pain. Although the pregnancy may continue normally, bleeding is associated with miscarriage and ectopic pregnancy. Further investigation is required, particularly if the bleeding is associated with lower abdominal pain.

### Lower abdominal pain

Lower abdominal pain may arise from the reproductive organs or the urinary or gastrointestinal tract or be musculoskeletal or neurological in origin (p. 108). Psychological and social factors may also contribute to the experience of pain.

To differentiate between the possible causes of lower abdominal pain, ask about:

- site of the pain (unilateral, bilateral or midline)
- onset (sudden or gradual, cyclical/related to menstruation or not).

Ovarian pain is often unilateral and can be physiological (*Mittelschmertz* is discomfort associated with ovulation). Ovarian cyst accidents involving torsion (twisting on the vascular pedicle

11

causing acute ischaemia), haemorrhage or rupture can lead to acute severe pain.

Primary dysmenorrhoea is pain arising from intense uterine contractions just before and during peak menstruation. Secondary or progressive dysmenorrhoea, due to underlying pathology such as endometriosis or chronic infection, often manifests as pain that lasts beyond the normal menstrual cycle. Infection, pelvic adhesions and endometriosis can cause generalised pain (Box 11.4).

Dyspareunia is pain during intercourse. Ask if it is felt around the vaginal entrance (superficial) or within the pelvis (deep). Pain due to an involuntary spasm of muscles at the vaginal entrance (vaginismus) may make intercourse impossible. Persistent deep dyspareunia suggests underlying pelvic pathology. Dyspareunia can be due to vaginal dryness following menopause.

Iliac fossa pain in early pregnancy is commonly associated with a corpus luteum cyst of the ovary but may indicate a tubal ectopic pregnancy. Ruptured ectopic pregnancy results in generalised abdominal pain, peritonism, haemodynamic instability and referred pain in the shoulder.

## Abdominal distension and bloating

Pelvic masses can cause non-specific symptoms like abdominal distension, bloating or urinary frequency due to pressure on the bladder. They may also be asymptomatic and picked up during routine abdominal or vaginal examination. Uterine masses include pregnancy and benign leiomyoma tumours (fibroids). Large ovarian cysts can also be midline, and malignant ovarian cysts are associated with ascites.

## Vaginal discharge

Discharge may be normal and variable during the menstrual cycle. Prior to ovulation, it is clear, abundant and stretches like egg white; after ovulation, it is thicker, does not stretch and is less abundant. Abnormal vaginal discharge occurs with infection. Ask about:

- consistency
- colour
- odour
- associated itch, pain or dysuria.

The most common non-sexually transmitted infection (caused by *Candida* species) gives a thick, white, curdy discharge often associated with marked vulval itching. Bacterial vaginosis is a common, non-sexually acquired infection caused by multiple bacteria, particularly *Gardnerella vaginalis*, producing a watery, fishy-smelling discharge. The pH of normal vaginal secretions is usually <4.5, but in bacterial vaginosis, it is >5. Sexually transmitted infections (STIs) can cause discharge, vulval ulceration or pain, dysuria, lower abdominal pain and general malaise. They may also be asymptomatic.

## Urinary incontinence

Inappropriate and involuntary voiding of urine is severe in 10% of cases, and its prevalence increases with age.

Stress incontinence occurs on exertion, coughing, laughing or sneezing and is associated with pelvic floor weakness.

Urge incontinence is an overwhelming desire to urinate when the bladder is not full due to detrusor muscle dysfunction.

## Prolapse

In 30% of patients, the pelvic contents bulge into the vagina (Fig. 11.20). They feel something 'coming down', particularly when standing or straining. Uterine prolapse is associated with previous childbirth and is classified as:

- Grade 1: halfway to the hymen.
- Grade 2: at the hymen.
- Grade 3: beyond the hymen.
- Grade 4 (procidentia): external to the vagina (Fig. 11.21).

### 11.4 Characteristics of pelvic pain

| | Uterine pain | Ovarian pain | Adhesions or pelvic infection | Endometriosis |
|---|---|---|---|---|
| Site | Midline | Left or right iliac fossa | Generalised lower abdomen; more on one side | Variable |
| Onset | Builds up before period | Sudden, intermittent | Builds up, acute on chronic | Builds up, sudden |
| Character | Cramping | Gripping | Shooting, gripping | Shooting, cramping |
| Radiation | Lower back and upper thighs | Groin; if free fluid, to shoulder | – | – |
| Associated symptoms | Bleeding from vagina | Known cyst, pregnancy, irregular cycle | Discharge, fever, past surgery | Infertility |
| Timing | With menstruation | May be cyclical | Acute, may be cyclical | Builds up during period |
| Exacerbating factors | – | Positional | Movement, examination | Intercourse, cyclical |
| Severity | Variable in spasms | Intense | Intense in waves | Variable |

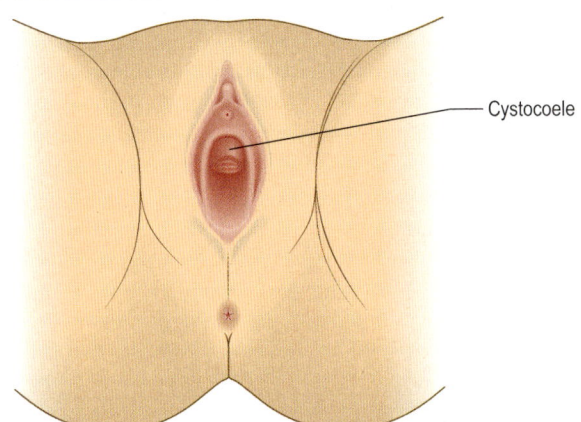

**Fig. 11.20** Anterior vaginal wall prolapse.

**Fig. 11.21** External prolapse of the uterus.

The top of the vagina (vault) can also prolapse after a previous hysterectomy. More commonly, the bulge relates to the vaginal wall. A cystocoele is a bulge on the anterior wall containing the bladder (see Fig. 11.20), and a rectocoele is a bulge on the posterior wall containing the rectum. An enterocoele is a bulge of the distal wall posteriorly containing the small bowel and peritoneum.

## Drug history

Tamoxifen has oestrogenic effects in postmenopausal patients, antibiotics can cause vaginal candidiasis, antipsychotic drugs can cause hyperprolactinaemia, and antiepileptic or antituberculous drugs may reduce the effectiveness of oral contraceptives.

## Family and social history

Family and social history, including smoking status and lifestyle, may also have an impact on gynaecological conditions. For

example, obesity is associated with an increased risk of gynaecological malignancy.

| **11.5 Taking a sexual history** |
| :--- |
| • Are you currently in a sexual relationship? |
| • How long have you been with your partner? |
| • Have you had any (other) sexual partners in the last 12 months? |
| • How many were male? How many were female? |
| • When did you last have sex with: |
|   • Your partner? |
|   • Anyone else? |
| • Do you use barrier contraception—sometimes, always or never? |
| • Have you ever had a sexually transmitted infection? |
| • Are you concerned about any sexual issues? |

## Sexual history

Sometimes a sexual history is required, but people often find it difficult to talk about sexual matters. It is important for you to be at ease and ask questions in a straightforward manner. Explain why you need to enquire, use clear, unambiguous questions (Box 11.5) and be non-judgemental. The sexual partners of patients with STIs should be informed and treated to prevent further transmission and reinfection of the treated person. Confidentiality is paramount, so do not give information to a third party. Do not perform a pelvic examination on someone who has not been sexually active.

## The physical examination

A vaginal examination is required to perform a routine cervical smear. Otherwise, the focus of gynaecological examination is to detect abnormalities that could explain the symptoms or alter treatment options (e.g. body mass index (BMI) and blood pressure assessment affect the use of the contraceptive pill). Signs of gynaecological disease are not limited to the pelvis, and a general, as well as a pelvic, examination is required (Box 11.6). You should offer a chaperone and record this in the records. The examination area should be private, with appropriate equipment and an adjustable light source available. The patient should have an empty bladder and remove their clothing from the waist down, along with any sanitary protection. Give them privacy to do this.

## Passing a speculum

Explain what you are going to do and why it is necessary, and obtain verbal consent. Use a vaginal speculum to see the cervix and the vaginal walls, carry out a cervical smear and take swabs if required. Specula are metal or plastic and come in various sizes and lengths. Metal specula may be sterilised and reused; plastic specula are always disposable. A metal speculum is cold, so

**11**

### 11.6 Focus of the gynaecological examination

| Clinical feature | General examination | Pelvic examination |
|---|---|---|
| Abnormal bleeding | Anaemia<br>Underweight (hypogonadotrophic hypogonadism)<br>Galactorrhoea, visual field defects (hyperprolactinaemia)<br>Hirsutism, obesity, acanthosis nigricans (PCOS) | Enlarged uterus (fibroids, pregnancy)<br>Abnormal cervix<br>Open cervical os (miscarriage)<br>Vaginal atrophy (most common cause of PMB) |
| Pain | Abdominal tenderness | Uterine excitation (acute infection or peritonism)<br>Fixed uterus (adhesions or endometriosis)<br>Adnexal mass (ovarian cyst) |
| Vaginal discharge | Rash (associated with some STIs) | Clear from cervix (chlamydia)<br>Purulent from cervix (gonorrhoea)<br>Frothy with strawberry cervix (trichomoniasis) |
| Urinary incontinence | Obesity, chronic respiratory signs (stress incontinence)<br>Neurological signs (urge incontinence) | Demonstrable stress incontinence<br>Uterine or vaginal wall prolapse |
| Abdominal distension or bloating | Ascites, weight loss, lymphadenopathy, hepatomegaly (malignancy)<br>Pleural effusion (some malignant or benign ovarian cysts) | Pelvic mass (uterine, ovarian or indiscriminate)<br>Fixed uterus and adnexae<br>Abnormal vulva (skin disease or malignancy) |

*PCOS,* Polycystic ovary syndrome; *PMB,* postmenopausal bleeding; *STI,* sexually transmitted infection.

warm it under the hot tap. Most patients find a speculum examination mildly uncomfortable, so always use a small amount of lubricating gel on the tip of each blade. Clean your hands and put on medical gloves. Ask the patient to lie on their back on the couch, covered with a modesty sheet to the waist, with their knees bent and apart (Fig. 11.22).

## Examination sequence (Videos 22 and 22A)

- Look at the perineum for any deficiency associated with childbirth; note abnormal hair distribution and clitoromegaly (associated with hyperandrogenism). Note any skin abnormalities, discharge or swellings of the vulva, such as the Bartholin's glands on each side of the fourchette (Fig. 11.23).
- Ask the patient to cough while you look for any prolapse or incontinence.
- Gently part the labia using your left hand (Fig. 11.24). With your right hand, gently insert a lightly lubricated bivalve speculum (Figs 11.25–11.26A), with the blades vertical, fully into the vagina, rotating the speculum through 90 degrees so that the handles point anteriorly and the blades are now horizontal (see Fig. 11.26B). Someone who has been pregnant may need a larger or longer speculum or a bolster under the sacrum if the cervix is very posterior. If they find the examination difficult, ask them to try to insert the speculum themself.
- Slowly open the blades and see the cervix between them. If you cannot see it, reinsert the speculum at a more downward angle, as the cervix may be behind the posterior blade. Note any discharge or vaginal or cervical abnormalities.
- Open the blades a little during the initial removal of the speculum to avoid catching and pulling on the cervix.

**Fig. 11.22** Position for pelvic examination.

## To assess prolapse (Video 22B)

- Ask the patient to lie on their left side and bring their knees up to their chest.
- Use a univalve Sims speculum, placing a small amount of lubricating jelly on the blade.

**Fig. 11.23** Bartholin's abscess.

**Fig. 11.24** Inspection of the vulva.

**Fig. 11.25** Bivalve speculum.

A

B

**Fig. 11.26** Bivalve speculum examination. A Insertion of the speculum. B Visualisation of the cervix after rotation through 90 degrees.

- Insert the blade to hold back the posterior wall.
- Ask them to cough while you look for uterine descent and the bulge of a cystocoele (Fig. 11.27).
- Repeat, using the speculum to hold back the anterior vaginal wall to see a rectocoele or enterocoele.

## Taking a cervical smear

There are two ways of taking a smear:

- using liquid-based cytology
- using a microscope slide.

**Fig. 11.27** Examination in the left lateral position using a Sims speculum.

A

Cytology specimen jar

B

Glass slide

**Fig. 11.28** Taking a cervical smear. **A** Liquid-based cytology. **B** Using a spatula.

Liquid-based cytology is increasingly common, as it allows for efficient processing and gives fewer inadequate smears. Many screening services now test these for human papilloma virus (HPV) rather than performing routine cytology.

### Examination sequence (Video 22C)

- Always label the cytological medium or slide and ask the questions required to fill in the request form before starting the examination to avoid mixing specimens.
- Clearly visualise the entire cervix.

#### Liquid-based cytology
- Insert the centre of the plastic broom into the cervical os.
- Rotate the broom 5 times through 360 degrees (Fig. 11.28A).
- Push the broom 10 times against the bottom of the specimen container.
- Twirl 5 times through 360 degrees to dislodge the sample.
- Firmly close the lid.

#### Conventional smear
- Insert the longer blade of the spatula into the cervical os.
- Rotate the spatula through 360 degrees (see Fig. 11.28B).
- Spread once across the glass slide.
- Place the slide immediately into fixative (methylated spirits) for 3–4 minutes.
- Remove it and leave it to dry in the air.

## Bimanual examination

### Examination sequence (Video 22D)

- Apply gloves and lubricate your right index and middle finger with gel.
- Gently insert them into the vagina and feel for the firm cervix. The uterus is usually anteverted (Fig. 11.29A), and you can feel its firmness anterior to the cervix. If the uterus is retroverted and lying over the bowel (15%; Fig. 11.29B), you will feel the firmness posterior to the cervix.
- Push your fingers into the posterior fornix and lift the uterus while pushing on the abdomen with your left hand.
- Place your left hand above the umbilicus and bring it down, palpating the uterus between both hands and note its size, regularity and any discomfort (Fig. 11.30).

A                                                           B

**Fig. 11.29** Coronal section. **A** Anteverted uterus. **B** Retroverted uterus.

**Fig. 11.30** **Bimanual examination of the uterus.** Use your vaginal fingers to push the cervix back and upwards, and feel the fundus with your abdominal hand.

**Fig. 11.31** **Palpating an adnexal mass.**

- Move your vaginal fingers into the anterior fornix and palpate the anterior surface of the uterus, holding it in position with your abdominal hand.
- Move your fingers to the lateral fornix and, with your left hand above and lateral to the umbilicus, bring it down to assess any adnexal masses between your hands on each side (Fig. 11.31).
- If urinary leakage occurs when the patient coughs, try lifting the anterior vaginal wall with your fingers and ask them to cough again. This stops genuine stress incontinence.

The normal cervix os may be a slit after childbirth. The vaginal squamous epithelium and the endocervical columnar epithelium meet on the cervix. The position of this squamo-columnar junction varies considerably, so the cervix can look very different in individual people. If the transition zone is on the cervix, this is called an ectopy and looks red and friable; there may be small cysts called Nabothian follicles. The normal uterus should feel regular and be mobile and the size of a plum. The Fallopian tubes cannot be felt, and normal ovaries are palpable only in the very slim.

Vulval changes include specific skin diseases, infections such as herpes or thrush, and malignancy. Visual abnormalities of the cervix such as ulceration or bleeding suggest cervical pathology, including polyps or malignancy. Tender nodules in the posterior fornix suggest endometriosis, and both endometriosis and pelvic adhesions cause fixation of the uterus. Acute pain when touching the cervix (cervical excitation) suggests an acute pelvic condition such as infection, cyst accident or tubal rupture.

Fibroids can cause uterine irregularity and enlargement. The size is related to that of the uterus in pregnancy. A tangerine-sized uterus is 6 weeks, an apple at 8 weeks, an orange at 10 weeks and a grapefruit at 12 weeks. After 12 weeks, the uterus can be palpated suprapubically on abdominal palpation. A large midline mass may be ovarian or uterine. Push the mass upwards with your left hand and feel the cervix with your right hand; if the mass moves without the cervix, this suggests it is ovarian.

## Investigations

Common gynaecological investigations are summarised in Box 11.7. Patients of reproductive age should be considered potentially pregnant, and a pregnancy test is routine. The mainstay of gynaecological investigation is a pelvic ultrasound scan, which can be carried out abdominally or transvaginally (Fig. 11.32). Endometrial biopsy is a common test, particularly for PMB, and is performed during vaginal examination using a suction catheter (Pipelle, Fig. 11.33). When a couple presents with subfertility, the key female investigations are serum progesterone 1 week before expected menses to confirm ovulation and a test of tubal patency (Fig. 11.34).

**11**

## 11.7 Investigations in gynaecological disease

| Clinical feature | Investigations | Diagnosis |
|---|---|---|
| Abnormal bleeding | Full blood count | Anaemia |
| | Ultrasound scan | Fibroids, endometrial polyp or pregnancy outcome and location |
| | Endometrial biopsy | Endometrial hyperplasia or carcinoma |
| | Hysteroscopy | Intrauterine polyps or fibroids |
| | Colposcopy | Cervical premalignant and malignant changes |
| | Gonadotrophins, sex steroids and prolactin | PCOS, premature ovarian insufficiency, hyperprolactinaemia or hypogonadotrophic hypogonadism |
| Pain | White blood count | Infection |
| | C-reactive protein | Acute inflammation |
| | High vaginal and endocervical swabs | Pelvic and vaginal infections, chlamydia or gonorrhoea |
| | Midstream specimen of urine | Urinary tract infection |
| | Ultrasound scan | Ovarian cysts, tubo-ovarian abscesses or intraperitoneal bleeding |
| | Laparoscopy | Pelvic adhesions and endometriosis |
| | Serial serum HCG | Ectopic pregnancy |
| Vaginal discharge | High vaginal and endocervical swabs | Pelvic and vaginal infections, chlamydia or gonorrhoea |
| Urinary incontinence | Midstream specimen of urine | Urinary tract infection |
| | Urodynamic studies | Degree of stress or urge incontinence |
| Abdominal distension or bloating | Ultrasound | Ovarian cysts, fibroids, pregnancy and ascites |
| | CT/MRI scan | Staging of pelvic malignancy |
| | Serum CA-125 | Ovarian tumour marker |
| | Renal and liver function tests | Systemic effects of pelvic masses |
| | Direct or ultrasound-guided biopsy | Diagnosis of potential malignancy |

*CA-125,* Cancer antigen 125; *CT,* computed tomography; *HCG,* human chorionic gonadotrophin; *MRI,* magnetic resonance imaging; *PCOS,* polycystic ovary syndrome.

# OBSTETRIC HISTORY AND EXAMINATION: THE BOOKING VISIT

In the UK, pregnant patients are seen at approximately 10 antenatal visits; the visits may either be conducted by a midwife alone or be shared with an obstetrician. Care is individualised depending on maternal age, past medical history and general health, as well as any complications that develop as the pregnancy proceeds.

The booking (first) visit takes place at 8–12 weeks' gestation.

## The history

Take a complete medical history and record details of any previous pregnancies (Boxes 11.8–11.9). Establish the date of the LMP (Box 11.10).

### Past medical history

Ask about:

- all past medical and surgical events
- diseases that may be affected by pregnancy: for example, asthma may improve during pregnancy while inflammatory bowel disease may worsen postnatally

- diseases that cause an increased risk in pregnancy, such as diabetes, cardiac disease or Systemic Lupus Erythematosus (SLE).

### Drug history

Ask about:

- prescribed medications
- over-the-counter drugs and 'natural' remedies

Find out at what gestation any drugs were taken. Check that pregnant patients are taking 400 µg of folic acid daily until 12 weeks gestation to reduce the incidence of neural tube defects (some higher-risk patients need a higher dose of 5 mg, for example, patients taking anti-epileptic medication or those with pre-existing diabetes).

### Family history

To explore possible inherited conditions, take a complete family history of both the pregnant patient and the father (Boxes 11.11 and 11.12).

**Fig. 11.32 Pelvic ultrasound.** **A** Transvaginal scan of the uterus. **B** Scan showing an ovarian cyst.

**Fig. 11.33** Pipelle for endometrial biopsy.

**Fig. 11.34 Hysterosalpingogram.** The scan assesses the uterus and bilateral tubal patency.

11

### 11.8 Checklist for the obstetric history

- Age
- Parity
- Menstrual history, last menstrual period, gestation, expected date of delivery
- Presenting symptom
- Past obstetric history
- Past medical and surgical history
- Drug history
- Family history
- Social history

### 11.9 Information to be recorded for previous pregnancies

- Date and gestation of delivery
- Indication for and mode of delivery (e.g. spontaneous vaginal delivery, operative vaginal delivery (forceps or ventouse) or Caesarean section)
- Singleton or multiple pregnancy
- Any pregnancy complications (take a full history)
- Duration of first and second stage of labour
- Weight and sex of the baby
- Health at birth, mode of infant feeding
- Postnatal information about mother and baby

## Social history

Enquire about the use of alcohol, tobacco and illegal drugs. Check a carbon monoxide level to detect the level of smoking. Advise all smokers to stop and offer referral to smoking cessation support. Advise all pregnant persons to avoid alcohol.
Ask:

- who the patient's partner/support is
- how stable the relationship is

### 11.10 Definitions

| Term | Definition |
|------|------------|
| LMP | First date of the last menstrual period (LMP) |
| EDD | Estimated date of delivery: 40 weeks from LMP. Fewer than 5% of babies deliver on their due date; the majority deliver between 37 and 42 completed weeks–this period is called term. Estimated Date of Delivery (EDD) is most accurately calculated from an ultrasound scan measurement of the foetal crown–rump length or head circumference done at the end of the first trimester |
| Parity | Number of previous births. Written in the format x + y, where x is the number of live births and any births over 24 weeks, and y is the number of all other pregnancies–babies born before 24 weeks with no signs of life, ectopic pregnancy, miscarriage and termination of pregnancy. Multiple pregnancy counts as one delivery–the number refers to pregnancies delivered and not to the number of foetuses/babies |
| Gestation | Number of weeks + days of pregnancy counted from LMP (although not conceived till ovulation approximately 2 weeks later or 14 days before the next period is due) |
| Trimester | The 40 weeks of pregnancy are divided into three trimesters of approximately 13 weeks each |
| Liquor or amniotic fluid | Fluid surrounding the fetus in utero |
| Oligohydramnios, polyhydramnios | Too little and excess amniotic fluid, respectively |
| Miscarriage | Expulsion of a fetus prior to viability |
| Live birth | Birth of a baby with signs of life |
| Still birth | Birth of a potentially viable baby without signs of life–in the UK, any that occur above 24 weeks; in Australia and other places, 20 weeks and above |
| Puerperium | The 6-week period after birth |
| Linea nigra | A dark line of discoloration in the midline of the abdominal skin |
| Striae gravidarum | Stretch marks–those from the current pregnancy appear white and those from any previous pregnancy are more silvery |

### 11.11 Examples of single-gene disorders that can be detected antenatally

**Autosomal dominant**
- Huntington's chorea
- Myotonic dystrophy

**Autosomal recessive**
- Cystic fibrosis
- Thalassaemia
- Sickle cell disease

**X-linked**
- Duchenne muscular dystrophy
- Haemophilia

### 11.12 Age-related risk of Down's syndrome (trisomy 21)

| Maternal age | Risk |
|--------------|------|
| 20 | 1 in 1500 |
| 30 | 1 in 900 |
| 35 | 1 in 400 |
| 40 | 1 in 100 |
| 45 | 1 in 30 |

and liver (high vitamin A content). Domestic violence can start or escalate in pregnancy and is associated with an increased risk of maternal death. All patients must be seen alone (without their partner) on at least one antenatal visit to allow this to be explored.

## Occupational history

Ask the patient about their occupation and whether they plan to continue it. Occupations involving exposure to ionising radiation pose specific risks to the foetus or mother, so their job plan may require modification for safety reasons. There is no definitive evidence of a link between heavy work and preterm labour or pre-eclampsia.

## Examination sequence

- Calculate BMI (weight/height$^2$).
- Obtain a midstream specimen of urine for microscopy, culture and sensitivities.
- Measure blood pressure.
- Do not perform a routine full physical examination (including breast and vaginal examination) in healthy pregnant patients. It is unnecessarily intrusive and has a low sensitivity for disease identification. However, you should perform a full examination, including cardiac auscultation, of any patient with poor general health.

## Investigations

Routine investigations are required at the booking visit (Box 11.13).

- if the patient is not in a relationship, who will give support during and after the pregnancy
- whether the pregnancy was planned; if unplanned, find out how they feel about it.

Lower socioeconomic status is linked with increased perinatal and maternal mortality.

Encourage regular exercise and avoidance of certain foods, such as tuna (high mercury content), soft cheeses (risk of *Listeria*)

## 11.13 Antenatal investigations

| Investigation | Timing | Indication/comment |
|---|---|---|
| Mid-stream specimen urine (MSU) for culture | Booking; always sent | Detects asymptomatic bacteriuria (and group B streptococcus) |
| Urinalysis | Every visit | Trace or + proteinuria: send MSU, ask about symptoms of urinary tract infection |
| | | ++ Proteinuria: consider pre-eclampsia or, rarely, underlying renal disorder |
| | | Glycosuria: consider random blood glucose or glucose tolerance test |
| Full blood count | Booking, 28 weeks, 36 weeks | If haemoglobin is <105 g/L, treat; consider checking haematinics |
| Haemoglobin electrophoresis | Booking | To check for sickle cell disease and thalassaemias |
| Blood group and antibody screen | Booking, 28 weeks | More often if advised by laboratory |
| Hepatitis B | Booking | If the patient is a previous intravenous drug abuser or is known to be HIV- or hepatitis B-positive, also carry out hepatitis C screening |
| HIV | Booking | Unless the patient opts out |
| Syphilis | Booking | |
| Plasma glucose | Booking | |
| Carbon monoxide level | Every visit for smokers | Advice and referral for cessation, growth scans |
| Combined biochemical screening and nuchal translucency measurement for trisomy 21 | 11–14 weeks | Detects 80–90% of affected pregnancies |
| First-trimester ultrasound scan | 6–13 weeks | Viability, gestational age ±7 days, fetal number, some major anomalies (e.g. anencephaly) |
| Detailed ultrasound scan | 18–22 weeks | Detects 90% of major congenital abnormalities and placental site |
| Placental site | If low at 20 weeks, recheck later at about 34 weeks | If there is an anterior placenta in a woman who has had a previous Caesarean section, recheck the scan at 28 weeks to consider the risk of placenta acreta |
| Growth scan | After 24 weeks; can be as often as 2–4 weekly | Previous growth-restricted baby, other risk factors, measurement of a small-for-dates baby, reduced foetal movements |
| Presentation scan | After 36 weeks | If there is concern that presentation is not cephalic |
| Amniocentesis | 15 weeks onwards | For fetal karyotype; 0.5–1% risk of miscarriage |
| Chorionic villus biopsy | 10 weeks onwards | For fetal karyotype, single-gene disorder; 2% risk of miscarriage |
| Free foetal DNA maternal test (non-National Health Service) | End of first trimester | To detect trisomy: current guidance advocates use as a screening test only |

*DNA*, Deoxyribonucleic acid; *HIV*, human immunodeficiency virus.

# ROUTINE ANTENATAL CHECK IN LATER PREGNANCY

## The history

Ask about:

- any new symptoms
- symptoms relevant to ongoing conditions unrelated to pregnancy
- the mother's perception of foetal movements.

Fetal movements are initially felt at 16–20 weeks' gestation. Their frequency increases until about 32 weeks to an average of 30 movements per hour, and this level remains unchanged until delivery. The 'classic' fetal movement is a kick, but any perceived fetal activity counts as movement. Movements may decrease if the mother is given sedative drugs and may be felt less if the placenta is anterior. They also may decrease with intrauterine compromise, which may precede stillbirth.

## Common presenting symptoms

### Physiological symptoms

- Breast tenderness: often the earliest symptom of pregnancy and may occur even before a missed period.
- Mild dyspnoea: may be due to increased respiratory drive early in pregnancy or diaphragmatic compression by the growing uterus late in pregnancy.
- Heartburn: gradually increases in prevalence, affecting up to three-quarters of patients by the third trimester. It results from relaxation of the gastro-oesophageal sphincter and acid reflux.
- Constipation, urinary frequency, nausea and vomiting (which usually resolve by 16–20 weeks).
- Aches and pains, especially backache, carpal tunnel syndrome and pubic symphyseal discomfort.

These physiological symptoms affect patients to different degrees and will occasionally merit examination and investigation to exclude other problems. Secondary amenorrhoea is the most obvious symptom of early pregnancy.

### Reduced fetal movements

This is a common emergency presentation or reason for referral to a hospital by a midwife, and merits a full history, examination and fetal monitoring. It can be a sign of fetal compromise.

### Vaginal bleeding in pregnancy

Vaginal bleeding in pregnancy before viability may herald a miscarriage; after 24 weeks, it is called an antepartum haemorrhage. It can be a sign of a placental abruption, where the placenta prematurely separates, or of a low-lying placenta. At term, light vaginal bleeding can also be a sign of labour. Vaginal bleeding is never considered normal in pregnancy and always merits hospital review with a full history and examination. Painless bleeding is more typical of local causes, such as a cervical polyp, or a low-lying placenta, whereas painful bleeding is more in keeping with placental abruption. It is imperative to always consider venous access and send blood for blood count and cross-matching in any pregnant woman presenting with vaginal bleeding.

### Abdominal pain

Abdominal pain is common in pregnancy. It can be caused by benign physiological issues such as constipation and is also a common presenting feature of labour when patients are contracting in established labour or tightening in early labour. It can also be caused by polyhydramnios or placental abruption.

Any condition causing abdominal pain can present coincidentally in pregnancy, however. A common example is urinary tract infection; less common causes include appendicitis, ovarian cyst accidents, sickle cell crisis or inflammatory bowel disease. It is critical to take a complete history of a pregnant patient with abdominal pain and to perform a full obstetric and abdominal examination, including renal angle palpation. This becomes more difficult as pregnancy progresses, and the expanding uterus makes palpation of other organs and masses difficult. Ultrasound or MRI scanning may aid diagnosis.

### Pre-eclampsia

Pre-eclampsia is a multifactorial syndrome comprised of high blood pressure, proteinuria and placental compromise, and is a significant cause of maternal and foetal morbidity. It is often asymptomatic and detected by blood pressure monitoring and urinalysis, although some patients develop generalised headaches and rapidly worsening peripheral oedema. A history focused on headaches, worsening oedema and upper abdominal pain should be taken. The examination is that of a routine antenatal assessment but should also include a check for hyperreflexia and ankle clonus.

### Pruritus

Pruritus (itching) affects one-quarter of pregnant patients. Rarely, it is associated with liver cholestasis, in which case it is generalised, and there is no rash.

### Breathlessness

Mild breathlessness is physiological in pregnancy. In rare circumstances, increased breathlessness is due to pulmonary oedema in pre-eclampsia or exacerbation of heart disease. If breathlessness is associated with chest pain, a pulmonary embolism (p. 85) should be considered. The chest should be examined, and oxygen saturation and respiratory rate measured. An electrocardiogram is helpful, and the risks/ benefits of radiological imaging should be assessed. Consideration should be given to an echocardiogram to exclude unknown congenital or acquired heart disease (e.g. cardiomyopathy).

## The physical examination

### Examination sequence (Videos 23 and 23A)

- Before examining the patient, ask them to empty their bladder (perform urinalysis). They should lie with their head on a low pillow, with their abdomen exposed from the symphysis pubis to the xiphisternum.
- Examine patients in late pregnancy in the left lateral position or semirecumbent, 15 degrees to the horizontal, to avoid

A             B             C

**Fig. 11.35 Abdominal examination.** **A** Palpate the fundal area to identify which pole of the fetus (breech or head) is occupying the fundus. **B** Slip your hands gently down the sides of the uterus to identify which side the firm back and knobbly limbs of the fetus are positioned on. **C** Turn to face the patient's feet and slide your hands gently on the lower part of the uterus.

**11**

vena cava compression, which can cause hypotension for the mother and hypoxia for the foetus.

- Measure blood pressure.
- Note their general demeanour. Are they at ease or distressed by physical pain?
- On inspection, look for signs of pregnancy, such as the linea nigra (a dark discoloration of the midline of the abdominal skin) and striae gravidarum (stretch marks).
- Look for any scars, particularly from a previous Caesarean section. Note the swelling of the uterus arising from the pelvis and any other swellings. You may also see fetal movements.

## Uterine examination (Video 23B) ▶

- Ask the patient to report any tenderness and observe their facial and verbal responses constantly.
- Place the flat of your hand on the uterine swelling. Gently flex your fingers to palpate the upper and lateral edges of its firm mass. Note any tenderness, rebound or guarding outside the uterus. Palpate lightly to avoid triggering myometrial contraction, which makes fetal parts difficult to feel. Avoid deep palpation of any tender areas of the uterus. Note any contractions and any foetal movements.
- Face the patient's head. Place both your hands on either side of the fundus and feel the fetal parts. Estimate if the liquor volume is normal. Assess how far from the surface the fetal parts are. If you can feel them only on deep palpation, this implies large amounts of fluid (Fig. 11.35A).
- With your right hand on the patient's left side, feel down both sides of the uterus. The fuller side suggests the location of the fetal back (see Fig. 11.35B).
- Now face the patient's feet. Place your hands on either side of the uterus, with your left hand on the left side, and feel the lower part of the uterus to try to identify the presenting part. Ballott the head by pushing it gently from one side to the other and feel its hardness move between your fingers (see Fig. 11.35C).
- The size of the uterus increases as pregnancy advances (Fig. 11.36). At 20 weeks, the uterine fundus is at the umbilicus; by 36 weeks, it reaches the xiphisternum. The distance

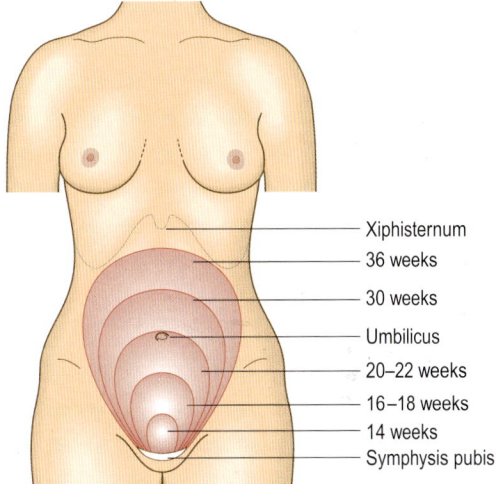

Xiphisternum
36 weeks
30 weeks
Umbilicus
20–22 weeks
16–18 weeks
14 weeks
Symphysis pubis

**Fig. 11.36 Approximate fundal height with increasing gestation.**

from the pubic symphysis to the top of the uterine fundus is the symphyseal fundal height (SFH). In a singleton pregnancy, if the baby is growing well, the SFH in centimetres approximates the duration of pregnancy in weeks. In multiple pregnancies, the fundus will measure larger at each stage. After 20 weeks, measure the SFH in centimetres. With a tape measure, fix the end at the highest point on the fundus (not always in the midline) and measure to the top of the symphysis pubis. To avoid bias, place the blank side of the tape facing you, lift the tape and read the measurement on the other side. The SFH is measured at every visit and recorded on a SFH centile chart in the maternal handheld record. In tall or thin patients, the SFH may be smaller than expected; in obese patients, it may be larger. After 25 weeks gestation, a difference of 3 or more between the number of completed weeks of pregnancy and the SFH in centimetres may suggest that the baby is small or large for dates. If this discrepancy occurs or if the SFH centile is static or falling, the patient should be referred for a growth scan (Fig 11.37).

- In late pregnancy or labour, you need to assess the fetal lie, fetal presentation and engagement of the head in the maternal pelvis. The lie describes the longitudinal axis of the fetus related to the longitudinal axis of the mother's uterus. Most fetuses have a longitudinal lie in the third trimester (Fig. 11.38). From 36 weeks, a position other than longitudinal is abnormal and requires further investigation.
- The presentation is the part of the fetus's body that is expected to deliver first. With a longitudinal lie, there is either a cephalic or a breech presentation. Finally, assess whether more than 50% of the presenting part has entered the bony pelvis. This is usually the head, which is then said to be engaged (Fig. 11.39).
- Percussion of the pregnant abdomen is unnecessary.
- Listen for the fetal heart if you cannot feel fetal movements. A hand-held Doppler machine can be used from 14 weeks.

From 28 weeks, the Doppler machine is held over the anterior shoulder of the foetus.

- Do not perform a vaginal examination routinely in pregnancy unless there is a specific indication. Never perform a vaginal examination after 20 weeks unless the placental location is known, as there is a risk of severe bleeding if it is low.

Abdominal organs are displaced during pregnancy. For example, in the case of ovarian cysts or an inflamed appendix, the pain and tenderness may not be in the usual sites. The kidneys and liver cannot normally be palpated and listening for bowel sounds may be difficult in late pregnancy. Ultrasound scanning is now used routinely to assess fetal development (Figs 11.40 and 11.41).

## Investigations

Routine investigations are required at specific antenatal visits (see Box 11.13).

**Fig. 11.37** **International symphysis-fundal height standards.** University of Oxford.

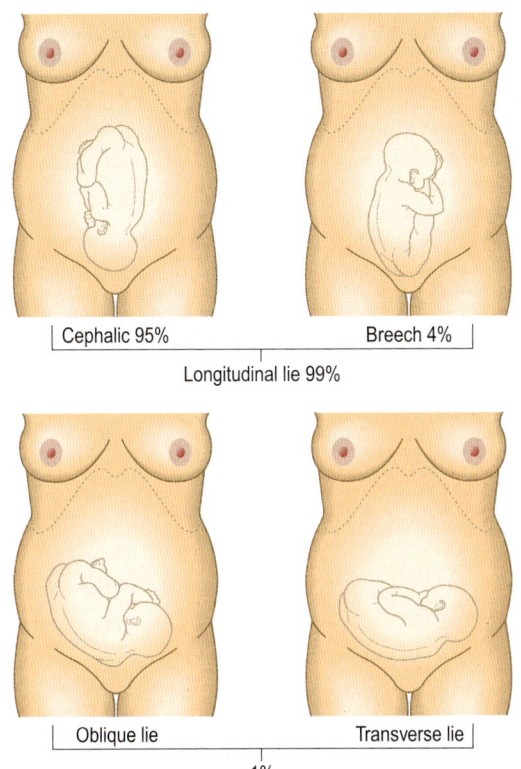

Cephalic 95% | Breech 4%

Longitudinal lie 99%

Oblique lie | Transverse lie

1%

**Fig. 11.38** The lie and presentation of the foetus at term.

**Fig. 11.40** Ultrasound scan at 12 weeks showing a twin pregnancy.

11

**Fig. 11.41** Ultrasound scan at 13 weeks showing crown–rump measurement.

Perform dipstick urinalysis at each visit, looking for glycosuria or proteinuria. Protein of ≥1+ may indicate a urinary tract infection or pre-eclampsia. Glycosuria requires a formal test for gestational diabetes.

| Completely above | Sinciput +++ Occiput ++ | Sinciput ++ Occiput + | Sinciput + Occiput just felt | Sinciput + Occiput not felt | None of head palpable |
|---|---|---|---|---|---|
| 5/5 | 4/5 | 3/5 | 2/5 | 1/5 | 0/5 |
| Free, above the brim | 'Fixing' | Fixed, not engaged | Just engaged | Engaged | Deeply engaged |

Level of pelvic brim

**Fig. 11.39** Descent of the fetal head.

# MALE REPRODUCTIVE SYSTEM

## Anatomy and physiology

The male genitalia include the testes, epididymides and seminal vesicles, penis, scrotum and prostate gland (Fig. 11.42).

The testes develop intra-abdominally near the kidneys and migrate through the inguinal canal into the scrotum by birth. They have their own blood, lymphatic and nerve supply, so testicular problems may cause abdominal pain and enlargement of the para-aortic lymph nodes. The scrotum is a pouch with thin, pigmented, wrinkled skin that helps to regulate the temperature of the testes (Fig. 11.43), as sperm production is most efficient below body temperature. The left testis lies lower than the right. Each testis is oval, 3.5–5 cm long, and covered by the tunica albuginea, which forms the posterior wall of the tunica vaginalis. This is a prolongation of the peritoneal tube that forms as the testis descends during development. If it persists, it may be associated with an indirect inguinal hernia sac or a congenital hydrocoele. Along the posterior border of each testis is the epididymis.

The testes produce sperm and testosterone, starting at puberty (10–15 years of age; see Fig. 15.19). Sperm mature in the epididymis and pass down the vas deferens to the seminal vesicles. They are ejaculated from the urethra, together with prostatic and seminal vesicle fluid, at orgasm.

The penis has two cylinders of endothelium-lined spaces surrounded by smooth muscle, the corpora cavernosa (Fig. 11.44). These are bound with the bulbospongiosus surrounding the urethra, which expands into the glans penis. The penile skin is reflected over the glans, forming the prepuce (foreskin). Sexual arousal causes a parasympathetically mediated increased blood flow into the corpora cavernosa with erection to enable vaginal penetration. Continued stimulation causes sympathetic-mediated contraction of the seminal vesicles and prostate, closure of the bladder neck and ejaculation. Following orgasm, a reduction in blood inflow causes detumescence.

The prostate and seminal vesicles contribute to seminal fluid. After age 40, the prostate develops a trilobar structure because

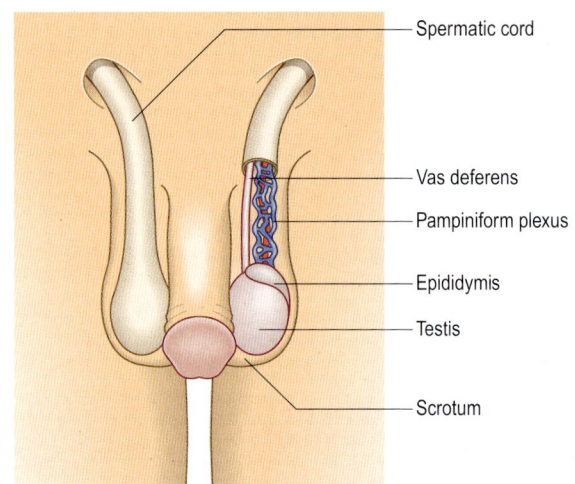

**Fig. 11.43** The scrotum and its contents.

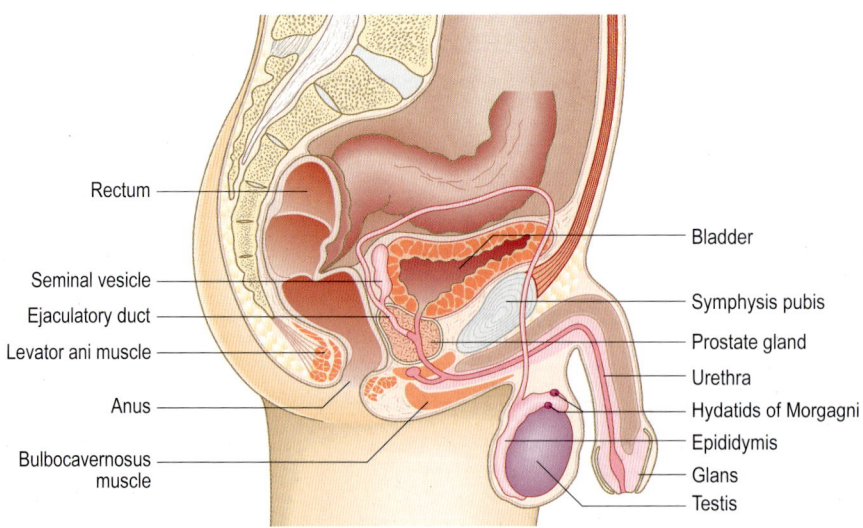

**Fig. 11.42** **Anatomy of the male genitalia.** The male genitalia include the external organs, seminal vesicles and prostate gland.

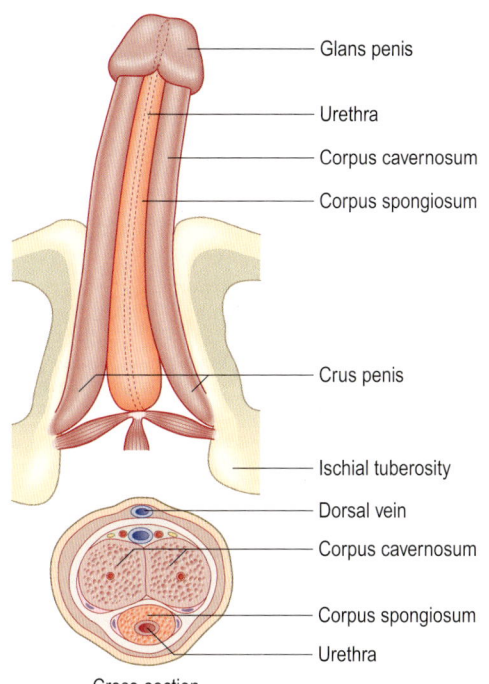

**Fig. 11.44 Anatomy of the penis.** The shaft and glans penis are formed from the corpus spongiosum and the corpus cavernosum.

of benign enlargement. Two lateral lobes and a variable median lobe protrude into the bladder and may cause urethral and bladder outflow obstruction. Prostate cancer develops in the peripheral tissue of the lateral lobes and sometimes may be detected by digital rectal examination. Only the posterior aspect and the lateral lobes of the prostate can be felt by rectal examination (p. 111).

# The history

Disorders of the male genitals may present as urinary symptoms, genital or pelvic pain, genital swellings, sexual dysfunction or infertility.

In addition to documenting the patient's main genital or urinary problems, be sure to ask about:

- the timescale of their development
- how they affect lifestyle and any sexual activity
- sexual function, if appropriate
- past conceptions or problems with fertility
- general urological symptoms:
  - genital swelling
  - genital or pelvic pain
  - lower urinary tract symptoms
  - urethral discharge.

There may be associated systemic upset or clinical signs associated with urological disease; a complete history and examination are therefore important.

## Common presenting symptoms

### Urinary symptoms

Urinary symptoms are a common presentation of genital or lower urinary tract dysfunction. Dysuria (see below), voiding symptoms and haematuria are covered in Chapter 12.

### Penile discharge or dysuria

Ask about:

- the duration of discharge or dysuria
- whether these are new or recurrent symptoms
- any other urinary symptoms
- the sexual history
- any systemic upset.

These symptoms usually represent urethritis which is the result of either an STI or a urinary tract infection. They may precede and lead to epididymo-orchitis (see later) or prostatitis. Prostatitis is associated with pelvic, perineal or scrotal pain, fever and systemic upset in acute bacterial prostatitis, or may lead to chronic pain and urinary symptoms in chronic prostatitis.

### Scrotal swelling or pain

Patients often present acutely with scrotal pain and swelling together; they may also, however, present with either symptom alone.

Ask about:

- duration of the swelling
- whether it is unilateral or bilateral
- association with pain
- onset of pain: sudden or gradual
- character and duration of the pain
- radiation of the pain
- any history of trauma
- any associated symptoms:
  - systemic upset (nausea, vomiting, fever or weight loss)
  - urinary symptoms
  - urethral discharge
- sexual history (see Box 11.5).

There are many causes of scrotal swelling or pain, but a patient with sudden-onset unilateral scrotal pain should be considered to have testicular torsion until proven otherwise. Testicular torsion occurs most commonly between the ages of 10 and 30 years and is very rare over the age of 40. Pain is usually of acute onset and excruciating; it is not relieved by lying still. It is often associated with nausea and vomiting but not usually fever, lower urinary tract symptoms or urethral discharge.

11

| Normal | Hydrocoele | Epidydimal cyst |
| Epididymitis | Varicocoele | Tumour of testis |

**Fig. 11.45** Swellings of the scrotum.

Epididymo-orchitis is the most common differential diagnosis. The pain of epididymo-orchitis is often more insidious in onset compared to testicular torsion, and the patient may report a dull ache initially. There may be associated fevers, dysuria or urethral discharge, suggesting underlying STI or urinary tract infection. The discomfort is often worse when standing or moving around and may be relieved when lying still. On examination, it is usually possible to distinguish the tender, inflamed epididymis from the adjacent testis. If testicular torsion cannot be excluded on history and examination, urgent testicular exploration is warranted, as torsion will cause loss of a testis if not relieved within 4–6 hours. While an ultrasound examination may be used to confirm a diagnosis of epididymo-orchitis, it should never be requested to assess for torsion.

Other scrotal swellings include hernias, varicocoele, hydrocoele, epididymal cysts and testicular tumours. These are usually painless, although vague or constant dull aches may be described (Fig. 11.45). Examination findings can usually differentiate these diagnoses (Box 11.14).

## Penile skin lesions

Ask about:

- location, duration and progression of the lesion
- any pain
- any problem retracting the prepuce
- any associated systemic upset
- any urinary symptoms
- any history of dermatological disease
- sexual history.

The inability to retract the foreskin (phimosis) is a common symptom in the urology clinic. Phimosis may be normal, 95% of babies are born with a non-retractile prepuce, but this usually resolves by the age of 16 years, when only 1% of boys have

### 11.14 Summary of examination findings in common scrotal pathologies

**Inguinoscrotal: unable to 'get above'**

**Inguinoscrotal hernia**
- May be reducible and have a cough impulse
- Does not transilluminate
- May be associated with bowel sounds on auscultation

**Hydrocoele**
- Is not reducible
- Transilluminates
- Not associated with bowel sounds
- It is possible to palpate the normal cord above some hydrocoeles

**Scrotal mass: able to 'get above'**

**Epididymal cyst**
- Firm, well circumscribed and separate from testicular body
- Transilluminates

**Testicular tumour**
- A hard, mass that may be well circumscribed or ill defined, arising from the testicular body
- Does not transilluminate

**Varicocoele**
- Described as feeling like a 'bag of worms' around the cord
- Present on standing or with a Valsalva manoeuvre but usually resolves on lying flat

persistent phimosis. This may produce balanitis (recurrent infection of the glans penis), posthitis (infection of the prepuce) or both (balanoposthitis).

If a tight foreskin is retracted and is not replaced, swelling and pain ensue, resulting in paraphimosis due to the tight preputial band (Fig. 11.46).

Dermatological conditions and drug reactions may affect the genital skin. Painful genital ulcers are usually caused by herpes simplex; painless ulcers occur in reactive arthritis (p. 293), lichen simplex and (rarely) syphilis. Genital warts may also be present, as well as penile carcinoma.

## Erectile dysfunction

Erectile dysfunction (ED) is the consistent or recurrent inability to attain and/or maintain a penile erection sufficient for penetrative intercourse.

Clarify from the history:

- Is the problem failure to gain or maintain an erection, painful erection, penile deformity on erection or a combination of these?
- How long has ED been a problem?
- Has the patient ever been able to gain a rigid erection?
- Do they ever have morning erections on waking?
- Are they able to gain an erection under any circumstances, such as masturbation?
- Do their problems prevent penetrative intercourse?

**Fig. 11.46** Paraphimosis. Oedema of the foreskin behind an encircling constriction ring caused by the foreskin not being replaced–in this case, after catheterisation.

- Are there any other symptoms of sexual dysfunction, including reduced libido, problems achieving orgasm, premature ejaculation or failure to ejaculate?

Consider possible precipitating events: for example, relationship difficulties or trauma. Assess cardiovascular, neurological and psychiatric comorbidities, as well as take drug history.

If the patient has never had an erection, they may have primary ED due to an anatomical abnormality. Secondary ED is more common and may be psychological or organic in aetiology. Psychological ED may have a precipitating event, and loss of erection occurs in some but not all situations; early-morning erections or erections with masturbation usually remain unaffected. Organic ED affects all erections and is often associated with medical comorbidities, including diabetes mellitus, cardiovascular disease, hypertension, peripheral vascular disease, endocrine disorder or neurological disorder. ED is a common early symptom of metabolic syndrome and should precipitate screening for cardiovascular disease and diabetes.

If erections are painful or associated with deformity, the likely diagnosis is Peyronie's disease. This is a fibrotic condition of the penile shaft, of unknown aetiology, producing painful curvature, narrowing or shortening of the corpora cavernosa with erection.

If the problem is a prolonged erection (priapism), establish the duration and whether it is painful. Particular attention should be paid to drug history, history of perineal trauma or past medical history of haematological, neurological or oncological disease. Painful (low-flow or ischaemic) priapism is a urological emergency which requires urgent treatment to prevent permanent ED.

## Past medical history

Ask about previous urological procedures, including neonatal surgery. Record relevant general surgical procedures, particularly pelvic operations that may contribute to lower urinary tract symptoms, or ED. Cardiovascular, endocrine, neurological, renal and psychiatric diseases may predispose or contribute to both urinary tract symptoms and ED.

## Drug history

Ask about previous urological drug treatments and obtain a full list of all medications and drugs taken recreationally. In particular, note drugs such as:

- diuretics: contribute to urinary symptoms
- alpha-blockers: may cause retrograde ejaculation
- antihypertensive agents: may cause erectile dysfunction
- vasoactive drugs, such as alprostadil: may result in a prolonged erection
- antidepressants or antipsychotics: may affect urinary and sexual function.

## Social history

Smoking, drinking alcohol and recreational drugs can affect fertility and sexual function. Smoking is a significant risk factor for urological cancers.

## The physical examination

Ensure privacy. Use a warm, well-lit room with a moveable light source. Explain what you are going to do and why it is necessary, and offer a chaperone. Record the chaperone's name; if the offer is refused, record the fact. Apply alcohol gel and put on gloves. Allow the patient privacy to undress.

Ask the patient to stand and expose the area from the lower abdomen to the top of the thighs. Initially, examine the patient standing before asking them to lie on their back to re-examine any scrotal swellings while lying down.

## Skin

### Examination sequence

- Look in turn at the groin, skin creases, perineum and scrotal skin for redness, swellings or ulcers. Note the hair distribution.
- If you see any swellings in the groin, palpate these and define them using 'SPACESPIT' (see Box 3.8 in the 14th edition).

A general examination may reveal a lack of secondary sexual characteristics suggestive of hypogonadism (p. 231). There may be alopecia or an infestation. Patients who shave their pubic hair may have dermatitis or folliculitis (infection around the base of the hairs), causing an irritating red rash. Intertrigo (infected eczema)

11

occurs in the skin creases, and lymphadenopathy may stem from local or general causes.

Scrotal oedema can be caused by systemic or local diseases. Heart and liver dysfunction may lead to significant genital oedema, as may nephrotic syndrome and lymphoedema due to pelvic lymphadenopathy.

## Penis

### Examination sequence

- Look at the shaft and check the position of the urethral opening to exclude hypospadias (urethra opening partway along the shaft of the penis; see Fig. 15.11A in the 14th edition).
- Palpate the shaft for fibrous plaques (usually on the dorsum). Palpate any other lesions to define them.
- Retract the prepuce and inspect the glans for red patches or vesicles.
- Always draw the foreskin forward after examination to avoid a paraphimosis.
- Take a urethral swab if your patient has a discharge or is having sexual health screening.

Normal enlarged follicles may mimic warts. Numerous uniform, pearly penile papules around the corona of the glans are normal.

Warts, sebaceous cysts, or a hard plaque of Peyronie's disease may occur on the shaft and phimosis, adhesions, inflammation or swellings on the foreskin or glans may be noted.

## Scrotum

Examine the scrotum with the patient standing. Then ask them to lie down if you find swelling you cannot 'get above'. Ask the patient whether they have any genital pain. If they are cold or apprehensive, the dartos muscle contracts, and you will not be able to palpate the scrotal contents properly.

### Examination sequence

- Inspect the scrotum for redness, swelling or ulcers, lifting it to inspect the posterior surface.
- Note the position of the testes and any paratesticular swelling and tenderness.
- Palpate the scrotum gently, using both hands. Check that both testes are present. If they are not, examine the inguinal canal and perineum, checking for undescended or ectopic testes.
- Place the fingers of both your hands behind each testis, in turn, to immobilise it, and use your index finger and thumb to palpate the body of the testis methodically. Feel the anterior surface and medial border with your thumb and the lateral border with your index finger (Fig. 11.47).
- Check the size and consistency of the testis. Note any nodules or irregularities. Measure the testicular size in centimetres from one to the other.
- Palpate the spermatic cord with your right hand. Gently pull the testis downward and place your fingers behind the neck

Fig. 11.47 Palpation of the testis.

of the scrotum. Feel the spermatic cord and within it the vas, like a thick piece of string.

- Decide whether a swelling arises in the scrotum or from the inguinal canal. If you can feel above the swelling, it originates from the scrotum; if you cannot, the swelling usually originates in the inguinal region (Fig. 11.48).
- Check any inguinoscrotal swelling for a cough impulse and auscultate for bowel sounds.
- Place the bright end of a torch against a scrotal swelling (transillumination; Fig. 15.9). Fluid-filled cysts allow light transmission, and the scrotum glows bright red. This is an inconsistent sign, which does not differentiate a hydrocoele from other causes of intrascrotal fluid, such as a large epididymal cyst. With thick-walled cysts, transillumination may be absent.

The right testicle is usually closer to the inguinal canal than the left, but the testes may be highly mobile (retractile). A normal testis is 5 cm long. The normal epididymis is barely palpable, except for its head (Fig. 11.49), which feels like a pea separate from the superior pole of the body of the testicle.

Sebaceous cysts are common in the scrotal skin. If you can get above a scrotal swelling, it is a true scrotal swelling. If not, it may be a varicocoele, hydrocele or inguinal hernia that has descended into the scrotum (see Fig. 11.45).

## Varicocoele

A varicocoele is a dilatation of the veins of the pampiniform plexus and feels like a 'bag of worms' in the cord when the patient is standing and should disappear when he lies down. If it does not, particularly on the left where the gonadal (testicular) vein inserts into the renal vein, consider a retroperitoneal mass such as renal cancer compressing the testicular veins.

## Hydrocoele

These are swellings caused by fluid in the tunica vaginalis. They are usually idiopathic but may be secondary to inflammatory conditions or tumours. They can be limited to the scrotum or extend into the inguinal canal.

A  Fingers can 'get above' mass      B  Fingers cannot 'get above' mass

**Fig. 11.48** **Testing for scrotal swellings.** [A] It is possible to 'get above' a true scrotal swelling. [B] This is not possible if the swelling is caused by an inguinal hernia that has descended into the scrotum. A hydrocele may also extend into the inguinal region.

11

**Fig. 11.49** **Palpation of the epididymis.** The epididymis is readily felt only at the top of the testis.

**Fig. 11.50** **Left testicular torsion.** There is shortening of the cord with retraction of the testis and global swelling of the scrotal contents. Refer the patient urgently to a surgeon for scrotal exploration.

## Epididymal cyst

Swellings of the epididymis that are felt to be completely separate from the body of the testis are epididymal cysts. They are isolated and adherent to the epididymis alone; they transilluminate and are never malignant. Painful swellings at the superior pole of the testis or adjacent to the head of the epididymis, are usually due to torsion of a paramesonephric duct remnant, the hydatids of Morgagni. This is more common in infancy and is often associated acutely with a blue discoloration on the skin, referred to as the 'blue dot sign'.

## Testicular tumour

Testicular tumours cause painless, hard swellings of the body of the testis. Around 15% of tumours may occur close to the rete testis and may give rise to epididymal swelling and pain.

## Epididymitis

Inflammation of the epididymis produces painful epididymal swelling, most often caused by an STI in young patients, or a coliform urinary infection in the elderly.

## Testicular torsion

A retracted or high-lying testicle, accompanied by acute pain and swelling, occurs in testicular torsion (Fig. 11.50). A palpable twist in the cord may be identified behind the testis on examination although patients are often in too much pain to allow full examination.

## Single testis

This may be due to incomplete testicular descent of the 'missing' testis through the inguinal canal or an ectopic testis in the groin. Ask about previous surgery for a testicular tumour or testicular maldescent. Unilateral testicular atrophy may result from a mumps infection, torsion, vascular compromise after inguinal hernia repair, or from a late orchidopexy for unde-scended testis.

## Bilateral testicular atrophy

This suggests primary, or secondary, hypogonadism (p. 231) or primary testicular failure. Look for hormonal abnormalities or signs of anabolic steroid usage and check the development of secondary sexual characteristics (see Fig. 15.20).

## Prostate

Ask the patient to lie in the left lateral position.

## Examination sequence

- Perform a rectal examination (p. 111).
- Palpate the prostate through the anterior rectal wall.
- Note any tenderness.
- Assess size, symmetry and consistency. Is it hard or boggy?
- Feel for any nodules.
- Withdraw your finger. Give the patient tissues to clean themself and privacy in which to get dressed.

The prostate is normally smooth, rubbery, non-tender and about the size of a walnut. It has defined margins with an indentation, or sulcus, between the two lateral lobes. Sometimes the seminal vesicles are felt above the prostate.

Tenderness or soft 'bogginess' suggests prostatitis or pros-tatic abscess.

Prostate cancer may cause a discrete nodule, a craggy mass or obliteration of the midline sulcus, and the prostate may feel fixed to the lateral pelvic sidewall.

## Investigations

The relevant urological investigations depend on the clinical problem revealed on history and examination. First-catch urine can be tested for both *Chlamydia trachomatis* and *Neisseria gonorrhoeae* from a single specimen using nucleic acid amplifi-cation tests, and this should be performed for all patients pre-senting with urethritis or acute scrotal pain suspected to be due to epididymo-orchitis. Scrotal ultrasound is the gold standard for confirming the clinical diagnosis of scrotal swelling or pain, with the exception of testicular torsion.

When prostate cancer is suspected, a prostate-specific anti-gen (PSA) blood test should be requested. PSA is raised in prostate cancer but also increases with age, prostatic volume, following prostatic trauma (including prostate examination or urinary tract instrumentation) and urinary tract infection. If the PSA is elevated, a multiparametric MRI scan of the prostate may be considered with subsequent prostate biopsy to investigate for prostate carcinoma.

Early-morning testosterone should be measured in all patients with erectile dysfunction to assess for hypogonadism. Serum alpha-f-etoprotein, beta-HCG and lactate dehydrogenase are tumour markers that may be raised in the presence of testicular cancer.

---

### OSCE example 1: Breast examination

Ms McIntyre, 27 years old, presents with a 6-week history of a lump in her right breast.

#### Please examine her breast

- Introduce yourself and clean your hands.
- Obtain verbal consent for the examination from the patient.
- Offer a chaperone.
- Ask her to undress to the waist and sit on the edge of the bed.
- Inspect for asymmetry, skin or nipple changes, or obvious lumps.
- Ask her to put her hands on her hips and push in while you look for changes in the breast.
- Ask her to lie on the couch with her upper body at 45 degrees. Palpate her breasts, noting the characteristics of any lumps.
- Examine her axillae and supraclavicular fossae.
- Thank the patient and clean your hands.

#### Summarise your findings

There is a firm, mobile, non-tender lump about 2 cm in diameter at 11 o'clock in the right breast, 5 cm from the nipple. There are no overlying skin changes, and the lump is not tethered. I could feel no lymphadenopathy in the neck or axilla.

#### Suggest a diagnosis
One possible diagnosis is breast cancer. The differential includes fibrocystic disease, a breast cyst or an abscess.

#### Suggest investigations
Triple assessment: clinical assessment, ultrasound scan and ultrasound-guided core biopsy.

## OSCE example 2: Scrotal pain history

Mr Atkins, 20 years old, presents to the emergency department with scrotal pain.

### Please take a focused history

- Introduce yourself and clean your hands.
- Obtain verbal consent to take a history from the patient.
- Ask an open question about why this person has come to the emergency department.
- Explore the symptoms offered at presentation—in this case, scrotal pain:
  - time of onset and duration
  - severity of pain
  - exacerbating/relieving factors
  - constant or intermittent nature
  - radiation to groin or loin
  - any precipitating event such as trauma
  - associated urinary symptoms, urethral discharge, swelling, fever, nausea or weight loss
  - sexual history
  - past medical history, including undescended testes
  - drug history
  - social history.

### Summarise your findings

The patient reports a gradual onset of aching testicular and scrotal pain with some associated urethral discharge and fever.

### Suggest a differential diagnosis

This history is most suggestive of epididymo-orchitis. The differential includes testicular torsion and testicular cancer.

### Suggest initial investigations

Ultrasound may confirm epididymo-orchitis, but if testicular torsion cannot be excluded on history and examination, urgent testicular exploration is required.

11

## OSCE example 3: Gynaecological examination

Samantha Turner is a 38-year-old presenting for her routine cervical smear test.

### Please talk to the patient and take a cervical smear and perform a pelvic examination from the manikin.

- Introduce yourself to the patient
- Confirm it is the correct patient
- Explain the procedure and obtain verbal consent
- Obtain focused history to allow completion of the request form (e.g. LMP, previous smear and results)
- Ensure chaperone present
- Ask patient to empty bladder
- Allow privacy to remove bottom half of clothing, lie on examination couch and cover with modesty blanket
- Ensure adequate lighting and equipment available
- Clean hands and apply gloves
- Ask chaperone assistant to help with fixative and check it with you
- Inspect the perineum
- Insert speculum and inspect vagina and cervix
- Take cervical smear
- Remove speculum
- Perform bimanual examination
- Thank patient and clean hands
- Give privacy to change and ensure all paperwork and records are completed

### Presentation to examiner

On inspection, the perineum was normal. On speculum examination, there was no discharge, and the vaginal walls were healthy. The cervix was normal with round cervical os and small ectopy. There was no contact bleeding on taking the cervical smear. On bimanual examination, the uterus was anteverted, mobile, non-tender and normal size. There were no adnexal masses, the abdomen was non-tender, and neither ovary could be palpated. In summary, the pelvic examination was normal.

# The renal system

Anatomy and physiology 272

The history 272

Common presenting symptoms 272
Past medical history 277
Drug history 277
Family history 277
Social history 278

The physical examination 278

General appearance 278
Assessment of fluid balance 279

Abdominal examination 280
Targeted examination of other systems 281

Interpretation of the findings 281

Investigations 281

Urinalysis 281
Investigation of renal function 282

OSCE example 1: renal history 284

OSCE example 2: renal examination 285

Integrated examination sequence for renal disease 286

## Anatomy and physiology

The kidneys lie posteriorly in the abdomen, retroperitoneally on either side of the spine at the T12–L3 level, and are 11–14 cm long (Fig. 12.1). The right kidney lies 1.5 cm lower than the left because of the liver. The liver and spleen lie anterior to the kidneys. The kidneys move downwards during inspiration as the lungs expand.

Together, the kidneys receive approximately 25% of cardiac output, and account for nearly 10% of basal metabolic rate. Each kidney contains about 1 million nephrons, each comprising a glomerulus, proximal tubule, loop of Henle, distal tubule, and collecting duct (Fig. 12.2). Urine is formed by glomerular filtration, modified by complex processes of secretion and reabsorption in the tubules and then enters the calyces and the renal pelvis.

The primary functions of the kidneys are:

- Excretion of waste products of metabolism, such as urea and creatinine
- Maintenance of salt, water, and electrolyte homeostasis
- Regulation of blood pressure via the renin–angiotensin-aldosterone system
- Endocrine functions related to erythropoiesis and vitamin D metabolism

The renal capsule and ureter are innervated by T10–12/L1 nerve roots; pain from these structures is felt in these dermatomes.

The bladder acts as a reservoir. As it fills, it becomes ovoid and rises out of the pelvis in the midline towards the umbilicus, behind the anterior abdominal wall. The bladder wall contains a layer of smooth muscle, the detrusor, which contracts under parasympathetic control, allowing urine to pass through the urethra (micturition). The conscious desire to micturate occurs when the bladder holds approximately 250–350 mL of urine. The male urethra runs from the bladder to the tip of the penis and has three parts: prostatic, membranous and spongiose (Fig. 12.3).

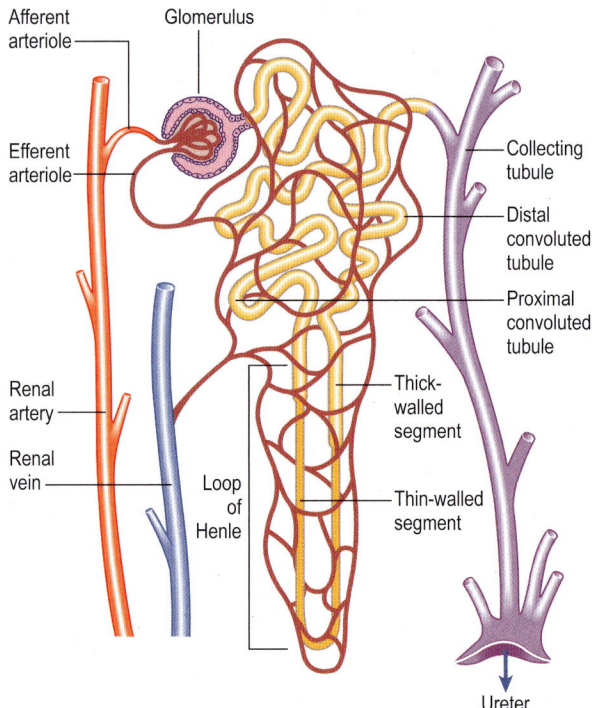

**Fig. 12.2** A single nephron.

The female urethra is much shorter, with the external meatus situated anterior to the vaginal orifice and behind the clitoris (Fig. 12.4). Two muscular rings acting as valves (sphincters) control micturition:

- The internal sphincter is at the bladder neck and involuntary.
- The external sphincter surrounds the membranous urethra and is under voluntary control; it is innervated by the pudendal nerves (S2–4).

The anatomy and physiology of the prostate are covered in more detail on page 268.

## The history

Renal disease may be asymptomatic, or present with non-specific symptoms, such as lethargy or breathlessness. It is usually only after initial investigation that the history-taking can be focused on the possible renal causes.

## Common presenting symptoms

### Dysuria

Dysuria (pain or discomfort during urination) is a common symptom of urinary tract infection (UTI). There is usually associated urinary frequency, urgency and suprapubic discomfort

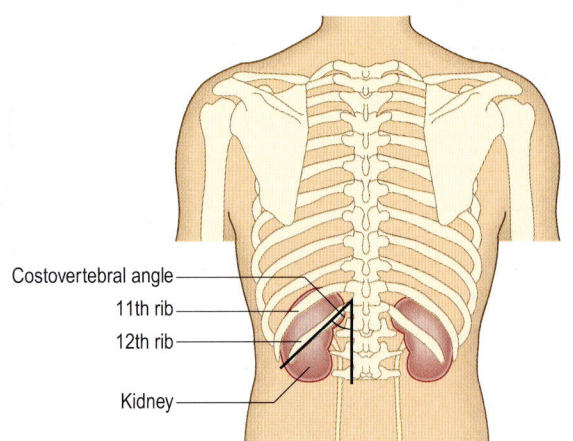

**Fig. 12.1** The surface anatomy of the kidneys from the back.

(cystitis). Other causes include urethritis and acute prostatitis (which may be associated with severe perineal or rectal pain).

Ask about:

- Systemic upset with fever and suprapubic discomfort. Pyelonephritis is suggested by a history of significant fever (>38.0°C), rigors, vomiting and flank pain. There may not always be symptoms of a preceding UTI.
- Symptoms of urine outflow obstruction (slow flow, hesitancy, incomplete emptying, dribbling, nocturia).
- History of sexual contacts.

## Loin pain

Severe loin pain is usually due to ureteric obstruction; renal calculi are the most common cause. The pain often comes in waves and is described as 'colicky'. The patient is unable to find a comfortable position and will move around the bed (unlike a patient with peritonism, who lies still).

Ask about:

- Location of the pain: Is it just in the loin (pelvic/upper ureter obstruction), or does it radiate into the testicle or labium (lower ureter obstruction)?
- Presence of fever, rigors and dysuria: these may suggest infection
- Previous episodes of loin pain

Loin pain may also occur due to bleeding from a renal or ureteric tumour or due to infection. Non-renal causes of loin pain, such as a leaking aortic aneurysm (in older patients with vascular

**12**

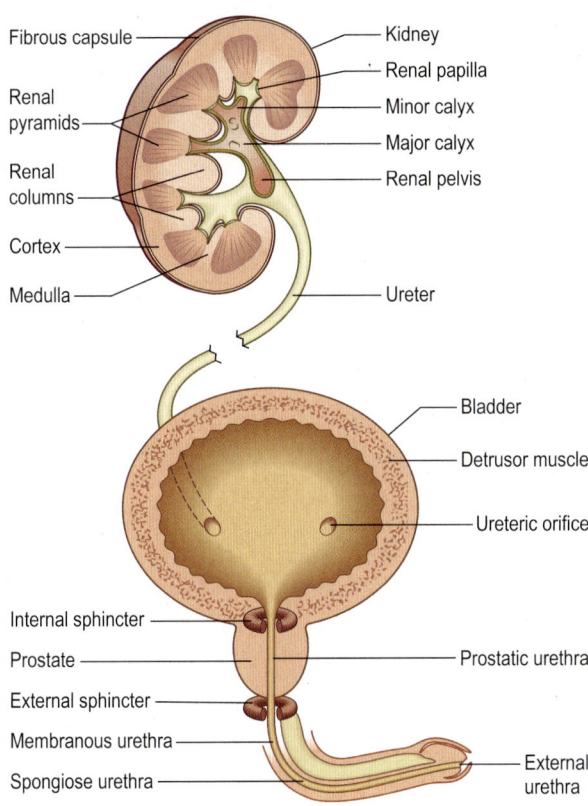

Fibrous capsule — Kidney
Renal pyramids — Renal papilla
— Minor calyx
Renal columns — Major calyx
Cortex — Renal pelvis
Medulla — Ureter
— Bladder
— Detrusor muscle
— Ureteric orifice
Internal sphincter —
Prostate —
External sphincter — Prostatic urethra
Membranous urethra —
Spongiose urethra — External urethra

**Fig. 12.3** The male urinary tract.

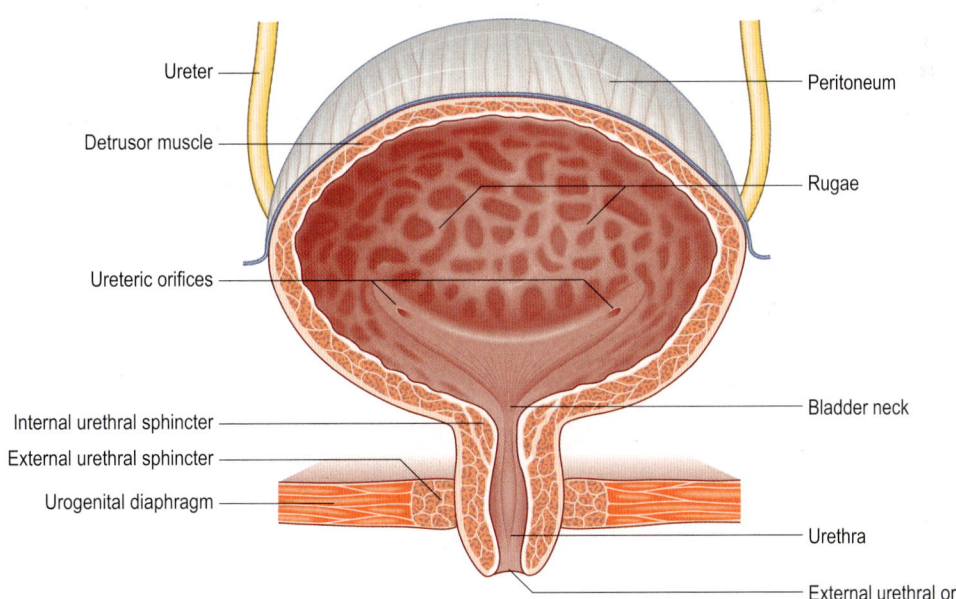

Ureter — Peritoneum
Detrusor muscle — Rugae
Ureteric orifices — Bladder neck
Internal urethral sphincter —
External urethral sphincter —
Urogenital diaphragm — Urethra
— External urethral orifice

**Fig. 12.4** The female urinary tract.

disease) and ectopic pregnancy (in women of child-bearing age), should be considered.

## Voiding symptoms

Symptoms are usually due to either bladder storage or voiding-phase problems.

Ask about:

- Urgency, frequency, nocturia and urge incontinence (storage symptoms)
- Hesitancy, poor stream, straining to void and terminal dribbling (voiding symptoms); these symptoms may be followed by a sense of incomplete emptying

Storage symptoms are usually associated with bladder, prostate or urethral problems, such as UTI, tumour, urethral calculi or obstruction from prostatic enlargement, or are caused by neurological disease, such as multiple sclerosis.

Voiding symptoms are often the result of bladder outflow obstruction from prostatic enlargement (in men) or urethral obstruction or genital prolapse (in women).

In women, incontinence is the most common symptom. Stress incontinence is urine leakage with increased abdominal pressure (such as when coughing or sneezing or due to weakened pelvic floor muscles), and urge incontinence is the urge to pass urine followed by involuntary leakage. These symptoms can occur separately or together, and increase with age. Overflow incontinence occurs without warning, often on changes in position, and is painless.

Polyuria, the passing of higher volumes of urine, has a number of causes, including excess water intake, osmotic diuresis (as in diabetes mellitus) and diabetes insipidus (inadequate secretion or action of vasopressin [antidiuretic hormone, ADH]).

Oliguria (passing of less than 500 mL of urine per day) and anuria (complete absence of urine) may be due to either very low fluid intake, mechanical obstruction or loss of kidney function (see later.)

Pneumaturia, passing gas bubbles in the urine, is suggestive of a fistula between the bladder and the colon from a diverticular abscess, malignancy or inflammatory bowel disease.

## Hematuria

The presence of blood in the urine is common. It may either be seen by the patient (visible haematuria) or be identified by urinalysis or microscopy (non-visible).

### Visible haematuria

Visible haematuria will be described as pink, red or brown in colour. Ask about previous episodes, their time course and whether they were persistent or intermittent. Haematuria can be due to an underlying problem anywhere along the renal tract from the glomerulus to the bladder (Fig. 12.5). Immunoglobulin A (IgA) nephropathy is the most common glomerular cause, which is often preceded by a non-specific upper respiratory tract infection. The haematuria associated with bladder

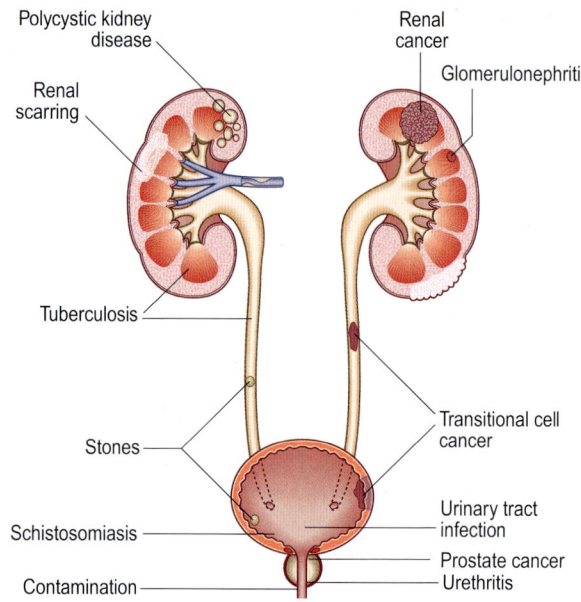

**Fig. 12.5** Principal sources of haematuria.

tumours is usually painless and intermittent. This is the most important cause to exclude in patients over 45 years of age without a UTI.

Ask about:

- Loin pain, as this may indicate ureteric obstruction due to blood, calculi, or a tumour; flank pain and haematuria may be features of renal cell carcinoma.
- Fever, dysuria, suprapubic pain and urinary frequency, which may indicate urinary infection.
- Family history of renal disease; polycystic kidney disease can present with visible haematuria due to cyst rupture.

### Non-visible haematuria

Non-visible (or microscopic) haematuria is a dipstick urinalysis abnormality, with 1+ considered positive. It can indicate renal or urinary tract disease. Non-visible haematuria in women of reproductive age is most commonly due to contamination by menstrual blood.

## Proteinuria and nephrotic syndrome

Proteinuria is the excretion of more than 150 mg of protein in the urine per day. It is usually asymptomatic but, if persistent, may indicate underlying renal disease.

Nephrotic syndrome is characterised by the combination of heavy proteinuria (>3.5 g/24 hours), hypoalbuminaemia and oedema. Nephrotic syndrome may come on over a few weeks (as in minimal change disease) and cause acute kidney injury (AKI), or it can evolve over many months (as in membranous nephropathy), giving a picture of chronic kidney disease (CKD). The most common cause of nephrotic syndrome is diabetes mellitus. Patients may notice that the urine is frothy due to the proteinuria; hyperlipidaemia, hypercoagulability, and an increased risk of infection may also develop.

Ask about:

- Weight loss, altered bowel habit, cough, back pain or chronic inflammatory conditions such as rheumatoid arthritis, inflammatory bowel disease or bronchiectasis (in particular if undertreated). The latter cause nephrotic syndrome as a result of renal AA amyloid deposition.
- Ankle swelling (pitting oedema): Younger patients may also notice facial swelling and puffy eyelids, especially first thing in the morning.
- Breathlessness (pleural effusions).
- Abdominal swelling (ascites).

## Acute kidney injury

AKI (Box 12.1) covers a range of presentations from relatively mild changes in kidney function to dialysis-requiring kidney failure. The typical presentation is with a recently identified rise in serum creatinine. AKI may have prerenal, renal or postrenal causes (Box 12.2); there is an increased risk in patients with pre-existing CKD. The history should focus on differentiating between these.

### Prerenal acute kidney injury

This is almost always due to volume depletion (hypovolaemia).

Ask about:

- Fluid losses, such as vomiting, diarrhoea or bleeding, and inadequate oral intake due to nausea or delirium.
- Recent operations or investigations that may be associated with increased fluid losses or reduced intake (fasting, bowel preparation).

- Any features of infection, such as fever, sweats, productive cough or dysuria.

Establish whether there is an underlying condition that may predispose to a reduction in renal blood flow.

Ask about:

- History of heart failure or liver disease.
- Recent drug prescriptions, such as those that block the renin–angiotensin-aldosterone system (e.g. angiotensin-converting enzyme inhibitors), other antihypertensive agents, diuretics (such as furosemide or spironolactone) and non-steroidal anti-inflammatory drugs (NSAIDs); NSAIDs can also cause intrinsic renal disease, such as interstitial nephritis and minimal change disease

### 12.1 Definition of acute kidney injury

| RIFLE[a] AKIN[b] | Serum creatinine criteria | Urine output criteria |
|---|---|---|
| Risk AKIN stage 1 | Increase>50% | < 0.5 mL/kg/h for 6 hours |
| Injury AKIN stage 2 | Increase>100% | <0.5 mL/kg/h for 12 hours |
| Failure AKIN stage 3 | Increase>200% or serum creatinine >350 μmol/L (3.96 mg/dL) | 0.3 mL/kg/h for 24 hours or anuria for 12 hours |
| Loss | Renal replacement therapy for >4 weeks | – |
| End-stage kidney disease | Renal replacement therapy for >3 months | – |

[a]Risk, injury, failure, loss, end-stage kidney disease
[b]Acute kidney injury network

### 12.2 Causes of acute kidney injury

**Prerenal**

- Hypovolaemia (e.g. blood loss, diarrhoea, vomiting, diuresis or inadequate oral intake)
- Relative hypovolaemia (e.g. heart failure or nephrotic syndrome)
- Sepsis
- Drugs (e.g. antihypertensives, diuretics or non-steroidal anti-inflammatory drugs)
- Renal artery stenosis or occlusion
- Hepatorenal syndrome

**Intrarenal**

- Glomerular disease (e.g. immunoglobulin A nephropathy, systemic vasculitis or systemic lupus erythematosus)
- Interstitial nephritis (drug-induced)
- Acute tubular necrosis/injury (may follow a prerenal cause)
- Multiple myeloma
- Rhabdomyolysis
- Intrarenal crystal deposition (e.g. urate nephropathy or ethylene glycol poisoning)
- Thrombotic microangiopathy (e.g. haemolytic uraemic syndrome or scleroderma renal crisis)
- Accelerated-phase hypertension
- Cholesterol emboli

**Postrenal**

- Renal stones (in papilla, ureter, or bladder)
- Papillary necrosis
- Ureteric or bladder transitional cell carcinoma
- Intraabdominal or pelvic malignancy (e.g. cervical carcinoma)
- Retroperitoneal fibrosis
- Blood clot
- Bladder outflow obstruction (e.g. prostatic enlargement)
- Neurogenic bladder
- Urethral stricture
- Posterior urethral valves
- Iatrogenic (e.g. ureteric damage at surgery, blocked urethral catheter)

12

## Intrinsic acute kidney injury

The most common cause in the hospital setting will be acute tubular injury (ATI), which may lead to acute tubular necrosis (ATN). This usually follows renal hypoperfusion when any of the causes identified above results in ischaemia–reperfusion injury. A less common cause is rhabdomyolysis, which is suggested by a history of prolonged immobilisation, such as following a fall. ATI normally recovers, but this can take days to weeks. AKI can also be the first clinical presentation of a systemic disease that affects the kidney (such as myeloma, infective endocarditis, vasculitis or systemic lupus erythematosus).

Ask about:

- Recent illnesses or operations.
- Drug history and any recent changes in medications; several commonly prescribed medications (such as antibiotics, NSAIDs or proton pump inhibitors) are recognised as causing an allergic interstitial nephritis, but almost any drug can be implicated.
- Symptoms of systemic disease: weight loss, fever, night sweats, tiredness, arthralgia, myalgia, bony pain, numbness, weakness, rashes, cough and breathlessness.

Occasionally, AKI can be the result of a primary glomerulonephritis. IgA nephropathy is the most common cause in the northern and western hemispheres. This classically presents with visible haematuria following an upper respiratory tract infection–so-called 'synpharyngitic haematuria'.

Ask about:

- Prior episodes.
- Loin pain and haematuria.
- Previous sore throat; a similar clinical illness can occur in postinfectious glomerulonephritis due to preceding beta-haemolytic streptococcal infection of the throat or skin.

## Postrenal acute kidney injury

This is usually due to any cause of obstruction from the renal pelvis to the urethra. The most common cause is bladder outflow obstruction; in men, this is often due to prostatic hypertrophy, either benign or malignant.

Ask about:

- Urinary urgency, frequency, nocturia and incontinence.
- Poor urine stream and terminal dribbling.
- Previous prostatic assessments, including prostate examination and measurements of prostate-specific antigen.
- Suprapubic pain.
- Leg weakness, perineal numbness or faecal incontinence (may indicate a spinal cord lesion).

In acute urinary retention there is usually a complete inability to pass urine and associated suprapubic discomfort. Chronic urinary retention is usually painless.

For ureteric disease to cause AKI, both kidneys need to be affected (or the patient has a single functioning kidney). Ureteric obstruction is most commonly due to malignancy, such as that of the bladder, cervix, ovary or uterus. These conditions are usually painless. The history should explore any previous diagnosis and recent operations and treatment, including radiotherapy.

## ▌ Chronic kidney disease

CKD is defined by degree of renal dysfunction and/or the presence of proteinuria (Boxes 12.3 and 12.4); these need to be present for at least 3 months. The diagnosis of CKD therefore requires preceding biochemical data to enable its distinction from AKI. Most patients with CKD have few symptoms until they have kidney failure.

### 12.3 Definition of chronic kidney disease

| CKD stage | eGFR (mL/min/1.73 m$^2$) | Description | Management |
|---|---|---|---|
| 1 | ≥90 | Kidney damage with normal or ↑ GFR | Observe; control blood pressure and risk factors |
| 2 | 60–89 | Kidney damage with mild ↓ GFR | |
| 3A | 45–59 | Moderate ↓ GFR | |
| 3B | 30–44 | | |
| 4 | 15–29 | Severe ↓ GFR | Prepare for kidney failure |
| 5 | <15 | Kidney failure | Dialysis, transplantation or conservative care |

p: the addition of p to a stage (e.g. 2p, 3Bp) means that there is significant proteinuria. Proteinuria is quantified on the basis of an albumin:creatinine (ACR) or protein:creatinine (PCR; see Box 12.4).
T: the addition of T to a stage (e.g. 4T) indicates that the patient has a renal transplant.
D: the addition of D to stage 5 CKD (i.e. 5D) indicates that the patient is on dialysis.

(e)GFR, (estimated) glomerular filtration rate.

### 12.4 Quantification of proteinuria using either urine albumin:creatinine ratio or protein:creatinine ratio

| ACR (mg/mmol) | PCR (mg/mmol) | Interpretation |
|---|---|---|
| >2.5/3.5[a] | >15 | Abnormal; adequate to define CKD stages 1 and 2; start ACE inhibitor or angiotensin-receptor blocker if diabetes is present |
| 30 | >50 | Use ACE inhibitor or angiotensin-receptor blocker if blood pressure is elevated; suffix 'p' on CKD stage |
| 70 | 100 | Requires tight blood pressure control |
| >250 | >300 | Nephrotic-range proteinuria |

[a]Values for males/females
ACE, Angiotensin-converting enzyme; CKD, chronic kidney disease.

The key in earlier stages is to ask about:

- Underlying conditions that may explain the aetiology of CKD, including diabetes mellitus, vascular disease (evidence of previous myocardial infarction, stroke or peripheral vascular disease), hypertension, hyperlipidaemia, episodes of acute glomerulonephritis (such as IgA nephropathy) or nephrotic syndrome (such as membranous disease)
- Previous incidental urine abnormalities, such as proteinuria or non-visible haematuria that may suggest a preceding glomerular disease.

A number of genetic diseases can present with CKD, so a detailed family history is required (see later).

## Kidney failure and uraemia

Occasionally, patients will present with symptoms of uraemia. This is most common in patients with known end-stage kidney disease once the estimated glomerular filtration rate (eGFR) is <10 mL/min/1.73 m$^2$. The symptoms are often nonspecific.

Ask about:

- Anorexia, nausea and vomiting.
- Lethargy.
- Poor concentration.
- Pruritus
- Breathlessness, which may occur due to fluid overload, worsening acidosis and/or anaemia.
- Peripheral oedema.

Less commonly, uraemia may present with features of pericarditis or peripheral neuropathy.

## The patient with a renal transplant

Identifying the fact that a patient has had a kidney transplant is important early in the history. The main presenting problems are a decline in kidney function (usually identified by routine blood tests), infection or malignancy. The risks of the latter two are increased by immunosuppression. Infections in renal transplant patients may be masked by immunosuppression. Lymphoma, in particular, needs to be considered post-transplantation.

Ask about:

- Date of transplant operation; organ rejection is more common in the first few weeks.
- Current and previous immunosuppression and any recent changes in treatment that may increase the risk of rejection; any intercurrent illness that may have contributed to AKI.
- Fever, weight loss, cough, breathlessness, dysuria and tenderness over the graft.

## The dialysis patient

There are two main forms of dialysis: haemodialysis and peritoneal dialysis. Each group can have specific presentations. Haemodialysis is delivered via an arteriovenous fistula or tunnelled vascular access catheter. A fistula has an obvious thrill (p. 278), and the patient may complain that this has been lost. This is usually due to thrombosis and needs urgent attention from a vascular surgeon. The most common problem with vascular access catheters is infection. Peritoneal dialysis involves a tunnelled catheter, and infection is also a common presentation. Ask about fever and rigors (and their relation to haemodialysis), abdominal pain and peritoneal dialysate fluid appearance (Has it become 'cloudy?').

## Other presenting symptoms

Finally, hypertension, anaemia and electrolyte disorders are other common features of renal disease.

## Past medical history

Ask the patient about their past medical history, including hypertension, vascular disease, diabetes mellitus, inflammatory diseases (such as rheumatoid arthritis, inflammatory bowel disease, chronic infections), urinary tract stones or surgery and previous evidence of renal disease, which may include dialysis and renal transplantation.

## Drug history

Enquire about long-term medication, any recent changes in treatment, recent courses of antibiotics and use of non-prescription medications, such as NSAIDs and herbal remedies.

## Family history

Document any family history of renal disease, hypertension, stroke, diabetes or deafness. If the parents are deceased, ask at what age and if the cause of death is known. The most common inherited renal conditions are autosomal dominant polycystic kidney disease (ADPKD) and Alport syndrome (hereditary nephritis). ADPKD usually affects members in each generation, and both males and females are affected. However, around 10% of those affected have no preceding family history, possibly because family members died

12

before the diagnosis was made. There is an association with berry aneurysms, so enquire about a history of subarachnoid haemorrhage in family members. Alport syndrome is caused by abnormalities in type IV collagen and can be associated with early-onset deafness. It is genetically heterogeneous, but the X-linked form is the most common. The typical presentation is with non-visible haematuria in childhood or more significant renal disease in the late teenage and early adult years.

## Social history

Ask about smoking, alcohol intake and recreational drug use. Ask about the patient's social support (family, housing and social work input) and occupation. Enquire as to how independent they are in their activities of daily living and how their illness has affected their work.

## The physical examination

The renal system can affect many aspects of the physical examination, but this may also be relatively normal, even with significant disease.

## General appearance

Advanced CKD is most likely to alter the general appearance. The patient may look unwell with pallor; the skin may have scratch marks from pruritus, and in severe cases there may be drowsiness, myoclonic twitching (p. 153) or asterixis (p. 118). In marked uraemia the patient's skin may appear yellow, but this is a late feature. Hiccupping may occur. Breathlessness may represent fluid overload or hyperventilation due to metabolic acidosis.

### Hands

Examine the hands, looking for pallor of the palmar creases suggestive of anaemia. Inspect the nails, looking for Muehrcke's lines (Fig. 12.6), which may be a sign of hypoalbuminaemia (nephrotic syndrome) or the half-and-half (Lindsay's) nails of CKD (proximal half white, distal half red or brown; Fig. 12.7).

### Dialysis access

Examine the arms for an arteriovenous fistula. This will look like prominent blood vessels on the forearm or upper arm (Fig. 12.8); there may be scars from previous fistulae on either arm. A functioning fistula will have a readily palpable fluid thrill (a continuous buzzing feel). A tunnelled venous access catheter may be seen exiting the anterior chest wall; the line can be followed under the skin before it enters the internal jugular vein (Fig. 12.9).

### Face

Inspect the face for rashes, which may indicate underlying connective tissue disease: the butterfly rash of systemic lupus

**Fig. 12.6** Muehrcke's lines. *(From Short N, Shah C. Muehrcke's lines. Am J Med. 2010;123(11):991–992, Elsevier.)*

**Fig. 12.7** Half-and-half (Lindsay's) nails.

erythematosus, for example. Look for conjunctival pallor, as anaemia is common in CKD. An inflamed eye, seen with scleritis and/or uveitis, may occur in systemic vasculitis. Fundoscopy may reveal changes of diabetic or hypertensive retinopathy (see Figs 8.17 and 8.18). Most patients with CKD due to diabetes mellitus will have evidence of retinal disease. The presence of hypertensive retinopathy (such as arteriolar narrowing, arteriovenous nipping, cotton-wool exudates or blot haemorrhages) indicates end-organ damage due to high blood pressure; more severe fundoscopy signs, such as flame haemorrhages and papilloedema, may indicate accelerated-phase hypertension, which can cause AKI. Inspection of the mouth may reveal gingival hyperplasia caused by calcineurin inhibitors (such as ciclosporin or tacrolimus). Uraemic fetor may be present.

### Skin

Inspect the skin more generally for rashes, bruising, scratch marks and excoriations. A vasculitic rash will appear as purpura,

**Fig. 12.8** Haemodialysis fistula.

**Fig. 12.9** Tunnelled venous access catheter.

**Fig. 12.10** Vasculitic rash.

rashes will be harder to identify on darker skin tones, so ask about changes in skin appearance.

## Assessment of fluid balance

### Examination sequence (Video 1)

An accurate check on fluid balance is critical to assessing renal disease and can be completed as a single sequenced process.

### General appearance

Does the patient look hypovolaemic or fluid-overloaded? In a dehydrated patient, the eyes may appear sunken and the mucous membranes, dry. Pinch the skin over the anterior chest wall (rather than forearms) to determine if there is reduced skin turgor (elasticity). These features, although relatively insensitive, are most common when there has been significant salt and water loss, as occurs with vomiting or diarrhoea. A patient with fluid overload may be breathless due to pulmonary oedema or pleural effusions, and there may be obvious signs of peripheral oedema.

### Pulse and blood pressure

Measure pulse and blood pressure (avoiding an arm with an arteriovenous fistula). Hypertension is common in renal disease. Is there evidence of hypovolaemia (tachycardia or hypotension)? Ascertaining whether blood pressure falls when the patients stands or sits upright is a sensitive indicator of hypovolaemia.

most commonly on the legs (Fig. 12.10), and may be due to systemic vasculitis, Henoch-Schönlein purpura or cryoglobulinaemia, all of which can cause AKI and CKD. A drug rash increases the likelihood of an allergic interstitial nephritis. All these

## Jugular venous pressure

Assess the jugular venous pressure (JVP; p. 57). The JVP may be elevated due to fluid overload or, rarely, due to cardiac tamponade from uraemic pericarditis.

## Examination of the chest

Examine the chest for signs of pulmonary oedema and/or pleural effusion (p. 98); both are features of fluid overload. Auscultate the heart (p. 50), listening for a third heart sound, which provides further evidence of fluid overload. A fourth heart sound may indicate left ventricular stiffening due to hypertension. A flow murmur may be present in anaemia of chronic renal disease. Quiet heart sounds suggest a pericardial effusion. A pericardial rub may occur in uraemia.

## Peripheral oedema

Examine for pitting oedema at the base of the spine (sacral oedema, common in bed-bound patients) and in the legs, starting at the ankles and noting the highest level at which oedema can be identified (such as midcalf, knees, or mid-thigh). In severe cases, oedema can extend into the scrotum or labia. Significant oedema is a hallmark of nephrotic syndrome.

## Weight

Look for sequential measures of a patient's weight, as this will provide an accurate assessment of fluid loss or gain over the short term.

## Fluid balance charts

The physical examination should be complemented, where possible, by measurement of fluid input (oral and intravenous) and output (urine volumes and other losses).

### Abdominal examination

### Examination sequence (Video 6G) ▶

Ask the patient to lie flat with their arms by their sides. Expose the abdomen fully down to the level of the anterior iliac spine.

### Inspection

- Look for abdominal distension in the flanks (which may indicate ascites, a further marker of fluid overload, or large polycystic kidneys). Look for operative scars, such as those relating to a renal transplant in the left or right iliac fossa, extending inferiorly to the midline (Fig. 12.11) and those of a previous nephrectomy in the left or right flank. A nephrectomy is often needed in patients with ADPKD to make space for a subsequent renal transplant. In addition, look for the presence of a peritoneal dialysis catheter.

**Fig. 12.11** Renal transplant scar in the right iliac fossa.

### Palpation

- Kneel beside the bed and use your right hand, keeping the palmar surface flat. Observe the patient's face for signs of discomfort throughout. Palpate each region in turn, beginning with light palpation followed by deeper palpation (p. 106 and Fig. 6.1C).* Describe any masses you feel. Examine for abdominal aortic aneurysm (p. 73).
- Significantly enlarged kidneys are palpable as masses in the flanks. You should be able to 'get above' the mass. Identification of less obviously enlarged kidneys requires deeper palpation and a ballotting technique. Starting on the right side, your left hand should be placed under the patient's back, with your index finger against the 12th rib in the paramedian position; the right pushes firmly down on the anterior abdominal wall. Ask the patient to take a deep breath, and push up by flexing the fingers of your left hand (Fig. 12.12A). The kidney can be felt against the fingers of the right hand. The same procedure is followed on the left side with your left hand under the patient and your little finger against the 12th rib (see Fig. 12.12B). The procedure is otherwise identical. ADPKD is the most common cause of palpable kidneys.
- A transplanted kidney may be palpated as a mass (usually 12–14 cm in length) in either iliac fossa, although the right is more common. Any tenderness should be noted, as this may indicate graft pyelonephritis or rejection.
- A palpable bladder may be felt as a soft, midline, suprapubic mass that you cannot 'get below'. In acute retention, palpation will worsen discomfort.
- When pyelonephritis is suspected, tenderness in the renal angle should be determined. If this is nontender on palpation, you may sit the patient up and percuss with a closed fist over both renal angles.

### Percussion

- Ascites should be assessed using the standard technique for shifting dullness or a fluid thrill (p. 124). Peritoneal dialysis fluid is also evident as a fluid level determined by percussion. To identify an enlarged bladder, you should percuss over the midline from a resonant area at the umbilicus, moving

A  B

**Fig. 12.12** Palpation of the kidney. **A** Right kidney. **B** Left kidney.

inferiorly to identify where the percussion note becomes dull. The percussion note should be resonant over enlarged kidneys.

### Auscultation

- Listen for abdominal bruits over the epigastrium and both renal arteries (p. 272). This may be a sign of renovascular disease or atheromatous disease in other arteries.

## Targeted examination of other systems

The kidneys are involved in many multisystem diseases. Renal impairment itself may also affect other systems. The history will help direct the examination to these elements.

### Joints

Examine for inflammation and swelling of joints, which can occur in systemic vasculitis. The presence of a chronic arthritis, such as rheumatoid disease, may lead to amyloid (a cause of nephrotic syndrome), and medication used to treat arthritis, such as NSAIDs, can cause AKI. Examine for areas of bony tenderness in the spine; this may be a feature of myeloma.

### Nervous system

Examine for a peripheral neuropathy (sensory and/or motor), which can occur with a systemic vasculitis. In diabetes mellitus, the presence of neuropathy is common in those with CKD.

### Prostate

Physical examination of the prostate is covered on pages 126 and 128.

## Interpretation of the findings

Renal disorders may come to light because of patient symptoms or abnormalities on biochemical investigation. Clinical assessment will be dictated by the scenario; focus on the relevant positive and negative findings when describing the case.

In patients with an acute presentation, the key element is to begin with a description of the patient's general appearance and fluid status. This should summarise whether they are clinically euvolaemic, hypovolaemic or fluid-overloaded. Are there any features of a multisystem disease (such as rash, joint swelling, or eye inflammation) or any signs in the abdomen that suggest renal disease (such as enlarged kidneys, renal transplant, renal bruits or enlarged bladder) that may point to a diagnosis? Urinalysis (see below) should be used to identify infection or intrinsic renal diseases, such as glomerulonephritis or nephrotic syndrome.

In patients with CKD, fluid balance assessment should be presented in the same way. The examination findings should focus on whether there is evidence of an underlying disease that may explain CKD: for example, diabetes mellitus (retinopathy, neuropathy), hypertension (retinopathy), ADPKD (enlarged kidneys, previous surgery), renovascular disease (renal bruits) or previous renal transplantation. In addition, include any features of the adverse effects of CKD, such as anaemia, skin excoriations from pruritus or weight loss, in your presentation.

## Investigations

### Urinalysis

Urinalysis should be considered an essential part of the renal examination. Urine should be obtained as a midstream specimen so it can be optimally used for subsequent investigations (see later). Urine abnormalities may reflect:

- Abnormally high levels of a substance in the blood exceeding the capacity for normal tubular reabsorption, such as glucose, ketones, conjugated bilirubin and urobilinogen.
- Altered kidney function: for example, proteinuria or failure to concentrate urine.
- Abnormal contents, such as blood arising at any point between the kidney and the urethra.

The urine dipstick test uses chemical reagents, which change colour when they are immersed and then removed from urine, to detect abnormalities. Urine test strips contain up to 10 of these chemical pads; however, not all are used in the assessment of renal disease. The key elements are described in Box 12.5.

Normal fresh urine is clear but varies in colour. Cloudy fresh urine is usually due to the presence of leucocytes (pyuria). Discoloration of the urine can occur due to drugs (e.g. rifampicin), foods (e.g. beetroot) or metabolites (e.g. bilirubin). Strong odours can be due to infections; some foods, like asparagus, impart a characteristic smell to the urine.

## Investigation of renal function

Functional studies may be useful in patients with voiding symptoms (Box 12.6). In addition to urinalysis, there are a number of other blood and urine tests (Box 12.7), as well as imaging studies (Box 12.8), that may help in the assessment of the patient with renal disease.

### 12.5 Key elements of urine dipstick test

| Investigation | Comment |
|---|---|
| Specific gravity | Reflects urine solute concentration; varies between 1.002 and 1.035; raised when kidneys actively reabsorb water (e.g. in fluid depletion or renal failure due to decreased perfusion) abnormally low values indicate failure to concentrate urine |
| pH | Normally 4.5–8.0; in renal tubular acidosis, pH never falls to <5.3 despite acidaemia |
| Glucose | Small amounts may be excreted by normal kidneys. Glycosuria may indicate poorly controlled diabetes mellitus. It may occur in intrinsic renal disease when tubular glucose reabsorption is impaired. |
| Ketones | Test is specific for acetoacetate and does not detect other ketones (e.g. β-OH butyrate, acetone). Ketonuria occurs in diabetic ketoacidosis, starvation, alcohol use and very-low-carbohydrate diets. |
| Protein | Varies between trace and 4+. The greater the degree of proteinuria, the more likely there is to be significant renal disease. Most patients with nephrotic syndrome will have 4+ protein. The presence of both blood ($\geq$2+) and protein ($\geq$2+)—an 'active urinary sediment'—often indicates intrinsic renal disease. As urinalysis is semiquantitative, confirmatory laboratory quantification should be undertaken using either a urine albumin:creatinine or protein:creatinine ratio (see Box 12.4) |
| Blood | $\geq$1+ is positive for non-visible haematuria. The test does not differentiate between haemoglobin and myoglobin. If you suspect rhabdomyolysis, measure myoglobin with a specific laboratory test. |
| Bilirubin and urobilinogen | Bilirubin is not normally present. Urobilinogen may be up to 33 μmol/L in health. Abnormalities of bilirubin and urobilinogen require investigation for possible haemolysis or hepatobiliary disease. |
| Leucocyte esterase | Indicates the presence of neutrophils in urine; seen in urinary tract infection or inflammation, stone disease and urothelial cancers |
| Nitrite | Most gram-negative bacteria convert urinary nitrate to nitrite. A positive result indicates bacteriuria, but a negative result does not exclude its presence. |

### 12.6 Functional assessment of the lower urinary tract

**Frequency/volume chart**

- Chart is used to monitor micturition patterns, including nocturia, and fluid intake.
- The patient collects their urine, measures each void and charts it against time over 3–5 days.

**Urine flow rate**

- The patient voids into a special receptacle that measures the rate of urine passage.
- A low flow does not differentiate between poor detrusor contractility and bladder outlet obstruction.

**Urodynamic tests**

- Invasive tests necessitating the insertion of bladder and rectal catheters to measure total bladder pressure and abdominal pressure and to allow bladder filling.
- Filling studies determine detrusor activity and compliance.
- Low detrusor pressures with low urine flow suggest detrusor function problems.
- High detrusor pressures with low flow suggest bladder outlet obstruction.

## 12.7 Blood and urine investigations in renal and urological disease

| Investigation | Indication/comment |
|---|---|
| Serum urea/creatinine | Levels generally ↑ as GFR ↓, but values are affected by diet and muscle mass, and do not measure renal function accurately |
| eGFR | Usually provided by the laboratory and is based on the serum creatinine<br>Usually reported as 'normal' if ≥60 mL/min/1.73 m$^2$<br>CKD is classified on the basis of the eGFR (see Box 12.3) |
| Creatinine clearance | A good measurement of GFR but requires a 24-hour urine collection and blood sample |
| Plasma electrolytes | ↑ Potassium (↓ excretion) in AKI and advanced CKD<br>↓ Bicarbonate (↓ H$^+$ excretion) common in AKI and CKD<br>↓ Calcium (impaired renal vitamin D$_3$ activation) and ↑ phosphate (↓ excretion) in CKD<br>↑ Urate common in CKD (may be associated with gout) |
| Plasma and urine osmolality | A measure of renal concentrating ability in unexplained hyponatremia. If the plasma osmolality is low, the urine osmolality should be lower still (<150 mosmol/kg); in the absence of hypovolaemia, any other finding is consistent with syndrome of inappropriate ADH (vasopressin) secretion<br>In patients with unexplained polyuria, test the concentrating ability of the kidneys by an overnight fluid deprivation test. In healthy people, urinary osmolality should rise to >600 mosmol/kg; any other finding suggests lack of ADH or renal tubular unresponsiveness to ADH. |
| Alkaline phosphatase and parathyroid hormone | ↑ in secondary hyperparathyroidism related to ↓ calcium and ↑ phosphate levels |
| Antinuclear factor and ANCA | Systemic lupus erythematosus and vasculitis may affect the kidney. |

*ADH*, Antidiuretic hormone (vasopressin); *AKI*, acute kidney injury; *ANCA*, antineutrophil cytoplasmic antibody; *CKD*, chronic kidney disease; *(e)GFR*, (estimated) glomerular filtration rate.

**12**

## 12.8 Imaging for the investigation of renal and urological disease

| Investigation | Indication/comment |
|---|---|
| Ultrasound scan | Assesses kidney size/shape/position; evidence of obstruction; renal cysts or solid lesions; stones; ureteric urine flow; gross abnormality of bladder, postmicturition residual volume<br>Used to guide kidney biopsy |
| Doppler ultrasound of renal vessels | Assesses renovascular disease, renal vein thrombosis<br>Arterial resistive index may indicate obstruction |
| Computed tomography of the kidney ureter bladder (CT KUB) | Renal colic; renal, ureteric or bladder stones |
| CT urogram | Frank haematuria; renal or bladder malignancy |
| Angiography/CT or magnetic resonance angiography | Hypertension ± renal failure, renal artery stenosis; angioplasty and/or stenting |
| Isotope scan | Suspected renal scarring (e.g. reflux nephropathy) diagnosis of obstruction<br>Assessment of glomerular filtration rate (GFR) in each kidney—measures renal uptake and excretion of radiolabelled chemicals |
| Renal biopsy | Used to diagnose parenchymal renal disease |

## OSCE example 1: renal history

Ms Measham, 60 years old, is attending to discuss the results of her recent blood tests. She has presented with a 3-month history of tiredness, and you know that her renal function was normal 1 year ago.

### Investigations

Haemoglobin: 101 g/L (10.1 g/dL) (reference range: female
115–165 g/L (11.5–16.5 g/dL); male 130–180 g/L (13.0–18.0 g/dL))
White cell count: $8.9 \times 10^9$/L (normal range: $4.0$–$11.0 \times 10^9$/L)
Platelet count: $510 \times 10^9$/L (normal range: $150$–$400 \times 10^9$/L)
Potassium: 5.2 mmol/L (normal range: 3.5–5.0 mmol/L)
Urea: 14.5 mmol/L (40.6 mg/dL; normal range: 3.0–7.0 mmol/L
(8.4–19.6 mg/dL))
Creatinine: 163 μmol/L (1.84 mg/dL; normal range:
60–120 μmol/L (0.68–1.36 mg/dL))
Dipstick urinalysis: blood: 3+, protein 3+

### Take a history from the patient

- Introduce yourself to the patient, and clean your hands.
- Obtain consent to take a history.
- Establish that the patient was well until 3 months ago and that the main symptoms are tiredness and breathlessness on exertion.
- Ask about:
  - Weight loss, appetite and bowel motions
  - Peripheral oedema
  - Haemoptysis
  - Urinary symptoms: dysuria, nocturia, urgency, hesitancy, incontinence, loin pain
  - Back pain, fevers and rigors
- Confirm details of the past medical history.
- Document current medication and any relevant recent changes.
- Determine how symptoms are affecting the patient's lifestyle: both work and leisure.
- Establish the family history.
- Thank the patient and clean your hands.

### Summarise your findings

The patient has presented with 3 months of lethargy, and investigations reveal that he has anaemia in the context of renal impairment.

### Suggest a differential diagnosis

The most likely diagnosis is an intrinsic renal disease, probably a glomerulonephritis, which may be part of a multisystem disorder. Infection is also possible.

### Suggest additional investigations

Relevant further investigations might include erythrocyte sedimentation rate, C-reactive protein, vasculitis and myeloma screens, and iron stores. Renal ultrasound, chest X-ray and midstream urine for microscopy and culture could be considered. The patient would benefit from a referral to a nephrologist. They may require a renal biopsy.

## OSCE example 2: renal examination

Mr. Silva, 45 years old, is known to have adult polycystic kidney disease and has a history of intermittent loin pain and hypertension.

### Please examine the abdomen

- Introduce yourself and clean your hands.
- Obtain permission to examine the patient.
- Perform a peripheral examination, including hands, arms and face. Look for leuconychia, pallor and an arteriovenous fistula for haemodialysis (if functioning, it will have a palpable thrill).
- Measure the blood pressure.
- Inspect the abdomen. Examine for scars from a previous nephrectomy (increasingly, these will be laparoscopic rather than scars from an open nephrectomy) or from a current or previous renal transplant in the right or left iliac fossa and a distended abdomen if polycystic kidneys are large.
- Ask if the abdomen is painful. Start with light palpation and then proceed more deeply across all abdominal regions. Assess for specific organomegaly, including liver, spleen, kidneys and bladder. Findings may include an irregular enlarged liver (polycystic liver) or palpable masses in one or both flanks (polycystic kidneys; it is key to distinguish these from the liver or spleen). Remember to ballott both kidneys.
- Percuss over any mass.
- Assess for shifting dullness due to ascites.
- Auscultate over the abdomen and over masses.

### Summarise your findings

This man has bilateral flank masses, which are ballottable. I can get above the masses, and the percussion note over them is resonant. These are most likely to represent bilaterally enlarged kidneys. The patient also has a functioning left arteriovenous fistula, most likely for haemodialysis.

### Suggest a diagnosis

The most likely cause is autosomal dominant polycystic kidney disease.

### Suggest initial investigations

An ultrasound scan would be the simplest test to show the presence of cysts. Magnetic resonance imaging would provide more detail about renal size.

### Advanced level comments

In addition to hypertension and renal failure, complications of APCKD include cyst haemorrhage and infection and subarachnoid haemorrhage due to a ruptured berry aneurysm.

12

## Integrated examination sequence for renal disease

- Position the patient: Start with patient at a 45-degree angle.
- Examine the general appearance:
  - Uremic facies
  - Myoclonus
  - Scratch marks
  - Dyspnoea, hyperventilation
- Check the hands, arms and face:
  - Splinter haemorrhages
  - Arteriovenous fistulae and scars
  - Tunnelled vascular access catheter
  - Pallor, eye inflammation
  - Examine skin for vasculitic (purpuric) rash
- Assess fluid balance:
  - Pulse, blood pressure, skin turgor and jugular venous pressure
  - Heart sounds
  - Chest examination: percussion and auscultation to assess for pleural effusions or pulmonary **oedema**
  - Sacral and ankle oedema
- Reposition the patient: supine with their arms at their sides.
- Perform an abdominal examination:
  - Inspection: peritoneal dialysis catheter, abdominal distension due to ascites or enlarged kidneys, scars from a renal transplant
  - Palpation: ballot for enlarged kidneys, palpate the suprapubic area for the bladder and any renal transplant in the right or left iliac fossa
  - Percussion: shifting dullness for ascites, enlarged kidneys resonant to percussion, suprapubic dullness indicating bladder enlargement
  - Auscultation: abdominal bruits
- Other:
  - In men with a history of urinary outflow problems, perform a rectal examination of the prostate.
  - Perform dipstick urinalysis.

**Jane Gibson**
**Phil Walmsley**

# The musculoskeletal system

**The history 288**
Common presenting symptoms 288
Past medical history 292
Drug history 292
Family history 292
Social history 293

**The physical examination 293**
General principles 293
General examination 293

**Detailed examination of the musculoskeletal system 296**
Gait 296

Spine 297
Upper limb 302
Lower limb 309

**Fractures, dislocations and trauma 319**
The history 319
The physical examination 319

**Investigations 320**

**OSCE example 1: Right shoulder pain 322**

**OSCE example 2: Painful hands 322**

**Integrated examination sequence for the locomotor system 323**

# The history

## Common presenting symptoms

### ▍Pain

In musculoskeletal pain, the acronym SOCRATES (see Box 2.2, p. 12) suggests questions that help reveal useful diagnostic clues.

### Site

Fig. 13.1 illustrates the anatomy of a typical joint. Determine which component is painful: the joint (arthralgia), muscle (myalgia) or other soft tissue. Pain may be localised and may suggest the diagnosis, for example, a red, hot, tender first metatarsophalangeal joint in gout (Fig. 13.2), or swelling of several joints suggesting inflammatory arthritis. Causes of arthralgia and myalgia are shown in Boxes 13.1 and 13.2.

### Onset

Pain from traumatic injury is usually immediate and exacerbated by movement. An affected joint may develop haemarthrosis (bleeding into the joint). Inflammatory arthritis can develop over 24 hours or more insidiously. Crystal arthritis (gout and pseudogout) causes acute, severe pain that develops quickly, often overnight. Joint sepsis causes pain that develops over 1–2 days.

### Character

Bone pain can be described as a 'deep ache' or 'penetrating' and is characteristically worse at night. Common causes of localised pain are tumours, osteomyelitis (infection), osteonecrosis or osteoid osteoma (a benign bone tumour). Generalised bony conditions, such as osteomalacia, more commonly cause diffuse pain.

Pain from fractures is usually sharp and stabbing, aggravated by any movement and relieved by rest and splintage.

Muscle pain may be described as 'stiffness' or 'aching' and is aggravated by use of the affected muscle(s).

**Fig. 13.1** Structure of a joint and surrounding tissues.

Bone — Skin and subcutaneous tissue
— Bursa
Capsule — Tendon
Synovium — Tendon sheath
Fibrocartilage pad — Ligamentous thickening of capsule
Joint space — Muscle
Articular cartilage — Bursa

**Fig. 13.2 Acute gout of the first metatarsophalangeal joint.** This causes swelling, erythema, and extreme pain and tenderness (podagra). *From Colledge NR, Walker BR, Ralston SH, eds. Davidson's Principles and Practice of Medicine. 21st ed. Edinburgh: Churchill Livingstone; 2010.*

| **13.1 Common causes of arthralgia (joint pain)** |
| --- |
| **Infective** |
| • Viral (e.g. rubella, parvovirus B19, mumps, hepatitis B, chikungunya) |
| • Bacterial (e.g. staphylococci, Mycobacterium tuberculosis, Borrelia) |
| • Fungal |
| **Postinfective** |
| • Rheumatic fever |
| • Reactive arthritis |
| **Inflammatory** |
| • Rheumatoid Arthritis |
| **Degenerative** |
| • Osteoarthritis |
| **Tumour** |
| • Primary (e.g. osteosarcoma, chondrosarcoma) |
| • Metastatic (e.g. from lung, breast, prostate) |
| • Systemic tumour effects (e.g. hypertrophic pulmonary osteoarthropathy) |
| **Crystal formation** |
| • Gout, pseudogout |
| **Trauma** |
| • For example, Road traffic accidents |
| **Others** |
| • Chronic pain disorders (e.g. fibromyalgia (usually diffuse pain)) |
| • Hypermobile Ehler's Danlos syndrome |

## 13.2 Causes of muscle pain (myalgia)

**Infective**

- Viral: Coxsackie, cytomegalovirus, echovirus, dengue, SARS CoV2
- Bacterial: *Streptococcus pneumoniae*, *Mycoplasma*
- Parasitic: schistosomiasis, toxoplasmosis

**Traumatic**

- Tears
- Haematoma
- Rhabdomyolysis

**Inflammatory**

- Polymyalgia rheumatica
- Myositis
- Dermatomyositis

**Drugs**

- Alcohol withdrawal
- Statins
- Triptans

**Metabolic**

- Hypothyroidism
- Hyperthyroidism
- Addison's disease
- Vitamin D deficiency
- Neuropathic

## 13.3 Common patterns of referred and radicular musculoskeletal pain

| Site where pain is perceived | Site of pathology |
| --- | --- |
| Occiput | C1, 2 |
| Interscapular region | C3, 4 |
| Tip of shoulder, upper outer aspect of arm | C5 |
| Interscapular region or radial fingers and thumb | C6, 7 |
| Ulnar side of forearm, ring and little fingers | C8 |
| Medial aspect of upper arm | T1 |
| Chest | Thoracic spine |
| Buttocks, knees, legs | Lumbar spine |
| Lateral aspect of upper arm | Shoulder |
| Forearm | Elbow |
| Anterior thigh, knee | Hip |
| Thigh, hip | Knee |

pain, early-morning stiffness and loss of function is likely to be inflammatory arthritis. 'Flitting' pain, starting in one joint and moving to others over a period of days, is a feature of rheumatic

'Shooting' pain is often caused by impingement of a peripheral nerve or nerve root; for example, buttock pain, which 'shoots down the back of the leg', is caused by lumbar disc protrusion.

Progressive joint pain in patients over 40 years old is most commonly caused by osteoarthritis.

Fibromyalgia, a chronic pain syndrome, causes widespread, constant pain with little diurnal variation, which is poorly controlled by conventional analgesic/anti-inflammatory drugs.

### Radiation

Pain from nerve compression radiates to the distribution of the affected nerve or nerve root (see Fig. 7.26), such as lower leg pain in intervertebral disc prolapse or hand pain in carpal tunnel syndrome. Neck pain radiates to the shoulder or scalp. Hip pain is commonly felt in the groin but may radiate to the thigh or knee. Common patterns of radiation are summarised in Box 13.3.

### Associated symptoms

For example, swelling and redness of a joint indicate inflammatory arthritis.

### Timing (frequency, duration and periodicity of symptoms)

A history of several years of pain with a normal examination suggests fibromyalgia (Box 13.4). A history of several weeks of

## 13.4 Clinical vignette: arthralgia and fatigue

A 34-year-old mother-of-two presents to her General Practitioner (GP) with a 1-year history of gradually worsening pain and persistent fatigue. The pain moves around and involves the back, neck, shoulders, elbows, hands and knees. All joints are described as swollen, particularly her hands, which swell 'all over'. Further history reveals poor sleep, with the patient wakening every 2 hours and feeling unrefreshed in the morning. She has a difficult social background and a past history of depression and irritable bowel syndrome. Examination shows no skin or joint abnormality but there is widespread tenderness, particularly across her shoulders, in her neck and down her back (see figure). Blood tests are all normal. She is diagnosed with fibromyalgia.

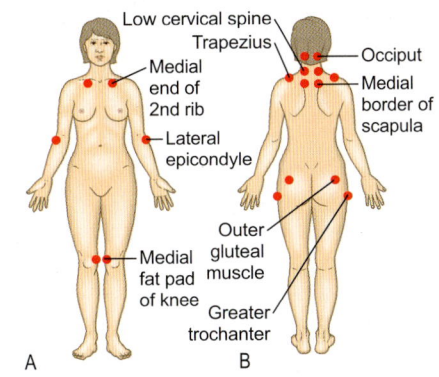

**Typical tender points in fibromyalgia.** **A** Anterior view. **B** Posterior view.

fever and gonococcal arthritis. If intermittent, with resolution between episodes, it may be palindromic rheumatism.

### Exacerbating/relieving factors

Pain from joints damaged by intra-articular derangement or osteoarthritic degeneration worsens with exercise. Pain from inflammatory arthritis worsens with rest. Pain from a septic joint is present both at rest and with movement.

### Severity

Apart from trauma, the most severe joint pain occurs in septic and crystal arthritis. Disproportionately, severe pain is seen acutely in compartment syndrome (increased pressure in a fascial compartment, compromising perfusion and viability of compartmental structures) and chronically in complex regional pain syndrome. Neurological involvement in diabetes mellitus, leprosy, syringomyelia and syphilis (tabes dorsalis) may impair joint sensation, reducing pain despite obvious pathology on examination. Grossly abnormal joints may even be pain-free (e.g. Charcot joints, Fig 10.14C, p. 237). Partial muscle tears are painful; a complete rupture may be less so.

### Patterns of joint involvement

Different patterns of joint involvement aid the differential diagnosis (Fig. 13.3). Are the small or large joints of the arms or legs affected? How many joints are involved? Involvement of one joint is called monoarthritis; 2–4 joints, oligoarthritis; and more than 4, polyarthritis.

- Predominant involvement of the small joints of the hands and feet suggests inflammatory arthritis, such as rheumatoid arthritis or systemic lupus erythematosus (SLE).
- Medium- or large-joint swelling is more likely to be degenerative (osteoarthritis) or seronegative arthritis (such as psoriatic arthritis).
- Nodal osteoarthritis particularly affects the distal interphalangeal (DIP) joints of the hands and the carpometacarpal (CMC) joint of the thumb.

## Stiffness

Ask what the patient means by stiffness. Is it:

- restricted range of movement?
- difficulty moving, but with a normal range?
- painful movement?
- localised to a particular joint or more generalised?

There are characteristic differences between inflammatory and non-inflammatory presentations of joint stiffness. Inflammatory arthritis causes early-morning stiffness that takes at least 30 minutes to wear off with activity. Non-inflammatory, mechanical arthritis causes stiffness after rest that eases rapidly on movement.

Disease of the soft tissues rather than the joint itself may cause stiffness. In polymyalgia rheumatica, stiffness commonly affects the shoulder and pelvic areas.

## Swelling

Ask about the site, extent and time course of the swelling.

Rheumatoid arthritis

A

Psoriatic arthritis

B

Axial spondyloarthritis

C

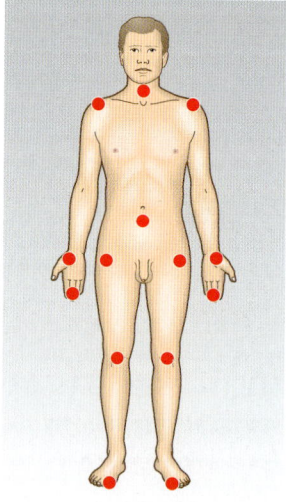
Osteoarthritis

D

**Fig. 13.3 Contrasting patterns of joint involvement in polyarthritis.** [A] Rheumatoid arthritis (symmetrical, small and large joints, upper and lower limbs). [B] Psoriatic arthritis (asymmetrical, large > small joints, swelling of a whole digit – dactylitis, enthesitis). [C] Axial spondyloarthritis (spine and sacroiliac joints, asymmetrical peripheral arthritis, large > small joints, enthesitis). [D] Osteoarthritis (symmetrical, small and large joints, base of thumb, distal interphalangeal joints).

The speed of onset of swelling is a clue to the diagnosis:

- Rapid (<30 minutes), severe swelling suggests a haemarthrosis (Fig. 13.4B). This occurs when vascular structures such as bone or ligament are injured and becomes worse in the presence of anticoagulants or bleeding disorders.
- Swelling over hours, or days, post injury suggests traumatic effusion, such as with a meniscal tear or articular cartilage abrasion.
- Septic arthritis develops over a few hours up to two days with pain, marked swelling, tenderness, redness and extreme reluctance to move the joint actively or passively. Concurrent glucocorticoid or non-steroidal anti-inflammatory drug therapy suppresses these features.
- Crystal-induced arthritis (gout or pseudogout) can mimic septic arthritis. It commonly starts overnight or early in the morning due to the rise in serum urate following the evening meal.

A

B

**Fig. 13.4** A Olecranon bursitis. B Right-knee haemarthrosis.

## Erythema and warmth

Erythema (redness) can occur with infective, traumatic and crystal-induced conditions and may be present in inflammatory arthritis. All affected joints will be warm. Erythema associated with DIP joint swelling helps to distinguish DIP joint psoriatic arthritis from the Heberden's nodes of osteoarthritis.

## Weakness

Weakness suggests joint, neurological or muscle disease. The problem may be focal or generalised.

Joint disorders can cause weakness, either by inhibition of function due to pain or by disruption of the joint and its supporting structures. Nerve entrapment may be a cause, for example, carpal tunnel syndrome at the wrist. Muscle disorders can produce widespread weakness associated with pain and fatigue, such as in myositis, and with a rash, as in dermatomyositis. Proximal muscle weakness can occur in endocrine disorders: for example, hypothyroidism or excess of glucocorticoids.

## Locking and triggering

'Locking' is an incomplete range of movement at a joint because of an anatomical block. It may be associated with pain. Patients use 'locking' to describe various problems, so clarify exactly what they mean.

True locking is a block to the normal range of movement caused by mechanical obstruction, typically preventing full extension, for example from a loose body or torn meniscus, within the joint. The patient may be able to 'unlock' the joint by trick manoeuvres.

Pseudolocking is a loss of the range of movement due to pain.

Triggering is a block to the extension of a finger, which then 'gives' suddenly when extending from a flexed position. In adults, it normally affects the ring or middle fingers and is caused by nodular or fibrous thickening of the flexor sheath due to chronic low-grade trauma. The cause may be occupational or associated with inflammatory arthritis. Triggering can also be congenital, in which case, it usually affects the thumb.

## Extra-articular symptoms

Patients may present with extra-articular features of a disease (Box 13.5) that they may not connect with musculoskeletal problems.

Ask about:

- Rashes: occur with psoriasis, vasculitis, viral infections, connective tissue diseases, sarcoidosis and auto-inflammatory disease. Ask whether they are photosensitive (SLE, Box 13.6).
- Weight loss, low-grade fever and malaise: associated with rheumatoid arthritis and SLE. High-spiking fevers in the evening, accompanied by a rash, occur in adult-onset Still's disease.

13

## 13.5 Extra-articular signs in rheumatic conditions

| Condition | Extra-articular signs |
|---|---|
| Rheumatoid arthritis | Rheumatoid nodules, palmar erythema, episcleritis, dry eyes, interstitial lung disease, pleural ± pericardial effusion, small-vessel vasculitis, Raynaud's phenomenon, low-grade fever, weight loss, lymphadenopathy, splenomegaly, leg ulcers |
| Psoriatic arthritis | Psoriasis, nail pitting, onycholysis, enthesitis, dactylitis, episcleritis |
| Reactive arthritis | Urethritis, mouth and/or genital ulcers, conjunctivitis, iritis, enthesitis (inflammation of tendon or ligament attachments) (e.g. Achilles enthesitis/plantar fasciitis, rash (keratoderma blennorrhagica)) |
| Axial spondyloarthritis | Inflammatory bowel disease, psoriasis, enthesitis, iritis, episcleritis, aortic regurgitation, apical interstitial fibrosis |
| Septic arthritis | Fever, malaise, source of sepsis (e.g. skin, throat, gut) |
| Gout | Tophi, signs of renal failure or alcoholic liver disease, obesity |
| Sjögren's syndrome | 'Dry eyes' (keratoconjunctivitis sicca), xerostomia (reduced or absent saliva production), salivary gland enlargement, Raynaud's phenomenon, neuropathy |
| Systemic lupus erythematosus | Photosensitive rash, especially on face, mucocutaneous ulcers, alopecia, fever, pleural ± pericardial effusion, diaphragmatic paralysis, pulmonary fibrosis (rare), Raynaud's phenomenon, lymphopenia |
| Systemic sclerosis | Skin tightening (scleroderma, see Fig. 3.30C), telangiectasia, Raynaud's phenomenon, calcific deposits in fingers, dilated nail-fold capillaries, pulmonary fibrosis |
| Vasculitis | Rash, fever, malaise, neuropathy, tender cranial arteries in giant cell arteritis, nasal crusting and saddle nose in granulomatous polyangiitis |
| Auto-inflammatory Diseases | Rash, recurrent fever, serositis, aphthous ulceration, hepatomegaly, splenomegaly, deafness |
| Other | Erythema nodosum of shins in sarcoidosis and Behçet's disease, viral rashes, drug rashes, oral and genital ulceration in Behçet's disease |

• Headache, jaw pain on chewing (claudication) and scalp tenderness: features of temporal arteritis.

Connective tissue disease may present with multiple extra-articular features:

• Raynaud's phenomenon.
• Sicca symptoms (dryness of mouth and eyes).
• Rashes.
• Gastrointestinal problems, including dysphagia and mouth ulcers.
• Respiratory problems, including dyspnoea from interstitial lung disease, or pleural pain or effusions associated with rheumatoid arthritis or connective tissue disease.
• Back pain and stiffness or arthritis associated with abdominal pain, diarrhoea, bloody stool and mouth ulcers. They may suggest arthritis associated with inflammatory bowel disease.

## Past medical history

Note past episodes of musculoskeletal involvement, extra-articular diseases as listed in the previous section, fractures and possible complicating comorbidities such as diabetes or obesity.

## Drug history

Many drugs have side effects that may either worsen or precipitate musculoskeletal conditions (Box 13.7).

## 13.6 Clinical vignette: joint pain and rash

A 32-year-old woman is seen in the outpatient clinic with fatigue and intermittent pain and swelling in her hands, which she has had for the last year. She noticed a rash across her cheeks and on her arms while she was on holiday in Spain recently, and this seems to have sparked off painful mouth ulcers and worsening joint pain. She has no other relevant history. Examination shows a 'butterfly' rash across the cheeks and nose, several mouth ulcers and two swollen metacarpophalangeal joints. Blood tests reveal anaemia, lymphopenia, positive antinuclear antibody and raised anti-double-stranded deoxyribonucleic acid antibodies.
A diagnosis of systemic lupus erythematosus is made.

## Family history

Inflammatory arthritis is more common if a first-degree relative is affected. Osteoarthritis, osteoporosis and gout are heritable in a variable polygenic fashion. Spondyloarthritis is more common in patients with human leucocyte antigen B27. A single-gene defect (monogenic inheritance) is found in hereditary sensorimotor neuropathy (Charcot–Marie–Tooth disease), osteogenesis imperfecta, Ehlers–Danlos syndrome, Marfan's syndrome and muscular dystrophies.

**13.7 Drugs associated with adverse musculoskeletal effects**

| Drug | Possible adverse musculoskeletal effects |
|---|---|
| Glucocorticoids | Osteoporosis, myopathy, osteonecrosis, infection |
| Statins | Myalgia, myositis, myopathy |
| Angiotensin-converting enzyme inhibitors | Myalgia, arthralgia, positive antinuclear antibody |
| Antiepileptics | Osteomalacia, arthralgia |
| Immunosuppressants | Infections |
| Quinolones | Tendinopathy, tendon rupture |

## Social history

Identify functional difficulties, including the ability to use pens, tools and cutlery. How does the condition affect the patient's activities of daily living, such as washing, dressing and toileting? Can they use the stairs, and do they need walking aids? Ask about functional independence, especially cooking, housework and shopping.

Ask about current and previous occupations. Is the patient working full- or part-time, on sick leave or receiving benefits? Has the patient had to take time off work because of the condition and is their job at risk? Litigation may be pending following injury and in occupational disorders such as repetitive strain disorder, hand vibration syndrome and fatigue fractures.

Smoking is a risk factor for rheumatoid arthritis and possibly other inflammatory arthritides. High alcohol intake contributes to gout and falls that may result in fracture. It can also cause myopathy, neuropathy and rhabdomyolysis.

Some conditions are seen in certain ethnic groups; for example, sickle cell disease may present with bone and joint pain in African patients. Osteomalacia is more common in Asian patients. Bone and joint tuberculosis is more common in African and Asian patients.

A sexual history may be relevant (Chapter 2, p. 17) since sexually transmitted diseases are associated with musculoskeletal problems, such as reactive arthritis, gonococcal arthritis, human immunodeficiency virus infection and hepatitis B.

## The physical examination

Practise examining as many joints as possible to become familiar with normal appearances and ranges of movement.

### General principles

Firstly, examine the patient's overall appearance for features such as pallor, rash, skin tightening and hair changes.

### Look – feel – move

Follow a process of observation, palpation and movement for each joint or group of joints in turn.

Look at the skin, subcutaneous tissues and bony outline of each area. Before palpating, ask the patient which area is painful or tender. Feel for warmth, swelling, stability and deformity. Assess if the deformity is reducible or fixed. Assess active before passive movement. Do not cause the patient additional pain. Compare one limb with the opposite side. Always expose the joint above and below the affected one. In suspected systemic disease, examine all joints and systems fully.

Use standard terminology to describe position and movement. Describe movements from the neutral position:

- flexion: bending at a joint from the neutral position
- extension: straightening a joint towards the neutral position
- hyperextension: moving beyond the normal neutral position (indicating a torn ligament or ligamentous laxity, such as Hypermobile Ehler's Danlos syndrome)
- adduction: moving towards the midline of the body (finger adduction is movement towards the axis of the limb)
- abduction: moving away from the midline.

To describe altered limb position due to joint/bone deformity, use:

- valgus: the distal part deviates away from the midline
- varus: the distal part deviates towards the midline.

In the wrist and hand, use:

- radial deviation: the distal part deviates towards the radial side
- ulnar deviation: the distal part deviates towards the ulnar side.

## General examination

### Skin, nail and soft tissues

The skin and nails are common sites of associated lesions. Skin changes of psoriasis may be hidden in the umbilicus, natal cleft or scalp (Fig. 14.3B, p. 329), for example. The rash of SLE is found across the cheeks and bridge of the nose. Nail pitting and onycholysis occur in psoriasis (Fig. 3.7A, p. 27).

Small, dark-red spots due to capillary infarcts occur in rheumatoid arthritis, SLE and systemic vasculitis. Common sites are the nail folds (Fig. 13.5, often seen in rheumatoid arthritis) and the lower legs in systemic vasculitis (fig 14.7, p. 331).

In systemic sclerosis, the thickened, tight skin produces a characteristic facial appearance (see Fig. 3.30C on p. 39). In the hands, flexion contractures, calcium deposits in the finger pulps (Fig. 13.6) and tissue ischaemia leading to ulceration may occur. The telangiectasias of systemic sclerosis are purplish, blanch with pressure and are most common on the hands and face. In the fingers, the pallor of Raynaud's phenomenon, pulp atrophy or ulceration may be evident.

Reactive arthritis is associated with conjunctivitis, urethritis, circinate balanitis (painless superficial ulcers on the prepuce and glans) and superficial mouth ulcers.

**13**

Fig. 13.5 Nail-fold infarcts caused by small-vessel vasculitis.

A

B

Fig. 13.6 Systemic sclerosis in the hand. **A** Calcium deposits ulcerating through the skin. **B** x-ray showing calcium deposits. *(A) From Forbes CD, Jackson WF. Colour Atlas of Clinical Medicine. 3rd ed. Edinburgh: Mosby; 2003.*

## Nodules

The firm, non-tender, subcutaneous nodules of rheumatoid arthritis most commonly occur on the extensor surface of the forearm (Fig. 13.7), sites of pressure or friction such as the sacrum or Achilles tendon, or in the lungs. Multiple small nodules can occur

Fig. 13.7 Rheumatoid nodules at the olecranon and ulnar border.

in the hands. Rheumatoid nodules are strongly associated with a positive anti-cyclic citrullinated peptide (anti-CCP) antibody or rheumatoid factor.

Bony nodules in osteoarthritis affect the lateral aspects of the DIP joints (Heberden's nodes) or the proximal interphalangeal (PIP) joints (Bouchard's nodes, Fig. 13.8). They are smaller and harder than rheumatoid nodules.

Gouty tophi are firm, irregular subcutaneous crystal collections (monosodium urate monohydrate). Common sites are the olecranon bursa, helix of the ear and the fingers (Fig. 13.9), hands, knees and toes. If superficial, they may appear white, and may ulcerate, discharge crystals and become secondarily infected.

## Eyes

Redness of the eyes may be due to conjunctivitis in reactive arthritis or 'dry eyes' in Sjögren's syndrome, rheumatoid arthritis and other connective tissue disorders. Scleritis and episcleritis occur in rheumatoid arthritis and psoriatic arthritis. An acutely painful, very red eye due to iritis occurs in axial spondyloarthritis (Fig. 13.13, p. 298). The sclerae are blue in certain types of osteogenesis imperfecta (see Fig. 3.30A on p. 39) and in the scleromalacia of longstanding rheumatoid arthritis.

## General features

Weight loss, muscle loss, fever and lymphadenopathy are all features of systemic involvement in inflammatory arthritis and connective tissue disease.

## Joints: the GALS screen

GALS (gait, arms, legs, spine) is a rapid screen for musculo-skeletal and neurological deficits and for functional ability; it helps identify joints that require more detailed examination, as described later.

### Initial questions

- Do you have any pain or stiffness in your muscles, joints or back?
- Do you have difficulty dressing yourself?

**Fig. 13.8 Osteoarthritis of the hand** Heberden's (single arrow) and Bouchard's (double arrow) nodes.

**Fig. 13.9** Gouty tophi.

• Do you have difficulty walking up and down the stairs?

If all three replies are negative, the patient is unlikely to have a significant musculoskeletal problem; otherwise, perform the GALS screen.

## Examination sequence (Video 24)

Ask the patient to undress to their underwear and stand in front of you. Demonstrate actions to the patient rather than simply telling them what to do. Any asymmetry, reduced range of movement, pain or deformity demands a detailed examination.

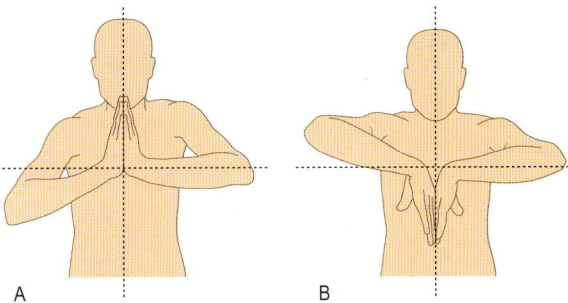

**Fig. 13.10 Assessing the wrist.** **A** Extension. **B** Flexion. There is a reduced range of movement at the right wrist.

### Gait
• Ask the patient to walk ahead in a straight line, then turn and walk back towards you. Look for smoothness and symmetry of the gait.

### Arms
• Stand in front of the patient.
• Inspect the dorsum of the hands and check for full extension at the metacarpophalangeal (MCP), PIP and DIP joints.
• Gently squeeze across the MCP joints. Tenderness suggests inflammation, as in rheumatoid arthritis.
• Ask the patient to:
• Clench their fists and then open their hands flat.
• Squeeze your index and middle fingers.
• Touch each of their fingertips with the thumb.
• Make a 'prayer sign', with their elbows as high as possible. Then reverse this with the backs of their hands together and elbows low (Fig. 13.10).
• Put their arms straight out in front of their body.
• Bend their arms up to touch their shoulders.
• Place their elbows by the side of their body, bent at 90 degrees. Turn their palms up and down.
• Put their hands behind their head, with their elbows back.
• Put their hands behind their back.

### Legs
• Ask the patient to lie supine on the couch.
• Palpate each knee for warmth, swelling and patellar tap.
• Flex each hip and knee with your hand on the patient's knee. Feel for crepitus in the patellofemoral joint and knee.
• Unless contraindicated, perform Thomas's test for fixed flexion deformity on both hips (see Fig. 13.35).
• Flex the patient's knee and hip to 90 degrees, and passively rotate each hip internally and externally.
• Look at the feet for any abnormality. Examine the soles, looking for calluses and ulcers, indicating abnormal load bearing.
• Gently squeeze across the metatarsal heads for tenderness.

### Spine
• Stand behind the patient. Assess the straightness of the spine, muscle bulk and symmetry in the trunk, legs, ankle and foot.
• Stand beside the patient. Ask them to bend down and try to touch their toes, while you look for abnormal spinal curvature or limited hip flexion.

**13**

| 13.8 The Beighton scoring system to assess hypermobility | |
|---|---|
| **Ask the patient to** | **Score** |
| Bring the thumb to touch the forearm, with the wrist flexed | 1 point each side |
| Extend the little finger >90 degrees, with the hand in a neutral position | 1 point each side |
| Extend the elbow >10 degrees | 1 point each side |
| Extend the knee >10 degrees | 1 point each side |
| Touch the floor, with the palms of hands and the knees straight | 1 point |
| A score of ≥4 indicates hypermobility | |

Reproduced from Beighton P, Solomon L, Soskolne CL. Articular mobility in an African population. *Ann Rheum Dis*. 1973; 32(5):413, with permission from BMJ Publishing Group.

- Stand behind the patient, hold their pelvis, and ask them to turn from side to side without moving their feet.
- Ask them to slide their hand down the lateral aspect of their leg towards their knee.
- Stand in front of the patient. Ask them to put their ear to each shoulder in turn.
- Ask the patient to look down to the floor and then up to the ceiling.
- Ask them to open their jaw wide and move it from side to side.

### Hypermobility

Some patients have a greater than normal range of joint movement. If this is severe, patients may present with recurrent dislocations or sensations of instability. Milder cases may develop arthralgia or be symptom-free. Mild hypermobility is normal, but Marfan's and Hypermobile Ehler's Danlos syndromes (Box 13.8) cause significant hypermobility.

## Detailed examination of the musculoskeletal system

The GALS screen provides a rapid but limited assessment. This section describes the detailed examination required for thorough evaluation.

### Gait

Gait is the cyclical pattern of musculoskeletal motion that carries the body forwards. Normal gait is smooth, symmetrical and ergonomically economical, with each leg 50% out of phase with the other. It has two phases: stance and swing. The stance phase is from initial contact to toe-off, when the foot is on the ground and load-bearing. The swing phase is from toe-off to initial contact when the foot is off the ground. When both feet are on the ground, this is a double stance.

A limp, or antalgic gait, is an abnormal gait due to pain, structural change or spasticity.

## Examination sequence (Video 24A)

- Ask the patient to walk barefoot in a straight line. Then repeat in shoes.
- Observe the patient from behind, in front and from the side.
- Evaluate what happens at each level (foot, ankle, knee, hip and pelvis, trunk and spine) during both stance and swing phases.

### Pain

An antalgic gait is one altered to reduce pain. Pain in a lower limb is usually aggravated by weight bearing, so minimal time is spent in the stance phase on that side. This results in a 'dot–dash' mode of walking. If the source of pain is in the spine, axial rotatory movements are decreased, resulting in a slow gait with small paces. Patients with hip pain may lean towards the affected side, as this decreases the joint reaction force in the hip joint.

### Structural change

Patients with limb-length discrepancy may limp or walk on tiptoe on the shorter side, with compensatory hip and knee flexion on the longer side. Assess for limb-length discrepancy (see Fig. 13.36). Other structural changes producing an abnormal gait include joint fusion, bone malunion and contracture.

### Weakness

This may be due to nerve or muscle pathology or altered muscle tone. In a normal gait, the hip abductors of the stance leg raise the contralateral hemipelvis. In Trendelenburg gait, abductor function is poor when weight-bearing on the affected side, so the contralateral hemipelvis falls (see Fig. 13.37).

Common causes of a Trendelenburg gait are:

- painful hip joint problems, as in osteoarthritis
- weak hip abductors, as in poliomyelitis or after hip replacement
- structural hip joint problems, as in congenital dislocation.

A high-stepping gait occurs in foot drop due to common peroneal nerve palsy. The knee is raised high to bring the weak foot off the ground.

### Increased tone

This occurs with upper motor neurone lesions, such as cerebrovascular accident (stroke) or cerebral palsy. The gait depends on the specific lesion, contractures and compensatory mechanisms (see Box 7.7 on p. XXX).

# Spine

The spine is divided into the cervical, thoracic, lumbar and sacral segments (Fig. 13.11). Most spinal diseases affect multiple segments, causing altered posture or function of the whole spine. Spinal disease may occur without local symptoms, presenting with referred pain, neurological symptoms or signs in the trunk or limbs. Common causes of spinal pain are shown in Box 13.9.

## Definitions

Scoliosis is the lateral curvature of the spine (Fig. 13.12A).

Kyphosis is the curvature of the spine in the sagittal (anterior–posterior) plane, with the apex posterior (see Fig. 13.12B). The thoracic spine normally has a mild kyphosis.

Lordosis is the curvature of the spine in the sagittal plane, with the apex anterior (see Fig. 13.12C).

Gibbus is a spinal deformity caused by an anterior wedge deformity of a single vertebra, producing localised angular flexion (see Fig. 13.12D).

## Cervical spine

### Anatomy and physiology

Head nodding occurs at the atlanto-occipital joint, and rotational neck movements mainly at the atlantoaxial joint. Flexion, extension and lateral flexion occur mainly at the mid-cervical level. The

| 13.9 Common spinal problems |
| --- |
| • Mechanical back pain |
| • Prolapsed intervertebral disc |
| • Spinal stenosis |
| • Axial Spondyloarthritis |
| • Compensatory scoliosis from leg-length discrepancy |
| • Cervical myelopathy |
| • Pathological pain/deformity (e.g. osteomyelitis, tumour, myeloma) |
| • Osteoporotic vertebral fracture resulting in kyphosis (or rarely lordosis), especially in the thoracic spine with loss of height |
| • Cervical rib |
| • Scoliosis |
| • Spinal instability (e.g. spondylolisthesis) |

**13**

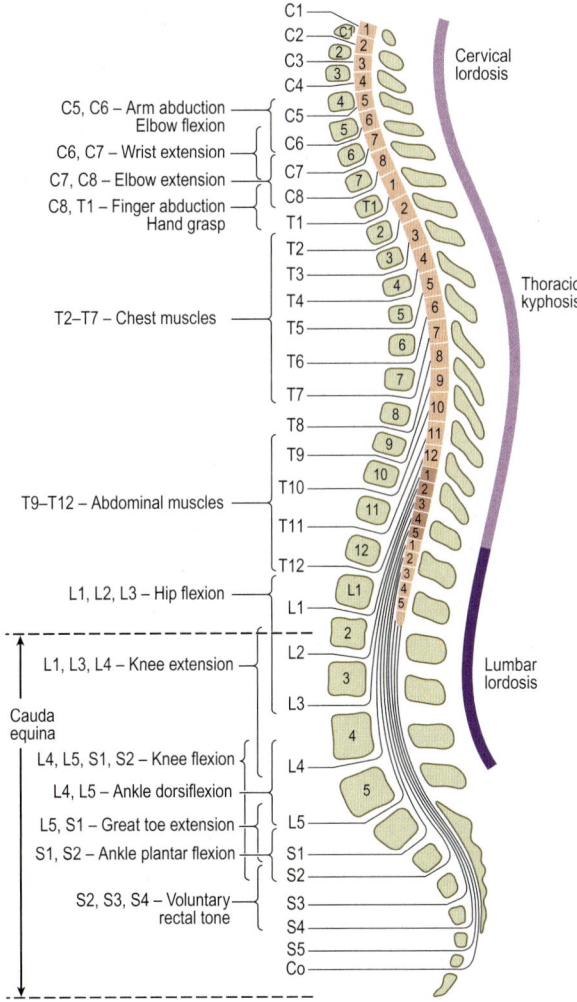

**Fig. 13.11** The normal spinal curves and root innervations.

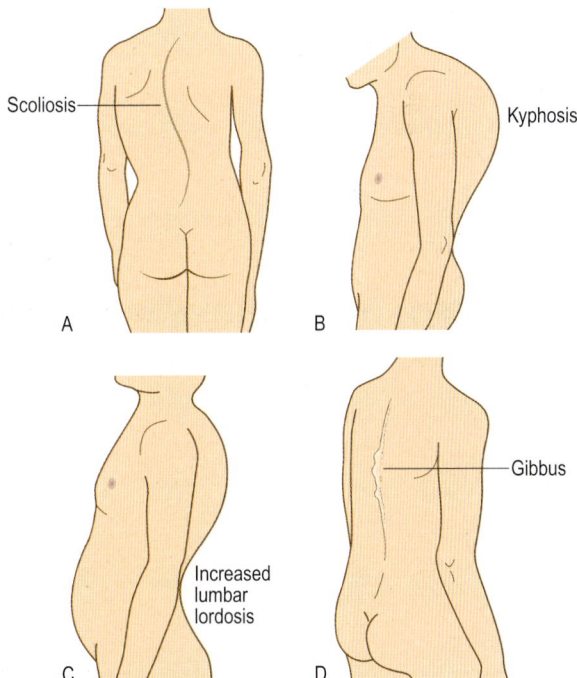

**Fig. 13.12** Spinal deformities.

neural canal contains the spinal cord and the emerging nerve roots, which pass through the exit foramina bounded by the facet joints posteriorly and the intervertebral discs and neuro-central joints anteriorly. The nerve roots, particularly in the lower cervical spine, may be compressed or irritated by lateral disc protrusion or by osteophytes arising from the facet or neuro-central joints. Central disc protrusions may press directly on the cord (see Fig. 7.30 on p. 166).

### The history

The most common symptoms are pain and difficulty turning the head and neck. Neck pain is usually felt posteriorly but may be referred to the head, shoulder, arm or interscapular region. Cervical disc lesions cause radicular pain in one arm or the other, roughly following the dermatomes of the affected nerve roots (see Box 13.3). If the spinal cord is compromised (cervical myelopathy), upper motor neurone leg weakness, altered sensation and sphincter disturbance may occur.

### The physical examination

Be particularly careful when examining patients with rheumatoid arthritis, as atlantoaxial instability can lead to spinal cord damage when the neck is flexed.

In patients with neck injury, never move the neck. Splint it and check for abnormal posture. Check for neurological function in the limbs and x-ray or computed tomography (CT) to assess bony injury.

## Examination sequence (Video 25) ▶

Ask the patient to remove enough clothing for you to see their neck and upper thorax, then direct them to sit on a chair.

### Look
- Face the patient. Observe the posture of their head and neck. Note any abnormality (Box 13.10), such as loss of lordosis (usually due to muscle spasm).

### Feel
- Feel the midline spinous processes from the occiput to T1 (usually the most prominent).

| 13.10 Causes of abnormal neck posture |
|---|
| **Loss of lordosis or flexion deformity** |
| • Acute lesions, rheumatoid arthritis, trauma |
| **Increased lordosis** |
| • Axial Spondyloarthritis |
| **Torticollis (wry neck)** |
| • Sternocleidomastoid spasm, contracture, trauma |
| • Pharyngeal/parapharyngeal infection |
| **Lateral flexion** |
| • Erosion of lateral mass of atlas in rheumatoid arthritis |

- Feel the paraspinal soft tissues.
- Feel the supraclavicular fossae for cervical ribs or enlarged lymph nodes.
- Feel the anterior neck structures, including the thyroid.
- Note any tenderness in the spine, trapezius, interscapular and paraspinal muscles.

### Move
Assess active movements (Fig. 13.13).
Ask the patient to:
- Look down to the floor so you can assess forward flexion. The normal range is 0 (neutral) to 80 degrees. Record the decreased range as the chin–chest distance.
- Look upwards at the ceiling as far back as possible, to assess extension. The normal range is 0 (neutral) to 50 degrees. The combined flexion–extension arc is normally approximately 130 degrees.
- Put their ear on to their shoulder so that you can assess lateral flexion. The normal range is 0 (neutral) to 45 degrees.
- Look over their right/left shoulder. The normal range of lateral rotation is 0 (neutral) to 80 degrees.

If any of the active movements are reduced, gently perform passive movements. Confirm whether the end of a range has a sudden or gradual resistance, plus whether it is pain or stiffness that restricts movement. Pain or paraesthesiae in the arm on passive neck movement suggests nerve root involvement.

## Thoracic spine

### Anatomy and physiology

This segment of the spine is the least mobile and maintains a physiological kyphosis throughout life. Movement is mainly rotational with a very limited amount of flexion, extension and lateral flexion.

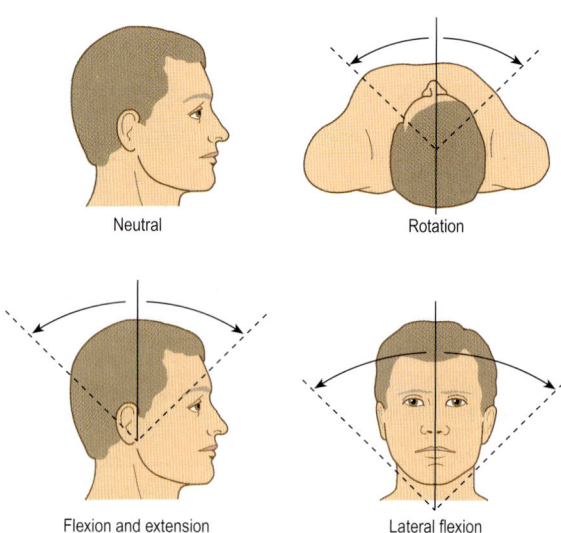

Neutral

Rotation

Flexion and extension

Lateral flexion

**Fig. 13.13** Movements of the cervical spine.

### The history

Presenting symptoms in the thoracic spine are: localised spinal pain (Box 13.11), pain radiating round the chest wall or, less frequently, signs of cord compression – upper motor neurone leg weakness (paraparesis), sensory loss, and loss of bladder or bowel control. Thoracic spine disc lesions are rare but may cause pain radiating around the chest, mimicking cardiac or pleural disease. Osteoporotic vertebral fractures can present with acute pain or painless loss of height with increased kyphosis.

Vertebral collapse from malignancy may cause cord compression. Infection causes acute pain, often with systemic upset or fever. With poorly localised thoracic pain, consider intrathoracic causes such as myocardial ischaemia or infarction, oesophageal or pleural pain, and aortic aneurysm.

### The physical examination

**Examination sequence (Video 26)**

Ask the patient to undress to expose their neck, chest and back.

#### Look
- With the patient standing, inspect their posture from behind, from the side and the front, noting any deformity, such as a rib hump or abnormal curvature (see Fig. 13.12).

#### Feel
- Palpate the midline spinous processes from T1 to T12. Feel for increased prominence of one or more posterior spinal processes, implying an anterior wedge-shaped collapse of the vertebral body.
- Feel the paraspinal soft tissues for tenderness.

#### Move
- Ask the patient to sit with their arms crossed. Ask them to twist round both ways and look behind.

## Lumbar spine

### Anatomy and physiology

The surface markings are the spinous process of L4, which is level with the pelvic brim, and the 'dimples of Venus', overlying the sacroiliac joints. The normal lordosis may be lost in disorders such as axial spondyloarthritis and lumbar disc protrusion.

| 13.11 Causes of thoracic spine pain | |
|---|---|
| **Adolescents and young adults** | |
| • Scheuermann's disease | • Disc protrusion (rare) |
| • Axial spondyloarthritis | |
| **Middle-aged and elderly** | |
| • Degenerative change | • Osteoporotic fracture |
| • Dissecting aortic aneurysm | |
| **Any age** | |
| • Tumour | • Infection |

The principal movements are flexion, extension, lateral flexion and rotation. In flexion, the upper segments move first, followed by the lower segments, to produce a smooth lumbar curve. However, even with a rigid lumbar spine, patients may be able to touch their toes if their hips are mobile.

In an adult, the spinal cord ends at L2. Below this, only the spinal nerve roots may be injured by disc protrusion.

### The history

Low back pain is an extremely common symptom. Most commonly this is 'mechanical' and caused by degenerative changes in discs and facet joints (spondylosis).

Analyse the symptoms using 'SOCRATES'. For back pain, ask specifically about:

- occupational or recreational activity that may strain the back
- additional clinical features suggesting significant spinal pathology (Box 13.12)
- prior treatment with glucocorticoids.

Radicular pain, caused by sciatic nerve root compression, radiates down the posterior aspect of the leg to the lower leg or ankle (sciatica). Groin and thigh pain in the absence of hip abnormality suggests referred pain from L1 to L2.

Consider also abdominal and retroperitoneal pathology, such as abdominal aortic aneurysm.

Mechanical low back pain is common after standing for too long or sitting in a poor position. Symptoms worsen as the day progresses and improve after resting.

**13**

| 13.12 Important features for history-taking in acute low back pain |
|---|
| **Features that may indicate serious pathology and require urgent referral** |
| **History** |
| • Age <20 years or >55 years<br>• Recent significant trauma (fracture)<br>• Pain:<br>  ◦ Non-mechanical (infection/tumour/pathological fracture)<br>• Fever (infection)<br>• Difficulty in micturition | • Faecal incontinence<br>• Motor weakness<br>• Sensory changes in the perineum (saddle anaesthesia)<br>• Sexual dysfunction (e.g. erectile/ejaculatory failure)<br>• Gait change (cauda equina syndrome)<br>• Bilateral 'sciatica' |
| **Past medical history** |
| • Cancer (metastases)<br>• Previous glucocorticoid use (osteoporotic collapse) |
| **System review** |
| • Weight loss/malaise without obvious cause (e.g. cancer) |
| **Psychosocial factors associated with greater likelihood of long-term chronicity and disability** |
| • A history of anxiety, depression, chronic pain, irritable bowel syndrome, chronic fatigue, social withdrawal<br>• A belief that the diagnosis is severe (e.g. cancer). Faulty beliefs can lead to 'catastrophisation' and avoidance of activity<br>• Lack of belief that the patient can improve leads to an expectation that only passive, rather than active, treatment will be effective<br>• Ongoing litigation or compensation claims (e.g. work, road traffic accident) |

Insidious onset of back or buttock ache and stiffness in an adolescent or young adult suggests inflammatory disease of the sacroiliac joints and lumbar spine (axial spondyloarthritis, Box 13.13). Symptoms are worse in the morning or after inactivity and ease with movement. Morning stiffness is more marked than in osteoarthritis or mechanical pain, lasting at least 30 minutes. Other clues to the diagnosis are peripheral joint involvement, extra-articular features or a positive family history.

Acute onset of low back pain in a young adult, often associated with bending or lifting, is typical of an acute disc protrusion (slipped disc). Coughing or straining to open the bowels exacerbates the pain. There may be symptoms of lumbar or sacral nerve root compression. Cauda equina syndrome occurs when a central disc prolapses or another space-occupying lesion compresses the cauda equina. There are features of sensory and motor disturbance, including diminished perianal sensation and disturbance of bladder function. The motor disturbance may be profound, as in paraplegia. Cauda equina syndrome and spinal cord compression are neurosurgical emergencies.

Acute back pain in the middle-aged, elderly or those with risk factors, such as glucocorticoid therapy, may be due to osteoporotic fracture. This is eased by lying, exacerbated by spinal flexion and not usually associated with neurological symptoms.

Acute onset of severe progressive pain, especially when associated with malaise, weight loss or night sweats, may indicate pyogenic or tuberculous infection of the lumbar spine or sacroiliac joint. The infection may involve the intervertebral discs and adjacent vertebrae and may track into the psoas muscle sheath, presenting as a painful flexed hip or groin swelling.

Consider a malignant disease involving a vertebral body in patients with unremitting spinal pain of recent onset that disturbs sleep. Other clues are a previous history of cancer, and systemic symptoms or weight loss.

Chronic intermittent pain in the lumbar spine is typical of degenerative disc disease. There is stiffness in the morning or after immobility. Pain and stiffness are relieved by gentle activity but recur with, or after, excessive activity.

Diffuse pain in the buttocks or thighs brought on by standing too long or walking is the presenting symptom of lumbosacral spinal stenosis. This can be difficult to distinguish from intermittent claudication (Chapter 4, p. 70). The pain may be accompanied by tingling and numbness. Typically, it is relieved by rest or spinal flexion. Stooping or holding on to a supermarket trolley may increase exercise tolerance.

### The physical examination

## Examination sequence

Ask the patient to stand with their back fully exposed.

### Look
- Look for obvious deformity (decreased/increased lordosis, scoliosis) and soft-tissue abnormalities such as a hairy patch or lipoma that might overlie a congenital abnormality, for example, spina bifida.

### Feel
- Palpate the spinous processes and paraspinal tissues. Note overall alignment and focal tenderness.
- After warning the patient, lightly percuss the spine with your closed fist and note any tenderness.

### Move (Fig. 13.14)
- Flexion: ask the patient to try to touch their toes with their legs straight. Record how far down the legs they can reach. Some of this movement depends on hip flexion. Usually, the upper segments flex before the lower ones, but the progression should be smooth.
- Extension: ask the patient to straighten up and lean back as far as possible (normal 10–20 degrees from a neutral erect posture).
- Lateral flexion: ask them to reach down to each side, touching the outside of their leg as far down as possible while keeping their legs straight.

---

### 13.13 Clinical vignette: back pain

A 34-year-old man attends his general practitioner's surgery with back pain. He first developed pain in his late teens, but it improved for a few years. He has had persistent pain in his lower back and sometimes in his buttocks for 5 years now. It wakes him from sleep, and he can be very stiff in the mornings, although this eases as the morning progresses. There is no radiation to the leg. He is stiff after sitting or driving. He has always put it down to his occupation. He has used ibuprofen to good effect but has had diarrhoea and abdominal pain recently, which he attributes to this drug. Examination in the outpatient clinic shows a thin man with reduced lumbar mobility (modified Schober's index, reduced at 2 cm; see Fig. 13.15), pain on sacroiliac joint compression, and tenderness at his Achilles insertion. Investigations show him to have a raised C-reactive protein, an anaemia of chronic disease, a positive human leucocyte antigen B27 and a raised faecal calprotectin, suggesting inflammatory bowel disease. Magnetic resonance imaging confirms bilateral sacroiliitis and inflammatory changes in the lumbar spine.
A diagnosis of axial spondyloarthritis is made.

**Axial spondyloarthritis.** The patient trying to touch his toes.

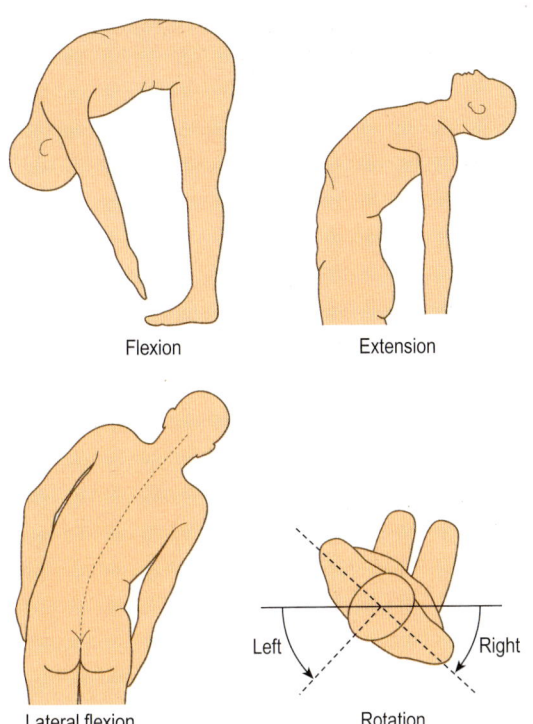

Flexion                    Extension

Lateral flexion            Rotation

Left        Right

**Fig. 13.14** Movements of the lumbar and dorsal spine.

### Special tests

Schober's test for forward flexion

## Examination sequence (Video 26A)

- Mark the skin in the midline at the level of the posterior iliac spines (L5) (Fig. 13.15; mark A).
- Use a tape measure to draw two more marks: one 10 cm above (mark B) and one 5 cm below this (mark C).
- Place the end of the tape measure on the upper mark (B). Ask the patient to touch their toes. The distance from B to C should increase from 15 to more than 20 cm.

In this test, the distance between the two points should increase by at least 5 cm. An increase of less than 5 cm indicates restriction in the lumbar spine that may be due to axial spondyloarthritis.

### Root compression tests

Intervertebral disc prolapses causing nerve root pressure occurs most often in the lower lumbar region, leading to compression of the corresponding nerve roots.

The sciatic nerve (L4–5; S1–3) runs behind the pelvis, so straight-leg raising stretches the L4, L5 and S1 nerve roots (affected by L3/4, L4/5 and L5/S1 disc prolapse, respectively).

B
10 cm
A
5 cm
C

20+ cm

**Fig. 13.15** Schober's test. When the patient bends forward maximally with the knees straight, distance BC should increase by at least 5 cm.

The femoral nerve (L2–4) lies anterior to the pubic ramus, so straight-leg raising or other forms of hip flexion do not pull on its roots. Problems with the femoral nerve roots may cause quadriceps weakness and/or diminished knee jerk on that side.

Sciatic nerve stretch test (L4–S1)

## Examination sequence (Videos 26B and 26C)

- With the patient lying supine, lift their foot to flex the hip passively, keeping the knee straight.
- When a limit is reached, raise the leg to just less than this level, and dorsiflex the foot to test for nerve root tension (Fig. 13.16).

Femoral nerve stretch test (L2–4)

## Examination sequence (Video 26D)

- With the patient lying on their front (prone), flex their knee and extend the hip (Fig. 13.17). This stretches the femoral nerve. A positive result is when pain is felt in the back or the front of the thigh. This test can, if necessary, be performed with the patient lying on their side (with the test side uppermost).

Flip test for functional overlay

## Examination sequence

- Ask the patient to sit on the end of the couch with their hips and knees flexed to 90 degrees (Fig. 13.18A).
- Examine the knee reflexes.
- Extend the patient's knee, as if to examine the ankle jerk. If achieved, this puts the straight leg at 90 degrees of hip flexion (see Fig. 13.18B) and excludes sciatic nerve root compression; patients with root compression will lie back ('flip').

### Sacroiliac joints

In general, examination of the sacroiliac joints is unreliable.

**13**

A

B

C

D

**Fig. 13.16 Stretch test: sciatic nerve.** [A] Straight-leg raising limited by the tension of the root over a prolapsed disc. [B] Tension is increased by dorsiflexion of the foot (Bragard's test). [C] Root tension is relieved by flexion at the knee. [D] Pressure over the centre of the popliteal fossa bears on the posterior tibial nerve, which is 'bowstringing' across the fossa, causing pain locally and radiation into the back.

A

B

**Fig. 13.17 Stretch test: femoral nerve.** [A] Pain may be triggered by knee flexion alone. [B] Pain may be triggered by knee flexion in combination with hip extension.

A

B

Negative

**Fig. 13.18 Sciatic nerve: 'flip' test.** [A] Divert the patient's attention to the tendon reflexes. [B] The patient with physical nerve root compression cannot permit full extension of the leg.

## Examination sequence

• Lay the patient supine, flex the hip to 90 degrees and press down on the knee to transfer pressure through to the sacroiliac joints. This may cause pain in the buttock or lower back if the sacroiliac joint is inflamed.

## Upper limb

The prime function of the upper limb is to position the hand appropriately in space. This requires intact shoulder, elbow and wrist movements. The hand may function in both precision and power modes, with the intrinsic muscles of the hand providing grip and fine manipulative movements, and the forearm muscles supplying power and stability.

It is important to distinguish between systemic and local pathology. Systemic pathology, such as rheumatoid arthritis, usually affects several sites. Local conditions should be differentiated from referred or radicular pain and establish whether the condition is inflammatory or not from the pattern of diurnal stiffness and pain.

## Hand and wrist

The wrist joint has metacarpocarpal, intercarpal, ulnocarpal and radiocarpal components. Together, they provide a wide range of possible movements, including flexion, extension, adduction (deviation towards the ulnar side), abduction (deviation towards the radial side) and composite movement of circumduction (the hand moves in a conical fashion on the wrist). Always name the affected digit (index, middle, ring, little fingers and thumb) in documentation to avoid confusion. The PIP and DIP joints are hinge joints and allow only flexion and extension. The MCP joints allow flexion and extension, and some abduction/adduction, which is greatest when the MCP joints are extended.

Motor and sensory innervation of the hand is shown in Fig. 7.27 on page 163.

### The history

The patient will often localise symptoms of pain, stiffness, loss of function, contractures, disfigurement and trauma. If symptoms are vague or diffuse, consider referred pain or a compressive neuropathy such as carpal tunnel syndrome (see Box 7.11 on p. 164). If PIP or MCP joint swelling is prominent, consider inflammatory arthritis.

Painful, swollen and stiff hand joints are common and important presenting symptoms and scoring systems (Box 13.14) are used to define the presence of rheumatoid arthritis.

### The physical examination

**Examination sequence (Video 27)**

Seat the patient facing you, with their arms and shoulders exposed. Start by examining the hand and fingers, then move proximally.

### Look

- Erythema suggests acute inflammation caused by soft-tissue infection, septic arthritis, tendon sheath infection or crystal arthritis. Palmar erythema is associated with rheumatoid arthritis.
- Swelling of MCP joints due to synovitis produces loss of interknuckle indentation on the dorsum of the hand, especially when the MCP and interphalangeal joints are fully flexed (loss of the normal 'hill–valley–hill' aspect; Fig. 13.19A). 'Spindling' (swelling at the joint, tapering proximally and distally; Fig. 13.19B) is seen when the PIP joints are affected.
- Deformity of phalangeal fractures may produce rotation. Ask the patient to flex the fingers together (Fig. 13.20) and then in turn. Normally, with the MCP and interphalangeal joints flexed, the fingers should not cross and should point to the scaphoid tubercle in the wrist.
- The fingers are long in Marfan's syndrome (arachnodactyly, Fig. 3.21B on p. 33).
- Boutonnière (or buttonhook) deformity is a fixed flexion deformity at the PIP joint with hyperextension at the DIP joint. 'Swan neck' deformity is hyperextension at the PIP joint with flexion at the DIP joint (Fig. 13.21).
- A 'mallet' finger (see Fig. 13.21) is a flexion deformity at the DIP joints that is passively correctable. This is usually caused by minor trauma disrupting the extensor expansion at the base of the distal phalanx, with or without bony avulsion.
- There may be subluxation and ulnar deviation at the MCP joints in rheumatoid arthritis (Fig. 13.22).
- Bony expansion of the DIP, PIP joints of the fingers and CMC joint of the thumb is typical of osteoarthritis (see Fig. 13.8).
- Anterior (or volar) displacement (partial dislocation) of the wrist may be seen in rheumatoid arthritis.

### 13.14 American College of Rheumatology/European League Against Rheumatism classification criteria for rheumatoid arthritis, 2010

| Criteria | Score |
|---|---|
| **Duration of symptoms (as reported by patient)** | |
| <6 weeks | 0 |
| >6 weeks | 1 |
| **Joint distribution (0–5)** | |
| 1 large joint[a] | 0 |
| 2–10 large joints | 1 |
| 1–3 small joints[b] (large joints not counted) | 2 |
| 4–10 small joints (large joints not counted) | 3 |
| >10 joints (at least 1 small joint) | 5 |
| **Serology (0–3)** | |
| Negative RF and negative ACPA | 0 |
| Low positive RF or low positive ACPA | 2 |
| High positive RF or high positive ACPA | 3 |
| **Acute-phase reactants** | |
| Normal CRP and normal ESR | 0 |
| Abnormal CRP or abnormal ESR | 1 |

Patients must have at least 1 swollen joint not better explained by another disease.

A score of ≥6 classifies the patient as having definite rheumatoid arthritis. A score of 4–5 is probable rheumatoid arthritis (i.e. a patient may have clinical rheumatoid arthritis but not fulfil all criteria).

[a]Large joints: shoulders, elbows, hips, knees and ankles
[b]Small joints: all metacarpophalangeal and proximal interphalangeal joints, thumb interphalangeal joint, wrists and 2nd–5th metatarsophalangeal joints.

*ACPA,* Anti-cyclic citrullinated peptide antibody; *CRP,* C-reactive protein; *ESR,* erythrocyte sedimentation rate; *RF,* rheumatoid factor.

Reproduced from Aletaha D, Neogi T, Silman AJ, et al. Rheumatoid arthritis classification criteria: an American College of Rheumatology/ European League Against Rheumatism collaborative initiative. *Arthritis Rheumatol.* 2010; 62(9): 2569–2581, with permission from John Wiley and Sons.

**13**

### Extra-articular signs

- Dupuytren's contracture affects the palmar fascia, resulting in fixed flexion of the MCP and PIP joints of the little and ring fingers (see Fig. 3.5).
- Wasting of the interossei occurs in inflammatory arthritis and ulnar nerve palsy. Carpal tunnel syndrome causes wasting of the thenar eminence. T1 nerve root lesions (Fig. 13.23) cause wasting of all small hand muscles.
- Look for nail-fold infarcts, telangiectasia, palmar erythema, psoriasis, scars of carpal tunnel decompression, tendon transfer or MCP joint replacement.

A

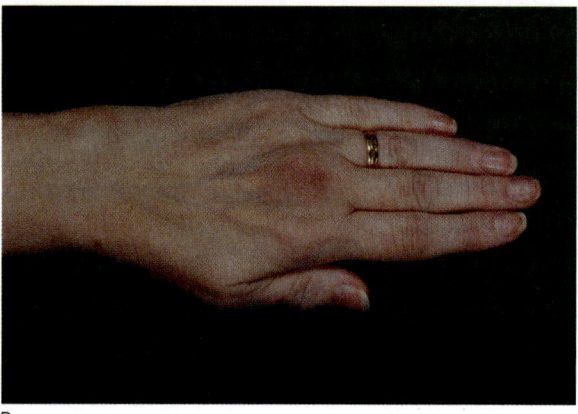

B

**Fig. 13.19** **Swelling of the metacarpophalangeal (MCP) and proximal interphalangeal (PIP) joints.** [A] Ask the patient to make a fist. Look at it straight on to detect any loss of the 'hill–valley–hill' aspect. [B] Swelling and erythema of the middle finger MCP joint and index and middle finger PIP joints. Note also small muscle wasting.

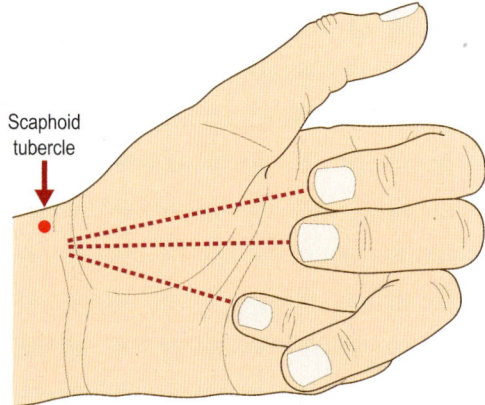

**Fig. 13.20** Flexion of the fingers showing rotational deformity of the ring finger.

- Nail changes, such as pitting and onycholysis (separation of the nail from its bed), occur in psoriatic arthritis (see Fig. 3.7A on p. 27).

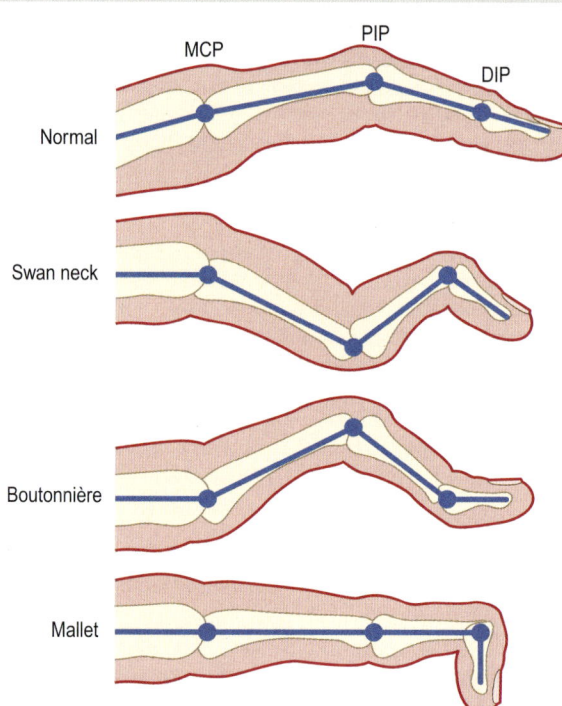

**Fig. 13.21** **Deformities of the fingers.** Swan neck and boutonnière deformities occur in rheumatoid arthritis. Mallet finger occurs with trauma. *DIP,* Distal interphalangeal; *MCP,* metacarpophalangeal; *PIP,* proximal interphalangeal.

**Fig. 13.22** **Advanced rheumatoid arthritis.** Small muscle wasting, subluxation and ulnar deviation at the metacarpophalangeal joints, boutonnière deformities at the ring and little fingers, and swelling and deformity of the wrist.

## Feel

- Hard swellings usually arise from bone; soft swellings suggest synovitis.
- Palpate above and below the interphalangeal joints with your thumb and index finger to detect sponginess.

**Fig. 13.23** **T1 root lesion (cervical rib) affecting the right hand.** Wasting of the thenar eminence and interossei, and flexed posture of the fingers due to lumbrical denervation.

- Test the MCP joints by examining for sponginess and squeeze gently across them for pain.
- Palpate the flexor tendon sheaths in the hand and fingers to detect swelling or tenderness. Ask the patient to flex and then extend their fingers to establish whether there is triggering.
- De Quervain's tenosynovitis causes swelling, tenderness and crepitus (a creaking sensation that may even be audible) of the tendon sheaths of abductor pollicis longus and extensor pollicis brevis. Symptoms are aggravated by movements of the wrist and thumb.
- Crepitus may also occur with movement of the radiocarpal joints in osteoarthritis, most commonly secondary to old scaphoid or distal radial fractures.

## Move

### Active movements

- Ask the patient to make a fist and then extend their fingers fully.
- Flexor digitorum profundus: ask the patient to flex the DIP joint while you hold the PIP joint in extension (Fig. 13.24A).
- Flexor digitorum superficialis: hold the patient's other fingers fully extended (to eliminate the action of the flexor digitorum profundus, as it can also flex the PIP joint) and ask the patient to flex the PIP joint in question (see Fig. 13.24B).
- Extensor digitorum: ask the patient to extend their fingers with the wrist in the neutral position (see Fig. 13.24C).
- Flexor and extensor pollicis longus: hold the proximal phalanx of the patient's thumb firmly and ask them to flex and extend the interphalangeal joint (see Fig. 13.24D).
- Extensor pollicis longus: ask the patient to place their palm on a flat surface and to extend their thumb like a hitch-hiker (see Fig. 13.24E). Pain occurs in de Quervain's disease.
- Insert your index and middle finger from the thumb side into the patient's palm and ask them to squeeze them as hard as possible to test their grip.
- Ask the patient to put the palms of their hands together and extend their wrists fully in the 'prayer sign' (normal is 90 degrees of extension, Fig. 13.10A).

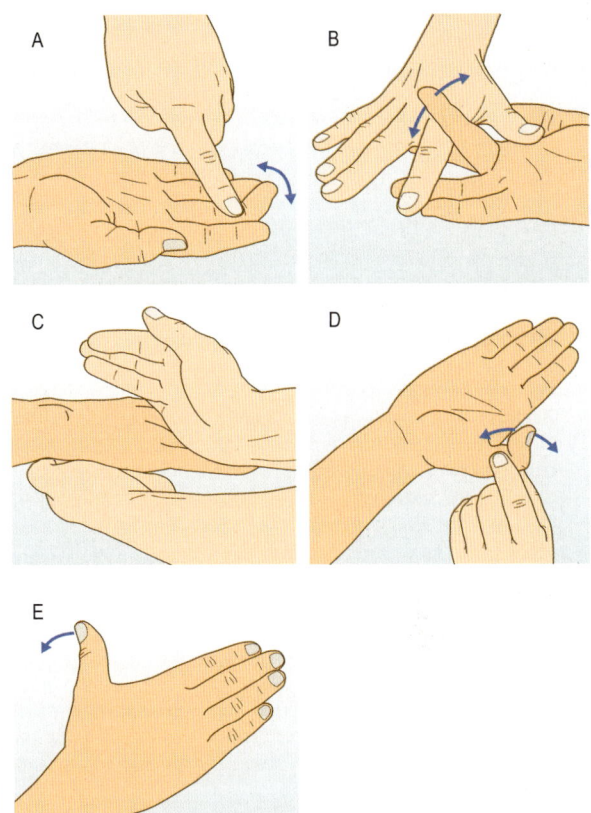

**Fig. 13.24** **Testing the flexors and extensors of the fingers and thumb.** **A** Flexor digitorum profundus. **B** Flexor digitorum superficialis. **C** Extensor digitorum. **D** Flexor pollicis longus. **E** Extensor pollicis longus.

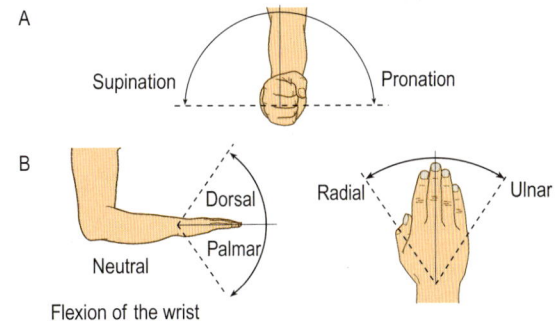

**Fig. 13.25** Terms used to describe upper limb movements.

- Ask the patient to put the backs of their hands together and flex their wrists fully – the 'reverse prayer sign' (normal is 90 degrees of flexion, Fig. 13.10B).
- Check pronation and supination, flexion and extension, and ulnar and radial deviation (Fig. 13.25).

13

### Passive movements

- Move each of the patient's fingers through flexion and extension and notice any loss of range of movement.
- Fully flex and extend the patient's wrist and note the range of movement and end-feel. Check for radial and ulnar deviation.

### Radial, ulnar and median nerve motor function

- Use 'Paper – scissors – stone – OK' as an *aide-mémoire* (Fig. 13.26).
- Radial nerve (wrist and finger extensors): ask the patient to extend the wrist and fingers fully ('paper sign').
- Ulnar nerve (hypothenar muscles, interossei, two medial lumbricals, adductor pollicis, flexor carpi ulnaris and the ulnar half of flexor digitorum profundus): ask the patient to make the 'scissors sign'.
- Median nerve (thenar muscles that abduct and oppose the thumb, the lateral two lumbricals, the medial half of flexor digitorum profundus, flexor digitorum superficialis, flexor carpi radialis, palmaris longus and pronator teres): ask the patient to clench the fist fully ('stone sign'). The best test of median nerve motor function is the ability to abduct the thumb away from the palm because of inconstant crossover in the nerve supply to the thenar eminence muscles other than abductor pollicis brevis. However, clenching the fist fully also depends on median function because of its flexor supply.
- Anterior interosseous nerve (flexor pollicis longus, the index finger flexor digitorum profundus and pronator quadratus): ask the patient to make the 'OK' sign. This depends on the function of both flexor pollicis longus and index finger flexor digitorum profundus.

### Examining the wrist and hand with a wound

Test the tendons, nerves and circulation in a patient with a wrist or hand wound. The wound site and the hand position at the

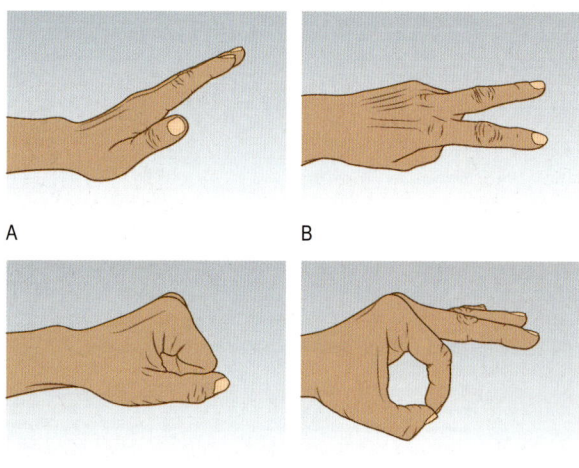

A              B

C              D

**Fig. 13.26 Rapid assessment of the motor functions of the radial, ulnar and median nerves.** A Paper (radial). B Scissors (ulnar). C Stone (median). D OK (median – anterior interosseus).

time of injury indicate which structures may be potentially damaged. Remember, normal movement may still be possible even with 90% division of a tendon, so surgical exploration is often needed for correct diagnosis and treatment. Sensory aspects of nerve injury are covered on Chapter 7, page 164.

## Elbow

### Anatomy and physiology

The elbow joint has humeroulnar, radiocapitellar and superior radioulnar articulations. The medial and lateral epicondyles are the common flexor and extensor origins, respectively, for the forearm muscles. These two prominences and the tip of the olecranon should be easily palpated. They form an equilateral triangle when the elbow is flexed to 90 degrees, and a straight line when the elbow is fully extended. A subcutaneous bursa overlies the olecranon and may become inflamed or infected (bursitis). Elbow pain may be localised or referred from the neck. Inflammatory arthritis and epicondylitis are common causes of elbow pain.

### The physical examination

## Examination sequence

### Look

- Look at the overall alignment of the extended elbow. There is normally a valgus angle of 11–13 degrees with the elbow fully extended (the 'carrying angle').
- Look for:
- the swelling of synovitis between the lateral epicondyle and olecranon, resulting in a block to full extension
- Skin changes of psoriasis, olecranon bursitis, tophi or nodules
- rheumatoid nodules on the proximal extensor surface of the forearm (see Fig. 13.7).

### Feel

- Palpate the bony contours of the lateral and medial epicondyles and olecranon tip.
- Feel for sponginess, suggesting synovitis, on either side of the olecranon when the elbow is fully extended.
- Feel for focal tenderness over the lateral or medial epicondyle (see 'Special tests' below).
- Feel for olecranon bursa swelling, nodules and tophi.
- Feel for rheumatoid nodules on the proximal extensor surface of the forearm.

### Move

- Assess the extension–flexion arc: ask the patient to touch their shoulder on the same side and then straighten the elbow as far as possible. The normal range of movement is 0–145 degrees; a range of less than 30–110 degrees will cause functional problems.
- Assess supination and pronation: ask the patient to put their elbows by the sides of their body and flex them to 90 degrees. Now ask them to turn their palms upwards (supination: normal range 0–90 degrees) and then downwards (pronation: normal range 0–85 degrees).

## Special tests

Tennis elbow (lateral epicondylitis)

### Examination sequence

- Ask the patient to flex their elbow to 90 degrees and pronate and flex the hand/wrist fully.
- Support the patient's elbow. Ask them to extend their wrist against your resistance.
- Pain is produced at the lateral epicondyle and may be referred down the extensor aspect of the arm.

Golfer's elbow (medial epicondylitis)

### Examination sequence

- Ask the patient to flex their elbow to 90 degrees and supinate the hand/wrist fully.
- Support the patient's elbow. Ask them to flex their wrist against your resistance.
- Pain is produced at the medial epicondyle and may be referred down the flexor aspect of the arm.

## Shoulder

### Anatomy and physiology

The shoulder joint consists of the glenohumeral joint, acromio-clavicular joint and subacromial space. Movement also occurs between the scapula and the chest wall. The rotator cuff is composed of the supraspinatus, subscapularis, teres minor and infraspinatus muscles. They and their tendinous insertions assist stability and movement, particularly abduction at the gleno-humeral joint.

### The history

Pain is a common symptom (Boxes 13.15 and 13.16) and is frequently referred to in the upper arm. Glenohumeral pain may occur over the anterolateral aspect of the upper arm. Pain felt at the shoulder may also be referred from the cervical spine or diaphragmatic and subdiaphragmatic peritoneum via the phrenic nerve. The most common cause of referred pain is cervical spondylosis, where disc-space narrowing and osteophytes cause nerve root impingement and inflammation.

Stiffness and limitation of movement around the shoulder, caused by adhesive capsulitis of the glenohumeral joint, is common after immobilisation or disuse following injury or stroke. This is also termed 'frozen shoulder'. However, movement can still occur between the scapula and chest wall.

Some rotator cuff disorders, especially impingement syndromes and tears, present with a painful arc where abduction of the arm between 60 and 120 degrees causes discomfort (Fig. 13.27).

| **13.15 Causes of shoulder girdle pain** | |
|---|---|
| **Rotator cuff** | |
| • Degeneration | • Tendonitis |
| • Tendon rupture | • Calcification |
| **Subacromial bursa** | |
| • Inflammation due to inflammatory arthritis, injury or overuse | • Calcification |
| **Capsule** | |
| • Inflammation (Adhesive capsulitis, polymyalgia rheumatica) | |
| **Head of humerus** | |
| • Tumour | • Fracture/dislocation |
| • Osteonecrosis | |
| **Joints** | |
| • Glenohumeral, sternoclavicular: <br>  ○ Inflammatory arthritis, osteoarthritis, dislocation, infection | • Acromioclavicular: <br>  ○ Subluxation, osteoarthritis |

**13**

| **13.16 Common conditions affecting the shoulder** | |
|---|---|
| **Non-trauma** | |
| • Rotator cuff syndromes( e.g. supraspinatus) infraspinatus tendonitis | • Adhesive capsulitis ('frozen shoulder') |
| • Impingement syndromes (involving the rotator cuff and subacromial bursa) | • Calcific tendonitis |
| | • Bicipital tendonitis |
| | • Inflammatory arthritis |
| | • Polymyalgia rheumatica |
| **Trauma** | |
| • Rotator cuff tear | • Fracture of the clavicle |
| • Glenohumeral dislocation | • Fracture of the head or neck of the humerus |
| • Acromioclavicular dislocation | |

### The physical examination

### Examination sequence (Video 28)

Ask the patient to sit or stand and expose their shoulder completely.

### Look

Examine from the front and back, and in the axilla, for:
- Deformity: Deformities of the anterior glenohumeral and complete acromioclavicular joint dislocation should be visible (Fig. 13.28), but the shoulder contour in posterior gleno-humeral dislocation may appear abnormal only when you stand above the seated patient and look down on the shoulder.

**Fig. 13.27** Painful arc.

**Fig. 13.28 Right anterior glenohumeral dislocation.** Loss of the normal shoulder contour.

- Swelling.
- Muscle wasting, especially of the deltoid, supraspinatus and infraspinatus. Wasting of the supraspinatus or infraspinatus indicates a chronic tear of their tendons.
- Size and position of the scapula: assess whether it is elevated, depressed or 'winged' (Fig. 13.29).

## Feel
- Palpate from the sternoclavicular joint along the clavicle to the acromioclavicular joint.
- Palpate the acromion and coracoid (2 cm inferior and medial to the clavicle tip) processes, the scapula spine and the biceps tendon in the bicipital groove.
- Extend the shoulder to bring the supraspinatus anterior to the acromion process, allowing palpation of the supraspinatus tendon.

**Fig. 13.29 'Winging' of the left scapula.** This caused by paralysis of the nerve to serratus anterior.

## Move
### Active movements (Fig. 13.30)
- Ask the patient to flex and extend their shoulder as far as possible.
- Abduction: ask the patient to lift their arm away from their side.
- Palpate the inferior pole of the scapula between your thumb and index finger to detect scapular rotation and determine how much movement occurs at the glenohumeral joint. The first 0–15 degrees of abduction are produced by the supraspinatus. The middle fibres of the deltoid are responsible for the next 15–90 degrees. Past 90 degrees, the scapula needs to be rotated to achieve abduction, which is carried out by the trapezius and serratus anterior muscles (Fig. 13.31). If the glenohumeral joint is excessively stiff, movement of the scapula over the chest wall will predominate. If there is any limitation or pain (painful arc) associated with abduction, test the rotator cuff.
- Internal rotation: with the patient's arm by their side and the elbow flexed at 90 degrees, ask them to put their hand behind their back and feel as high up the spine as possible. Document the highest spinous process that they can reach with the thumb.
- External rotation: in the same position, with the elbow tucked against their side, ask them to rotate their hand outwards.
- Deltoid: ask the patient to abduct their arm out from their side, parallel to the floor, and resist while you push down on the humerus. Compare both sides.

### Rotator cuff muscles
To test the component muscles of the rotator cuff, the effect of other muscles crossing the shoulder needs to be neutralised.
- Internal rotation of the shoulder – subscapularis and pectoralis major:
- To isolate subscapularis, place the patient's hand behind their back. If they cannot lift it off their back, it suggests a tear (Gerber test).
- Pain on forced internal rotation suggests tendonitis.

**Fig. 13.30** Movements of the shoulder.

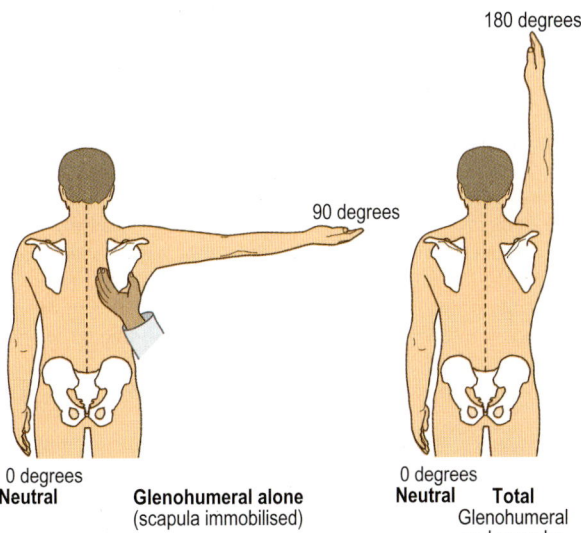

**Fig. 13.31** Contribution of the glenohumeral joint and scapula to shoulder abduction.

- Abduction of the arm – supraspinatus:
- With the patient's arm by their side, test abduction. Full abduction requires both glenohumeral and scapular components.
- Loss of power suggests a tear.
- Pain on forced abduction at 60 degrees suggests tendonitis.
- Determine the degree of glenohumeral abduction by holding the inferior pole of the scapula and asking them to abduct. Abduction should reach 90 degrees before scapular rotation occurs
- External rotation – infraspinatus and teres minor:
- Test external rotation with the arm in the neutral position and at 30 degrees to reduce the contribution of the deltoid. Loss of power suggests a tear.
- Pain on forced external rotation suggests tendonitis.
- No movement or fixed internal rotation suggests a frozen shoulder.

### Bicipital tendonitis

- Palpate the long head of the biceps in its groove on the head of the humerus, noting any tenderness. Ask the patient to supinate their forearm and then flex the arm against resistance. Pain occurs in bicipital tendonitis. A rupture of the long head of biceps causes the muscle to bunch distally (the Popeye sign).

### Impingement (painful arc)

- Passively and fully abduct the patient's arm
  Ask them to lower (adduct) it slowly.
- Pain occurring between 60 and 120 degrees of abduction occurs in painful arc.
- Passively abduct the internally rotated arm to 30–45 degrees.
- Ask them to continue to abduct their arm.
  Pain on active movement, especially against resistance, suggests impingement.

### Special tests for impingement

#### Neer test

The patient sits in a relaxed position with their elbow fully extended. Scapular rotation is prevented with one hand while the other abducts the arm in internal rotation. This causes the greater tuberosity to impinge against the acromion. A positive test is indicated by pain.

#### Hawkins–Kennedy test (Fig. 13.32)

The patient is examined while sitting or standing, with their shoulder flexed at 90 degrees and their elbow flexed at 90 degrees, supported by the examiner to ensure maximal relaxation. The examiner forcefully rotates the arm internally. Reproduction of the patient's pain is a positive sign.

## Lower limb

### Hip

#### Anatomy

The hip is a ball-and-socket joint which allows flexion, extension, abduction, adduction, internal/external rotation and the combined movement of circumduction (Fig 13.33).

**13**

## The history

Pain is usually felt in the groin but can be referred to the anterior thigh, the knee or the buttock. Ask the patient to point to their

**Fig. 13.32** Hawkins–Kennedy test for shoulder impingement.

A

B

**Fig. 13.34** Fracture of the neck of the right femur. [A] Shortening and external rotation of the leg. [B] x-ray showing translation and angulation.

site of pain. Hip pain is usually exacerbated by activity. However, osteonecrosis and tumours may cause pain both at rest and at night. Lateral hip or thigh pain, aggravated when lying on that side, suggests trochanteric pain syndrome. Fracture of the neck of the femur is common following relatively minor trauma in postmenopausal women and all patients aged over 70 years. The classical appearance is a shortened, externally rotated leg (Fig. 13.34); if the fracture is only minimally displaced or impacted, some patients may be able to weight-bear.

Distinguish pain arising from the hip or pelvis (Box 13.17) from:

- lumbar nerve root irritation (Chapter 4, p. 71)
- spinal or arterial claudication (p. 64)
- abdominal causes such as hernia (p. 97).

Ask how the pain restricts activities. Record walking ability in terms of the time and distance the patient is able to manage (e.g. outside and on stairs, and note whether any walking aids are used).

Anterior superior iliac spine

Rectus femoris

Acetabular labrum

Head of femur

Pubic tubercle

Iliofemoral ligament

Lesser trochanter

Greater trochanter

**Fig. 13.33** Anteriorly, the hip joint is covered by an inverted Y-shaped iliofemoral ligament and the pubofemoral ligament. From Angerame MR, Dennis DA. Anatomy of the hip. In: Berry DJ, Lieberman JR, eds. Surgery of the Hip. Philadelphia: Elsevier; 2020:158–167.

## 13.17 Causes of musculoskeletal pelvic pain

- Inflammation
  - hip joint (e.g. Rheumatoid Arthritis)
  - sacro-iliac joints in axial spondyloarthritis
  - bursitis in inflammatory arthritis
- Degeneration
  - Osteoarthritis of hip
  - Labral tear
- Fracture
  - Trauma
  - Primary or secondary tumour
  - Osteomalacia
  - Paget's disease
  - Renal osteodystrophy
  - Stress fractures in female athlete triad
  - Osteogenesis imperfecta
- Overuse
  - Tendonitis, bursitis
  - Gilmore's groin
- Metabolic / Other
  - Paget's disease
  - Osteonecrosis
  - Chronic pain
  - Inguinal hernia

### *The physical examination*

### Examination sequence (Video 29) ▶

Patients should undress to their underwear and remove socks and shoes. You should be able to see the iliac crests.

### Look

- Assess gait.
- Carry out a general inspection: ask the patient to stand.
- From the front, check if:
- stance is straight and symmetrical
- shoulders lie parallel to the ground and symmetrically over the pelvis (this may mask a hip deformity or true shortening of one leg)
- hips, knees, ankles or feet are deformed
- muscles are wasted (from neuromuscular disease or disuse secondary to arthritis).
- From the side, look for:
- a stoop or increased lumbar lordosis (both may result from limited hip extension)
- scars, sinuses or skin changes around the hip.
- From behind, assess:
- whether the spine is straight or curved laterally (scoliosis)
- the relative positions of the shoulders and pelvis

- any difference in leg lengths
- for any gluteal atrophy.

### Feel

- Palpate for tenderness over the greater trochanter, suggesting trochanteric pain syndrome.
- Feel the anterior superior iliac crest for enthesitis.
  This is a good time to check for leg shortening (see 'Special tests').

### Move

Position the patient supine on the couch and check and ensure that the pelvic brim is perpendicular to the spine.
- Check the range of flexion of each hip in turn.

**Fig. 13.35** Testing hip movement. [A] Abduction. [B] Flexion. [C] Extension.

- Abduction and adduction: stabilise the pelvis by placing your left hand on the opposite iliac crest. With your right hand, abduct the patient's leg until you feel the pelvis start to tilt (normal 45 degrees). Test adduction by crossing one of the patient's legs over the other and continuing to move it medially (normal 25 degrees) (Fig. 13.35A).
- Internal and external rotation: with the patient's leg in full extension, roll it on the couch and watch the foot to indicate the range of rotation. Test with the knee (and hip) flexed at 90 degrees. Move the foot medially to test external rotation and laterally to test internal rotation (normal 45 degrees for each movement) (see Fig. 13.35B).
- Extension: ask the patient to lie prone on the couch. Place your left hand on the pelvis to detect any movement. Lift

**Fig. 13.36 Thomas test.** A Passively flex both legs as far as possible. B Extend the test leg. Limitation indicates fixed flexion deformity.

each of the patient's legs in turn to assess the range of extension (normal range is 0–20 degrees) (see Fig. 13.35C).

## Thomas test (Video 29A)

This reveals any fixed flexion deformity (incomplete extension) that may be masked by compensatory movement in the lumbar spine or pelvis and increased lumbar lordosis.

- Place your left hand under the patient's back (to detect any masking of hip limitation by movement of the pelvis and lumbar spine).
- Passively flex both legs (hips and knees) as far as possible (Fig. 13.36A).
- Keep the non-test hip maximally flexed and, by feeling with your left hand, confirm that the lordotic curve of the spine remains eliminated.
- Ask the patient to extend the test hip. Incomplete extension in this position indicates a fixed flexion deformity at the hip (see Fig. 13.36B).
- If the contralateral hip is not flexed sufficiently, the lumbar lordosis will not be eliminated, and fixed flexion deformity of the ipsilateral knee confuses the issue. In this case, perform the test with the patient lying on their side.
- Do not perform the test if the patient has a hip replacement on the non-test side, as forced flexion may cause dislocation.

### Special tests

#### Shortening

Shortening occurs in the hip and other lower limb conditions (Box 13.18). Apparent shortening is present if the affected limb appears shortened but is not, usually because of an adduction or flexion deformity at the hip.

## Examination sequence (Video 29B)

- Ask the patient to lie supine and stretch both legs out as far as possible equally, to eliminate any soft-tissue contracture/abnormal posture.
- Measure with a tape:
- from umbilicus to medial malleolus: the apparent length
- from anterior superior iliac spine to medial malleolus: the 'true length' (Fig. 13.37).

### 13.18 Causes of true lower limb shortening

**Hip**

- Fractures (e.g. neck of femur)
- Following total hip arthroplasty
- Slipped upper femoral epiphysis
- Perthes' disease (juvenile osteochondritis)
- Unreduced hip dislocation
- Septic arthritis
- Loss of articular cartilage (arthritis, joint infection)
- Congenital coxa vara
- Missed congenital dislocation of the hip

**Femur and tibia**

Growth disturbance secondary to:
  Juvenile Idiopathic Arthritis
  Poliomyelitis
  Cerebral palsy
  Fractures
  Osteomyelitis
  Septic arthritis
  Growth-plate injury
  Congenital causes

- Confirm any limb length discrepancy by 'block testing':
- Ask the patient to stand with both feet flat on the ground.
- Raise the shorter leg, using a series of blocks of graduated thickness until both iliac crests feel level.

Trendelenburg's sign

## Examination sequence (Video 29C)

- Stand in front of the patient.
- Palpate both iliac crests and ask the patient to stand on one leg for 30 seconds.
- Repeat with the other leg.
- Watch and feel the iliac crests to see which moves up or down.
- Normally, the iliac crest on the side with the foot off the ground should rise. The test is abnormal if the unsupported hemipelvis falls below the horizontal (Fig. 13.38). This may result from gluteal weakness or inhibition from hip pain caused by osteoarthritis or structural abnormality of the hip joint, such as in coxa vara or developmental hip dysplasia.

## ▌Knee

### Anatomy

The knee is a complex hinge joint with tibiofemoral and patellofemoral articulations. It has a synovial capsule that extends under the quadriceps muscle (the suprapatellar pouch), reaching 5 cm above the superior edge of the patella. The joint is largely subcutaneous, allowing easy palpation of the patella, tibial tuberosity, quadriceps tendon, patellar tendon, tibial plateau margin

**Fig. 13.37** True and apparent lengths of the lower limbs.

Apparent length of leg
Anterior superior iliac spine
True length of leg
Medial malleolus

**Fig. 13.38 Trendelenburg's sign.** Powerful gluteal muscles maintain the position when standing on the left leg. Weakness of the right gluteal muscles results in pelvic tilt when standing on the right leg.

and femoral condyles. The knee depends on its muscular and ligamentous structures for stability (Fig. 13.39).

The hamstring muscles are primary flexors of the knee. Extension is provided by the extensor apparatus, comprising quadriceps muscles, quadriceps tendon, patella, patellar tendon and tibial tuberosity. Any disruption of this 'extensor apparatus' prevents straight-leg raising or produces an extensor lag (a difference between active and passive ranges of extension).

The medial and lateral collateral ligaments resist valgus and varus stress, respectively. The anterior cruciate ligament (ACL) prevents anterior subluxation of the tibia on the femur, and the posterior cruciate ligament resists posterior translation. The medial and lateral menisci are crescentic fibrocartilaginous structures that lie between the tibial articular surface and the femoral condyles. There are several important bursae around the knee:

- anteriorly: the suprapatellar, prepatellar (between the patella and the overlying skin) and infrapatellar bursae (between the skin and the tibial tuberosity/patellar ligament)
- posteriorly: several bursae lie in the popliteal fossa (see Fig. 13.39D).

### The history

#### Pain

Generalised knee pain is likely to originate from pathology in the tibiofemoral joint. Anterior knee pain, particularly after prolonged sitting or going downstairs, suggests patellofemoral joint pathology. Medial or lateral pain could come from the collateral ligaments or meniscal tears.

Keep in mind that pain in the knee may be referred pain from the hip.

Take a detailed history of the mechanism of any injury. The direction of impact, load and deformation predict which structures are injured.

#### Swelling

The normal volume of synovial fluid is 1–2 mL and is clinically undetectable. An effusion indicates intra-articular pathology. Haemarthrosis (bleeding into the knee) is caused by injury to a vascular structure within the joint, such as a torn cruciate ligament or an intra-articular fracture. The menisci are predominantly avascular and do not cause a haemarthrosis, unless torn at their periphery or in conjunction with some other internal derangement. The speed of onset of any effusion is important in suggesting a potential cause.

#### Locking

Common causes of locking in the knee are a meniscal tear, a loose body (e.g. from osteochondritis dissecans), osteoarthritis or synovial chondromatosis. Bucket-handle and anterior beak meniscal tears are especially associated with locking. Posterior horn tears commonly cause pain and limit movement in the last few degrees of flexion. Meniscal tears also cause local joint-line tenderness. Congenital discoid meniscus may present with locking and clunking.

#### Instability ('giving way')

Any of the four main ligaments may rupture from trauma or become incompetent with degenerative disease. The patella is prone to dislocation laterally because the normal knee has a valgus angle.

**13**

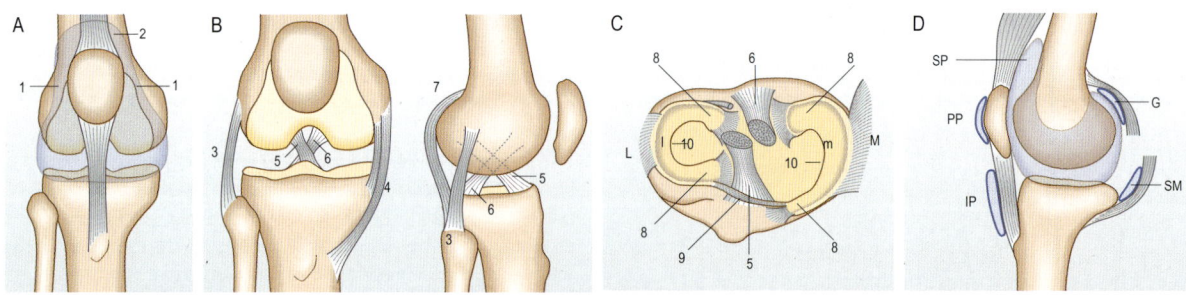

**Key**

| | | | | | |
|---|---|---|---|---|---|
| G | Bursa under the medial head of gastrocnemius | 1 | Extensions of synovial sheath on either side of patella | 7 | Posterior ligament |
| IP | Infrapatellar bursa | 2 | Extension of synovial sheath at upper pole of patella | 8 | Horns of lateral (l) and medial (m) menisci |
| L | Lateral tibiofemoral articulation | | | 9 | Connection of anterior horns |
| M | Medial tibiofemoral articulation | 3 | Lateral ligament | 10 | Unattached margin of meniscus |
| PP | Prepatellar bursa | 4 | Medial ligament | | |
| SM | Semimembranosus bursa | 5 | Anterior cruciate ligament | | |
| SP | Suprapatellar pouch (or bursa) | 6 | Posterior cruciate ligament | | |

**Fig. 13.39** **Structure of the right knee.** A Anterior view, showing the common synovial sheath. B Anterior and lateral views, showing the ligaments. C Plan view of the menisci. D Bursae.

## *The physical examination*

Observe the patient walking and standing as for gait. Note posture and deformities such as genu valgum (knock knee) or genu varum (bow legs).

### Look

Ask the patient to lie supine on the couch. Expose both legs fully and look for:

- Scars, sinuses, erythema or skin pathology.
- Muscle wasting: quadriceps wasting is almost invariable with inflammation, internal derangement or chronic pain, and develops within days. Measure the thigh circumference in both legs at 20 cm above the tibial tuberosity.
- Leg length discrepancy.
- Flexion deformity: if the patient lies with one knee flexed, this may originate from the hip, the knee or be a combined problem.
- Swelling: look for an enlarged prepatellar bursa ('housemaid's knee') and any knee joint effusion. Large effusions form a horseshoe-shaped swelling above the knee. Swelling extending beyond the joint margins suggests infection, major injury or rarely a tumour.
- Baker's cyst: bursa enlargement in the popliteal fossa.

### Feel (Videos 30A and 30B) ▶

- Warmth: compare both sides.
- Effusion.
- Patellar tap:
- With the patient's knee extended, empty the suprapatellar pouch by sliding your left hand down the thigh until you reach the upper edge of the patella.
- Keep your hand there and, with the fingertips of your right hand, press briskly and firmly over the patella (Fig. 13.40).
- In a moderate-sized effusion, you will feel a tapping sensation as the patella strikes the femur.
- 'Bulge' or 'ripple' test (Fig. 13.41):

**Fig. 13.40** Testing for effusion by the patellar tap.

Sweep upwards

Slide hand down suprapatellar pouch

Extend fingers and sweep down lateral side

Medial    Lateral

Look for fluid bulge on medial side

**Fig. 13.41** Bulge or ripple test to detect small knee effusions.

- Extend the patient's knee and, with the quadriceps muscles relaxed, empty the medial compartment into the suprapatellar bursa and lateral side by stroking the medial side of the knee (see Fig. 13.41A).
- Empty the suprapatellar bursa by sliding your hand down the thigh to the patella (see Fig. 13.41B).
- Without lifting your hand off the knee, extend your fingers (or thumb) to stroke the lateral side of the knee (see Fig. 13.41C).
- The test is positive if a ripple or bulge of fluid appears on the medial side of the knee. It is useful for detecting small amounts of fluid but may produce a false negative if a tense effusion is present.
- Synovitis: with the patient's knee extended and the quadriceps relaxed, feel for sponginess on both sides of the quadriceps tendon.
- Joint lines: feel the medial and lateral joint lines. If there is tenderness, localise this as accurately as possible. In adolescents, localised tibial tuberosity tenderness suggests Osgood–Schlatter disease, a traction apophysitis.

## Move
### Active flexion and extension
- With the patient supine, ask them to flex their knee up to their chest and then extend the leg back down to lie on the couch (normal range 0–140 degrees).
- Feel for crepitus between the patella and femoral condyles, suggesting chondromalacia patellae (more common in younger female patients) or osteoarthritis.
- Record the range of movement: if there is a fixed flexion deformity of 15 degrees and flexion is possible to 110 degrees, record this as a range of movement of 15–110 degrees.
- Ask the patient to lift their leg and note any extensor lag.

### Passive flexion and extension
- Normally, the knee can extend so that the femur and tibia are in longitudinal alignment. Record full extension as 0 degrees. A restriction to full extension occurs with meniscal tears, osteoarthritis and inflammatory arthritis. To assess hyperextension in the patient, lift both of the patient's legs by the feet.

Hyperextension (genu recurvatum) is present if the knee extends beyond the neutral position. Up to 10 degrees is normal.
- Test the extreme range of knee flexion with the patient face down on the couch, which makes comparison with the contralateral side easy. A block to full flexion is often caused by a tear of the posterior horn of the menisci.

## Ligament testing
### Collateral ligament
With the knee fully extended, abduction or adduction should not be possible. If either ligament is lax or ruptured, movement can occur. If the ligament is strained (partially torn) but intact, pain will be produced but the joint will not open.

### Examination sequence (Video 30C)
- With the patient's knee fully extended, hold their ankle between your elbow and side. Use both hands to apply a valgus and then a varus force to the knee.
- Use your thumbs to feel the joint line and assess the degree to which the joint space opens. Major opening of the joint indicates collateral and cruciate injury (Fig. 13.42A).
- If the knee is stable, repeat the process with the knee flexed to 30 degrees to assess minor collateral laxity. In this position, the cruciate ligaments are not taut.

### Anterior cruciate ligament

### Examination sequence
### Anterior drawer test
- Flex the patient's knee to 90 degrees and maintain this position using your thigh to immobilise the patient's foot.
- Check that the hamstring muscles are relaxed and look for posterior sag (posterior subluxation of the tibia on the femur).

**13**

**Fig. 13.42** Testing the ligaments of the knee. [A] Collateral ligaments. [B] Cruciate ligaments.

This causes a false-positive anterior drawer sign that should not be interpreted as ACL laxity.
- With your hands behind the upper tibia and both thumbs over the tibial tuberosity, pull the tibia anteriorly (see Fig. 13.42B). Significant movement (compared with the opposite knee) indicates that the ACL is lax. Movement of >1.5 cm suggests ACL rupture. There is often an associated medial ligament injury.

### Lachman test
- Flex the knee at 20–30 degrees with the patient supine. Place one hand behind the tibia and grasp the patient's thigh with the other hand. Pull the tibia forward to assess the amount of anterior motion of the tibia in comparison to the femur. An intact ACL should prevent forward translational movement ('firm endpoint'), while a deficient ACL will allow increased forward translation without a decisive 'endpoint'.

### Posterior drawer test
- Push backwards on the tibia. Posterior movement of the tibia relative to the femoral condyles suggests posterior cruciate ligament laxity.

#### Tests for meniscal tears

Meniscal tears in younger, sporty patients usually result from a twisting injury to the weight-bearing leg. In middle-aged patients, degenerative, horizontal cleavage of the menisci is common, with minimal or no history of trauma. Meniscal injuries commonly cause slow-onset effusions, especially on weight bearing or after exercise. Associated joint-line tenderness is common.

A simple test for a meniscal tear is to extend the patient's knee rapidly from 30 degrees of flexion to full extension. If the patient experiences medial or lateral pain, this suggests a tear, and formal testing should take place.

Meniscal provocation test (McMurray test)

### Examination sequence (Video 30D)

Ask the patient to lie supine on the couch. Test the medial and lateral menisci in turn.

### Medial meniscus
- Passively flex the patient's knee to its full extent.
- Externally rotate the patient's foot and abduct the upper leg at the hip, keeping the foot towards the midline (that is, creating a varus stress at the knee).
- Extend the patient's knee smoothly. In medial meniscus tears, a click or clunk may be felt or heard, accompanied by discomfort.

### Lateral meniscus
- Passively flex the patient's knee to its full extent.
- Internally rotate the patient's foot and adduct the leg at the hip (that is, creating a valgus stress at the knee).
- Extend the patient's knee smoothly. In lateral meniscus tears, a click or clunk may be felt or heard, accompanied by discomfort.

*Patella*

### Examination sequence (Video 30E)

- Look for prepatellar bursa swelling.
- Feel around the patella for tenderness suggestive of enthesitis or tendonitis.

### Patellar apprehension test
- With the patient's knee fully extended, push the patella laterally and flex the knee slowly. If the patient actively resists flexion, this suggests previous patellar dislocation or instability.

Other tests for patellofemoral pathology are unreliable and may be positive in normal individuals.

## Ankle and foot

### Anatomy

The ankle is a hinge joint. The talus articulates with a three-sided mortise made up of the tibial plafond and the medial and lateral malleoli. This allows principally dorsiflexion and plantar flexion, although some axial rotation can occur at the plantar-flexed ankle. The bony mortise is the major factor contributing to stability, but the lateral, medial (deltoid) and inferior tibiofibular ligaments are also important (Fig. 13.43).

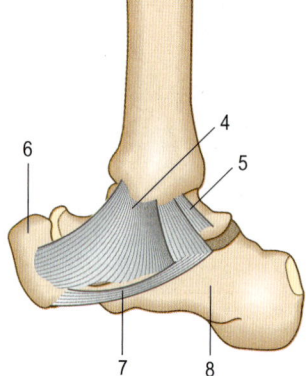

1 Lateral malleolus
2 Medial malleolus
3 Lateral (external) ligament
4 Medial ligament
5 Deep fibres of medial ligament
6 Navicular
7 Spring ligament
8 Calcaneus
9 Talus

**Fig. 13.43** Ankle ligaments.

Movements of the ankle and foot are summarised in Fig. 13.44. Foot movements are inversion and eversion, principally occurring at the mid-tarsal (talonavicular/calcaneocuboid) and subtalar (talocalcaneal) joints.

## The history

A 'twisted' ankle is a very common injury, and is usually related to a sporting injury, such as stepping off a kerb or a stair awkwardly. Establish the exact mechanism of injury and the precise site of pain. Frequently, there has been a forced inversion injury, stressing the lateral ligament. A sprain occurs when some fibres are torn but the ligament remains structurally intact. A complete ligament tear allows excessive talar movement in the ankle mortise with instability.

Achilles tendon rupture is associated with sudden plantar flexion at the ankle against resistance (e.g. in jumping or lunging). It is common in middle-aged patients doing unaccustomed activities such as squash, and it is associated with some medications such as oral glucocorticoids and fluoroquinolone antibiotics. Sudden pain occurs above the heel and there is often a sensation or noise of a crack. Patients may feel as if they have been kicked or even shot.

Forefoot pain, often localised to the second metatarsal, after excessive activity such as trekking, marching or dancing, suggests a stress fracture (Fig. 13.45). Symptoms are relieved by rest and aggravated by weight bearing.

### Non-traumatic conditions

Anterior metatarsalgia with forefoot pain is common, especially in middle-aged women. Acute joint pain with swelling suggests an inflammatory arthropathy such as rheumatoid arthritis or gout. In severe cases, the metatarsal heads become prominent and walking feels like walking on pebbles or broken glass.

Plantar surface heel pain that is worse in the foot-strike phase of walking may be caused by plantar fasciitis and tends to affect middle-aged patients and those with seronegative arthritides.

Posterior heel pain may be caused by Achilles tendonitis or enthesitis.

Spontaneous lancinating pain in the forefoot radiating to contiguous sides of adjacent toes occurs with Morton's

**Fig. 13.45 Stress fracture of second metatarsal.** Fracture site and callus *(arrow)*.

neuroma. A common site is the interdigital cleft between the third and fourth toes. This occurs predominantly in women aged 25–45 years and is aggravated by wearing tight shoes.

## The physical examination

### Examination sequence (Video 31) ▶

Ask patients to remove their socks and shoes.

### Look

- Examine the soles of the shoes for abnormal patterns of wear.
- Assess gait. Look for:
- increased height of step, indicating 'foot drop'
- ankle movement (dorsiflexion/plantar flexion)
- position of the foot as it strikes the ground (supinated/pronated)
- hallux rigidus – loss of movement at the metatarsophalangeal (MTP) joints.
- From behind and with the patient standing:
- Observe how the heel is aligned (valgus/varus).
- From the side:
- Observe the position of the midfoot, looking particularly at the medial longitudinal arch. This may be flattened (pes planus – flat foot) or exaggerated (pes cavus).
- If the arch is flattened, ask the patient to stand on tiptoe. This restores the arch in a mobile deformity but not in a structural one.
- A 'splay foot' has widening at the level of the metatarsal heads, often associated with MTP joint synovitis.

**Fig. 13.44 Terminology used for movements of the ankle and foot.**

Neutral

Dorsiflexion (extension)

Plantar (flexion)

Eversion / Inversion

Forefoot adduction / Forefoot abduction

Flexion / Extension

13

**Fig. 13.46** Hallux valgus overriding the second toe.

- Examine the ankle and foot for scars, sinuses, swelling, bruising, callosities (an area of thickened skin at a site of repeated pressure), nail changes, oedema, deformity and position.
- Look for deformities of the toes such as hallux valgus (Fig. 13.46) or overriding toes.
- Observe any bunion (a soft-tissue bursal swelling) over the first metatarsal head that may be inflamed or infected.

## Feel
- Feel for focal tenderness and heat.
- In an acute ankle injury, palpate the proximal fibula, both malleoli, the lateral ligament and the base of the fifth metatarsal.
- Gently compress the forefoot. Assess the MTP joints for swelling and tenderness suggestive of inflammatory arthritis.

## Move (see Fig. 13.44)
### Active movements
- Assess plantar flexion/dorsiflexion at the ankle, inversion/eversion of the foot and flexion/extension of the toes.

### Passive movements
- Grip the patient's heel from below with the cup of your left hand, with your thumb and index finger on the malleoli.
- Put the foot through its arc of movement (normal range 15 degrees dorsiflexion to 45 degrees plantar flexion).
- If dorsiflexion is restricted, assess the contribution of the gastrocnemius (which acts across both knee and ankle joints) by measuring ankle dorsiflexion with the knee extended and flexed. If more dorsiflexion is possible with the knee flexed, this suggests a gastrocnemius contracture.

### Passive foot inversion/eversion
- Examine the subtalar joint in isolation by placing the foot into dorsiflexion to stabilise the talus in the ankle mortise.
- Move the heel into inversion (normal 20 degrees) and eversion (normal 10 degrees).
- Examine the combined mid-tarsal joints by fixing the heel with your left hand and moving the forefoot with your right hand into dorsiflexion, plantar flexion, adduction, abduction, supination and pronation.

### Passive hallux and lesser toe movements
- Assess flexion and extension at MTP and interphalangeal joints. Pain and stiffness at the first MTP joint suggest hallux rigidus.
- If there is toe deformity, assess impingement on the other toes. Claw toes result from dorsiflexion at MTP joints and

plantar flexion at PIP and DIP joints. Hammer toes are due to dorsiflexion at MTP and DIP joints and plantar flexion at PIP joints. Mallet toes describe plantar flexion at DIP joints.

## Special tests
Achilles tendon

Examination sequence

- Ask the patient to kneel with both knees on a chair.
- Palpate the gastrocnemius muscle and the Achilles tendon for focal tenderness and soft-tissue swelling. Achilles tendon rupture is often palpable as a discrete gap in the tendon about 5 cm above the calcaneal insertion (Fig. 13.47A).

A

B

**Fig. 13.47** Ruptured Achilles tendon. **A** Site of a palpable defect in the Achilles tendon *(arrow)*. **B** Thomson's test. Failure of the foot to plantar-flex when the calf is squeezed is pathognomonic of an acute rupture of the Achilles tendon.

Thomson's (Simmond's) test

## Examination sequence

Squeeze the calf just distal to the level of maximum circumference. If the Achilles tendon is intact, plantar flexion of the foot will occur (see Fig. 13.47B).

Mulder's sign for Morton's neuroma

## Examination sequence

- Squeeze the metatarsal heads together with one hand while at the same time putting pressure on the interdigital space with your other hand. The pain of the neuroma will be localised to the plantar surface of the interdigital space and may be accompanied by a 'clunk' as the neuroma slides between the metatarsal heads. Paraesthesia will radiate into the affected toes.

A

B

**Fig. 13.48 Colles' fracture.** [A] Clinical appearance of a dinner-fork deformity. [B] x-ray appearance.

# Fractures, dislocations and trauma

A fracture is a breach in the structural integrity of a bone. This may arise in:

- normal bone from excessive force
- normal bone from repetitive load-bearing activity (stress fracture)
- bone of abnormal structure with minimal or no trauma.

The epidemiology of fractures varies geographically. There is a predicted epidemic of osteoporotic fractures because of the increasing size of elderly populations. Although any osteoporotic bone can fracture, common sites are the distal radius (Fig. 13.48), neck of femur (see Fig. 13.34), proximal humerus and spinal vertebrae.

Fractures resulting from road traffic accidents and falls are decreasing because of legislative and preventive measures such as seat belts, air bags and improved roads. A fracture may occur in the context of severe trauma.

## The history

Establish the mechanism of injury. For example, a patient who has fallen from a height on to their heels may have obvious fractures of the calcaneal bones in their ankles but is also at risk of fractures of the proximal femur, pelvis and vertebral column.

## The physical examination

Use the 'Look – feel – move' approach. Observe patients closely to see if they move the affected part and are able to weight-bear.

## Examination sequence

### Look
- See if the skin is intact. If there is a breach in the skin and the wound communicates with the fracture, the fracture is open or compound; otherwise, it is closed.
- Look for associated bruising, deformity, swelling or wound infection (Fig. 13.49).

A

B

**Fig. 13.49 Ankle deformity.** [A] Clinical appearance. [B] Lateral x-ray view showing tibiotalar fracture dislocation.

**13**

## Feel

- Gently feel for local tenderness.
- Feel distal to the suspected fracture to establish if sensation and pulses are present.

## Move

- Establish whether the patient can move joints distal and proximal to the fracture.
- Do not move a fracture site to see if crepitus is present; this causes additional pain and bleeding.

Describe the fracture according to Box 13.19. Each suspected fracture requires an X-ray with orthogonal views, which involves two views (at least) at perpendicular planes of the affected bone. The joints above and below should also be imaged.

## Investigations

Common investigations in patients with musculoskeletal disease are summarised in Box 13.20.

### 13.19 Describing a fracture

- Which bone(s) is/are involved?
- Is the fracture open (compound) or closed?
- Is the fracture complete or incomplete?
- Where is the bone fractured (intra-articular/epiphysis/physis/metaphysis/diaphysis)?
- What is the fracture's configuration (transverse/oblique/spiral/comminuted (multifragmentary)/butterfly fragment)?
- What components of deformity are present?
  - Translation is the shift of the distal fragment in relation to the proximal bone. The direction is defined by the movement of the distal fragment (e.g. dorsal or volar) and is measured as a percentage of the overall diameter of the bone described.
  - Angulation is the angle formed by the deflection of the distal fragment relative to the proximal fragment, measured in degrees.
  - Rotation is measured in degrees along the longitudinal axis of the bone (e.g. for spiral fracture of the tibia or phalanges).
  - Shortening: proximal migration of the distal fragment can cause shortening (e.g. in an oblique fracture). Shortening may also occur if there has been impaction at the fracture site (e.g. a Colles' fracture of the distal radius).
- Is there distal nerve or vascular deficit?
- What is the state of the tissues associated with the fracture (soft tissues and joints [e.g. fracture blisters, dislocation])?

### 13.20 Common musculoskeletal investigations

| Investigation | Indication/comment |
|---|---|
| **Urinalysis** | |
| Protein | Glomerular disease (e.g. SLE, vasculitis) <br> Secondary amyloid in RA and other chronic arthropathies <br> Drug adverse effects (e.g. myocrisin, penicillamine) |
| Blood | Glomerular disease (e.g. SLE, vasculitis) |
| **Haematological** | |
| Full blood count | Anaemia in inflammatory arthritis, blood loss after trauma <br> Neutrophilia in sepsis and very acute inflammation, e.g. acute gout <br> Leucopenia in SLE, Felty's syndrome and adverse effects of antirheumatic drug therapy |
| Erythrocyte sedimentation rate/plasma viscosity | Non-specific indicator of inflammation or sepsis |
| C-reactive protein | Acute-phase protein |
| **Biochemical** | |
| Urea and creatinine | ↑ in renal impairment (e.g. secondary amyloid in RA or adverse drug effect) |
| Uric acid | May be ↑ in gout. Levels may be normal during an acute attack |
| Calcium | ↓ in osteomalacia; normal in osteoporosis |
| Alkaline phosphatase | ↑ in Paget's disease, metastases, osteomalacia and immediately after fractures |
| Angiotensin-converting enzyme | ↑ in sarcoidosis |
| Urinary albumin : creatinine ratio | Glomerular disease (e.g. vasculitis, SLE) |
| **Serological** | |
| Immunoglobulin M rheumatoid factor | ↑ titres in 60–70% of cases of RA; occasionally, low titres in other connective diseases. Present in up to 15% of normal population. Superseded by anti-cyclic citrullinated peptide antibodies |
| Anti-cyclic citrullinated peptide antibody (ACPA) | Present in 60–70% of cases of RA and up to 10 years before onset of disease. Highly specific for RA. Occasionally found in Sjögren's syndrome |

### 13.20 Common musculoskeletal investigations—cont'd

| Investigation | Indication/comment |
|---|---|
| Antinuclear factors | ↑ titres in most cases of SLE; low titres in other connective tissue diseases and RA |
| Anti-Ro, Anti-La | Sjögren's syndrome |
| Anti-double-stranded DNA | SLE |
| Anti-Sm | SLE |
| Anti-ribonucleoprotein | Mixed connective tissue disease |
| Lupus anticoagulant, anti-cardiolipin antibodies, anti-$\beta_2$ glycoprotein 1 | SLE, antiphospholipid syndrome |
| Antineutrophil cytoplasmic antibodies | Granulomatosis with polyangiitis, polyarteritis nodosa, Churg–Strauss vasculitis |
| **Other**<br>Schirmer tear test, salivary flow test | Keratoconjunctivitis sicca (dry eyes), Sjögren's syndrome |
| **Imaging**<br>Plain radiography (x-ray) | Fractures, erosions in RA and psoriatic arthritis, osteophytes and joint-space loss in osteoarthritis, bone changes in Paget's disease, pseudofractures (Looser's zones) in osteomalacia |
| Ultrasonography | Detection of effusion, synovitis, cartilage breaks, enthesitis and erosions in inflammatory arthritis. Double contour sign in gout |
|  | Detection of bursae, tendon pathology and osteophytes |
| Magnetic resonance imaging | Joint and bone structure; soft-tissue imaging |
| Computed tomography | High-resolution scans of thorax for pulmonary fibrosis, neck scan in trauma |
| Dual-energy x-ray absorptiometry | Gold standard for determining osteoporosis. Usual scans are of lumbar spine, hip and lateral vertebral assessment for fractures |
| Isotope bone scan | Increased uptake in Paget's disease, bone tumour, infection, fracture. Infrequently used due to high radiation dose. |
| **Joint aspiration/biopsy**<br>Synovial fluid microscopy | Inflammatory cells (e.g. ↑ neutrophils in bacterial infection) |
| Polarised light microscopy | Positively birefringent rhomboidal crystals – calcium pyrophosphate (pseudogout)<br>Negatively birefringent needle-shaped crystals – monosodium urate monohydrate (gout) |
| Bacteriological culture | Organism may be isolated from synovial aspirates |
| Biopsy and histology | Synovitis – RA and other inflammatory arthritides |

*RA,* Rheumatoid arthritis; *SLE,* systemic lupus erythematosus.

**13**

## OSCE example 1: Right shoulder pain

Mr Hunt, 38 years old, has a 2-month history of right shoulder pain, with no history of trauma.

### Please examine the shoulder

- Introduce yourself and clean your hands.
- Expose both of the patient's shoulders and arms.
- Comment on acromioclavicular deformity and muscle wasting; look for winging of the scapula.
- Compare the right shoulder to the normal left shoulder.
- Perform active and passive movements. In particular, look for frozen shoulder, which is diagnosed by limitation of external rotation and flexion.
- Finally, examine the arm, looking for conditions such as biceps rupture.
- If all movements of the shoulder are normal, conduct a full examination of the neck.
- Thank the patient and clean your hands.

### Summarise your findings

The patient reports pain between 120 and 60 degrees of abduction when lowering the abducted shoulder. Pain is reproduced upon abduction against resistance.

### Suggest a differential diagnosis

The most common cause of these symptoms is impingement syndrome, which can be confirmed by carrying out special tests (Neer and Hawkins–Kennedy). Differentials include frozen shoulder, calcific tendonitis, acromioclavicular joint pain, arthritis (osteoarthritis, rheumatoid arthritis or posttraumatic), long head of biceps rupture and referred pain from the neck.

### Suggested investigations

X-ray will reveal degenerative changes in osteoarthritis or tendon calcification. Ultrasound may demonstrate effusions, calcific deposits and tendon damage/rupture.

## OSCE example 2: Painful hands

Mrs Hill, 46 years old, presents with an 8-week history of insidious onset of pain, stiffness and swelling of her hands. She smokes 15 cigarettes per day.

### Please examine her hands

- Introduce yourself and clean your hands.
- Look:
  - In this case, there is swelling of two MCP joints on the right, and one PIP joint on the left.
  - Normal nails and skin (therefore psoriatic arthropathy is unlikely).
- Feel:
  - Ask first what is sore and seek permission to examine gently.
  - Tender, soft swelling of the MCP and PIP joints in the hands and left elbow.
  - In feet: tender across her MTP joints on squeeze test but no palpable swelling.
- Move:
  - Painful MCP joints in right hand on active and passive flexion, reducing handgrip and fine movements.
  - Left elbow does not fully straighten

### Summarise your findings

The patient has tender, soft swelling of two MCP joints and one PIP joint. There is pain associated with active and passive movement of the affected joints, resulting in limitation of hand and elbow function.

### Suggest a differential diagnosis

The pattern of joint involvement, patient's gender, duration of symptoms and history of smoking support a clinical diagnosis of rheumatoid arthritis. The differential diagnosis of psoriatic arthropathy is less likely because of her normal nails and lack of the typical skin changes of psoriasis.

### Suggest initial investigations

Full blood count, renal function tests, calcium, phosphate and liver function tests are carried out to assess for anaemia of chronic disease and to determine suitability for disease-modifying antirheumatic drugs; C-reactive protein to assess the degree of systemic inflammation; anti-CCP antibody to confirm whether seropositive rheumatoid arthritis is present; application of the 2010 American College of Rheumatology/European League Against Rheumatism criteria (see Box 13.14) for classification of rheumatoid arthritis; hand and foot X-rays to detect any bony erosions; chest x-ray to look for rheumatoid lung disease.

## Integrated examination sequence for the locomotor system

- Ask the patient to undress to their underwear.
- Ask the GALS (gait, arms, legs, spine) questions and perform the GALS screen.
- Identify which of the joints require more detailed examination:
  - What is the pattern of joint involvement?
  - Is it likely to be inflammatory or degenerative?
- Examine gait and spine in more detail first, if appropriate, then position the patient on the couch for detailed joint examination.
- Assess the general appearance:
  - Look for pallor, rashes, skin tightness, evidence of weight or muscle loss, obvious deformities.
  - Check the surroundings for a temperature chart, walking aids and splints, if appropriate.
- Examine the relevant joint, or all joints if systemic disease suspected:
  - Ask about tenderness before examining the patient.
  - Look at the skin, nails, subcutaneous tissues, muscles and bony outlines.
  - Feel for warmth, swelling, tenderness and reducibility of deformities.
  - Move:
  - Active movements first: demonstrate to the patient then ask them to perform the movements. Is there pain or crepitus upon movement?
  - Passive movements second: determine the patient's range of movement. Measure with a goniometer. What is the end-feel like? Describe the deformities.
- If systemic disease is suspected, go on to examine all other systems fully.
- Consider what investigations are required:
  - Basic blood tests.
  - Inflammatory markers.
  - Immunology.
  - Ultrasound.
  - x-rays, CT, MRI.
  - Special tests.
  - Joint aspiration for synovial fluid analysis or culture.

**13**

Michael J Tidman
Alice SM Tidman

14

# The skin, hair and nails

**Anatomy and physiology 326**
Skin 326
Hair 327
Nails 327

**The history 327**
Common presenting symptoms 327
Past medical and drug history 328
Family and social history 328

**The physical examination 328**
Distribution of a rash 328
Morphology of a rash 329

Colour 330
Specific features 332
Morphology of lesions 332
Mouth, hair and nail signs 335
Supplementary examination techniques 336

**Investigations 336**

**OSCE Example 1: Pruritus 337**

**OSCE Example 2: Pigmented lesion 337**

**Integrated examination sequence for the skin 337**

Dermatological conditions are very common (10–15% of general practice consultations) and present to healthcare professionals in all specialties. In the UK, 50% are lesions ('lumps and bumps'), including skin cancers, and most of the remainder are acute and chronic inflammatory disorders ('rashes'), including infections, with genetic conditions accounting for a small minority; this ratio will vary across the world, although the principles of skin assessment are the same globally.

Dermatological diagnosis can be challenging. Not only are there a vast number of distinct skin diseases, but also each may present with a great variety of morphologies and patterns determined by intrinsic genetic factors, including the degree of skin pigmentation, with the diagnostic waters muddied still further by external influences such as rubbing and scratching, infection, and well-meaning attempts at topical and systemic treatment. Even in one individual, lesions with the same pathology can have a very variable appearance (e.g., melanocytic naevi, seborrhoeic keratoses and basal cell carcinomas).

Many skin findings will have no clinical significance, but it is important to be able to examine the skin properly in order to identify tumours and rashes, and to recognise cutaneous signs of underlying systemic conditions. The adage that the skin is a window into the inner workings of the body is entirely true, and an examination of the integument will often provide the discerning clinician with important clues about internal disease processes, as well as information about the physical and psychological wellbeing of an individual.

## Anatomy and physiology

### Skin

The skin is the largest of the human organs, with a complex anatomy (Fig. 14.1) and a number of essential functions (Box 14.1). It has three layers, the most superficial of which is the epidermis, a stratified squamous epithelium containing melanocytes (pigment-producing cells) within its basal layer and Langerhans cells (antigen-presenting immune cells) throughout. The packaging and distribution of melanin within the epidermal cells determines the depth of skin pigmentation.

The dermis is the middle and most anatomically complex layer, containing vascular channels, sensory nerve endings, numerous cell types (including fibroblasts, macrophages, adipocytes and smooth muscle), hair follicles and glandular structures (eccrine, sebaceous and apocrine), all enmeshed in collagen and elastic tissue, within a matrix comprising glycosaminoglycan, proteoglycan and glycoprotein.

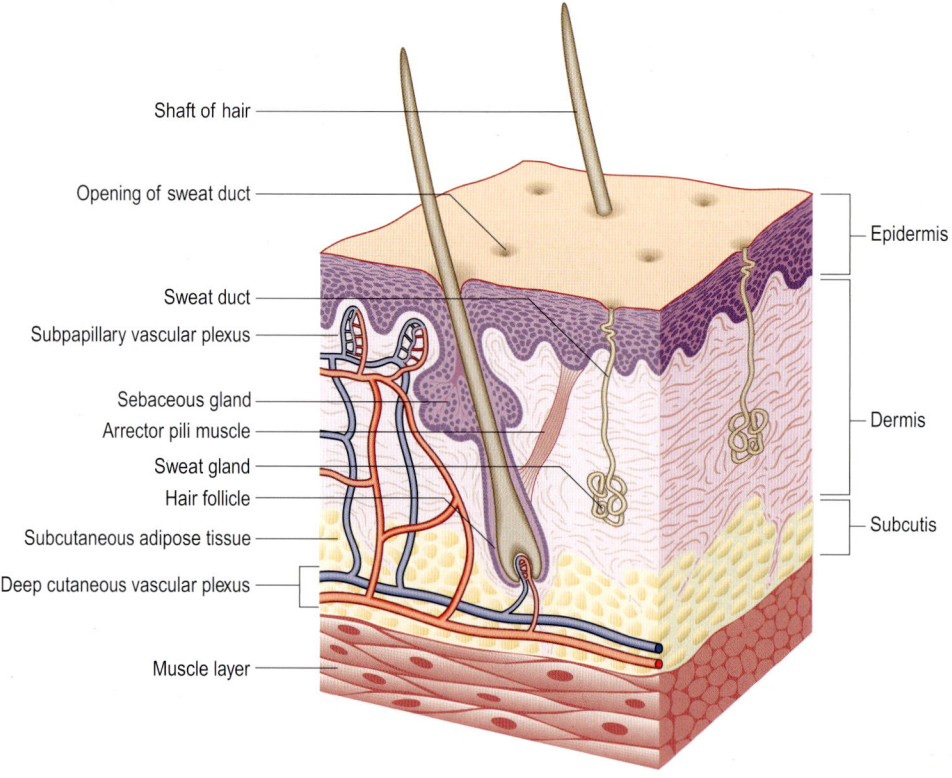

Shaft of hair

Opening of sweat duct

Sweat duct

Subpapillary vascular plexus

Sebaceous gland

Arrector pili muscle

Sweat gland

Hair follicle

Subcutaneous adipose tissue

Deep cutaneous vascular plexus

Muscle layer

Epidermis

Dermis

Subcutis

**Fig. 14.1** Structures of the skin.

## 14.1 Functions of the skin

- Protection against physical injury and injurious substances, including ultraviolet radiation
- Anatomical barrier against pathogens
- Immunological defence
- Retention of moisture
- Thermoregulation
- Calorie reserve
- Appreciation of sensation (touch, temperature, pain)
- Vitamin D production
- Absorption – particularly foetal and neonatal skin
- Psychosexual and social interaction

The deep subcutis contains adipose and connective tissue.

Dermatoses (diseases of the skin) may affect all three layers and, to a greater or lesser extent, the various functions of the skin.

## Hair

Hair plays a role in the protective, thermoregulatory and sensory functions of skin, and also in psychosexual and social interactions. There are two main types of hair in adults:

- Vellus hair, which is short and fine and covers most of the body surface.
- Terminal hair, which is longer and thicker and is found on the trunk and limbs, as well as the scalp, eyebrows, eyelashes, and pubic, axillary and beard areas.

Abnormalities in hair distribution can occur when there is transitioning between vellus and terminal hair types (e.g., hirsutism in women) or vice versa (androgenic alopecia). Hairs undergo regular asynchronous cycles of growth and, thus, in health, mass shedding of hair is unusual. Hair loss can occur as a result of disorders of hair cycling, conditions resulting in damage to hair follicles (such as scarring inflammatory processes), or structural (fragile) hair disorders.

## Nails

The nail is a plate of densely packed, hardened, keratinised cells produced by the nail matrix. It serves to protect the fingertip and aids grasp and fingertip sensitivity. The white lunula at the base of the nail is the visible distal aspect of the nail matrix (Fig. 14.2). Fingernail regrowth takes approximately 6 months, and toenail regrowth 12–18 months.

## The history

The possible diagnoses in dermatological conditions are broad and some diseases have pathognomonic features. Thus, in order to ensure that your history-taking is focused and relevant, it may be appropriate to ask to glimpse the lesion or rash before embarking on detailed enquiry.

## Common presenting symptoms

These include:

- A rash: scaly, blistering or itchy
- A lump or lesion
- Pruritus (itch)
- Hair loss or excess hair (hirsutism, hypertrichosis)
- Nail changes

Ask:

- When did the lesion appear, or the rash begin?
- Where is the rash/lesion?

14

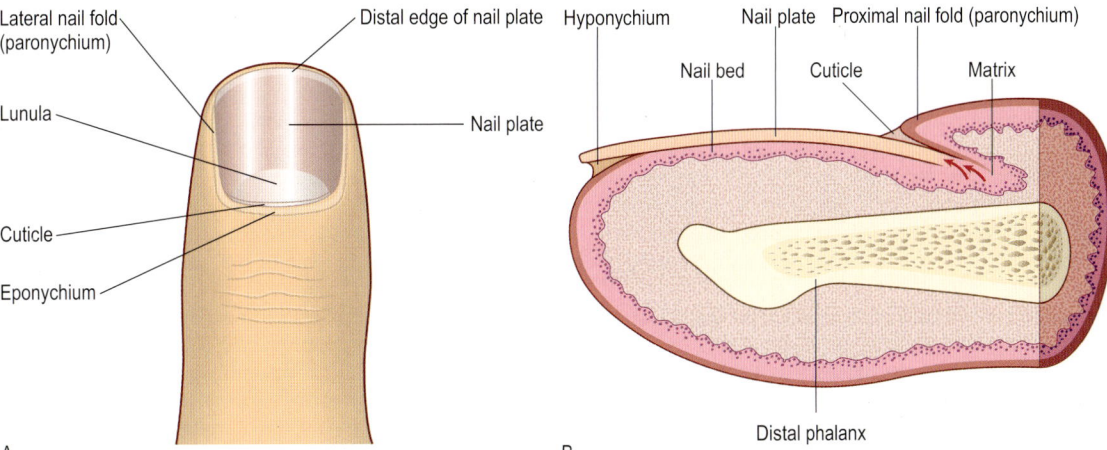

A     B

**Fig. 14.2 Structure of the nail.** A Dorsal view. B Cross-section.

- Has the rash spread, or the lesion changed, since its onset?
- Is the lesion tender or painful? Is the rash itchy? Is the itch intense enough to cause bleeding by scratching or to disturb sleep, as in atopic eczema and lichen simplex? Are there blisters?
- Do the symptoms vary with time? For example, the pruritus of scabies is usually worse at night, and acne and atopic eczema may show a premenstrual exacerbation.
- Were there any preceding symptoms, such as a sore throat in psoriasis, a severe illness in telogen effluvium, or a new oral medication in drug eruptions?
- Are there any aggravating or relieving factors? For example, exercise or exposure to heat may precipitate cholinergic urticaria.
- What, if any, has been the effect of topical or oral medications? Self-medication with oral antihistamines may ameliorate urticaria, and topical glucocorticoids may help inflammatory reactions.
- Are there any associated constitutional symptoms, such as joint pain (psoriasis), muscle pain and weakness (dermatomyositis), fever, fatigue or weight loss?
- Very importantly, what is the impact of the rash on the individual's quality of life?

## Past medical and drug history

Ask about general health and previous medical or skin conditions; a history of asthma, hay fever or childhood eczema suggests atopy. Coeliac disease is associated with dermatitis herpetiformis.

Take a full drug history, including any recent oral or topical prescribed or over-the-counter medications. Enquire about allergies not just to medicines but also to animals or foods.

## Family and social history

Enquire about occupation and hobbies, as exposure to chemicals may cause contact dermatitis. If a rash consistently improves when a patient is away from work, the possibility of industrial dermatitis should be considered. Ask about alcohol consumption and confirm smoking status.

Document foreign travel and sun exposure if actinic damage, tropical infections or photosensitive eruptions are being considered. The risk of squamous cell and basal cell cancers increases with total lifetime sun exposure, and intense sun exposures leading to blistering burns are a risk factor for melanoma. The susceptibility of an individual to sun-induced damage can be determined by defining their skin type using the Fitzpatrick scale (Box 14.2).

Ask about a family history of atopy and skin conditions.

The history of a skin disorder alone rarely enables a definite diagnosis, with perhaps the occasional exception: an itchy eruption that resembles a nettle rash, the individual components of which last less than 24 hours, is very likely to be urticaria; and an intensely itchy eruption that affects all body areas except the head (in adults) and is worse in bed at night should be considered to be scabies until proved otherwise.

---

### 14.2 Fitzpatrick scale of skin types

- Type 1: always burns, never tans
- Type 2: usually burns, tans minimally
- Type 3: sometimes burns, usually tans
- Type 4: always tans, occasionally burns
- Type 5: tans easily, rarely burns
- Type 6: never burns, permanent deep pigmentation

---

# The physical examination

Proper assessment of the skin involves all the human senses, with the exception of taste. Once we have listened to the patient's history, we look at the rash or lesion, touch the skin, and occasionally use our sense of smell to diagnose infection and metabolic disorders such as trimethylaminuria (fish odour syndrome). The increasing use of remote consultations ('teledermatology') in clinical practice introduces the risk of certain aspects of patient assessment being compromised, limiting the ability to make a precise diagnosis.

Examination of the skin should be performed under conditions of privacy in an adequately lit, warm room with, when appropriate, a chaperone present (p. 22). The patient should ideally be undressed to a degree that enables visualisation of all affected areas of the skin, but allowances should be made for modesty and religious practices. Routinely, the hair, nails and oral cavity (p. 213) should be examined, and the regional lymph nodes (p. 36) palpated. Assess skin type using the Fitzpatrick scale (see Box 14.2).

In documenting the appearance of a lesion or rash, use the correct descriptive terminology (Box 14.3); doing so often helps crystallise the diagnostic thought processes.

## Distribution of a rash

The distribution of dermatosis can be very informative. Is the eruption symmetrical? If so, it is likely to have a constitutional basis, and if not, it may well have an extrinsic cause. This golden rule has occasional exceptions (such as lichen simplex) but holds true in the majority of instances.

The pattern of a rash may immediately suggest a diagnosis: for example, the antecubital and popliteal fossae in atopic eczema (Fig. 14.3A); the extensor limb surfaces (see Fig. 14.3B), scalp, nails (see Fig. 3.7A) and umbilicus in psoriasis; the flexural aspects of the wrists and the oral mucous membranes in lichen planus (Fig. 14.4); the scalp, alar grooves and nasolabial folds in seborrhoeic dermatitis; and the sparing of covered areas in photosensitive eruptions. Does the rash follow a dermatome (as with shingles, see Fig. 7.9), or Langer's lines of skin tension (as with pityriasis rosea), or Blaschko (developmental) lines (as with certain genetic disorders)? The localisation of an eruption to fresh scars or tattoos may be a manifestation of sarcoidosis, and the anatomical location may provide a clue to diagnosis, such as the tendency of erythema

## 14.3 Descriptive terminology

| Term | Definition | Term | Definition |
|------|-----------|------|-----------|
| Abscess | A collection of pus, often associated with signs and symptoms of inflammation (includes boils and carbuncles) | Macule | A flat (impalpable) colour change |
| | | Milium | A keratin cyst |
| Angioedema | Deep swelling (oedema) of the dermis and subcutis | Naevus | A localised developmental defect (vascular, melanocytic, epidermal or connective tissue) |
| Annular | Ring-like | | |
| Arcuate | Curved | Nodule | A large papule (>0.5 cm) |
| Atrophy | Thinning of one or more layers of the skin | Nummular | Coin-shaped |
| Blister | A liquid-filled lesion (vesicles and bullae) | Onycholysis | Separation of the nail plate from the nail bed |
| Bulla | A large blister (>0.5 cm) | Papilloma | A benign growth projecting from the skin surface |
| Burrow | A track left by a burrowing scabies mite | Papule | An elevated (palpable) lesion, arbitrarily <0.5 cm in diameter |
| Callus (callosity) | A thickened area of skin that is a response to repeated friction or pressure | Patch | A large macule |
| Circinate | Circular | Pedunculated | Having a stalk |
| Comedo | A blackhead | Petechiae | Pinhead-sized macular purpura |
| Crust (scab) | A hard, adherent surface change caused by leakage and drying of blood, serum or pus | Pigmentation | A change in skin colour |
| | | Plaque | A papule or nodule that in cross-sectional profile is plateau-shaped |
| Cyst | A fluid-filled papular lesion that fluctuates and transilluminates | Poikiloderma | A combination of atrophy, hyperpigmentation and telangiectasia |
| Discoid | Disc-like | | |
| Ecchymosis (bruise) | A deep bleed in the skin | Purpura | Non-blanchable redness (also called petechiae) |
| | | Pustule | A papular lesion containing turbid purulent material (pus) |
| Erosion | A superficial loss of skin, involving the epidermis; scarring is not normally a result | Reticulate | Net-like |
| | | Scale | A flake on the skin surface, composed of stratum corneum cells (corneocytes), shed together rather than individually |
| Erythema | Redness of the skin that blanches on pressure | | |
| Erythroderma | Any inflammatory skin disease that affects >80% of the body surface | | |
| Exanthem | A rash | Scar | The fibrous tissue resulting from the healing of a wound, ulcer or certain inflammatory conditions |
| Excoriation | A scratch mark | | |
| Fissure | A split, usually extending from the skin surface through the epidermis to the dermis | Serpiginous | Snake-like |
| | | Stria(e) | A stretch mark |
| | | Targetoid | Target-like |
| Freckle | An area of hyperpigmentation that increases in the summer months and decreases during winter | Telangiectasia | Dilated blood vessels |
| | | Ulcer | A deep loss of skin, extending into the dermis or deeper; usually results in scarring |
| Furuncle | A boil | | |
| Gyrate | Wave-like | Umbilication | A depression at the centre of a lesion |
| Haematoma | A swelling caused by a collection of blood | Verrucous | Wart-like |
| Horn | A hyperkeratotic projection from the skin surface | Vesicle | A small blister (<0.5 cm) |
| Hyperkeratosis | Thickening of the stratum corneum | Wheal | A transient (<24 hours), itchy, elevated area of skin resulting from dermal oedema that characterises urticaria |
| Ichthyosis | Very dry skin | | |
| Keratosis | A lesion characterised by hyperkeratosis | Xerosis | Mild/moderate dryness of the skin |
| Lentigo | An area of fixed hyperpigmentation | | |
| Lichenification | Thickening of the epidermis, resulting in accentuation of skin markings; usually indicative of a chronic eczematous process | | |

**14**

nodosum (see Fig. 5.7B), pretibial myxoedema (see Fig. 10.2D) and necrobiosis lipoidica (Fig. 14.5) to involve the shins.

## Morphology of a rash

The morphology (shape and pattern) of a rash is equally important. Violaceous, polygonal, flat-topped papules, topped by a lacy

A

B

**Fig. 14.3 Distribution of rash.** A Atopic eczema localising to the flexural aspect of the knees. B Psoriasis involving the extensor aspect of the elbow.

patterning (Wickham's striae), are typical of lichen planus (see Fig. 14.4). The Koebner (isomorphic) phenomenon, where a dermatosis is induced by superficial epidermal injury, results in linear configurations (Fig. 14.6A), and occurs *par excellence* in psoriasis, lichen planus, viral warts and molluscum contagiosum. Linear or angular markings (erythema or scarring) raise the likelihood of artefactual (self-inflicted) damage to the skin. The presence of blisters limits the diagnostic possibilities to a relatively small number of autoimmune (such as dermatitis herpetiformis, pemphigoid (see Fig. 14.6B) and pemphigus), reactive (including erythema multi-forme, Stevens–Johnson syndrome and toxic epidermal necrolysis), infective (such as bullous impetigo and herpes simplex infection) and inherited (for example, epidermolysis bullosa) disorders. An annular (ring-like) morphology may be seen in granuloma annulare (see Fig. 14.6C), sarcoidosis, subacute cutaneous lupus erythe-matosus, and fungal infections ('ringworm'). Deeply pigmented skin types are frequently associated with follicular accentuation of in-flammatory processes as well as an increased tendency to scarring compared to lighter skin types (Fig. 14.7AB).

## Colour

The vascular contribution to the colour of a rash can be pivotal in diagnosis, particularly in light skin types, as redness can

A

B

C

**Fig. 14.4 Lichen planus.** A Discrete flat-topped papules on the wrist. B Wickham's striae, visible on close inspection. C A white lacy network of striae on the buccal mucosa.

**Fig. 14.5** Necrobiosis lipoidica diabeticorum: peripheral erythema and central yellow-coloured telangiectatic atrophic changes.

A

B

A

B

**Fig. 14.7** [A] Follicular eczema in dark skin. [B] Keloids due to inflammatory change in dark skin.

C

**Fig. 14.6 Rash morphology.** [A] Koebner response in psoriasis. [B] Tense bullae (blisters) in pemphigoid. [C] Annular lesions in granuloma annulare.

sometimes be difficult to assess in darker skin types. It is not sufficient to describe a rash as 'red' or 'pink'; it is essential to demonstrate whether or not a rash blanches on direct pressure or when the skin is stretched. Blanchable redness (erythema) indicates that the red blood cells causing the colour remain within blood vessels; non-blanchable redness (purpura) is the result of erythrocyte extravasation and entrapment in the collagen and elastic fibres of the dermis. Erythematous and purpuric eruptions usually have very different underlying causes.

The tint of the erythema may be helpful: a violaceous hue distinguishes lichen planus; a beefy-red or salmon-pink colour often typifies psoriasis; and a heliotrope (pink–purple) colour is a feature of dermatomyositis, especially on the eyelids.

Macular purpura may be the result of thrombocytopenia or capillary fragility (see Fig. 10.10D), but palpable purpura (often painful) usually indicates vasculitis (Fig. 14.8A) and necessitates exclusion of vasculitic inflammation in other organs. Purpura elicitable by pinching the skin ('pinch purpura') may be indicative of Amyloidosis light chain (AL) (see Fig. 14.8B).

In those individuals with skin pigmentation at the darker end of the spectrum, there is the added possibility of increased or decreased colour (hyper- or hypopigmentation) consequent to inflammation (Figs 14.9 and 14.10). Disorders characterised by reduced pigmentation, such as vitiligo (see Fig. 3.10), are more obvious in dark skin.

14

A                                                    B

**Fig. 14.8 Purpura.** ⟦A⟧ Cutaneous vasculitis. ⟦B⟧ AL (light chain) amyloidosis.

A

B

**Fig. 14.9** ⟦A⟧ Hyperpigmentation within antecubital fossa secondary to atopic eczema. ⟦B⟧ Post-inflammatory hypopigmentation in pityriasis alba on the cheek.

## Specific features

There are also a number of subtle clinical signs that can be of great diagnostic help in common rashes, such as the distinctive silver-coloured scale that appears when psoriasis is scratched (Fig. 14.11AB), the urtication that develops when the pigmented lesions of urticaria pigmentosa (a form of cutaneous mastocytosis) are rubbed (Darier's sign), the separation of the epidermis

A                                                    B

**Fig. 14.10** Pityriasis versicolor ⟦A⟧ in Caucasian skin (where affected skin is lightly pigmented). ⟦B⟧ in Afro-Caribbean skin (where affected skin is hypopigmented).

on applying a shearing force in pemphigus (Nikolsky's sign), and the very earliest lesions of lichen planus glinting in reflected light (see Fig. 14.11C).

Scratch marks (excoriations) indicate an itchy rash. In any pruritic eruption, it is prudent to look specifically for the burrows of scabies (Fig. 14.12AB) on the hands and feet, as well as to test for dermographism and examine for lymphadenopathy (p. 34), as urticaria and lymphoma are also important causes of itch.

## Morphology of lesions

Lesions should be measured and described according to their anatomical location, colour, symmetry, surface texture, consistency, demarcation of margin, tenderness and whether they are freely mobile or attached to underlying tissue (p. 329). Remember to examine the regional lymph nodes.

A

B

C

**Fig. 14.11** Specific signs [A] Psoriasis before surface rubbing. [B] After surface rubbing. [C] Lichen planus showing light reflection from small early lesions.

A

B

**Fig. 14.12** **Scabies burrows.** [A] A tortuous burrow. [B] Through the dermatoscope, individual mites are visible as small, dark arrowheads.

An irregularly roughened, jagged surface texture is often indicative of sunlight-induced damage (actinic keratosis), whereas the surface of a seborrhoeic keratosis (Fig. 14.13) has a smoother feel. The consistency of a lesion is often of diagnostic help: for example, the firm, button-like quality of a dermatofibroma is very characteristic; neurofibromas are rather soft (see Fig. 3.20); calcium deposits are hard; and cysts fluctuate and transilluminate. Basal cell carcinoma, the most common malignant tumour, is usually smooth (but may ulcerate); on inspection, it exhibits a milky, pearlescent colour (which may glint) and irregular telangiectasia (Fig. 14.14).

It is reassuring to see hair growing out of a pigmented lesion, as this usually indicates a benign process such as a melanocytic naevus. However, the possibility that a pigmented lesion is a malignant melanoma (Fig. 14.15), a potentially life-threatening cutaneous malignancy, should always be considered. The acronym ABCDE refers to features in a skin lesion that might suggest a melanoma:

- **A**symmetry
- **B**order irregularity
- **C**olour variation
- **D**iameter >6 mm, **D**ark or **D**ifferent
- **E**volving or changing

**Fig. 14.13** Seborrhoeic keratosis: multiple lesions over the temple and zygomatic regions.

**Fig. 14.15** Malignant melanoma.

A

B

**Fig 14.14** Basal cell carcinoma. **A** Viewed with the naked eye. **B** Dermatoscopy highlights distinctive telangiectasia.

Despite its origin from melanocytes, melanoma may occasionally lack pigment (amelanotic melanoma). The *ugly duckling* sign refers to pigmented lesions that immediately stand out as being different, and that therefore should be considered suspicious.

## Mouth, hair and nail signs

General physical examination of the skin should always include the oral cavity, hair and nails.

Inspection of the oral mucous membranes may reveal diagnostic clues such as the lace-like patterning of lichen planus (Fig. 14.4C), or the erosions of pemphigus. Gum hygiene may alert to the possibility of a nutritional deficiency such as scurvy (see Fig 3.19A).

Is there excess hair, either in a male pattern distribution (hirsutism) or not (hypertrichosis), or hair loss (alopecia)? Hirsutism may be a marker for hyperandrogenism. Hypertrichosis may be seen in malnutrition states, malignancy and porphyria cutanea tarda. Discrete, coin-sized areas of hair loss, with small 'exclamation mark' hairs at the periphery, are characteristic of alopecia areata (Fig. 14.16), an autoimmune disorder that may coexist with other autoimmune disorders. Diffuse, pronounced hair shedding (telogen effluvium) may be a physiological response to severe illness, major surgical operations, or childbirth and may be accompanied by transverse grooves on the fingernails, which gradually grow out normally (Beau's lines; see Fig. 3.7B).

Common abnormalities of the nails associated with underlying disease are covered on page 26 and in Box 3.3 and Fig. 3.7.

Some rare diseases produce specific nail appearances, such as the 'ragged cuticles' and abnormal capillary nail-bed loops associated with dermatomyositis (Fig. 14.17AB), and the progressive thickening and opacification of nails in yellow nail syndrome (Fig. 14.18).

**Fig. 14.16** Alopecia areata.

14

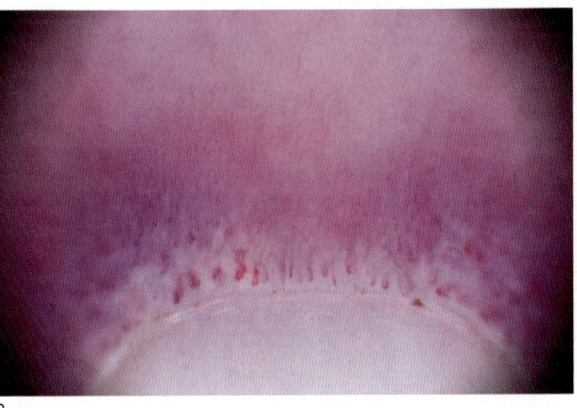

A

B

**Fig. 14.17** Nail appearances in systemic diseases. [A] The typical linear pattern of dermatomyositis with Gottren's papules on the dorsum of the hand. [B] Nail-fold telangiectasia in dermatomyositis, viewed through the dermatoscope.

**Fig. 14.18** Yellow nail syndrome in a patient with lymphoedema and pleural effusions.

**Fig. 14.19** Dermatoscope.

## Supplementary examination techniques

It is often necessary to complement naked-eye observation of the skin with assisted examination techniques, such as dermatoscopy, diascopy and Wood's lamp.

### Dermatoscopy

A dermatoscope consists of a powerful light source (polarised or non-polarised) and a magnifying lens, and enables considerably more cutaneous anatomical detail to be seen (Fig. 14.19).

Dermatoscopy is particularly useful in the assessment of pigmented lesions but is also often of great help in assessing other skin tumours, hair disorders and certain infections (scabies, viral warts and molluscum contagiosum).

### Diascopy

The pressure of a glass slide on the skin will compress the cutaneous blood vessels and blanch the area of contact. If blood is still visible through the glass, it is because red blood cells have extravasated (purpura). When granulomatous disorders (such as sarcoidosis or granuloma annulare) are diascoped, they typically manifest a green–brown ('apple jelly') colour.

### Wood's lamp

Examination of the skin using an ultraviolet light (Wood's lamp) is useful in two clinical situations: it enhances the contrast between normal skin and under - or over-pigmented epidermis (making conditions such as vitiligo and melasma easier to see); and it can identify certain infections by inducing the causative organisms to fluoresce (such as erythrasma, pityriasis versicolor and some ringworm infections).

## Investigations

After clinical examination, specific investigative techniques may be necessary in some cases to enable a precise diagnosis.

### Skin biopsy

This involves a sample of skin being removed under local anaesthesia and subjected to histological or immunohistochemical examination in the laboratory. However, clinicopathological correlation is usually necessary.

### Mycology

A fungal infection can be confirmed (or refuted) by scraping scale from the surface of a rash with a scalpel blade, clipping samples of nail or plucking hair, and undertaking microscopic examination and culture.

### Patch testing

Patch testing (Fig. 14.20) is performed to establish whether a contact allergy is the cause of an individual's rash. It involves applying putative allergens to the patient's skin, leaving the test patches undisturbed for 2 days, removing them and then reading the final result after 4 days. A positive result is indicated by an inflammatory reaction at the site of the patch.

**Fig. 14.20** Patch testing.

## OSCE Example 2: Pigmented lesion

Ms Forsythe, 55 years old, presents with a 6-week history of a changing pigmented lesion on her right calf.

### Please examine her skin

- Introduce yourself to the patient and clean your hands.
- Ask her to undress to underwear.
- Carry out a general inspection of the skin, estimating her Fitzpatrick skin type, and observing for signs of actinic damage and for other lesions that might require close assessment.
- Observe the lesion on her calf for size, symmetry, regularity of margins, variation of pigmentation and ulceration.
- Palpate the lesion.
- Examine for enlargement of regional lymph nodes.
- Examine the abdomen for an enlarged liver.
- Undertake a similar examination of any other suspicious lesions.
- Thank the patient and clean your hands.

### Suggest a differential diagnosis

Any changing pigmented lesion should raise suspicion of malignant melanoma, although melanocytic naevi, seborrhoeic keratoses, dermatofibromas, haemangiomas and pigmented basal cell carcinomas can cause diagnostic confusion.

### Suggested investigations

If, after examination, there is still suspicion regarding the malignant potential of the lesion, it should be excised for histological examination.

## OSCE Example 1: Pruritus

Mr Hassan, 45 years old, presents with a 4-month history of intense itch disturbing his sleep.

### Please examine his skin

- Introduce yourself to the patient and clean your hands.
- Ask him to undress to underwear.
- Carry out a general inspection, observing for the presence of a rash, scratch marks (and whether they are symmetrical), colour and dryness of the skin, pallor, jaundice, exophthalmos or goitre.
- Palpate the pulse for tachycardia and atrial fibrillation.
- Examine the hands and insteps for scabietic burrows, fine tremor, thyroid acropachy and koilonychia.
- Examine the abdomen for an enlarged liver or spleen.
- Examine the mouth for a smooth tongue or angular cheilitis.
- Test for dermographism.
- Examine for lymphadenopathy.
- Thank the patient and clean your hands.

### Suggest a differential diagnosis

Intense pruritus may be caused by dermatoses such as scabies and dermatitis herpetiformis but also by systemic disorders such as polycythaemia, iron deficiency, liver or renal dysfunction, hyper- or hypothyroidism, and lymphoma. The absence of a rash suggests a systemic cause for the itch.

### Suggest investigations

Full blood count; renal, liver and thyroid function tests; ferritin level and chest x-ray.

## Integrated examination sequence for the skin

- Prepare the patient:
  - Arrange for privacy.
  - Arrange for a chaperone, if necessary.
  - Remove sufficient clothing.
  - Remove makeup and wigs, if face and scalp are being examined.
- Carry out a general examination of the skin:
  - Look for excoriations, xerosis (dry skin), actinic damage and suspicious lesions, for example.
- Carry out a specific examination of a rash:
  - Extent.
  - Distribution: symmetry, pattern.
  - Morphology.
  - Colour.
  - Erythema/purpura.
  - Specific features, e.g. scale, signs of infection/infestation.
  - Mouth, hair and nails.
  - Regional lymph nodes.
- Carry out a specific examination of a lesion:
  - Site, size, colour.
  - Symmetry.
  - Surface texture.
  - Consistency.
  - Mobility.
  - Pattern of vasculature.
  - Regional lymph nodes.

# Section 3

## Applying history and examination skills in specific situations

15. Babies and children  341

16. Patients with mental illness and learning disability  367

17. The frail patient  379

18. The deteriorating patient  393

19. The dying patient  405

**Ben Stenson**
**Steve Cunningham**

# Babies and Children

**Babies 342**

**The history 342**
Maternal history 342
Pregnancy history 342
Birth history 342
Infant's progress 342
Presenting problems and definitions 342

**The physical examination of newborns 343**
Timing and efficacy of the routine neonatal examination 343
General examination 343
Cardiovascular examination 346
Respiratory examination 347
Abdominal examination 348
Neurological examination 349
Limbs 351
Weighing and measuring 352
Final inspection 352

**The physical examination of infants beyond the newborn period 352**

**Older children 353**

**The history 353**
Obtaining a history from children and young people compared with adults 353
Common presenting symptoms 353
Past medical history 356

Birth history 356
Vaccination history 356
Developmental history 356
Drug history 356
Family and social history 356
Systematic enquiry 357

**The physical examination 357**
Normal growth and development 357
Physical examination techniques in children and young people 359
The acutely unwell children and young people 360
General examination 360
Ears, nose and throat 361
Cardiovascular examination 362
Respiratory examination 362
Abdominal examination 362
Neurological examination 364
Spotting the sick children and young people 364

**Child protection 364**

**Remote consultation in paediatric practice 364**

**OSCE example 1: Diarrhoea 365**

**OSCE example 2: Chronic cough 365**

**Integrated examination sequence for the newborn child 366**

# BABIES

A baby is a neonate for its first 4 weeks and an infant for its first year. Neonates are classified by gestational age or birthweight (Box 15.1).

# The history

Ask the mother and look in the maternal notes for relevant history:

## Maternal history

Is there a family history of significant illness (e.g. diabetes, hereditary illnesses)? What were the outcomes of any previous pregnancies?

## Pregnancy history

How was the maternal health in pregnancy? Did the mother take medications or other drugs?

What did any antenatal screening tests show?

## Birth history

What was the birthweight, gestation at birth and mode of delivery? Was there prolonged rupture of the fetal membranes or maternal pyrexia? Was there a nonreassuring fetal status during delivery or meconium staining of the amniotic fluid? Was resuscitation required after birth? What were the Apgar scores (Box 15.2) and the results of umbilical cord blood gas tests?

## Infant's progress

Has the infant fed well? Has the infant passed meconium and urine since birth? In later infancy, what are the specific signs and systems and developmental progress, depending on the presenting problem?

### 15.1 Classification of newborn infants

**Birthweight**

- Extremely low birthweight (ELBW): <1000 g
- Very low birthweight (VLBW): <1500 g
- Low birthweight (LBW): <2500 g
- Normal: ≥2500 g

**Gestational age**

- Extremely preterm: <28 weeks
- Preterm: <37 weeks (<259th day)
- Term: 37–42 weeks
- Post-term: >42 weeks (>294th day)

### 15.2 Apgar score

| Clinical score | 0 | 1 | 2 |
|---|---|---|---|
| Heart rate | Absent | ≤100 bpm | >100 bpm |
| Respiratory effort | Absent | Slow and irregular | Good: strong |
| Muscle tone | Flaccid | Some flexion of arms and legs | Active movement |
| Reflex irritability | No responses | Grimace | Vigorous crying, sneeze or cough |
| Colour | Blue, pale | Pink body, blue extremities | Pink all over |

Add scores for each line; maximum score is 10.
*bpm,* Beats per minute.
Reproduced with permission: APGAR V, A proposal for a new method of evaluation of the newborn infant. *Curr Res Anesth Analg.* 1953;32(4):260–267.

## Presenting problems and definitions

Infants cannot report symptoms, so you must recognise the presenting problems and signs of illness, which are nonspecific in young infants. Always take the concerns of parents seriously.

### Pallor

Always investigate pallor in a newborn, as it implies anaemia or poor perfusion. Newborn infants have higher haemoglobin levels than older children and are not normally pale. Haemoglobin levels of less than 120 g/L (<12 g/dL) in the perinatal period are low. Preterm infants look red because they lack subcutaneous fat.

### Respiratory distress

Respiratory distress is tachypnoea (respiratory rate) greater than 60 breaths per minute, with intercostal and subcostal indrawing, sternal recession, nasal flaring and the use of accessory muscles.

### Cyanosis

Bluish discoloration of the lips and mucous membranes due to hypoxia is difficult to see in newborn infants unless oxygen saturation ($SpO_2$) is less than 80% (normal is ≥95%). Causes include congenital heart disease and respiratory disease. Cyanosis always needs investigation (p. 30).

### Acrocyanosis

Acrocyanosis is a bluish-purple discoloration of the hands and feet and is a normal finding, provided the newborn is centrally pink.

## Jaundice

Many newborns develop jaundice in the days after birth. Look for yellow sclerae in newborns with coloured skin, or you may miss it. Examine the baby in bright normal light. Normal physiological jaundice cannot be distinguished clinically from jaundice from a pathological cause. Newborn infants with jaundice require a bilirubin measurement to assess the need for further investigation and possible treatment.

## Jitteriness

Jitteriness is high-frequency tremor of the limbs and is common in term infants in the first few days. It is stilled by stimulating the infant and is not associated with other disturbance. If jitteriness is excessive, exclude hypoglycaemia, polycythaemia and neonatal abstinence syndrome (drug withdrawal). Infrequent jerks in light sleep are common and normal; regular clonic jerks are abnormal.

## Dysmorphism

Identifying abnormal body structure (dysmorphism) is subjective because of human variability. Individual features may be minor and isolated or may signify a major problem requiring investigation and management. A recognisable pattern of several dysmorphic features together may indicate a 'dysmorphic syndrome' such as Down's syndrome (p. 36). Use caution and sensitivity when discussing possible dysmorphism with parents of a newborn child.

## Hypotonia

Hypotonia (reduced tone) may be obvious when you handle an infant. Term infants' muscle tone normally produces a flexed posture at the hips, knees and elbows. Hypotonic infants may lack this flexion. Hypotonia can occur with hypoxia, hypoglycaemia or sepsis, or may be due to a specific brain, nerve or muscle problem. Preterm infants have lower tone than term infants and are less flexed.

## Apgar score

This first clinical assessment of a neonate is made immediately after birth. Tone, colour, breathing, heart rate and response to stimulation are each scored 0, 1 or 2 (see Box 15.2), giving a maximum total of 10. Healthy neonates commonly score 8 to 10 at 1 and 5 minutes. The score predicts the need for, and efficacy of, resuscitation. A low score should increase with time; a decreasing score is a cause for concern. Persistently low scores at 10 minutes predict death or later disability. Neonates with scores of less than 8 at 5 minutes require continued evaluation until it is clear they are healthy.

# The physical examination of newborns

## Timing and efficacy of the routine neonatal examination

Examine a newborn with the parents present. There is no ideal time. If it is performed on day 1, some forms of congenital heart disease may be missed because signs have not developed. If it is delayed, some babies will present before the examination with illness that may have been detectable earlier. Approximately 9% of neonates have an identifiable congenital abnormality, but most are not serious. Always record your examination comprehensively to avoid problems if illness or physical abnormality is identified later. Fewer than half of all cases of congenital heart disease or congenital cataract are detected by newborn examination.

## General examination

Examine babies and infants in a warm place on a firm bed or examination table. Have a system to avoid omitting anything, but avoid an overly rigid approach as you may be unable to perform key elements if you unsettle the baby. Do things that may disturb the baby later in the examination sequence.

## Examination sequence

- Observe whether the baby looks well and is well grown.
- Look for:
  - cyanosis
  - respiratory distress
  - pallor
  - plethora (suggesting polycythaemia).
- Note posture and behaviour.
- Note any dysmorphic features.
- Auscultate the heart and palpate the abdomen if the baby is quiet.
- If the baby cries, does the cry sound normal?

## Skin

### Normal findings

The skin may look normal, dry, wrinkled or vernix covered in healthy babies. There may be meconium staining of the skin and nails.

Prominent capillaries commonly cause pink areas called 'stork's beak marks' at the nape of the neck, eyelids and glabella (Fig. 15.1). Facial marks fade spontaneously over months; those on the neck often persist. Milia (fine white spots) and acne neonatorum (larger cream-coloured spots) are collected glandular secretions and disappear within 2 to 4 weeks. Erythema toxicum is a common fleeting, blanching, idiopathic maculopapular rash of no consequence, affecting the trunk, face and limbs in the first few days after birth.

15

**Fig. 15.1** Stork's beak mark.

**Fig. 15.2** Mongolian blue spot.

### Abnormal findings

Document any trauma such as scalp cuts or bruising.

Dense capillary haemangiomas (port-wine stains) will not fade. Referral to a dermatologist is advisable as laser treatment may help in some cases. Around the eye, they may indicate Sturge–Weber syndrome (a facial port-wine stain with an underlying brain lesion, associated with risk of later seizures, cerebral calcification and reduced cognitive function). Melanocytic naevi require follow-up and treatment by a plastic surgeon or dermatologist. A Mongolian blue spot (Fig. 15.2) is an area of bluish discolouration over the buttocks, back and thighs. Easily mistaken for bruising, it usually fades in the first year.

Subcutaneous fat necrosis causes palpable firm plaques, often with some erythema under the skin. If extensive, there can be associated hypercalcaemia that may require treatment. Blisters or bullae are usually pathological.

## Head

### Examination sequence

- Note the baby's head shape (Box 15.3) and any swellings.
- Feel the anterior fontanelle (Fig. 15.3). Is it sunken, flat or bulging?
- Palpate the cranial sutures.

### Normal findings

Transient elongation of the head is common from moulding during birth. Caput succedaneum is soft-tissue swelling over the vertex due to pressure in labour. Overriding cranial sutures have a palpable step.

### Abnormal findings

Cephalhaematoma is a firm, immobile, usually parietal swelling caused by a localised haemorrhage under the cranial periosteum. It may be bilateral, and periosteal reaction at the margins causes a raised edge. No treatment is required. Do not confuse this with the boggy, mobile, poorly localised swelling of subgaleal

| 15.3 Neonatal head shapes | |
|---|---|
| **Head shape** | **Description** |
| Microcephalic (small headed) | Small cranial vault |
| Megalencephalic (large headed) | Large cranial vault |
| Hydrocephalic (water headed) | Large cranial vault due to enlarged ventricles |
| Brachycephalic (short headed) | Flat head around the occiput |
| Dolichocephalic (long headed) | Head that looks long relative to its width |
| Plagiocephalic (oblique headed) | Asymmetrical skull |

haemorrhage (beneath the flat sheet of fibrous tissue that caps the skull), which can conceal a large blood loss and is life-threatening if unrecognised.

Separated cranial sutures with an obvious gap indicate raised intracranial pressure. Rarely, the cranial sutures are prematurely fused (synostosis), producing ridging, and the head shape is usually abnormal. Abnormal head size requires detailed investigation, including neuroimaging.

## Eyes

### Examination sequence

- Inspect the eyebrows, lashes, lids and eyeballs.
- Gently retract the lower eyelid, and check the sclera for jaundice.
- Test ocular movements and vestibular function:

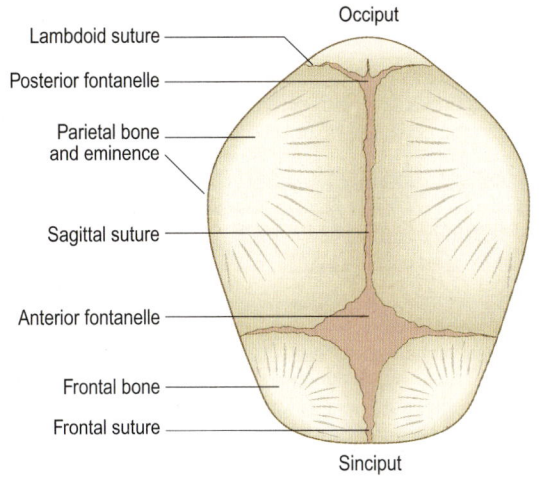

Fig. 15.3 The fetal skull from above.

- Turn the newborn's head to one side; watch as the eyes move in the opposite direction. These are called doll's-eye movements (see Fig. 8.15, p. 165).
- Hold the infant upright at arm's length and move them in a horizontal arc. The infant should look in the direction of movement and have optokinetic nystagmus. This response becomes damped by 3 months.

### Normal findings

Harmless yellow crusting without inflammation is common after birth in infants, due to narrow lacrimal ducts.

Term infants usually fix visually.

### Abnormal findings

Eye infection gives a red eye and purulent secretions. An abnormal pupil shape is usually a coloboma (a defect in the iris inferiorly that gives the pupil a keyhole appearance, Fig. 15.4). This can also affect deeper structures, including the optic nerve, and lead to visual impairment. It can be associated with syndromes, as can microphthalmia (small eyeballs). Large eyeballs that feel hard when palpated through the lids suggest congenital glaucoma (buphthalmos).

### *Ophthalmoscopy*

## Examination sequence

- Hold the baby in your arms. Turn your body from side to side, and the movement will encourage the baby to open their eyes.
- Look at each pupil from about 20 cm through the ophthalmoscope. You should see the red reflex of reflected light from the retina.

### Normal findings

Puffy eyes in the first days after birth impede the examination. If this happens, always examine again later because failure

Fig. 15.4 Coloboma.

to detect and treat a cataract will cause permanent amblyopia.

### Abnormal findings

An absent red reflex suggests cataract; refer to an ophthalmologist.

## Nose

## Examination sequence

- Exclude obstructed nostrils (choanal atresia) by blocking each nostril in turn with your finger to check that the infant breathes easily through the other.

## Mouth

## Examination sequence

- Gently press down on the lower jaw so that the baby will open the mouth.
- Shine a torch into the mouth and look at the tongue and palate. If you need to use a tongue depressor to obtain a clear view of the palate, it should be a sterile single-patient use item.
- Palpate the palate using your fingertip.

### Normal findings

Epstein's pearls are small, white mucosal cysts on the palate that disappear spontaneously.

White coating on the tongue that is easily scraped off with a swab is usually curdled milk.

### Abnormal findings

Ankyloglossia (tongue tie) is when the lingual frenulum joining the underside of the tongue to the floor of the mouth is so short that it interferes with feeding. It should not be diagnosed if feeding is

15

satisfactory. A white coating on the tongue, which is not easily removed and may bleed when scraped, is caused by *Candida albicans* (thrush). Macroglossia (a large protruding tongue) occurs in Beckwith–Wiedemann syndrome. A normal-sized tongue protrudes through a small mouth in Down's syndrome (glossoptosis).

Cleft palate may involve the soft palate or both hard and soft palates. It can be midline, unilateral or bilateral and may also involve the gum (alveolus). Cleft lip can appear in isolation or in association with it. Refer affected infants early to a specialist multidisciplinary cleft team. Micrognathia (a small jaw) is sometimes associated with cleft palate in the Pierre Robin syndrome, with posterior displacement of the tongue and upper airway obstruction.

A ranula is a mucous cyst on the floor of the mouth that is related to the sublingual or submandibular salivary ducts. Congenital ranulas may resolve spontaneously but sometimes require surgery.

Teeth usually begin to erupt at around 6 months but can be present at birth.

## Ears

### Examination sequence

- Note the size, shape and position.
- The helix should attach above an imaginary line around the head, level with the inner corners of the eyes.
- Check that the external auditory meatus looks normal.

#### Normal findings

The helix can be temporarily folded due to local pressure in utero. Preauricular skin tags do not require investigation.

#### Abnormal findings

Abnormal ear shape and position is a feature of some syndromes.

## Neck

### Examination sequence

- Inspect the neck for asymmetry, sinuses and swellings.
- Palpate any masses. Use 'SPACESPIT' (see Chapter 3, p. 34) to interpret your findings.
- Transilluminate swellings. Cystic swellings glow, as the light is transmitted through clear liquid. Solid or blood-filled swellings do not.

#### Normal findings

One-third of normal neonates have palpable cervical, inguinal or axillary lymph nodes. Neck asymmetry is often due to fetal posture and usually resolves.

#### Abnormal findings

A lump in the sternocleidomastoid muscle (sternomastoid 'tumour') is caused by a fibrosed haematoma with resultant muscle shortening. This may produce torticollis, with the head turned in the contralateral direction. Refer for physiotherapy.

## Cardiovascular examination

### Examination sequence

- Observe the baby for pallor, cyanosis and sweating.
- Count the respiratory rate.
- Palpate for the apex beat with your palm in the midclavicular line in the fourth or fifth intercostal space.
- Note if the heart beat moves your hand up and down (parasternal heave) or if you feel a vibration (thrill).
- Count the heart rate for 15 seconds, and multiply by 4.
- Feel the femoral pulses by placing your thumbs or fingertips over the midinguinal points while abducting the hips (Fig. 15.5).
- Auscultate the heart. Start at the apex using the stethoscope bell (best for low-pitched sounds). Then use the diaphragm in all positions for high-pitched sounds and murmurs (Fig. 15.6).
- Describe the heart sounds $S_1$ and $S_2$, any additional heart sounds and the presence of murmurs. The fast heart rate of a newborn makes it difficult to time additional sounds. Take time to tune into the different rate of the harsh breath sounds of a newborn, as they are easily confused with a murmur.
- Do not measure the blood pressure of healthy babies. In ill babies, cuff measurements overestimate the values when compared with invasive measurements. The cuff width should be at least two-thirds of the distance from the elbow to the shoulder tip.
- Palpate the abdomen for hepatomegaly (see later).

**Fig. 15.5 Palpating the femoral pulses.** The pulse can be difficult to feel at first. Use a point halfway between the pubic tubercle and the anterior superior iliac spine as a guide.

**Fig. 15.6 Auscultation positions in infants and children.** Recommended order of auscultation: **1**, apex; **2**, left lower sternal edge; **3**, left upper sternal edge; **4**, left infraclavicular; **5**, right upper sternal edge; **6**, right lower sternal edge; **7**, right mid-axillary line; **8**, right side of neck; **9**, left side of neck; **10**, posteriorly.

### Normal findings

In the early newborn period, the femoral pulses may feel normal in an infant who later presents with coarctation because an open ductus arteriosus can maintain flow to the descending aorta. Routine measurement of postductal oxygen saturation is increasingly popular as an additional newborn screening test for congenital heart disease. Lower limb $SpO_2$ should be 95% or higher.

Heart rates between 80 and 160 beats per minute (bpm) can be normal in the newborn, depending on the arousal state (Box 15.4).

### Abnormal findings

Infants with heart failure typically look pale and sweaty and have respiratory distress (p. 342).

If the apex beat is displaced laterally, there may be cardiomegaly, or mediastinal shift due to contralateral pneumothorax or pleural effusion.

Weak or absent femoral pulses suggest coarctation of the aorta. Radiofemoral delay is not identifiable in the newborn.

| 15.4 Normal ranges for heart and respiratory rate in the newborn | | |
|---|---|---|
| Sign | Preterm neonate | Term neonate |
| Heart rate (beats per minute) | 120–160 | 100–140 |
| Respiratory rate (breaths per minute) | 40–60 | 30–50 |

Patent ductus arteriosus may cause a short systolic murmur in the early days of life because the pulmonary and systemic blood pressures are similar, which limits shunting through the duct. As the pulmonary vascular resistance diminishes over subsequent weeks or months, the murmur progressively lengthens to become the continuous 'machinery' murmur recognised later in childhood.

Transient murmurs are heard in up to 2% of neonates, but only a minority have a structural heart problem. An echocardiogram is needed to make a structural diagnosis.

## Respiratory examination

### Examination sequence

- Note chest shape and symmetry of chest movement.
- Count the respiratory rate (for 15 seconds and multiply by 4).
- Listen for additional noises with breathing.
- Look for signs of respiratory distress: tachypnoea; suprasternal, intercostal and subcostal recession; flaring of the nostrils.
- Remember that percussion of the newborn's chest is not helpful.
- Use the diaphragm to auscultate anteriorly, laterally and posteriorly, comparing the sides. Breath sounds in the healthy newborn have a bronchial quality compared with older individuals (p. 98).

### Normal findings

Male and female newborn infants at term have small buds of palpable breast tissue. Small amounts of fluid are sometimes discharged from the nipple in the early days after birth.

### Abnormal findings

Stridor indicates large airway obstruction and is predominantly inspiratory (p. 210). Stridor and indrawing beginning on days 2 to 3 of life in an otherwise well baby may be due to laryngomalacia (softness of the larynx). Causes of respiratory distress include retained lung fluid, infection, immaturity, aspiration, congenital anomaly, pneumothorax, heart failure and metabolic acidosis.

**15**

## Abdominal examination

### Examination sequence

- Remove the nappy.
- Inspect the abdomen, including the umbilicus and groins, noting any swellings.
- From the infant's right side, gently palpate with the flat of your warm right hand. Palpate superficially before feeling for deeper structures.
- Palpate for splenomegaly. In the neonate the spleen enlarges down the left flank, not towards the right iliac fossa.
- Palpate for hepatomegaly:
  - Place your right hand flat across the abdomen beneath the right costal margin.
  - Feel the liver edge against the side of your index finger.
  - If you feel more than the liver edge, measure the distance in the mid-clavicular line from the costal margin to the liver edge. Describe it in fingerbreadths or measure it with a tape in centimetres.
- Check that the anus is present, patent and normally positioned.
- Digital rectal examination is usually unnecessary and could cause an anal fissure. Indications include suspected rectal atresia or stenosis and delayed passage of meconium. Put on gloves and lubricate your little finger. Gently press your fingertip against the anus until you feel the muscle resistance relax and insert your finger up to your distal interphalangeal joint.

### Normal findings

Abdominal distension from a feed or swallowed air is common.

You may see the contour of individual bowel loops through the thin anterior abdominal wall in the newborn, particularly with intestinal obstruction.

The umbilical cord stump usually separates after 4 to 5 days. A granuloma may appear later as a moist, pink lump in the base of the umbilicus. A small amount of bleeding from the umbilicus is common in the neonate.

The liver edge is often palpable in healthy infants.

In the neonate the kidneys are often palpable, especially if ballotted.

### Abnormal findings

In excessive umbilical bleeding, check that the infant received vitamin K and consider factor XIII deficiency. Spreading erythema around the umbilicus suggests infective omphalitis and requires urgent treatment.

Umbilical hernias are common; they are easily reduced, have a very low risk of complications and close spontaneously in infancy. An omphalocoele, or exomphalos (Fig. 15.7), is a herniation through the umbilicus containing intestines and other viscera, covered by a membrane that includes the umbilical cord. It may be associated with other malformations or chromosomal abnormality. Gastroschisis is a defect in the anterior abdominal wall with intestines herniated through it, without a covering

**Fig. 15.7** Small exomphalos with loops of bowel in the umbilicus. *From Lissauer T, Clayden G. Illustrated Textbook of Paediatrics. 2nd edn. Edinburgh: Mosby; 2001.*

**Fig. 15.8** Bilateral inguinal hernias in a preterm infant. An inguinal hernia is primarily a groin swelling; only when it is large does it extend into the scrotum. *From Lissauer T, Clayden G. Illustrated Textbook of Paediatrics. 2nd edn. Edinburgh: Mosby; 2001.*

membrane. The most common site is above and to the right of the umbilicus.

Inguinal hernias are common in the newborn, especially in boys and preterm infants (Fig. 15.8).

Meconium in the nappy does not guarantee that the baby has a patent anus because meconium can be passed through a rectovaginal fistula.

## Perineum

### Examination sequence

#### Female

- Abduct the legs, and gently separate the labia.
- In preterm infants the labia minora appear prominent, giving a masculinised appearance that resolves spontaneously over a few weeks. Milky vaginal secretions are normal. Later in the

first week, there is sometimes slight vaginal bleeding (pseudomenses) as the infant uterus 'withdraws' from maternal hormones. Vaginal skin tags are common and do not require treatment.

## Male

- Do not attempt to retract the foreskin. It is normal for it to be adherent in babies.
- Check that the urethral meatus is at the tip of the penis.
- Note the shape of the penis.
- Palpate the testes.
- If you cannot feel the testes in the scrotum, assess for undescended, ectopic or retractile testes. Palpate the abdomen for smooth lumps, moving your fingers down over the inguinal canal to the scrotum and perineum.
- A retractile testis just below the inguinal canal may be gently milked into the scrotum. Re-examine at 6 weeks if there is any doubt about the position of the testes.
- Transilluminate any large scrotal swellings using a torch to see if the light is transmitted through the swelling. This suggests a hydrocoele but can be misleading because a hernia of thin-walled bowel may transilluminate (Fig. 15.9).
- An inguinal hernia usually produces a groin swelling, but, if large, this may extend into the scrotum. Try to reduce it by gently pushing the contents upwards from the scrotum through the inguinal canal into the abdomen.

### Normal findings

The testes are smooth and soft and measure 0.7 × 1 cm across. The right testis usually descends later than the left and sits higher in the scrotum.

### Abnormal findings

A hydrocoele is a collection of fluid beneath the tunica vaginalis of the testis and/or the spermatic cord (p. 266). Most resolve spontaneously in infancy.

**Fig. 15.9 How to transilluminate a scrotal swelling.**

In hypospadias the meatal opening is on the ventral aspect of the glans, the ventral shaft of the penis or the scrotum or more posteriorly on the perineum (Figs 15.10 and 15.11A). In epispadias, which is rare, it is on the dorsum of the penis. Chordee is curvature of the penis and is commonly associated with hypospadias and tethering of the foreskin (see Fig. 15.11B).

## Spine and sacrum

### Examination sequence

- Turn the baby over.
- Inspect and palpate the entire vertebral column from neck to sacrum for neural tube defects.

### Normal findings

Sacral dimples are common and unimportant, provided the dimple base has normal skin and they are single, less than 5 mm in diameter and less than 2.5 cm from the anus.

### Abnormal findings

Pigmented patches may indicate spina bifida occulta. Dimples above the natal cleft, away from the midline, or hairy or pigmented patches with a base that cannot be visualised require further investigation.

## Neurological examination

This includes tone, posture, movement and primitive reflexes.

## General neurological assessment

### Examination sequence

- Look for asymmetry in posture and movement and for muscle wasting.
- To assess tone, pick the baby up and note if they are stiff or floppy. Note any difference between each side.
- Power is difficult to assess and depends on the state of arousal. Look for strong symmetrical limb and trunk movements and grasp.
- Tendon reflexes are of value only in assessing infants with neurological or muscular abnormalities.
- Check sensation by seeing whether the baby withdraws from gentle stimuli. Do not inflict painful stimuli or use a pin or needle.
- Check eyesight by carrying the alert baby to a dark corner. This normally causes the eyes to open wide. In a bright area the baby will screw up their eyes.

Ideally, electronic audiological screening should also be performed in the newborn period.

### Normal findings

Movements should be equal on both sides.
Tone varies and may be floppy after a feed.

15

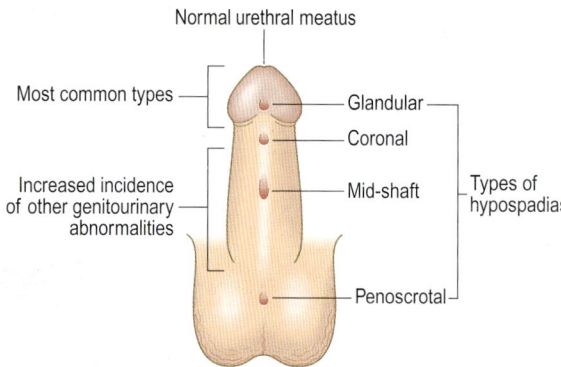

**Fig. 15.10** Varieties of hypospadias.

A                    B

**Fig. 15.11** **Hypospadias and chordee.** A Penile shaft hypospadias. B Lateral view showing the ventral curvature of the penis (chordee). *From Lissauer T, Clayden G. Illustrated Textbook of Paediatrics. 2nd edn. Edinburgh: Mosby; 2001.*

Reflexes are brisk in term infants, often with a few beats of clonus.

The plantar reflex is normally extensor in the newborn.

## Abnormal findings

Hypotonic infants may have a 'frog-like' posture with abducted hips and extended elbows. Causes include Down's syndrome, meningitis and sepsis.

Increased tone may cause back and neck arching and limb extension; the baby feels stiff when picked up. Causes include meningitis, asphyxia and intracranial haemorrhage.

Brachial plexus injuries include Erb's palsy, which affects brachial plexus roots C5 and C6, producing reduced movement of the arm at the shoulder and elbow, medial rotation of the forearm and failure to extend the wrist (Fig. 15.12). Klumpke's palsy may be seen after breech delivery due to damage to roots C8 and T1, with weakness of the forearm and hand. These injuries can be associated with ipsilateral Horner's syndrome and/ or diaphragmatic weakness in severe cases. Most perinatal brachial plexus injuries recover over subsequent weeks.

Facial nerve palsy causes reduced movement of the cheek muscles, and the side of the mouth does not turn down when the baby cries. Most cases are transient.

**Fig. 15.12** **Erb's palsy.** The right arm is medially rotated and the wrist is flexed. *From Lissauer T, Clayden G. Illustrated Textbook of Paediatrics. 2nd edn. Edinburgh: Mosby; 2001.*

## Primitive reflexes in newborn and young infants

The primitive reflexes are lower motor neurone responses that are present at birth but that become suppressed by higher centres by 4 to 6 months. They may be absent in infants with neurological depression or asymmetrical in infants with nerve injuries. Persistence into later infancy may indicate neurodevelopmental abnormality (p. 353). There are many examples, and there is no need to elicit them all because their individual value is limited.

## Examination sequence

### Grasp responses

- Gently stimulate the palm or sole with your finger to produce a palmar or plantar grasp.

### Ventral suspension/pelvic response to back stimulation

- Hold the baby prone, and look for neck extension. Stroke the skin over the vertebral column to produce an extensor response with pelvic elevation.

### Place-and-step reflexes

- Hold the baby upright, and touch the dorsum of the foot against the edge of a table. The baby will flex the knee and hip, placing the foot on the table (Fig. 15.13A).
- Lower the upright baby towards the table surface. When the feet touch the surface, a walking movement occurs.

**Fig. 15.13** **Primitive reflexes.** **A** Placing reflex. **B** The Moro reflex. **C** Tonic neck reflex.

## Moro reflex

- Support the supine baby's trunk and head in a semi-upright position. Let the head fall backwards slightly. The baby will quickly throw out both arms and spread the fingers (see Fig. 15.13B).

## Root-and-suck responses

- Gently stroke the baby's cheek. The baby turns to that side, and the mouth opens, as though looking for a nipple. This is 'rooting'. If you place your finger in a healthy infant's mouth, they will suck it vigorously.

## Asymmetric tonic neck reflex

- Turn the supine infant's head to the side. The arm and leg on the same side will extend, and the arm and leg on the opposite side will flex. This reflex is present at term and maximal at 1 month (see Fig. 15.13C).

## Limbs

### Examination sequence

- Inspect the limbs, and count the digits.
- If the foot is abnormally positioned, gently try to place it in a normal position. If the abnormal position is at all fixed, refer to a specialist.

- Examine the hips to check for developmental dysplasia of the hip (DDH):
- Lay the baby supine on a firm surface.
- Inspect the skin creases of the thighs for symmetry.
- Examine each hip separately. Hold the thigh with the knee and hip flexed and your thumb on the medial aspect of the thigh.
- Move the proximal end of the thigh laterally, and then push down towards the examining table (Barlow manoeuvre, Fig. 15.14A); a clunk indicates that the hip is dislocatable.
- Now abduct the thigh; if you feel a clunk, this is the head of the femur returning into the acetabulum (Ortolani manoeuvre, Fig. 15.14B). If the femoral head feels lax and you feel a clunk with an Ortolani manoeuvre without first performing the Barlow manoeuvre, then the hip was already dislocated.

### Normal findings

A small percentage of normal babies have single palmar creases, but this is also associated with Down's syndrome (see Fig. 3.31B, p. 40) and other chromosomal abnormalities. Tibial bowing is common in the newborn.

It is common to hear or feel minor ligamentous clicks during hip examination. These are of no consequence and feel quite different to the dislocation and relocation of developmental dysplasia of the hip (DDH). If in any doubt, obtain an expert opinion. Never use the term 'clicky hips'.

A                              B

**Fig. 15.14** Examination for developmental dysplasia of the hip. **A** The hip is dislocated posteriorly out of the acetabulum (Barlow manoeuvre). **B** The dislocated hip is relocated back into the acetabulum (Ortolani manoeuvre).

### Abnormal findings

Oligodactyly (too few digits), polydactyly (too many) or syndactyly (joined digits) may occur. In talipes equinovarus the foot is plantar-flexed and rotated, with the sole facing medially. In talipes calcaneovalgus the foot is dorsiflexed so that the heel is prominent and the sole faces laterally.

Many cases of DDH have associated risk factors, including a family history, breech delivery, positional talipes (especially calcaneovalgus) or oligohydramnios.

Some centres offer hip ultrasound screening.

## Weighing and measuring

### Examination sequence

- Weigh the infant fully undressed using electronic scales accurate to 5 g.
- Use a paper tape to measure the maximal occipitofrontal circumference round the forehead and occiput (Fig. 15.15). Repeat the measurement three times, noting the largest measurement to the nearest millimetre.
- Measure the crown–heel length using a neonatal stadiometer (Fig. 15.16). Ask a parent or assistant to hold the baby's head still, and stretch out the legs until the baby is fully extended (the least reproducible of the three measurements).
- Record the results on a centile chart appropriate to the infant's ethnic background.

### Final inspection

Perform a final top-to-toe inspection to avoid missing anything and to allow the parents a further opportunity to ask questions.

Occipital                              Frontal

**Fig. 15.15** Measurement of head circumference.

**Fig. 15.16** Measuring length accurately in infants.

## The physical examination of infants beyond the newborn period

Examination of young infants beyond the newborn period is similar to the newborn examination. Transient neonatal findings will no longer be present. Older infants are usually happier when examined on their parent's lap than on an examination table. The examination of the ears should include otoscopy (See Fig 15.23). You should check the hips whenever you examine an infant until they are walking normally. After the first few months the Ortolani and Barlow manoeuvres cannot be performed and the most important signs are limitation of abduction in the hip, and thigh skin crease asymmetry. Neurological history and examination should take account of the developmental stage of the child. The primitive reflexes disappear by 4 to 6 months. In later infancy, ask additional questions to obtain information about neurodevelopmental progress (Box 15.5).

## 15.5 Developmental attainment of preschool children at different ages*

| Skills | 4 months | 6 months | 10 months | 1–2 years | 2–3 years | 3–5 years |
|---|---|---|---|---|---|---|
| Gross motor | Has good head control on pull to sit<br>Keeps back straight when held in sitting position | Supports weight on hands when laid prone<br>Rolls front to back | Sits unsupported<br>Pulls to stand | Walks without support | Runs<br>Bounces on trampoline | Pedals a tricycle |
| Fine motor | Opens hands<br>Holds objects placed in hand | Transfers objects from hand to hand and to mouth | Uses pincer grip bilaterally without hand preference | Holds a crayon and scribbles | Can draw a circle | Can draw a cross, square, face/person |
| Personal social | Shows interest in toys<br>Laughs, vocalises | Has a variety of speech noises<br>Plays peep-bo | Starts to understand some words<br>Claps hands | Has 10–20 recognisable words | Can communicate verbally | Has 500–1500 words<br>Is dry by day |

Development is extremely variable and failure to attain only one milestone is of little significance, whereas failure to attain several milestones is cause for concern.

# OLDER CHILDREN

Individuals between 12 months and 16 years are known by nonspecific terms, including toddler, preschool, child, adolescent, teenager or young person. It is important to recognise and acknowledge age-related maturation, and a common phrase to span these years is 'children and young people' (CYP).

# The history

## Obtaining a history from children and young people compared with adults

There are many similarities in taking a history from CYP and from adults. Introduce yourself to the CYP and accompanying adult, and begin your observation of the CYP. Establish who the adult is (e.g. a parent, grandparent or carer), and begin to consider to what extent the CYP will be able to contribute to the history. Let the CYP become accustomed to you before asking specific questions.

Start with open-ended questions. Most often a parent will wish to explain their perspective on the CYP's problem, and it is important to enable them to do so. Young people in particular may wish to explain the problem from their perspective, and it is important to directly and openly engage with the CYP to give this opportunity. Once the presenting symptoms have been outlined, the history should focus on questions that aim to elucidate the differential diagnosis; a CYP is often good at helping with these more specific questions. Respect age and ability to recall events, and adopt a balanced perspective on whether responses from the parents or the CYP are more likely to be accurate for each question. Children younger than 6 years often provide little history, those aged 6 to 11 years can do so if they are sufficiently confident, and those aged 12 years and older should be able to provide a valuable history in the correct environment and with the use of questions that are framed in appropriate terminology. As

you would for adult history taking, include reflective summing up: for example, 'So what you are saying is that …'.

A paediatric history includes elements that are not part of the adult history (obstetric, developmental, immunisation histories), systematic enquiry has different components from those in adults (see later) and the differential diagnosis may include conditions seen only in children (e.g. abdominal migraine, toddler diarrhoea, croup, viral wheeze and febrile convulsion). Most other diagnoses also occur in adults.

## Common presenting symptoms

Diagnosis is built on patterns of symptoms; rarely will any one symptom or sign lead to a 'spot diagnosis'. The initial history suggests a differential diagnosis and prompts additional questions to assess the probability of particular diagnoses. As with adults, presenting symptoms should be described in terms of onset, frequency, severity, duration, aggravating and relieving factors, associated features and impact on function. Pain and the need for analgesia can be particularly difficult to assess in young children; objective scoring systems may help (Box 15.6).

The most common presenting problems in the child affect the respiratory, gastrointestinal and nervous systems (covered in Boxes 15.7–15.9) and the skin.

Skin symptoms can be acute or chronic. Acute-onset rash is common in children and can be described using the same terminology as for adults (see Chapter 14). Those who examine skin rashes in CYP should be able to describe the rash across all skin colours as appearances can be very different (Fig 15.17). An excellent resource (developed by a medical student) is the website www.blackandbrownskin.org.uk.

Most rashes are viral and resolve spontaneously. Rash with blistering is often itchy. It may be urticarial (with an environmental, viral, food or medicine trigger) or an insect bite. Blisters with associated yellow crusting may be infected bullous impetigo (most commonly caused by *Staphylococcus aureus*).

15

## 15.6 Pain assessment tool: FLACC scale

|  | 0 | 1 | 2 |
|---|---|---|---|
| Face | No particular expression or smile | Occasional grimace or frown, withdrawn, uninterested | Frequently or constantly quivering chin, clenched jaw |
| Legs | Normal position or relaxed | Uneasy, restless, tense | Kicking or legs drawn up |
| Activity | Lying quietly, normal position, moves easily | Squirming, shifting back and forth, tense | Arched, rigid or jerking |
| Cry | No cry (awake or asleep) | Moans or whimpers, occasional complaint | Crying steadily, screams or sobs, frequent complaints |
| Consolability | Content, relaxed | Reassured by occasional touching, hugging or being talked to, distractible | Difficult to console or comfort |

Each category is scored on a 0–2 scale to give a total score of 0–10: 0 = no pain; 1–3 = mild pain; 4–7 = moderate pain; 8–10 = severe pain.

## 15.7 Respiratory system

| Symptom[a,b] | Frequency | Diagnostic significance | Significance heightened if associated with | Differential diagnosis |
|---|---|---|---|---|
| **Acute** |  |  |  |  |
| Short of breath at rest (SOBar) | *** | High (indicates loss of all respiratory reserve) |  | LRTI, asthma, acute episodic wheeze, inhaled foreign body. Rarely, supraventricular tachycardia, congenital heart disease, heart failure or muscular weakness |
| Cough | *** | Low | SOBar, fever | LRTI, asthma, acute episodic wheeze, foreign body |
| Wheeze | *** | Moderate | SOBar, fever | LRTI, asthma, acute episodic wheeze, foreign body |
| Chest pain | * | High | Exercise Fever | Musculoskeletal pain, empyema, reflux oesophagitis, cardiac ischaemia |
| Stridor | *** | High | URTI, high fever, choking | Croup, foreign body, epiglottitis (if not immunised) |
| **Chronic** |  |  |  |  |
| Short of breath on exercise (SOBoe) | ** | Low | Cough, wheeze, failure to thrive | Lack of fitness, respiratory pathology, cardiac pathology, neurological weakness |
| Cough | *** | Low | Wheeze, SOBoe, failure to thrive | Isolated cough with sputum suggests infection, commonly bronchitis, rarely bronchiectasis, cystic fibrosis, inhaled foreign body. If also wheezy, consider asthma or viral-induced wheeze |
| Wheeze | *** | Moderate | SOBoe, failure to thrive | Isolated, persistent 'wheeze' usually arises from the nose (stertor (e.g. adenoidal hypertrophy)) or the largest airways (stridor (e.g. laryngomalacia)). Episodic wheeze with cough suggests asthma or viral-induced wheeze |
| Chest pain | * | High | Exercise | Nonspecific chest pain, musculoskeletal chest pain, very rarely cardiac ischaemia |

[a]Respiratory sounds: clarify what noise the parent or child is describing. The history sometimes reveals the source (e.g. nose (stertor), throat (stridor) or chest (rattle or wheeze)). A constant respiratory sound is more likely to be stertor, stridor or rattle (a sound associated with vibration of the chest). A very loud sound, such as one heard in the next room, is not genuine wheeze.
[b]Coexistent failure to thrive or weight loss always increases the significance of any symptom.

*LRTI/URTI,* Lower/upper respiratory tract infection.

Red, circular lesions with a pink centre are most often erythema multiforme (target lesions). Petechial or purpuric rashes that do not blanch with pressure are of most concern. These may be viral in origin but importantly can be an early sign of meningococcal disease (particularly if the CYP is febrile). A differential diagnosis of a purpuric rash is idiopathic thrombocytopenic purpura.

## 15.8 Gastrointestinal system

| Symptom | Frequency | Diagnostic significance | Significance heightened if associated with | Differential diagnosis |
|---|---|---|---|---|
| **Acute** | | | | |
| Vomiting | *** | Low: a very non-specific symptom in children | Fever, drowsiness, dehydration[a] | Acute gastritis/gastroenteritis, any infection (otitis media, pneumonia, urinary tract infection, meningitis), head injury, encephalitis |
| Diarrhoea | *** | Moderate | Fever, dehydration[a] | Acute gastroenteritis/colitis, appendicitis |
| Abdominal pain[b] | ** | Moderate | Fever, bloody stools | Acute gastroenteritis/colitis, acute surgical causes (e.g. appendicitis) intussusception |
| **Chronic** | | | | |
| Vomiting | *** | Moderate | Failure to thrive[c] Headache | Gastro-oesophageal reflux (rare in older children compared with infants), raised intracranial pressure, food allergy |
| Diarrhoea | *** | Moderate | Failure to thrive[c] | Commonly toddler's diarrhoea, also lactose intolerance. If failure to thrive, consider coeliac disease, inflammatory bowel disease |
| Abdominal pain[b] | *** | Low | Pain that is not periumbilical Headaches Diarrhoea and vomiting Failure to thrive[c] | If isolated and periumbilical, non-specific abdominal pain is common and other diagnoses include abdominal migraine, renal colic. If associated with other symptoms and/or failure to thrive, consider coeliac disease, inflammatory bowel disease, constipation |

[a]Symptoms of dehydration include dry mouth, foul-smelling breath, anuria and lethargy.
[b]Abdominal pain can be difficult to identify in young children who are not able to express themselves.
[c]Coexisting failure to thrive or weight loss always increases the significance of any symptom.

**15**

## 15.9 Nervous system

| Symptom | Frequency | Diagnostic significance | Significance heightened if associated with | Differential diagnosis |
|---|---|---|---|---|
| **Acute** | | | | |
| Headache | ** | Low | Vomiting, fever, neck stiffness, photophobia | Acute (simple) headache, migraine, meningitis/encephalitis |
| Unsteady gait | * | High | | Varicella encephalomeningitis, vestibular neuronitis |
| Seizure[a] | * | High | | Febrile seizure, meningitis/encephalitis Epilepsy, metabolic disorder |
| Disturbed level of consciousness | * | High | | Encephalitis, intoxication/drug ingestion (accidental/ deliberate) |
| **Chronic** | | | | |
| Headache[b] | ** | Low | Vomiting Abdominal pain | Brain tumour, migraine, chronic non-specific headache |
| Failure to pass developmental milestones | * | Moderate | Widening gap between age and age when 'normal' milestone should have been passed | Cerebral palsy, neglect |
| Developmental regression | * | High | | Muscular dystrophy, inborn error of metabolism, neurodegenerative conditions |
| Seizure | * | High | | Epilepsy; rarely, long QT syndrome or inborn error of metabolism |

[a]An acute seizure can be confused with a rigor in a febrile child. A seizure involves slow (1 beat per second), coarse, jerking that cannot be stopped, loss of consciousness and postictal drowsiness. A rigor is characterised by rapid (5 beats per second), fine jerking that can be stopped by a cuddle with no loss of consciousness. [b]Chronic headache can also arise from the mouth (e.g. dental abscess) or face.

**Fig. 15.17** **Appearance of measles rash in different skin colours.** *From Ottolini MG. Measles. In: Goldman-Cecil Medicine. 26th edn. Philadelphia: Elsevier; 2020.*

Chronic skin excoriation, most commonly in the flexures, suggests eczema, whereas plaques on the elbows/knees may indicate psoriasis.

Hair loss is distressing. If associated with itch, it is often due to tinea capitis; with a history of preceding illness, alopecia is a likely cause.

## Past medical history

Has the CYP regularly seen a healthcare professional (current or past) or are they currently taking any regular medication? Have they been in hospital before, and if so, why?

## Birth history

Was the CYP born at term or preterm (if so, at what gestation)?

- For those born at term, was the neonatal period normal? For example, did the child need to go to a special care baby unit?
- For those born preterm, take a full neonatal history to understand any potential impact and include time ventilated and in supplemental oxygen, time on feeding support, age at discharge from hospital and any neonatal follow-up.
- If the child is under 3 years of age: what was the birthweight, and were there any complications during pregnancy?

## Vaccination history

Are the CYP's immunisations up to date according to country-specific schedules? If not, explore why and consider how best to encourage catch-up.

## Developmental history

This is particularly important for children under 3 years of age or those with possible neurodevelopmental delay (see p. 353 and Box 15.5).

## Drug history

Prescribing errors often arise from poor reconciliation of medication lists between different healthcare professionals. It is a doctor's duty to ensure that medicines are accurately reconciled within documentation. Transcribe the medication, dose and frequency directly from the medication package or referral letter if possible. Enquire about any difficulties in taking medication to establish adherence. Clarify any adverse or allergic reactions to medications (including drug, date and reaction), and ensure this information is shared in the appropriate section of health records.

## Family and social history

The people whom a CYP may consider to be family can be diverse. It is important to establish who the family is and recognise that this may be in different households with different adults at different times. Children at risk of neglect may have complex domestic arrangements such as several caregivers; it is important that you understand these arrangements. Ask open and non-judgemental questions to understand:

- Who lives in the family home, and who cares for the child? Is there another household where the child spends regular time?
- Does anyone smoke in these places?
- Are there any pets? Are any symptoms associated with pet contact?

• Are there any similar symptoms in the child's first- or second-degree relatives?

Sketch a family tree, noting any step-parents, step-siblings or shared care arrangements. Consider parental consanguinity, which is not uncommon in some ethnic groups.

Occasionally, chronic symptoms are associated with anxiety or potential 'secondary' gain for the CYP; these may include chronic cough, abdominal pain and headache in a well-looking CYP in whom examination is normal. Look carefully at the CYP's facial expression, eye contact and body language when asking questions. Ask carefully but specifically about school (avoidance and bullying), social interactions (does the child have many friends?) and out-of-school activities. School avoidance should be addressed if it is related to anxiety or if the pretext of medical symptoms is used.

## Systematic enquiry

This screens for illnesses or symptoms that may be not recognised as important or relevant by the CYP or parents. For CYP aged over 12 years, the questions used for adults are appropriate. In younger children, ask age-related questions. Specific areas include:

• Ear, nose and throat: ask the parents about their perception of a child's hearing ability (reduced in chronic otitis media), repeated sneezing (rhinitis) or the presence of regular snoring with periods of struggling to breathe (symptomatic obstructive sleep apnoea).
• Gastrointestinal system: ask whether growth is as expected and whether there is recurrent abdominal pain or difficulty in opening the bowels (constipation).
• Respiratory system: ask whether the child has had a regular cough (particularly asleep) when otherwise well or had wheeze on a recurrent basis in response to triggers such as viral infection or exercise (consider asthma).
• Urinary system: 15% of children at 5 years of age will continue to have primary nocturnal enuresis. It is embarrassing for most children and frustrating to most parents, so be sensitive in your questioning on frequency and timing of events.

## The physical examination

## Normal growth and development

An understanding of CYP development is vital to identifying whether symptoms and signs are consistent with age.

For the first 2 years of life, children born prematurely should have their age adjusted to their expected date of delivery instead of their date of birth when assessing growth and development. Failure to make this correction would otherwise create a false impression of poor growth and developmental delay. Prematurely born infants can be at increased risk of impaired growth and development and merit increased surveillance, although most develop normally.

## Growth

Growth after infancy is extremely variable. Use gender- and ethnicity-specific growth charts (e.g. those shown in Fig. 15.18). CYP with Trisomy 21 have a differential growth trajectory, and specific charts to support growth monitoring are available online (https://www.cdc.gov/ncbddd/birthdefects/downsyndrome/growth-charts.html). Growth charts enable a comparison of the individual with the corresponding population normal range at a single time point. As important is the ability of growth charts to enable tracking of growth trajectories over time when a CYP is regularly measured. Each child should grow along a centile line for height and weight throughout childhood. Failure to thrive is failure to attain the expected growth trajectory. A child on the 0.4th centile for height may be thriving if this has always been their growth trajectory, while a child on the 50th centile for height may be failing to thrive if previously they were on the 99.6th centile.

A child's height is related to the average of their parents' height centile $\pm 2$ standard deviations. Parents whose average height lies on the 50th centile will have children whose height will normally lie between the 2nd and 98th centiles (approximately 10 cm above and below the 50th centile).

## Neurodevelopmental maturation

Normal development is heterogeneous within the population, which can make abnormalities difficult to identify. Important determinants are the child's environment and genetic potential. Developmental assessment requires patience, familiarity with children and an understanding of the range of normality for a given age.

### The preschool child (1 to 5 years)

At the younger end of this range, questions and observations relating to gross motor skills are most sensitive; as the child becomes older, questions and observations relating to fine motor and personal social skills become more meaningful. Delayed speech with normal attainment of motor milestones is not uncommon, particularly in boys, but should prompt hearing assessment (see Box 15.5).

### The school-age child (5+ years)

By this age, many neurodevelopmental problems have revealed themselves to parents, and relevant agencies, such as educational ones, may already be engaged. However, more subtle developmental problems such as dyslexia (learning disability affecting fluency and comprehension in reading) may remain unrecognised and can be a major handicap. Ask general questions such as, 'How is your child getting on at school?' and follow up by enquiring specifically about academic and social activity.

15

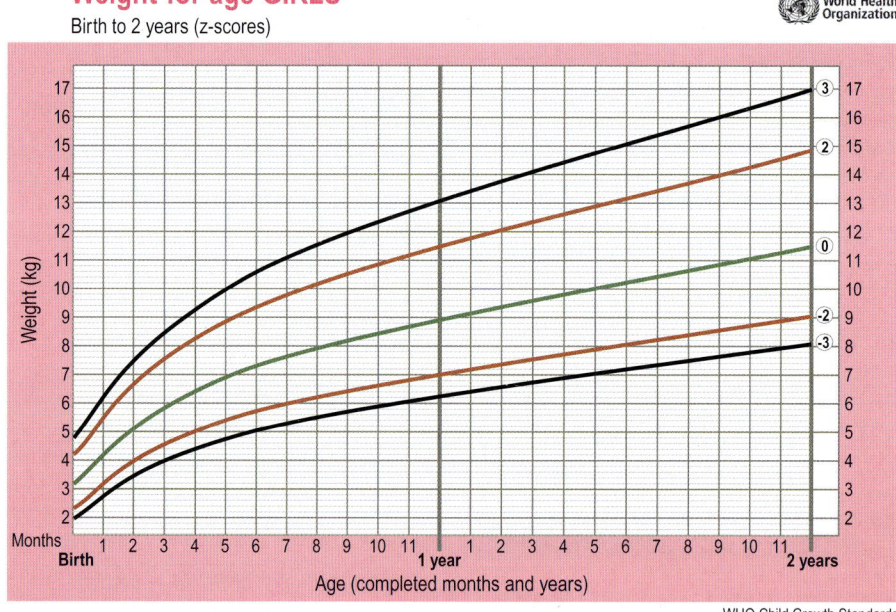

**Fig. 15.18** **Growth charts.** World Health Organization (WHO) standard centile charts for girls and boys. *From WHO Child Growth Standards. http://www.who. int/childgrowth/standards/weight_for_age/en/* © *World Health Organization 2017. All rights reserved.*

## Puberty

This stage of adolescence, when an individual becomes physiologically capable of sexual reproduction, is a time of rapid physical and emotional development. The age at the onset and end of puberty varies greatly but is generally 10 to 14 years for girls and 12 to 16 years for boys (Fig. 15.19). The average child grows 30 cm during puberty and gains 40 to 50% in weight.

**Female**

**Male**

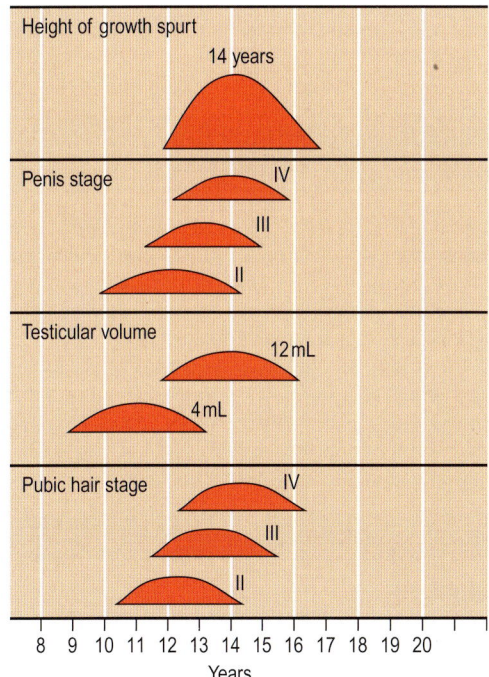

**Fig. 15.19** Timing of puberty in males and females.

If required, use a chart to stage puberty (Fig. 15.20). Pubertal staging has a wide normal range, with abnormalities apparent only on follow-up. Delayed or precocious puberty is not uncommon.

## Physical examination techniques in children and young people

CYP usually present with a symptom. Those with acute symptoms often have physical signs such as wheeze, but examination is normal in the majority who have chronic symptoms. Routine screening examination after infancy is unhelpful, as many paediatric diseases only produce signs late in the illness.

### Similarities in examination between children and young people and adults

The techniques used when examining CYP are the same as those in adults, with some exceptions. Examining CYP requires a range of skills that take time to learn. The key skills involve being:

- Observant during discussion or play, to identify elements of the examination that are naturally displayed and so can be partitioned from the formal examination process, reducing the duration of what is often a stressful encounter, particularly for younger children.
- Opportunistic, to examine systems as CYP present them. Chest and cardiac auscultation may be better earlier in the examination in younger children before they become restless or upset.
- Adaptive to CYP's mood and playfulness. A skilled practitioner can glean most examination findings from even the most uncooperative CYP. Usually the history suggests the diagnosis; the examination confirms it.

### Differences in examination between children and young people and adults

The appropriate approach varies with CYP's age.

#### 1 to 3 years

All children at this age can be reluctant to be approached by strangers and particularly dislike being examined. Early on, let children gradually become used to your presence and see that your encounter with their parents is friendly. Carefully observe the child's general condition, colour, respiratory rate and effort, and state of hydration while taking the history: that is, when the child is not focused on your close attention. For the formal examination, ask the parent to sit the child on the parent's knees. Examine the cardiorespiratory system and the abdomen with the young child sitting upright on the parent's knee. With patience, abdominal examination can be done with the child lying supine on the bed next to a parent or on the parent's lap. Taking your stethoscope from around your neck to use it can upset the child, so make slow, non-threatening moves. If the child starts crying,

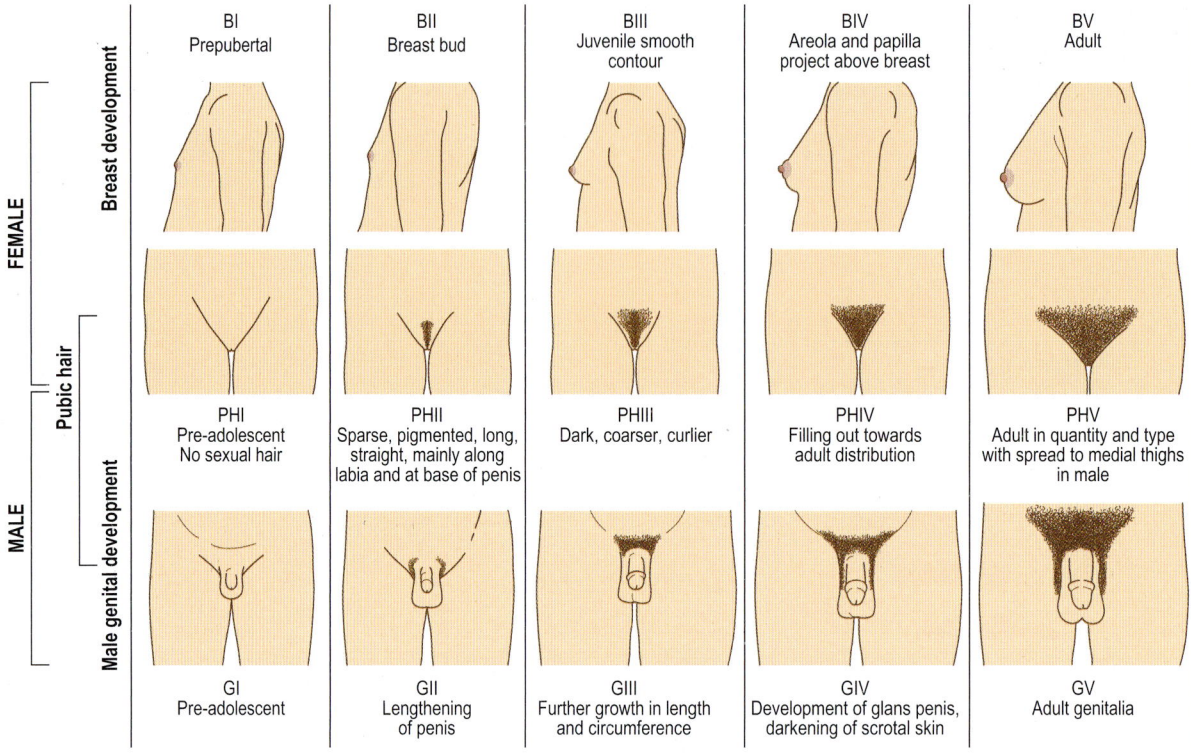

**Fig. 15.20 Stages of puberty in males and females.** Pubertal changes according to the Tanner stages of puberty.

chest auscultation and abdominal palpation become very difficult; take a pause. Ear, nose and throat examination often causes upset and is best left till last; suggesting that ear examination will tickle can help with older children.

### 3 to 5 years

Some children in this age range have the confidence and maturity to comply with many aspects of adult examination. They may cooperate by holding up their T-shirts for chest examination and turning round; if so, comment warmly on this cooperation and provide positive feedback on helpful behaviour. Children's social skills regress when they are unwell, and some are very apprehensive of strangers.

### 5+ years

The CYP may comply with a full adult-style examination. Although children under 11 years are often not able to express themselves well, those over 5 years are able to understand and comply with requests such as finger-to-nose pointing, heel-to-toe walking and being asked to 'sit forwards' and 'take a deep breath in and hold it'. Young people may find examination particularly embarrassing. Be aware and sensitive to this, and request permissions before proceeding.

## The acutely unwell children and young people

There are many nonspecific signs that are common to a range of conditions, from a simple cold to meningitis. These include a runny nose, fever, lethargy, vomiting, blanching rash and irritability. However, some signs are serious, requiring immediate investigation and management (Box 15.10).

CYP become ill quickly. If they have been unwell for less than 24 hours and initial examination reveals only nonspecific signs, they should ideally be reassessed in 1 to 2 hours if there is a high level of parental or clinical anxiety that the signs are out of keeping with a simple viral illness at that age.

## General examination

### Height

Use a stadiometer (Fig. 15.21).

### Vital signs

Normal ranges for vital signs vary according to age (Box 15.11).

## 15.10 Serious signs requiring urgent attention

- Poor perfusion with reduced capillary refill and cool peripheries (indicating shock)
- Listless, poorly responsive, whimpering child (suggesting sepsis)
- Petechial rash over the trunk (suggesting meningococcal sepsis)
- Headache with photophobia or neck stiffness (suggesting meningitis)
- Respiratory distress at rest (rapid rate and increased respiratory effort, indicating loss of respiratory reserve due to pneumonia or asthma)

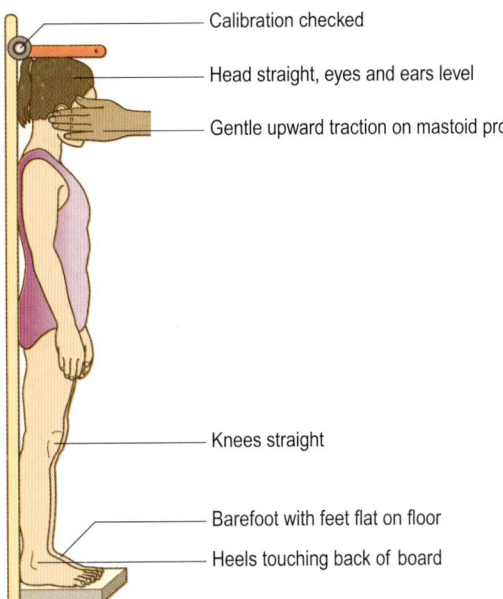

- Calibration checked
- Head straight, eyes and ears level
- Gentle upward traction on mastoid process
- Knees straight
- Barefoot with feet flat on floor
- Heels touching back of board

**Fig. 15.21** Stadiometer for measuring height accurately in children.

## 15.11 Physiological measurements in children of different ages

| Age (years) | Pulse (bpm) | Respiratory rate (breaths per minute) | Systolic blood pressure (mm Hg) |
|---|---|---|---|
| 0–1 | 110–160 | 30–60 | 70–90 |
| 2–5 | 60–140 | 25–40 | 80–100 |
| 6–12 | 60–120 | 20–25 | 90–110 |
| 13–18 | 60–100 | 15–20 | 100–120 |

*bpm,* Beats per minute.

# Ears, nose and throat

## The preschool child

### Throat

## Examination sequence

- Ask the parent to:
  - Sit the child on the parent's knees, both facing you.
  - Give an older child the opportunity to open the mouth spontaneously ('Roar like a lion!'). If this is not successful, proceed as described here.
  - Place one arm over the child's upper arms and chest (to stop the child pushing you away, Fig. 15.22).
  - Hold the child's forehead with their other hand (to stop the child pulling their chin down to their chest).
- Hold the torch in your non-dominant hand to illuminate the child's throat.
- Slide a tongue depressor inside the child's cheek with your dominant hand. The child should open their clenched teeth (perhaps with a shout), showing their tonsils and pharynx.

### Abnormal findings

Healthy tonsils and pharynx look pink; when inflamed, they are crimson–red.

Inspecting the throat (see Fig 15.22) reveals the presence, but not the cause, of the infection; pus on the tonsils and pharynx does not differentiate a bacterial from a viral infection (p. 210).

### Ears

## Examination sequence

- Ask the parent to:
  - Sit the child across the parent's knees with the child's ear facing you.
  - Place one arm around the child's shoulder and upper arm that are facing you (to stop them pushing you away, Fig. 15.23).
  - Place the parent's other hand over the parietal area above the child's ear that is facing you (to keep the child's head still).
- Use an otoscope with the largest speculum that will comfortably fit the child's external auditory meatus.
- To straighten the ear canal and visualise the canal and tympanic membrane, hold the pinna gently and pull it out and down in a baby or toddler with no mastoid development, or up and back in a child whose mastoid process has formed.

### Lymphadenopathy

#### Normal findings

Palpable neck and groin nodes are extremely common in children under 5 years of age. They are typically bilateral, less than

**15**

**Fig. 15.22** How to hold a child to examine the mouth and throat.

**Fig. 15.23** How to hold a child to examine the ear.

| 15.12 Causes of lymph node enlargement |
| --- |

**Cervical lymphadenopathy**

- Tonsillitis, pharyngitis, sinusitis
- 'Glandular fever' (infectious mononucleosis/cytomegalovirus)
- Tuberculosis (uncommon in developed countries)

**Generalised lymphadenopathy**

- Febrile illness with a generalised rash
- 'Glandular fever'
- Systemic juvenile chronic arthritis (Still's disease)
- Acute lymphatic leukaemia
- Drug reaction
- Mucocutaneous lymph node syndrome (Kawasaki disease)

symptoms such as weight loss, fevers or night sweats, these are typically a normal, healthy immune response to infection. Only rarely are they due to malignancy (Box 15.12).

## Cardiovascular examination

To assess the pulse (rate and volume), the brachial pulse in the antecubital fossa is best used for children below 2 to 3 years and the radial pulse in older CYP. Measure blood pressure using a cuff sized two-thirds the distance from elbow to shoulder tip. Repeat with a larger cuff if the reading is elevated. If in doubt, use a larger cuff, as smaller cuffs yield falsely high values.

## Respiratory examination

### Abnormal findings

The child under 3 years has a soft chest wall and relatively small, stiff lungs. When the lungs are made stiffer (by infection or fluid), the diaphragm must contract vigorously to draw air into the lungs. This produces recession (ribs 'sucking in'—tracheal, intercostal and subcostal) and paradoxical outward movement of the abdomen (wrongly called 'abdominal breathing'). These important signs of increased work of breathing are often noticed by parents. Older children may be able to articulate the accompanying symptom of dyspnoea.

In young children, their small, thin chests transmit noises readily, and the smaller airways are more prone to turbulence and added sounds. Auscultation may reveal a variety of sounds, including expiratory polyphonic wheeze (occasionally inspiratory too), fine end-expiratory crackles, coarse louder crackles transmitted from the larger airways and other sounds described as pops and squeaks (typically in the chest of recovering patients with asthma).

## Abdominal examination

In children aged 6 months to 3 years, examine the abdomen with the child sitting upright on the parent's knee. In the young child,

1 cm in diameter, hard and mobile with no overlying redness and can persist for many weeks. In the absence of systemic

**Fig. 15.24** NHS Scotland National Paediatric Early Warning Chart (PEWS) for children aged 2 to 4 years. For each domain, observations in the coloured areas contribute scores according to the legend in the R margin. The total score is recorded in the PEWS line. Used with the permission of Healthcare Improvement Scotland. *https:// ihub.scot/improvement-programmes/scottish-patient-safety-programme-spsp/spsp-programmes-of-work/maternity-and-children-quality-improvement-collaborative-mcqic/paediatric-care/pews/*.

splenic enlargement extends towards the left iliac fossa. In older children the enlarged spleen edge moves towards the right iliac fossa. Faecal loading of the left iliac fossa is common in constipation. Rectal examination is rarely indicated in CYP, but examination of the anus for fissures (common with constipation) can be helpful where appropriate.

## Neurological examination

Test power initially by watching the CYP demonstrate their strength against gravity. Ask them to lift their arms above their head, raise their leg from the bed while they are lying down and stand from a squatting position. If appropriate, test power against your strength.

Neck stiffness in CYP is usually apparent when you are talking to them or their parents. CYP with meningitis will not want to move, and if they are forced to do so, the neck remains aligned with the trunk. With a young child, move a toy to catch their attention and see if they move their head.

## Spotting the sick children and young people

It can be difficult to identify CYP with severe illness, particularly younger children. With experience you will learn to identify whether CYP are just miserable or really ill. Early-warning scores (e.g. Paediatric Early Warning Score (PEWS), Fig. 15.24) can help. Certain features correlate with severe illness (Box 15.13).

## Child protection

CYP who experience neglect or physical and/or emotional abuse are at increased risk of health problems. At-risk CYP may already be known to other agencies but do not assume this is the case when interagency communications are not available to you.

---

**15.13 Clinical signs associated with severe illness in children**

- Fever >38°C
- Drowsiness
- Cold hands and feet
- Petechial rash
- Neck stiffness
- Shortness of breath at rest
- Tachycardia
- Hypotension (a late sign in shocked children where blood pressure is initially maintained by tachycardia and increased peripheral vascular resistance)

---

**15.14 Signs that may suggest child neglect or abuse**

**Behavioural signs**

- 'Frozen watchfulness'
- Passivity
- Over-friendliness
- Sexualised behaviour
- Inappropriate dress
- Hunger, stealing food

**Physical signs**

- Identifiable bruises (e.g. fingertips, handprints, belt buckle, bites)
- Circular (cigarette) burns or submersion burns with no splash marks
- Injuries of differing ages
- Eye or mouth injuries
- Long-bone fractures or bruises in nonmobile infants
- Posterior rib fracture
- Subconjunctival or retinal haemorrhage
- Dirty, smelly, unkempt child
- Bad nappy rash

---

Injuries from physical abuse can often be detected visually. Consider nonaccidental injury if the history is not consistent with the injury or if the injury is present in unusual places such as over the back. It may be difficult to detect neglect during a brief encounter, but consider it if the child appears unkempt, has unexplained pain/discomfort or is socially withdrawn. The parent–child relationship gives insight into neglect; the child is apparently scared of the parent ('frozen watchfulness') or the parent appears oblivious to the child's attention (Box 15.14).

## Remote consultation in paediatric practice

The recent global pandemic has made necessary remote consultation. While this may become part of normal practice in future, it has significant limitations as well as advantages (see Chapter 21). There is a risk that remote consultation can adversely affect the appropriate assessment of CYP in communities or households where technology and access to WiFi do not enable a visual review of the child. Where video consultation is possible, always ensure that CYP are present at least at the start of the consultation so that you can ask specific questions of them and observe any specific signs that may help your clinical decision making. Younger CYP, in particular, get bored very easily during video consultation and tend to disappear off camera.

## OSCE example 1: Diarrhoea

Ismail, 4 months old, is brought in to see you by his mother. She is anxious as he has had diarrhoea for several days. He is breastfed.

### Please perform a newborn examination, focusing on the cardiovascular system

- Introduce yourself to the mother. Wash your hands thoroughly and wear personal protective equipment (PPE) as per local guidance.
- Carry out a general inspection:
  - Look at the general state of the infant. Are they alert and interested, or quiet and lethargic?
  - Examine for signs of dehydration:
    - Sunken eyes, sunken fontanelle, reduced skin turgor, dry mucous membranes
    - Measure capillary refill by pressing on the midsternum for 5 seconds and counting the time for refill
    - Count the respiratory rate over 1 minute to identify tachypnoea
    - Count the pulse rate and pulse volume in the brachial artery.
    - Measure the child's blood pressure.
    - Assess the child's neurological status (AVPU—alert, verbal, pain, unresponsive).
- Is there any associated infection/condition that might be causing them to have diarrhoea. Perform an examination of the systems to exclude additional diagnoses, i.e.
  - respiratory crackles of pneumonia
  - inflamed ear for otitis media
  - bulging fontanelle of meningitis
- Dispose of any PPE you have used, wash your hands and thank the parent and child.

### Suggest a diagnosis

Diarrhoea is common and, with it, dehydration. Most children can recover if an adequate assessment of dehydration is made and they are provided with rehydration. Learn how to assess degrees of dehydration (commonly classified as 5, 10 or 15% dehydration) and how to calculate volume of fluid to replace (body weight in kg × percent dehydration × 10 = volume in mL to be replaced). Fluid replacement is in addition to routine daily requirements. If there are continued diarrhoeal losses, fluids may need recalculated every 4 to 8 hours to take account of this.

### Suggest investigations

Heart rate, respiratory rate, blood pressure, pulse oximetry.

**15**

## OSCE example 2: Chronic cough

Joanne, 2 years old, who has had a problem with cough. The cough has been present for the past 8 weeks following a severe viral infection. The cough affects her sleep but not her appetite, weight or activities.

### Please perform a chest examination, focusing on the respiratory system

- Introduce yourself to the parent and child. Wash your hands thoroughly, and wear PPE as per local guidance. Ensure that you use a stethoscope that has been appropriately cleaned.
- Carry out a general inspection: are there any signs of acute or chronic respiratory distress?
- Look for chest wall deformity (pectus excavatum, Harrison's sulcus).
- Look for signs of respiratory distress (tachypnoea, indrawing, accessory muscle use).
- Count the respiratory rate over 1 minute.
- Look at the colour and perfusion of the patient (cyanosis, pallor, sweatiness).
- Look for finger clubbing and poor weight gain.
   The respiratory rate is 20 per minute (normal), and there are no other abnormal findings on inspection except that you can hear the child have an intermittent moist cough.
- Auscultate: warm the stethoscope.
  - Auscultate the respiratory system in all lung regions, anteriorly and posteriorly, with the chest fully exposed.
  - Low-pitch rhonchi are auscultated in all lung regions. No crepitations are heard. Air entry is normal.
  - Heart sounds are normal with no murmur.
- Palpate: consider palpation if there are chest-wall abnormalities or differential chest expansion on inspection, to look for differential chest-wall movement.
- Dispose of any PPE you have used, wash your hands and thank the parent and child.

### Summarise your findings

This child has moist cough with low-pitch rhonchi on auscultation but a normal respiratory rate and no respiratory distress.

*Continued*

## OSCE example 2: Chronic cough—cont'd

### Suggest a diagnosis

Postviral cough is common in young children. Cough usually resolves within 6 weeks. A prolonged cough, particularly if moist requires clinical review. Persistent bacterial bronchitis often self resolves in many children, but for some the recovery can be aided by a course of broad-spectrum antibiotics (i.e. amoxicillin). If the moist cough resolves but recurs on stopping antibiotics or fails to stop with antibiotics, then further investigation may be required.

### Suggest initial investigations

Chest x-ray if recurrence or non-improvement.

## Integrated examination sequence for the newborn child

- Perform a general examination:
  - Looks well and is well grown? Dysmorphic features? Posture and behaviour? Does the cry sound normal?
  - Skin: note cuts, bruising, naevi (haemangiomas or melanocytic), blisters or bullae.
  - Head: check shape, swellings, anterior fontanelle, cranial sutures.
  - Eyes: check for jaundice, ocular movements and vestibular function; perform ophthalmoscopy.
  - Nose: check patency.
  - Mouth: check mucosa, tongue, palate, jaw and any teeth.
  - Ears: note size, shape and position; check the external auditory meatus.
  - Neck: inspect and palpate for asymmetry, sinuses and swellings.
- Examine the cardiovascular system:
  - Inspect: pallor, cyanosis and sweating.
  - Palpate: apex, check for heave or thrill, count heart rate, femoral pulses, feel for hepatomegaly.
  - Auscultate: heart sounds I and II, any additional heart sounds or murmurs.
- Examine the respiratory system:
  - Inspect: chest shape, symmetry of movement, respiratory rate, respiratory distress: tachypnoea, suprasternal, intercostal and subcostal recession, flaring of nostrils.
  - Auscultate anteriorly, laterally and posteriorly, comparing sides.
- Examine the abdomen:
  - Inspect: abdomen, umbilicus, anus and groins, noting any swellings.
  - Palpate: superficial, then deeper structures. Spleen, then liver.
- Examine the perineum:
  - Both sexes: check normal anatomy.
  - Male: assess the penis, noting shape; check the urethral meatus is at the tip. Do not retract the foreskin. Palpate the testes, and the inguinal canal if the testes are not in the scrotum. Transilluminate scrotal swellings.
- Examine the spine and sacrum:
  - With the infant in the prone position, inspect and palpate the entire spine for neural tube defects.
- Examine the neurological system:
  - Inspect: asymmetry in posture and movement, any muscle wasting.
  - Pick the baby up to note any stiff or floppy tone.
  - Sensation: does the baby withdraw from gentle stimuli?
  - In dim light, the eyes should open; in bright light, babies screw up their eyes.
- Check the primitive reflexes:
  - Check grasp responses, ventral suspension/pelvic response to back stimulation, place-and-step reflexes, Moro reflex, root-and-suck responses.
- Inspect the limbs:
  - Inspect: limbs, counting digits and checking feet are, or can be, normally positioned.
  - Check hips for developmental dysplasia/dislocation.
- Weigh and measure:
  - Weigh the infant to the nearest 5 g.
  - Measure: occipitofrontal circumference, crown–heel length (neonatal stadiometer).
  - Record on a centile chart.

# Patients with mental illness and learning disability

**The history 368**

General approach 368
Sensitive topics 368
The uncooperative patient 368

**The mental state examination 368**

Appearance 369
Behaviour 369
Speech 369
Mood 369
Thought form 370
Thought content 370
Perceptions 371
Cognition 372

Insight 373
Risk assessment 373
Capacity 373

**The physical examination 373**

**Collateral history 374**

**Psychiatric rating scales 374**

**Putting it all together: clinical vignettes 374**

**OSCE example 1: Assessing suicidal risk 376**

**OSCE example 2: Assessing delirium 377**

**Integrated examination sequence for the psychiatric assessment 377**

Mental disorders are very common, frequently coexist with physical disorders and cause much mortality and morbidity. Psychiatric assessment is, therefore, a required skill for all clinicians. It consists of four elements: history, mental state examination (MSE), selective physical examination and collateral information. Each element can be expanded considerably, so the assessment must be adapted to its purpose. Is it a quick screening of a patient presenting with other problems, a confirmation of a suspected diagnosis or a comprehensive review for a second opinion?

# The history

## General approach

The distinction between symptoms and signs is less clear in psychiatry than in the rest of medicine. The psychiatric interview, which covers both, has several purposes: to obtain a history of symptoms, to assess the present mental state for signs and to establish rapport that will facilitate further management.

A comprehensive history covers a range of areas (Box 16.1), but the nature of the presenting problem and/or the referral question, and the setting in which the history is being taken, will determine the degree of detail needed for each. When seeing someone in the Emergency Department with a first episode of psychosis, the focus is on symptoms, recent changes in function, family history and drug use; when interviewing someone in an outpatient clinic with a possible personality disorder, assessment concentrates instead on their personal history, which is essentially a systematised biography (Box 16.2).

---

### 16.1 Content of a psychiatric history

- Referral source
- Reason for referral
- History of presenting symptom(s)
- Systematic enquiry into other relevant problems and symptoms
- Past medical/psychiatric history
- Prescribed and non-prescribed medication
- Substance use: illegal drugs, alcohol, tobacco, caffeine
- Family history (including psychiatric disorders)
- Personal history

---

### 16.2 Personal history

- Childhood development
- Losses and experiences
- Education
- Occupation(s)
- Financial circumstances
- Relationships
- Partner(s) and children
- Housing
- Leisure activities
- Hobbies and interests
- Forensic history

---

## Sensitive topics

Some subjects require a particular skill. The common theme is reluctance to disclose, which can arise because the information is private and disclosure is potentially embarrassing (such as sexual dysfunction), distressing (major previous traumatic experiences, such as rape, childhood sexual abuse, witnessing a death) or incriminating (illicit drug misuse, other crimes, homicidal ideas). For interviews undertaken in non-clinical settings, such as police stations or prisons, or for the provision of court reports, potentially incriminating disclosures are obviously especially pertinent, and it is important to be clear with the patient about any limits to confidentiality in your interview. Some disclosures, such as those relating to sexual orientation or gender identity, may expose patients to the real or perceived risk of hostility or discrimination.

Try to develop rapport early in the interview, if possible, and to consolidate it before raising a sensitive topic, although sometimes you must cover such material without delay. It is particularly important to ask about suicidal thoughts.

While clinicians should be able to interview patients regardless of their age, gender, ethnic origin or sexual orientation, the skills required may vary because patient attitudes may differ. For example, it may be more difficult for a male patient to discuss erectile dysfunction with a female than a male interviewer, or for an adolescent patient to relate to an interviewer in their late middle age than someone closer to their own years. Clinicians need to be aware of the potential effects of demographic and other differences between themselves and their patients.

## The uncooperative patient

Adapt your approach to a patient who is mute, agitated, hostile or otherwise uncooperative during the interview by relying more on observation and collateral information. The safety of the patient, other patients, staff and the wider public is paramount, so your initial assessment of an agitated or hostile patient may be only partial.

# The mental state examination

The MSE is a systematic evaluation of the patient's mental condition at the time of interview. The aim is to establish signs of mental disorder that, taken along with the history, enable you to make, suggest or exclude a diagnosis. While making your specific enquiries, you need to observe, evaluate and draw inferences in the light of the history. This may be daunting, but with good teaching, practice and experience, you will learn the skills.

The MSE incorporates elements of the history, observation of the patient, specific questions exploring various mental phenomena, and short tests of cognitive function. Like the history, its focus is determined by the potential diagnoses. For example, detailed cognitive assessment in an elderly patient presenting with confusion is crucial; similarly, you should carefully evaluate mood and suicidal thoughts when the presenting problem is depression.

## Appearance

Think of this as a written account of a still photograph, prepared for someone who cannot see it. Observe:

- general elements such as attire and signs of self-neglect
- facial expression
- tattoos and scars (especially any that suggest recent or previous self-harm)
- evidence of substance misuse (such as injection tracks from intravenous drug use; spider naevi and jaundice from alcoholic liver disease)
- possibly relevant physical disease (such as exophthalmos from thyrotoxicosis).

## Behaviour

Think of this as a written account of a video recording, observing such features as:

- cooperation, rapport, eye contact
- social behaviour (such as aggression, disinhibition, fearful withdrawal)
- apparent responses to possible hallucinations or unobserved stimuli
- over-activity (agitation, pacing, compulsive hand washing)
- under-activity (stupor, motor retardation)
- abnormal activity (posturing, involuntary movements, Box 16.3).

## Speech

Think of this as a written description of an audio recording. It is not a description of *what* the patient says (that is, content), but of *how* they say it (form). Assess:

- articulation (such as stammering, dysarthria)
- quantity (mutism, garrulousness)
- rate (pressured, slowed)
- volume (whispering, shouting)
- tone and quality (accent, emotionality)
- fluency (staccato, monotonous)
- abnormal language (neologisms, dysphasia, clanging, Box 16.4).

### 16.3 Behaviour: definitions

| Term | Definition |
|---|---|
| Agitation | A combination of psychic anxiety and excessive, purposeless motor activity |
| Compulsion | A stereotyped action that the patient cannot resist performing repeatedly |
| Disinhibition | Loss of control over normal social behaviour |
| Motor retardation | Decreased motor activity, usually a combination of fewer and slower movements |
| Posturing | The maintenance of bizarre gait or limb positions for no valid reason |

### 16.4 Speech: definitions

| Term | Definition |
|---|---|
| Clang associations | Thoughts connected by their similar sound rather than by meaning |
| Echolalia | Senseless repetition of the interviewer's words |
| Mutism | Absence of speech without impaired consciousness |
| Neologism | An invented word, or a new meaning for an established word |
| Pressure of speech | Rapid, excessive, continuous speech (due to pressure of thought) |
| Word salad | A meaningless string of words, often with loss of grammatical construction |

## Mood

Mood is the patient's pervasive emotional state, while affect is the observable expression of their emotions, which is more variable over time. Think of mood as the emotional climate, and affect as the weather. Both have elements of subjective experience (i.e. how the patient feels, according to their own report and your specific questions) and how the patient *appears* to feel, according to your objective observation. So, a depressed patient might describe feeling sad, hopeless and unable to enjoy any aspect of life, and at interview, appear downcast, withdrawn and tearful, with little brightening of mood, even when talking about their much-loved children.

Pervasive disturbance of mood is the most important feature of depression, mania and anxiety, but mood changes commonly occur in other mental disorders such as schizophrenia and dementia. You might ask patients, 'How has your mood been lately?', 'Have you noticed any change in your emotions recently?' and 'Do you still enjoy things that normally give you pleasure?' Abnormalities of mood include a problematic pervasive mood, an abnormal range of affect, abnormal reactivity and inappropriateness or incongruity. Some terms relating to mood are defined in Box 16.5.

**16**

### 16.5 Mood: definitions

| Term | Definition |
|---|---|
| Blunting | Loss of normal emotional sensitivity to experiences |
| Catastrophic reaction | An extreme emotional and behavioural over-reaction to a trivial stimulus |
| Flattening | Loss of the range of normal emotional responses |
| Incongruity | A mismatch between the emotional expression and the associated thought |
| Lability | Superficial, rapidly changing and poorly controlled emotions |

Some patients prompt affective responses in the interviewer via the process of countertransference. The elated gaiety of some hypomanic patients can be infectious, as can the hopeless gloom of some people with depression. Recognising these responses in yourself can be helpful in understanding how the patient relates to others, and vice versa.

## Thought form

As with speech, this is not an assessment of *what* the patient is thinking about, but *how* they think about it. Assess it by observing how thoughts appear to be linked together and the speed and directness with which the train of thought moves, considering rate, flow, sequencing and abstraction. Some terms relating to thought form are defined in Box 16.6.

Thinking may appear speeded up, as in hypomania, or slowed down, as in profound depression. The flow of subjects may be understandable but unusually rapid, as in the *flight of ideas* that characterises hypomania, or unduly 'single track' and perseverative, as in some cases of dementia. Sometimes thinking appears to be very circumstantial, and the patient is hard to pin down, even when asked simple questions.

More severe disruption of the train of thought is termed 'loosening of associations' or 'formal thought disorder', in which the patient moves from subject to subject via abrupt changes of direction that the interviewer cannot follow. This is a core feature of schizophrenia. Concrete thinking, in the sense of difficulty handling abstract concepts, is a common feature of dementia and can be assessed by asking the patients to explain the meaning of common proverbs.

It may help to illustrate your assessment with verbatim examples from the interview, chosen to illustrate the patient's manner of thinking and speaking.

## Thought content

Thought content refers to the main themes and subjects occupying the patient's mind. It will become apparent when taking the history but may need to be explored further via specific enquiries. It may broadly be divided into preoccupations, ruminations and abnormal beliefs. These are defined in Boxes 16.7 and 16.8.

## Preoccupations

Preoccupations occur in both normal and abnormal mood states. Dwelling sadly on the loss of a loved one is entirely normal in bereavement; persisting in disproportionate guilty gloom about the state of the world may be a symptom of depression.

| 16.7 Thought content: definitions | |
|---|---|
| **Term** | **Definition** |
| Hypochondriasis | Unjustified belief in suffering from a particular disease in spite of appropriate examination and reassurance |
| Morbid thinking | Depressive ideas, e.g. themes of guilt, burden, unworthiness, failure, blame, death, suicide |
| Phobia | A senseless avoidance of a situation, object or activity stemming from an irrational fear |
| Preoccupation | Beliefs that are not inherently abnormal but which have come to dominate the patient's thinking |
| Ruminations | Repetitive, intrusive, senseless thoughts or preoccupations |
| Obsessions | Ruminations that persist despite resistance |

| 16.6 Thought form: definitions | |
|---|---|
| **Term** | **Definition** |
| Circumstantiality | Trivia and digressions impairing the flow but not direction of thought |
| Concrete thinking | Inability to think abstractly |
| Flights of ideas | Rapid shifts from one idea to another, retaining sequencing |
| Loosening of associations | Logical sequence of ideas is impaired. Subtypes include knight's-move thinking, derailment, thought blocking and, in its extreme form, word salad |
| Perseveration | Inability to shift from one idea to the next |
| Pressure of thought | Increased rate and quantity of thoughts |

| 16.8 Abnormal beliefs: definitions | |
|---|---|
| **Term** | **Definition** |
| Delusion | An abnormal belief, held with total conviction, which is maintained in spite of proof or logical argument to the contrary and is not shared by others from the same culture or cultural sub-group |
| Delusional perception | A delusion that arises fully formed from the false interpretation of a real perception, e.g. a traffic light turning green, confirms that aliens have landed on the rooftop |
| Magical thinking | An irrational belief that certain actions and outcomes are linked, often culturally determined by folklore or custom, e.g. fingers crossed for good luck |
| Overvalued ideas | Beliefs that are held, valued, expressed and acted on, beyond the norm for the culture to which the person belongs |
| Thought broadcasting | The belief that the patient's thoughts are heard by others |
| Thought insertion | The belief that thoughts are being placed in the patient's head from outside |
| Thought withdrawal | The belief that thoughts are being removed from the patient's head |

## Ruminations

These are preoccupations that are, in themselves, abnormal – and therefore symptoms of mental disorder – by reason of *repetition* (as in obsessional disorders) or *groundlessness* (as in hypochondriasis).

## Abnormal beliefs

These beliefs fall into two categories: those that are not diagnostic of mental illness (such as overvalued ideas, superstitions and magical thinking) and those that invariably signify mental illness (that is, delusions).

The main difference between them is that, delusions either lack a cultural basis for the belief, or have been derived from abnormal psychological processes. Judging the former requires awareness of the way belief sets can vary between cultures and subgroups. What is commonplace in some groups within society is sometimes regarded by those in other groups as so bizarre that it amounts to prima facie evidence of mental illness. It may be necessary to have a patient assessed by a clinician from the same subgroup, if possible, to address any doubts. Failing that, the clinician should interview others from the same subgroup to calibrate the patient's belief-set against theirs.

## Overvalued ideas

These are usually beliefs of great personal significance. They fall short of being full delusions but are abnormal because of their effects on a person's behaviour or wellbeing. For example, in anorexia nervosa, people may still believe they are fat when they are seriously underweight – and then respond to their belief, rather than their measured weight, by further starving themselves.

## Delusional beliefs

Delusions are beliefs which are firmly held *despite clear evidence to the contrary* and which are out of keeping with the patient's cultural background. These beliefs matter greatly to the person holding them, resulting in powerful emotions and important behavioural consequences; they are always of clinical significance. They are classified by their content, such as:

- paranoid
- religious
- grandiose
- hypochondriacal
- of guilt
- of love
- of jealousy
- of infestation
- of thought interference (broadcasting, insertion and withdrawal)
- of control.

Bizarre delusions are easy to recognise, but not all delusions are in themselves unusual ideas: a spouse convinced that their partner is unfaithful may or may not be deluded. Even if a partner were unfaithful, it would still amount to delusional jealousy if the belief were held without evidence or for some unaccountable reason, such as finding a dead bird in the garden.

Delusions can sometimes be understood as the patient's way of trying to make sense of their experience, while the content of the delusions often gives a clue that may help type the underlying illness: for example, delusions of guilt suggest severe depression, whereas grandiose delusions typify mania.

Some delusions are characteristic of schizophrenia. They include a delusional perception (or primary delusion) and 'passivity phenomena': namely, the belief (linked to the experience) that thoughts, feelings or acts are no longer controlled by a person's own free will.

## Perceptions

People normally distinguish between their inner and outer worlds with ease: we know what is real, what reality feels like and what resides in our 'mind's eye' or 'mind's ear'. In mental illness, this distinction can become disrupted, so that normal perceptions become unfamiliar, while abnormal perceptions seem real.

Abnormal perceptions are assessed via the history and specific enquiries, backed up by observation. They fall into several categories, defined in Box 16.9.

Perceptions may be *altered* (as in sensory distortions or illusions) or *false* (as in hallucinations and pseudohallucinations). In a third category, what is altered is not a perception in a specific sensory modality but a general sense of disconnection and unreality in oneself (depersonalisation), the world (derealisation) or both.

People find depersonalisation and derealisation intensely unpleasant but hard to describe. They may occur in association with severe tiredness or intense anxiety, but can also arise in most types of mental illness. Ask, for example, 'Have you ever felt that you were not real or that the world around you wasn't real?'

**16**

| 16.9 **Perceptions: definitions** | |
|---|---|
| **Term** | **Definition** |
| Depersonalisation | A subjective experience of feeling unreal |
| Derealisation | A subjective experience that the surrounding environment is unreal |
| Hallucination | A false perception arising without a valid stimulus from the external world |
| Illusion | A false perception that is an understandable misinterpretation of a real stimulus in the external world |
| Pseudohallucination | A false perception that is perceived as part of one's internal experience |

With altered perceptions, there is a real external object, but its subjective perception has been distorted. Sensory distortions, such as unpleasant amplification of light (photophobia) or sound (hyperacusis), can occur in physical diseases but are also common in anxiety states and drug intoxication or withdrawal. Diminution of perceptions, including pain, can occur in depression and schizophrenia.

Illusions, in which, for example, a bedside locker is misperceived as a threatening animal commonly occur among people with established impairment of vision or hearing. They are also found in predisposed patients who are subjected to sensory deprivation, notably after dark in a patient with clouding of consciousness. They are suggestive of an organic illness such as delirium, dementia or alcohol withdrawal.

True hallucinations arise without external stimuli. They usually indicate severe mental illness, although they can occur naturally when going to sleep (hypnagogic) or waking up (hypnopompic). Hallucinations are categorised according to their sensory modality as auditory, visual, olfactory, gustatory or tactile.

Any form of hallucination can occur in any severe mental disorder. The most common are auditory and visual hallucinations, the former associated with schizophrenia and the latter with delirium. Some auditory hallucinations are characteristic of schizophrenia, such as voices discussing the patient in the third person or giving a running commentary on the person's activities ('Now he's opening the kitchen cupboard'). Ask, for example, 'Do you ever hear voices when nobody is talking?' and 'What do they say?'

Pseudohallucinations are common. The key distinction from a true hallucination is that they occur within the patient, rather than arising externally. They have an 'as if' quality and lack the vividness and reality of true hallucinations. Consequently, the affected person is not usually distressed by them, and does not normally feel the need to respond, as often happens with true hallucinations.

## Cognition

If the history and observations suggest a cognitive deficit, it must be evaluated by standard tests. History, observation, MSE and rating scales (see later) are then used together to diagnose and distinguish between the '3Ds' (dementia, delirium and depression), which are common in the elderly and in hospital inpatients.

Core cognitive functions include:

- level of consciousness
- orientation
- memory
- attention and concentration
- intelligence.

## Level of consciousness

Mental disorders are rarely associated with a reduced (or clouded) level of consciousness, such as drowsiness, stupor or coma. The exception is delirium (which is both a physical and a mental disorder), where it is common.

## Orientation

This is a key aspect of cognitive function, being particularly sensitive to impairment. Disorientation is the hallmark of the 'organic mental state' found in delirium and dementia. Abnormalities may be evident during the interview, but some patients are adept at hiding them in social interactions. Check the patient's orientation to time, place and person by evaluating their knowledge of the current time and date, recognition of where they are and identification of familiar people.

## Memory

Memory function is divided into three elements:

- Registration is tested by asking the patient to repeat, after you, the names of three unrelated objects (e.g. apple, table, penny); any mistake is significant. Alternatively, in the digit span test, ask the patient to repeat after you a sequence of random single-digit numbers. Make sure you speak slowly and clearly. A person with normal function can produce at least five digits.
- Short-term memory (where short-term is defined as a matter of minutes) is tested by giving the patient some new information; once this has registered, check retention after 5 minutes, with a distracting task in between. Do the same with the names of three objects; any error is significant. Alternatively, use a six-item name and address (in the format: first name, last name, house number, street name, street type, town: (for example, Premal Rahindran, 25 Green Street, Leeds). More than one error indicates impairment.
- Long-term memory is assessed mainly from personal history. Gaps and mistakes are often obvious, but some patients may confabulate (that is, fill in the gaps with plausible but unconsciously fabricated facts), so check the account with a family member or other informant if possible. Confabulation is a core feature of Korsakoff's syndrome, a complication of chronic alcoholism. Failing long-term memory is characteristic of dementia, although the store of knowledge can be remarkably intact in the presence of severe impairment of other cognitive functions.

## Impaired attention and concentration

These occur in many mental disorders and are not diagnostic. Impaired attention is observed as increased distractibility, with the patient responding inappropriately to intrusive internal events (memories, obsessions, anxious ruminations) or to extraneous stimuli, which may be either real (a noise outside the room) or unreal (auditory hallucinations).

Concentration is the patient's ability to persist with a mental task. It is tested by using simple, repetitive sequences, such as asking the patient to repeat the months of the year or days of the week in reverse, or to do the 'serial 7s' test, in which 7 is subtracted from 100, then from 93, then from 86 and so on. Note the finishing point, the number of errors and the time taken.

## Intelligence

This is estimated clinically from a combination of the history of educational attainment and occupations and the evidence provided at interview of vocabulary, general knowledge, abstract thought, foresight and understanding. If in doubt as to whether the patient has a learning disability, or if there is a discrepancy between the history and presentation, a psychologist should be asked to formally test IQ.

## Insight

Insight is the degree to which a patient agrees that they are ill. It can be broken down into the recognition that abnormal mental experiences are in fact abnormal, agreement that these abnormalities amount to a mental illness, and acceptance of the need for treatment. Insight matters, since a lack of it often leads to non-adherence, and sometimes to the need for compulsory detention. You might ask, 'Do you think anything is wrong with you' or 'If you are ill, what do you think needs to happen to make you better?'

## Risk assessment

Risk assessment is a crucial part of every psychiatric assessment. Consider:

- Who is at risk?
- What is the nature of the risk?
- What is the likelihood of the risk?

The person usually at risk, if anyone, is the patient themselves. The risk posed to others by people with mental disorder must be neither overstated nor ignored. Any others at risk are most likely to be family or, less commonly, specific individuals (such as celebrities, in cases of stalking) or members of specific groups (defined by age, ethnicity, occupation and so on). Sometimes the risk applies non-specifically to strangers or to anyone preventing the patient from achieving their goals.

There may be direct risk to life and limb (as in suicide, self-harm or violence to others), or it may be an indirect risk, either to health (through refusal of treatment for physical or mental illness) or welfare (through inability to provide basic care – food, warmth, shelter, hygiene – for oneself or one's dependents). The risk may be imminent, as in a patient actively attempting self-harm, or remote, as in a patient refusing prophylactic medical treatment. Direct risks tend to be imminent and indirect risks remote, although this is not always so. A patient declining renal dialysis because their depression makes them feel unworthy is at an imminent but indirect risk of death. Finally, the likelihood of the risk may range from near certainty to a hypothetical possibility.

A risk assessment should readily distinguish between cases where there is an imminent, direct and near-certain risk to the patient's life (such as a man actively trying to throw himself from the window to escape delusional persecutors) and those where any risks apply to the welfare of other people, at some point in the future, and amount to possibilities (such as a depressed woman who may be neglecting her frail elderly father, for whom she is the sole carer). The former case calls for urgent intervention, probably via mental health legislation; the latter requires engagement over time, preferably in a voluntary way.

While all psychiatric evaluations require some assessment of risk, it should be considered in depth whenever the presentation includes acts or threats of self-harm or reports of command hallucinations, the past history includes self-harm or violent behaviour, the social circumstances show a recent, significant loss, or the mental disorder is strongly associated with risk (as in severe depression).

Assessing suicidality is the element of risk assessment that is most often needed. If a patient presents after an act of self-harm or overdose, the questions arise naturally ('What did you want to happen when you took the tablets? Did you expect to die? Is that what you wanted? How do you feel about that now? Do you still feel you'd be better off dead? Have you had thoughts about doing anything else to harm yourself?').

In other circumstances, the subject will need to be introduced, but do not fear that you may be putting ideas in the patient's mind ('You've told me how bad you have been feeling. Have you ever felt life is not worth living? Have you had any thoughts about ending your life? How close have you come? What has stopped you acting on those thoughts so far?').

## Capacity

Assessing a patient's decision-making capacity, especially for decisions relating to medical treatment, is a skill required of all clinicians and should not be delegated to psychiatrists. The legal elements vary widely between jurisdictions, but there are key clinical principles in common. The first is the *presumption* of capacity: clinicians should treat patients as retaining capacity until it is proven that they have lost it. Secondly, capacity is *decision-specific*: patients may not be able to understand the risks and benefits of complex medical treatment options while retaining the ability to decide whether or not to enter a nursing home. Thirdly, residual capacity should be *maximised*: if a patient's ability to understand is impaired by sensory deficits or language barriers, these should be corrected as far as possible by glasses, hearing aids and interpreters.

The central matters to be assessed are essentially cognitive: can the patient make, understand, remember and communicate decisions about medical treatment or other options before them?

Determining that a patient lacks capacity for a particular decision leads to the next stage: making that decision on their behalf. The key principles here are to ensure that any treatment proposed must benefit the patient and be the least restrictive option available; it should take account of any wishes the patient has previously expressed, as well as the views of family members and any other relevant others.

## The physical examination

Physical and mental disorders are associated, so always consider the physical dimension in any patient presenting with a psychiatric disorder, and vice versa. The setting and the patient's

**16**

age, health and mode of presentation will determine the extent of physical assessment required.

In psychiatric settings, general physical observation, coupled with basic cardiovascular and neurological examination, will usually suffice. Bear in mind that some physical disorders can present with psychiatric symptoms (such as thyrotoxicosis manifesting as anxiety – look for exophthalmos, lid lag, goitre, tachycardia and so on). For older patients with multiple medical problems, or those with alcohol dependence and associated physical harm, a more detailed examination is clearly needed.

In primary care and acute hospital settings, patients will usually undergo physical examination tailored to the presenting problem, but it is important to be aware that some psychiatric disorders can present with physical symptoms, such as panic attacks manifesting as chest pain, shortness of breath and transient neurological symptoms.

## Collateral history

Collateral history is important whenever assessment is limited by:

- physical illness, acute confusional state or dementia
- severe learning disability or other mental disorder impairing communication
- disturbed, aggressive or otherwise uncooperative behaviour.

Sources of third-party information will usually include family and other carers, as well as past and present general practitioners and other health professionals. Previous psychiatric assessments are particularly valuable when a diagnosis of personality disorder is being considered, as this depends more on information about behaviour patterns over time than on the details of the current presentation (Box 16.10).

## Psychiatric rating scales

The use of psychiatric rating scales as clinical tools in psychiatric assessment is increasing. Most were developed in research studies to make a confident diagnosis or to measure a change in the severity of illness. Some require special training; all must be used sensibly. In general, scales are too inflexible and limited in scope to replace a well-conducted standard psychiatric interview, but they can be useful adjuncts for screening, measuring response to treatment or focusing on particular areas.

In routine practice, scales are most widely used to assess cognitive function when an organic brain disorder is suspected. They include:

- Abbreviated Mental Test (AMT): takes less than 5 minutes (Box 16.11)
- 4A's test (4AT): takes less than 2 minutes (the4at.com)
- Mini-Mental State Examination (MMSE) or Montreal Cognitive Assessment (MoCA): takes 5–15 minutes.

Well-known instruments assessing areas other than cognition include:

- general morbidity:
  - General Health Questionnaire (GHQ)
- mood disorder:
  - Hospital Anxiety and Depression Scale (HADS)
  - Beck Depression Inventory (BDI)
- alcohol:
  - CAGE questionnaire (Box 16.12)
  - FAST questionnaire (Box 16.13).

## Putting it all together: clinical vignettes

Examples in practice are provided in Boxes 16.14–16.17.

---

**16.11 The Abbreviated Mental Test**

- Age
- Date of birth
- Time (to the nearest hour)
- Year
- Hospital name
- Recognition of two people, e.g. doctor, nurse
- Recall address
- Dates of First World War (or other culturally appropriate significant event)
- Name of the monarch/prime minister/president or other culturally appropriate figure)
- Count backwards 20–1

Each question scores 1 mark; a score of 8/10, or less, indicates confusion.

From Hodkinson HM. Evaluation of a mental test score for assessment of mental impairment in the elderly. Age and Ageing 1972; 1(4):233–238, by permission of Oxford University Press.

---

**16.10 Personality disorder: definition**

Patterns of experience and behaviour that are:
- pathological (i.e. outside social norms)
- problematic (for the patient and/or others)
- pervasive (affecting most or all areas of a patient's life)
- persistent (adolescent onset, enduring throughout adult life and resistant to treatment)

---

**16.12 The CAGE questionnaire**

- Cut down: Have you ever felt that you should cut down on your drinking?
- Annoyed: Have people annoyed you by criticising your drinking?
- Guilty: Have you ever felt bad or guilty about your drinking?
- Ever: Do you ever have a drink first thing in the morning, to steady you or help a hangover (an 'eye opener')?

Positive answers to two or more questions suggest problem drinking; confirm this by asking about the maximum taken.

## 16.13 The Fast Alcohol Screening Test (FAST) questionnaire

For the following questions please circle the answer that best applies
1 drink = $^1/_2$ pint of beer, or 1 glass of wine, or 1 single measure of spirits.

1.  Men: How often do you have eight or more drinks on one occasion?
    Women: How often do you have six or more drinks on one occasion?
    - Never (0)
    - Less than monthly (1)
    - Monthly (2)
    - Weekly (3)
    - Daily or almost daily (4)

2.  How often, during the last year, have you been unable to remember what happened the night before because you had been drinking?
    - Never (0)
    - Less than monthly (1)
    - Monthly (2)
    - Weekly (3)
    - Daily or almost daily (4)

3.  How often, during the last year, have you failed to do what was normally expected of you because of drinking?
    - Never (0)
    - Less than monthly (1)
    - Monthly (2)
    - Weekly (3)
    - Daily or almost daily (4)

4.  In the last year, has a relative or friend, or a doctor or other health worker, been concerned about your drinking or suggested you cut down?
    - Never (0)
    - Yes, on one occasion (2)
    - Yes, on more than one occasion (4)

### Scoring FAST

**First stage**
- If the answer to question 1 is 'Never', then the patient is probably not misusing alcohol.
- If the answer is 'Weekly' or 'Daily or almost daily', then the patient is a hazardous, harmful or dependent drinker.
- 50% of people are classified using this one question.

**Second stage**
- Only use questions 2–4 if the answer to question 1 is 'Less than monthly' or 'Monthly':
- Score questions 1–3: 0, 1, 2, 3, 4
- Score question 4: 0, 2, 4
- Minimum score is 0
- Maximum score is 16
- Score for hazardous drinking is 3 or more

## 16.14 Clinical vignette: overdose

A 19-year-old woman attends the accident and emergency department after having taken a medically minor overdose. She has presented in this way three times in the last 2 years. She needs no specific medical treatment.

Your assessment should concentrate first on the circumstances of the overdose and her intentions at the time. Collateral information should include assessments after previous presentations and any continuing psychiatric follow-up. Mental state examination should screen for any new signs of mental disorder emerging since her last assessment, and in particular any mood problems or new psychotic symptoms. She will clearly have undergone a detailed physical assessment, but even if the overdose appears medically trivial, you need to undertake a risk assessment to judge the chances of further self-harm or completed suicide in the near future. She probably does not need a detailed cognitive assessment or psychiatric rating scales.

## 16.15 Clinical vignette: confusion, agitation and hostility

An 85-year-old man in a medical ward, where he is undergoing intra-venous antibiotic treatment for a chest infection, now appears confused, agitated and hostile, in a way not previously evident to his family.

You need to approach him carefully to establish rapport and to interview him as much as he will allow, while anticipating that you may have to rely heavily on collateral information and a mental state examination limited to observation of appearance and behaviour. It will be crucial to talk to his family to establish his normal level of cognition and independence, and to the nursing staff to establish the diurnal pattern of his problems. If there is any history of previous episodes, acquire the results of previous assessments. He will need a neurological examination and an assessment of his cognition via a standard scale. Risk assessment should focus on the indirect risks to his health if he tries to leave the hospital against advice, generating a view about his detainability under mental health legislation. A capacity assessment of his ability to consent to continuing antibiotic treatment is required and may result in the issue of an incapacity certificate.

## 16.16 Clinical vignette: fatigue

A 35-year-old woman attends her general practitioner, presenting with fatigue.

Assessment of possible physical causes is required, via history, examination and appropriate blood tests, but as these proceed, the interview should also cover possible symptoms of depression, previous episodes, family history and recent stressors. Mental state examination should concentrate on objective evidence of lowered mood. Formal assessment of cognition is probably not necessary, but a standard rating scale for mood disorder may help establish a diagnosis and a baseline against which to measure change. Risk assessment is not a prominent requirement, unless a depressive illness is suspected and she reports thoughts of self-harm or is responsible for young children, in which case the chance of direct or indirect harm to them needs to be considered.

## 16.17 Clinical vignette: paranoid thoughts

A 42-year-old man attends a psychiatric outpatient clinic for the first time, having been referred by his general practitioner for longstanding paranoid thoughts.

It will be particularly important to establish rapport with a patient who is likely to be very wary. The interview needs to cover the psychiatric history in some detail, considering substance misuse, family history of mental illness and a full personal history in particular. Mental state examination should explore the paranoid thoughts in detail, to establish whether they are preoccupations or overvalued ideas (suggesting a personality disorder) or delusions (suggesting a psychotic illness). Risk assessment should concentrate on the risk to others about whom the patient has paranoid fears. Neither a detailed cognitive assessment nor a specific rating scale is likely to add much to the initial assessment.

## OSCE example 1: Assessing suicidal risk

A 27-year-old woman presented to the Emergency Department the previous day after taking an overdose of paracetamol while intoxicated with alcohol. She has undergone treatment with acetylcysteine overnight and is now medically fit for discharge.

### Please assess her risk of self-harm and suicide

- Introduce yourself and clean your hands.
- Explain the purpose of your assessment; try to gain rapport.
- Enquire how she is feeling physically (specifically asking about nausea, vomiting and abdominal pain).
- Tactfully introduce the subject of the overdose.
- Establish the number and type of tablets taken.
- Establish how much alcohol she drank, whether this was with the tablets (to 'wash them down') or whether she was already intoxicated at the time of the overdose.
- Clarify the circumstances. Who else was present or expected? Did she write a note, or otherwise communicate, what she had done or was planning to do?
- Clarify how she was found and either came or was brought to hospital.
- Explore recent or chronic stressors.
- Establish her intent at the time of the overdose. Did she expect to die? Is that what she wanted?
- Confirm her view now. Does she still wish to die? Does she have any thoughts about another overdose or other form of self-harm?
- Establish relevant past history. Are there any previous overdoses? Any previous or continuing psychiatric follow-up?
- Confirm whether she has parental or caring responsibilities for young children. Tactfully enquire about any thoughts of harming them.
- Establish who will be with her when she leaves hospital.
- Thank the patient and clean your hands.

### Summarise your findings

The risk assessment should concentrate most on the short-term risk of suicide.

### Advanced level comments

More advanced students would be expected to tabulate short- and long-term risks of both suicide and further self-harm and to quote the risk of completed suicide in the first year after an act of self-harm (1–2%).

## OSCE example 2: Assessing delirium

An 82-year-old man is admitted to an orthopaedic ward after falling and breaking his hip. Forty-eight hours after surgery, he became restless and agitated overnight, pulling out his intravenous line. He is now settled and cooperative.

### Please assess the likely cause of this episode

- Introduce yourself and clean your hands.
- Explain the purpose of your assessment; try to establish rapport.
- Enquire how he is feeling physically (specifically asking about pain, fever, constipation, urinary and respiratory symptoms).
- Establish his awareness of where he is, why he is there and how long he has been in hospital.
- Ask how much he remembers of the night's events, and enquire specifically about any recollection of hallucinations or persecutory fears.
- Enquire about any continuing hallucinations or fears.
- Ask about any previous similar episodes.
- Clarify how active he was before his fall and whether there is any awareness of memory impairment leading up to it.
- Ask about alcohol intake.
- Administer simple tests of cognitive function, especially of attention and memory (advanced performers should know the Abbreviated Mental Test questions).
- Undertake a basic physical examination, assessing for tremor, ophthalmoplegia and nystagmus.
- Gain the patient's permission to speak to his next of kin, general practitioner and others.
- Thank the patient and clean your hands.

### Summarise your findings

The diagnosis is delirium, with further enquiries needed to establish the likely cause (which may be alcohol withdrawal, given the timing), as well as the possibility of pre-existing cognitive impairment as a vulnerability factor.

**16**

## Integrated examination sequence for the psychiatric assessment

- Review the relevant information to clarify the reason for referral or mode of self-presentation.
- Establish rapport to reduce distress and assist assessment.
- Cover the key headings for the history (presenting symptoms, systematic review, past medical and psychiatric history, current medication, substance misuse, family history, personal history).
- Cover the headings for the personal history (childhood development, losses and experiences, education, occupation, financial circumstances, relationships, partner(s) and children, housing, leisure activities, hobbies and interests, forensic history).
- Make the extent, order and content of the assessment appropriate to the presentation and setting.
- Observe closely to gain objective evidence of mental state, especially non-verbal information.
- Cover the headings for the mental state examination systematically (appearance and behaviour, speech, mood, thought form and content, perceptions, cognition and insight).
- Use brief formal tests to assess cognitive function (Abbreviated Mental Test, Mini-Mental State Examination, Montreal Cognitive Assessment).
- Consider your own emotional response to your patient.
- Consider standardised rating scales as a screening tool (and sometimes to monitor progress).
- Undertake physical examination as appropriate to the setting and the presentation.
- Gather further background information from other sources to the degree necessary (with permission).
- As well as a diagnosis and management plan, be sure to consider:
  - assessment of risk to self or others
  - capacity to take decisions
  - need to use mental health or incapacity legislation.

**Andrew Elder**
**Elizabeth MacDonald**

17

# The frail patient

The frail patient 380

Assessment of the frail patient 380
Factors influencing presentation and history 381

The history 382
The presenting symptoms 382
Common presenting symptoms 382
Past medical history 382
Drug history 382
Family history 383
Social and functional history 383

Systematic enquiry 384

The physical examination 384
General examination 385
Systems examination 385
Functional assessment   387

Interpretation of the findings 388

OSCE Example 1: History in a frail patient with falls 389

OSCE Example 2: Examination of an acutely confused frail patient 390

Integrated clinical examination for the frail patient 391

## The frail patient

A frail person typically suffers from multimorbidity (multiple illnesses) and has associated polypharmacy (multiple medications). They often have cognitive impairment, visual and hearing loss, low bodyweight, poor mobility due to muscular weakness, unstable balance and poor exercise tolerance. Their general functional reserve and the capacity of individual organs and physiological systems are impaired, making the individual potentially vulnerable to the effects of minor illnesses. Frailty is likely to be a response to chronic disease and the ageing process.

Whilst frailty increases with advancing age and is usually seen in older patients, it can also occur in younger people.

Identifying frailty proactively can help target those patients who will benefit from specialised assessment and management. There are many tools available to identify and stratify the level of frailty. One commonly used scale is the Clinical Frailty Scale, which uses an individual's functional ability and level of dependency to determine their degree of frailty (Fig. 17.1).

## Assessment of the frail patient

When an individual is identified as frail, Comprehensive Geriatric Assessment is an evidence-based process that improves outcomes. It involves taking a history from the patient and, with the patient's consent, from a carer or relative, followed by a systematic assessment of:

- cognitive function and mood
- nutrition and hydration
- skin
- pain
- continence
- hearing and vision
- functional status.

The extent and focus of the assessment depend on the clinical presentation. In non-acute settings such as general practice or the outpatient clinic or day hospital, focus on establishing what diseases are present, and also which functional impairments, symptoms and problems most affect the patient's life.

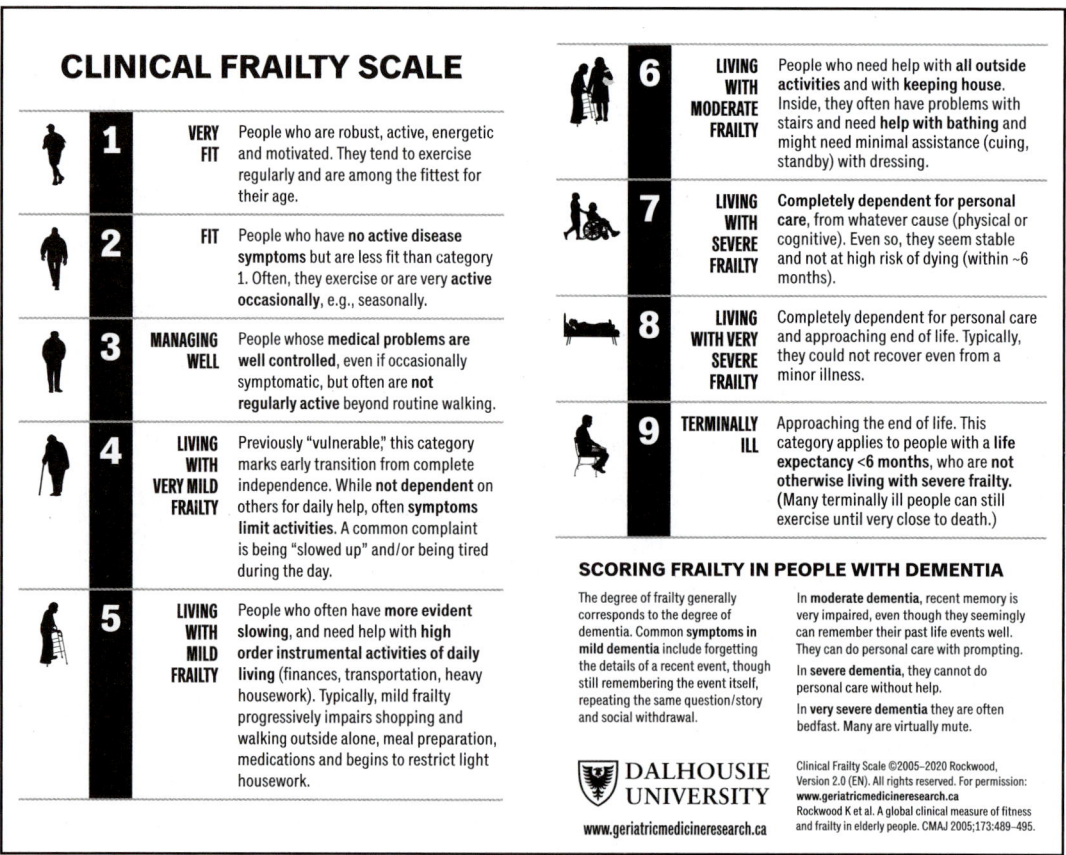

**Fig. 17.1** Clinical Frailty Scale v2.0. *From "Using the Clinical Frailty Scale in allocating scarce resources" by K Rockwood and O Theou, Canadian Geriatrics Journal, 23, p 211. Copyright 2020 by Kenneth Rockwood. Reprinted with permission.*

### 17.1 The multiprofessional team

| Professional | Key roles in assessment of |
|---|---|
| Physician | Physical state, including diagnosis and therapeutic intervention |
| Psychiatrist | Cognition, mood and capacity |
| Physiotherapist | Mobility, balance, gait and falls risk |
| Occupational therapist | Practical functional activities (self-care and domestic) |
| Nurse | Skin health, nutrition and continence |
| Dietician | Nutrition |
| Speech and language therapist | Speech and swallowing |
| Social worker | Social care needs |

In acute settings, such as following acute hospital referral, focus on what has changed or is new. Seek any new symptoms or signs of disease and any changes from baseline physical or cognitive function.

The complexity of the problems presented and the need for comprehensive and systematic analysis mean that assessment is divided into multiple components, undertaken at different times by different members of the multiprofessional team (Box 17.1).

## Factors influencing presentation and history

Classical patterns of symptoms and signs still occur in the frail patient, but modified or non-specific presentations are very common due to comorbidity, drug treatment and ageing itself. As the combination of these factors is unique for each individual, presentations will be different in each patient. Some general patterns can be recognised, however (Fig. 17.2). The first sign of new illness may be a change in functional status: typically, reduced mobility, altered cognition or impairment of balance leading to falls. Common precipitants are infections, changes in medication and metabolic derangements, but almost any acute medical illness can produce these non-specific presentations. Each of these presentations should

**Fig. 17.2** Functional decompensation in frail people.

be explored through careful history taking, physical examination and functional assessment.

## Communication difficulties, cognition and mood

Disorders of communication, cognition and mood are common and should always be considered at the start of the assessment of a frail adult.

Communication can be challenging for a variety of reasons (Box 17.2). As a result, the history can be incomplete, difficult to interpret or misleading, and the whole assessment, including physical examination, may be more time-consuming.

Whenever possible, assess the patient somewhere quiet with few distractions. Introduce yourself clearly, make your patient comfortable and ensure that they understand the purpose of your contact. Provide any glasses, hearing aids or dentures that they need and help them to switch on and adjust their hearing aid if necessary. If they still cannot hear you, use an electronic communicator, or if they can read easily, write down simple questions and instructions.

Cognitive function includes the processes of perception, attention, memory, reasoning, decision-making and problem solving (p. 320). Cognitive impairment increases with age and has implications for assessment, treatment, consent and prognosis. Consider cognitive impairment if a patient who appears to hear you has limited ability to cooperate with you, cannot recall their medical history or provides no specific symptoms. Other problems, including low mood or dysphasia, can mimic cognitive impairment. Some patients present with apparently good social skills or 'façade' and cover their impaired memory by diverting the conversation to another topic. Never ascribe changes in cognition to age alone, without excluding dementia or delirium (p. 377).

Depression is common in frail people and may be difficult to diagnose. Consider this if your patient struggles to concentrate, is withdrawn or is reluctant to interact. Standardised rating scales are available, such as the Geriatric Depression Scale. A formal psychiatric assessment may help.

Patients are often fearful that they will be admitted to the hospital or not return home after admission, and they may

### 17.2 Communication difficulties: the seven Ds

| Problem | Comment/causes |
|---|---|
| Deafness | Nerve or conductive |
| Dysphasia | Most commonly due to stroke disease but sometimes a feature of dementia |
| Dysarthria | Cerebrovascular disease, motor neuron disease, Parkinson's disease |
| Dysphonia | Parkinson's disease |
| Dementia | Global impairment of cognitive function |
| Delirium | Impaired attention, disturbance of arousal and perceptual disturbances |
| Depression | May mimic dementia or delirium |

17

understate their symptoms or functional limitations. Always try to corroborate the history from a partner, carer, relative or friend, with the patient's consent.

# The history

## The presenting symptoms

Frail patients often have multiple symptoms. Take time to detail each symptom and separate those arising from a new acute illness from those due to background disease and disabilities.

Ask:

- How long have you had a particular symptom?
- Has it changed recently?
- When were you last totally free of the symptom?

Try to establish what the patient's symptoms, functional abilities and mental status were before the new presenting problem. The Informant Questionnaire on Cognitive Decline in the Elderly (IQCODE) can help family members compare current with past cognition. This helps set realistic goals for treatment and rehabilitation.

The patient's perspective may vary from the clinician's, particularly in acute settings. For example, a patient referred following sudden loss of consciousness may be unconcerned by this but anxious about longstanding back pain. These symptoms should never be disregarded; if they are important to your patient, they should be important to you.

## Common presenting symptoms

### Decreased mobility

Ask about:

- the patient's usual mobility, when it changed and if the change was abrupt
- what factor, or factors, are causing the impaired mobility. Commonly, pain, weakness or loss of balance will be present, alone or in combination. Each may have a remediable cause.
- any falls
- use of walking aids
- history of recent head injury, fevers or rigors, dizziness or poor balance
- lower limb weakness, numbness or paraesthesia
- joint pain, especially in the back, neck or lower limbs
- any bladder or bowel symptoms
- current drug treatment and whether this has changed recently
- how the change in mobility is affecting their daily life.

### Confusion

Check that the patient can hear you clearly and ask if they would like a friend or relative to be with them. Although a confused patient may find it difficult to give an accurate history or a clear description of symptoms, never ignore what they tell you, as their perspective remains important to your care. Take a collateral history.

Establish:

- the person's normal cognitive state and whether the change has been abrupt or gradual (see earlier). Acute change, developing over hours or days, that fluctuates is suggestive of delirium
- any symptoms of common infections, such as urinary frequency, productive cough, fever or rigors, which can precipitate delirium
- whether the person has any pain, and if so, where
- current drug treatment and adherence, with any recent changes
- alcohol use.

If delirium is suspected, carry out a cognitive screening test, for example, 4A's test (4AT) (p. 377), to help confirm the diagnosis.

### Falls

A collateral history is helpful if a fall has been witnessed.

Establish:

- the patient's usual mobility
- how many falls they have had, over what time frame and whether injuries, including fractures or head injury, have been sustained
- whether the patient can rise from the floor unassisted
- whether the patient has a falls alarm or other means of calling for help
- the presence of dizziness or lightheadedness, and whether the problem is true vertigo or worse on standing (p. 194)
- the presence of palpitations, limb weakness, paraesthesia or any joint pain, especially in the back, neck or lower limbs
- quality of vision
- any problems with the feet
- any recent symptoms of infection
- current drug treatment and any recent changes.

## Past medical history

Detail the past history and known comorbidities from all available sources, including any previous records. Comorbidities may not be directly relevant to the current problem but may influence prognosis and the feasibility and appropriateness of potential investigations and treatments (Box 17.3).

## Drug history

Polypharmacy is associated with drug interactions, adverse events and difficulties with adherence. Take a detailed drug history, supplemented by the following:

- Identify all medications, including over-the-counter preparations.
- Ask whether any drugs have been started or stopped recently, or doses of regular medications altered.

## 17.3 How comorbidities or drugs can influence symptoms or clinical signs

| Comorbidity/drug | Effect of comorbidity or drug | Effect on presentation of new disease |
|---|---|---|
| Osteoarthritis of weight-bearing joint | Limited mobility | Patient does not experience exertional dyspnoea, resulting in late presentation of heart disease |
| Cognitive impairment | Poor recall or no recognition of symptoms | Patient does not describe symptoms of disease and diagnosis is not recognised |
| Anticholinergics<br>Diuretics<br>Some calcium antagonists | Dry mouth<br>Urinary frequency<br>Ankle swelling | A symptom is caused by drug treatment rather than disease |
| Vasodilators, diuretics<br>Beta-blockers<br>L-dopa (usually long-term) | Postural hypotension<br>Bradycardia<br>Dyskinetic limb movements | A sign is caused by drug treatment rather than disease |
| Beta-blockers | No tachycardia in gastrointestinal bleeding | An expected sign does not occur because of drug treatment |

- Ask the patient if they think any of their medications are causing any of their symptoms.
- Explore the patient's ability to self-administer drugs; ask if they use a dosette box or if a carer helps with administration.
- Explore the ability to read labels, open bottles or use inhalers correctly.
- If patients have their drugs with them, go through them together. Ask patients what they believe each one is for, how it affects them and how often they take it.
- Ask if there are any drugs that they sometimes omit, such as diuretics on days when they are going out.
- Ask carers if there are partially used supplies of drugs in the house.
- Clarify any 'allergies' or previous adverse events. Explore what symptoms the patient believes to be caused by their drugs, as some may be unrelated. If in doubt, regard the allergy as significant.
- Contact the prescriber, if necessary, to confirm details of the drug history.

## Family history

A first presentation of disease with a strong genetic basis is unlikely, but family history is still important to patients who have lost siblings or children to specific conditions and who may believe that their own symptoms are related.

## Social and functional history

Complement a comprehensive social history with information about the patient's functional ability, as this affects their capacity to cope at home and what assistance they need to support their function there. Try and get enough information to envisage, in your own mind, a typical day in the life of your patient.

Ask about:

- Their normal mobility and whether they transfer from chair to bed or toilet, and walk alone.
- Use of a walking aid and whether they can manage stairs.
- Their current level of function, what it was before, and the time course of any functional deterioration.
- How they manage day-to-day activities:
  - Can they wash and dress?
  - Do they do their own shopping and prepare their own meals?

Abrupt functional decline suggests a more acute underlying precipitant or disease. Insidious decline suggests alternate pathologies or progression of underlying chronic disease(s). Seek corroboration from a friend, relative or carer, but interpret all information obtained in association with objective functional assessment by yourself and other members of the multiprofessional team (see Box 17.1).

The frail patient's home environment is important:

- Does anyone else live with the patient? Patients who live alone often require more support.
- If they live alone, establish how long this has been the case.
- Have they lived in their current home for long?
- What is access like to the house/bedroom/toilets? Do they use stairs, inside or outside?
- What carer support does the patient have (home help, family or friends)? How often does any carer visit and what does each person do for the patient?
- If in sheltered accommodation:
  - Are meals provided?
  - Is there an on-site warden or are there personal safety alarms?
  - How does the patient feel about living there and do they wish to remain?

Most frail patients will not be in paid employment, but some may have informal roles supporting others in their home. If they

**17**

are retired, find out what they did, as it may be relevant to their condition and gives insight into their past life. Retirement can lead to social isolation, which contributes to mood disorders.

- Can the patient still get out by themselves or accompanied, or are they house-bound? How many visitors do they have?
- Establish if your patient is still driving, as there may be safety issues in the presence of visual or cognitive defects.
- Establish other lifestyle information. Alcohol overuse is not infrequent, and there may be many pack-years of cigarette use.

Get to know your patient when asking these questions and listening to the answers. Patient-centred care relies upon a good understanding of each patient's unique circumstances, concerns and perspectives.

## Systematic enquiry

Many diseases in frailer people present with non-specific functional deterioration such as immobility. The systematic enquiry is important as it may provide clues to specific underlying precipitants. Supplement the standard systematic enquiry with questions in the following areas:

- Cognition and mood: has the patient noticed any memory problems or has anyone else commented on their memory? Does anyone help them with letters and bills? Ask about how they sleep at night. How would they describe their mood and appetite? Are they still interested in previous pursuits, such as reading or watching favourite television programmes?
- Nutrition: has their weight been steady over the past few months? Have they noticed their clothes getting loose? How many meals do they have in the day and do they eat meat, fish, vegetables and fruit? Who prepares their meals? Do they have any problems with their teeth or gums? If they wear dentures, do they fit well? Is their mouth dry?
- Pain: always ask specifically about pain, as this may affect mobility and sleep.
- Continence: ask whether they ever notice incontinence or leakage from their bladder or bowels. Are they aware when they are about to pass urine or stool? Do they wear pads by day or by night? Do they ever find it hard to get to the toilet on time? Ask men about prostatic symptoms (p. 268) in particular. Do these problems stop them from doing other daily activities?
- Sensory impairment: ask about any problems with vision and whether they wear glasses. Can they see the television and read a newspaper? If they wear a hearing aid, find out if it is working and whether they are wearing it.
- Balance and falls: do they ever feel unsteady on their feet? Ask specifically about any falls in the past year and obtain a careful description of these (p. 194).

## The physical examination

It takes time and patience to perform a detailed assessment of a frail patient. Physical examination is easiest when your patient can comply with your instructions. All patients benefit from clear, careful instruction, and this is particularly important for the frail, who may have communication problems or find the examination routine demanding. Many have low levels of stamina and their movement may be limited. Integrate your physical examination to minimise movement for patients and maximise their understanding and cooperation. Help them to move around the room and to get on and off the examination couch. Remember that they will take longer to undress and dress. Most patients feel more comfortable if a family member, carer or friend is present, and always check if this is what they wish. If the patient has attended alone, always ask if they would like a chaperone to be present too.

Use the physical examination to find evidence of established comorbidities and explanations for functional problems, current symptoms, or concerns voiced by a carer. Some frail people have difficulty maintaining personal hygiene, grooming or appearance. Their hair and clothes may be unclean, nails unkempt and facial hair longer than in younger life. These findings may reflect underlying functional or cognitive impairment, social isolation or low mood and are relevant to the patient's overall functional status, condition and outlook, or need for social support.

Be aware of the common clinical signs found in frail patients. Just as the history uncovers multiple diverse and unexpected symptoms, a careful examination will often reveal many clinical signs in different clinical systems. In acute presentations, be alert to typical signs of acute illness that may be misleadingly absent in older patients (Box 17.4).

Document all examination findings, as this will help clinicians who assess the patient in the future. Assume that the physical

| 17.4 Modified signs in acutely unwell frail patients | | |
|---|---|---|
| **Feature** | **Clinical context** | **Modification** |
| Temperature | Possible sepsis | Systemic inflammatory response obtunded, may not mount pyrexia (or may become hypothermic) Core temperature normally lower and diurnal variation lost: ↑ temperature may occur but not > 37°C |
| Pulse rate | Volume status, response to sepsis or pain | Altered baroreceptor function may attenuate the rise in heart rate typically associated with these stressors |
| Blood pressure | Volume status, response to sepsis or pain | Altered baroreceptor function may modify blood pressure response to acute illness |
| Postural hypotension | Volume status | May be found in volume-replete patients due to primary autonomic dysfunction. Less reliable indicator of volume depletion |
| Skin turgor | Hydration | ↓ but less specific because of reduction in subcutaneous fat |

signs you find are due to disease, which may be treatable, rather than ageing, which is not.

## General examination

### Hydration and nutrition

Disorders of hydration are common in frail patients, but accurate clinical assessment is difficult and classical signs less reliable (Box 17.5).

Undernutrition and low bodyweight are common features of frailty that may develop rapidly in hospitalised patients. Screening tools are used to assess the risk of malnutrition (Fig. 17.3). Seek reversible causes. Consider chronic diseases such as chronic obstructive pulmonary disease, new serious diseases such as cancer, poor social support or isolation and depression, as these may present with low bodyweight. Other factors that may contribute include poor oral health, poor function (being unable to obtain or prepare food) and cognitive impairment (being unable to prepare food or remember to eat it).

### The skin

Bruising may suggest glucocorticoid use but is often simply age-related and caused by the reduction in subcutaneous supporting tissue. Rarely, it is due to scurvy (p. 32). Soft-tissue infections often cause functional decompensation and confusion, immobility and falls (see Fig. 17.2). Leg ulcers are common and frequently have multifactorial causes (p. 326). Pain from ulcers may reduce mobility. On admission to hospital, many frail patients have skin wounds that have been dressed in the community. Always remove these dressings with the help of a nurse, and assess the underlying lesion.

Frail patients with limited mobility are vulnerable to the rapid development of pressure sores, particularly when acutely ill. Standardised assessment scores such as the Waterlow score help identify patients at risk of skin breakdown.

| 17.5 Assessment of dehydration | |
|---|---|
| **Classical feature of dehydration** | **Interpretation in frail patients** |
| Postural hypotension | Less specific than in younger patients; may be caused by drugs, disease or age-related abnormal autonomic responses to postural change |
| Decreased skin turgor | Decreased collagen elasticity and reduced subcutaneous fat can mimic reduced turgor. Best assessed at the sternum |
| Impaired capillary refill time | Less reliable in the frail because less specific |
| Dry mouth | A non-specific finding caused by other problems, such as anticholinergic drugs or mouth breathing |
| Tachycardia in hypovolaemia | Less sensitive due to drug- or age-related abnormal autonomic responses |

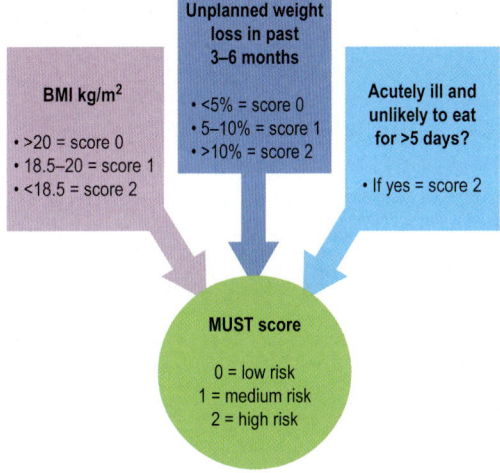

**Fig. 17.3 The Malnutrition Universal Screening Tool (MUST) score for assessment of risk of malnutrition.** *BMI*, body mass index. *The 'Malnutrition Universal Screening Tool' ('MUST') is reproduced here with the kind permission of BAPEN (British Association for Parenteral and Enteral Nutrition). For further information on 'MUST' see* www.bapen.org.uk. *Copyright © BAPEN 2012 (licence number LIC2206).*

### Pain behaviour

In patients with impairment of communication or cognition, always look for pain-related behaviour, as the patient may not volunteer or admit to pain or discomfort (Box 17.6).

### Vision and hearing

Hearing loss and visual symptoms, including impairment of visual acuity, are common (Box 17.7) but often overlooked, and this can adversely affect communication, interaction and function.

Use a Snellen chart or ask the patient to read from a newspaper to assess their vision. Hearing loss may be misinterpreted as cognitive impairment and vice versa. Make sure that the external auditory meatus is not blocked with wax. Ensure that patients wear their hearing aids with a functioning battery. Assess hearing using the whispered voice test if they do not have hearing aids (p. 197).

## Systems examination

Fully examine each system as outlined in previous chapters, and be aware of differences found in the frail older patient compared to younger patients.

**17**

## 17.6 Signs and behaviour associated with pain

| Type | Description |
|------|-------------|
| Autonomic changes | Pallor, sweating, tachypnoea, altered breathing patterns, tachycardia, hypertension |
| Facial expressions | Grimacing, wincing, frowning, rapid blinking, brow raising, brow lowering, cheek raising, eyelid tightening, nose wrinkling, lip corner pulling, chin raising, lip puckering |
| Body movements | Altered gait, pacing, rocking, hand wringing, repetitive movements, increased tone, guarding,[a] bracing[b] |
| Verbalisation/ vocalisation | Sighing, grunting, groaning, moaning, screaming, calling out, aggressive/offensive speech |
| Interpersonal interactions | Aggression, withdrawal, resistance |
| Changes in activity patterns | Wandering, altered sleep, altered rest patterns |
| Mental status changes | Confusion, crying, distress, irritability |

[a]Guarding = abnormal stiff, rigid or interrupted movement while changing position.
[b]Bracing = a stationary position in which a fully extended limb maintains and supports an abnormal weight distribution for at least 3 seconds.

## 17.7 Sensory problems

| Sensory modality | Underlying disease process |
|------------------|---------------------------|
| **Visual** | |
| Loss of near vision (presbyopia) | Common in older age because lens is less pliable |
| Loss of central vision | Macular degeneration |
| Loss of peripheral vision | Glaucoma Stroke disease (homonymous hemianopia) |
| Glare from lights at night | Cataracts |
| Eye pain | Glaucoma |
| **Auditory** | |
| High-frequency loss | Presbyacusis Conductive deafness more common due to otosclerosis |
| Generalised loss | Conductive – otosclerosis, wax Nerve – Paget's disease, drug-induced ototoxicity, acoustic neuroma |

## Cardiovascular examination

Corneal arcus (see Fig. 4.6C) increases in prevalence in the older adult but is an unreliable sign of dyslipidaemia. A widened pulse pressure occurs because there is decreased arterial compliance. Isolated systolic hypertension and postural hypotension occur more frequently. The latter may result from age-related baroreceptor reflex change, disease or drugs. It may not be symptomatic but increases the risk of a fall.

Medial sclerosis and arterial calcification can make it difficult to feel peripheral pulses but do not cause impaired perfusion and circulation in isolation. The carotid artery may become more tortuous and its pulsations more easily visible. This can create a false impression of arterial dilatation.

Atrial contribution to left ventricular filling increases with age, partly due to diastolic dysfunction of the heart, and a fourth heart sound ($S_4$) is more commonly heard.

## Respiratory examination

Localised crackles are common, and although they may not represent acute disease, you should never disregard new respiratory pathology as a possible cause.

## Gastrointestinal examination

Dry mouth and tongue are common side effects of drugs and may affect taste and swallowing. Abnormal dentition, oral thrush or mouth ulcers may reduce oral intake and nutrition.

## Neurological examination

Cognitive impairment may reduce the accuracy of the history and affect consent for investigation and treatment. Impaired vibration and position sense occur in old age and may impair balance and increase the risk of falls. Always exclude correctable causes such as vitamin $B_{12}$ deficiency. Bilateral absent ankle reflexes may be normal, but unilateral loss is likely to indicate pathology.

Asymmetry of tone, reflexes or power may relate to cerebrovascular disease. If tone is increased, look for additional tremors and the variation in tone on passive movement (cogwheeling) that might indicate extrapyramidal disease. Tremors and other involuntary movements are common, with essential tremors and extrapyramidal disease being the most frequent causes.

## Musculoskeletal examination

Low muscle mass is a frailty indicator and a risk factor for falls. Osteoarthritic changes in the hands and weight-bearing joints may predispose to falls or unsteadiness, even if relatively asymptomatic or painless. Gouty tophi may be asymptomatic and reflect underlying renal dysfunction and influence the choice of drug therapy. Kyphosis often occurs from painless osteoporotic vertebral collapse and may affect postural stability and respiratory function.

Always examine the feet. Bunions, onychomycosis with or without nail overgrowth, and foot ulcers are common. All can compromise mobility and stability, be a source of sepsis or pain, and affect gait. Observe your patient walking. A wide variety of pathologies can produce distinctive abnormalities in gait, including Parkinson's disease (see Fig. 7.17). Gait abnormalities are a risk factor for falls and can exacerbate joint problems.

## Functional assessment (Video 32)

Functional assessment is divided into an analysis of:

- mobility
- ability to undertake activities of daily living (ADLs):
  - personal ADLs: washing, dressing, feeding and toileting
  - domestic ADLs: preparing food, laundering clothes and cleaning the house.

Mobility is a key determinant of physical function. Many different pathologies can impair mobility, including neurological, muscular or joint disease. Frailty itself causes generally impaired muscle strength, function and poor mobility without specific clinical findings on examination of muscles, nerves, joints or gait.

Standardised rating scales are used to assess components of function and include the modified Barthel Index for ADLs and the Elderly Mobility Score. The Timed Get Up and Go Test is easy to perform and assesses both mobility and falls risk (Fig. 17.4). Use these scales to describe the patient's abilities succinctly and, using sequential recording over time, objectively assess improvement or deterioration.

### Examination sequence

### The frail person with decreased mobility

- General examination: look particularly for signs of acute illness (see Box 17.4). If the patient is able to walk, assess the posture and gait and any inappropriate footwear. Are they visually impaired (see Box 17.7)? Are there signs of sepsis or a distended bladder?
- Cardiovascular system: check for postural hypotension.
- Nervous system: note any neurological signs, particularly in the lower limbs, and look for evidence of Parkinson's disease (see Chapter 7).
- Musculoskeletal system: look for muscle wasting or fasciculation, joint abnormality and foot deformity.
- Consider specific investigations (Box 17.8).

### Delirium in a frail person

- If patients have problems with vision or hearing, ensure that they wear their glasses or a working hearing aid.
- Look for signs of acute illness (see Box 17.4) and pain (see Box 17.6).

**17.8 Specific investigations in the frail**

| Presentation | Investigations |
| --- | --- |
| Immobility and/or falls | Septic screen – include urinalysis and WCC<br>Electrolytes and renal function<br>Mental state assessment (p. 368)<br>CT head[a]<br>MRI spine[b] |
| Confusion | Septic screen – include urinalysis and WCC<br>Electrolytes and renal function<br>Mental state assessment (p. 368)<br>CT head[a] |
| Urinary incontinence | Urinalysis, urine culture<br>Voiding chart (frequency and volume)<br>Bladder ultrasound (postresidual volume)<br>Consider prostate-specific antigen in men |
| Faecal incontinence | Stool culture if diarrhoea<br>Abdominal X-ray if high impaction is suspected |

[a]If new neurological signs or head injury are suspected.
[b]If cord pathology is suspected.

*CT*, Computed tomography; *MRI*, magnetic resonance imaging; *WCC*, white cell count.

| Begin timing → | Rising from standard armchair | Walk to line on floor approximately 3 metres away | Turn and return to chair | Sit down on chair |

The normal time to finish the test is between 7 and 10 seconds.
Patients who cannot complete the task in that time probably have some mobility problems, especially if they take more than 20 seconds.

**Fig. 17.4** The Timed Get Up and Go Test.

- Examine the skin, large joints, lungs, heart valves, prostheses and abdomen for signs of sepsis.
- Examine for any new neurological features.
- Perform pulse oximetry ($SpO_2$).
- Feel for a distended bladder.
- Consider a rectal examination (p. 126) to check for faecal impaction.
- Consider specific investigations (see Box 17.8).

## The frail person with falls

- Look for signs of bony or soft-tissue injury and acute illness such as sepsis (see Box 17.4).
- Cardiovascular system: check for postural hypotension, arrhythmias and aortic stenosis.
- Nervous system: are there neurological signs in the lower limbs or evidence of Parkinson's disease (Chapter 7)? Is there visual impairment?
- Musculoskeletal system: look for joint or muscle abnormality and foot deformity. Is the footwear appropriate? Note any posture or gait abnormality (see Fig. 7.17).
- Consider specific investigations (see Box 17.8).

## The frail person with incontinence

- Observe whether the patient can mobilise or transfer to the toilet.
- Are they cognitively impaired? Is there any evidence of neurological disease?
- Abdomen: palpate for any abnormal abdominal masses. Is the bladder palpable?
- Examine the perineal skin and see if it is intact. Perform a rectal examination for anal fissures, haemorrhoids or other local diseases. Note if the rectum is empty or impacted with faeces; assess anal tone and sensation. In a man, assess prostate enlargement; in a woman, look for vaginal prolapse or atrophy.
- Consider specific investigations (see Box 17.8).

## Interpretation of the findings

Comprehensive geriatric assessment requires excellent communication among members of the multiprofessional team. A problem-based approach helps assimilate all the information and facilitate a clear and individualised management plan.

Start by creating a list to summarise all identified problems. Generate a provisional list after speaking with the patient and refine it after interviewing carers, undertaking the physical examination, and hearing the outcome of functional assessments. Do not confine the list to medical diagnoses but include symptoms, laboratory results and presenting features (Box 17.9).

The problem list builds a complete picture of the patient and alerts you to how the different problems may interact. If a problem has several contributing factors, list them all. Use the list to develop a management plan addressing each problem and contributing factor. Include actions such as diagnostic investigations, treatment of identified disease, alteration of drug therapy and rehabilitation. Tailor your management plan specifically to the individual, considering the outcome goals you have agreed with the patient. Explain the proposed management plan to your patient and ensure that they understand and agree.

### 17.9 A problem-based approach in a frail patient with immobility and confusion

| Problem | Potential contributory factors | Management plan |
|---|---|---|
| Urinary incontinence | Urinary tract infection<br>Faecal impaction | Perform urinalysis<br>Send a midstream specimen of urine to confirm<br>Carry out a rectal examination |
| Hyponatraemia | Bendroflumethiazide | Withhold bendroflumethiazide<br>Monitor serum sodium |
| Confusion with features of delirium | Urinary infection<br>Hyponatraemia<br>Underlying dementia | As above plus:<br>Check Mini Mental State Examination<br>Obtain a collateral history from a carer<br>Check thyroid function<br>Arrange an occupational therapy review |
| Foot ulcer | Absent pedal pulses | Check ankle: brachial pressure index<br>Discuss a dressing with the nurse |
| Poor mobility | Urinary infection<br>Hyponatraemia<br>Pain from foot ulcer<br>Underlying cerebrovascular disease | As above plus:<br>Prescribe simple analgesia<br>Carry out a full neurological/gait examination<br>Assess vascular risk factors<br>Arrange a physiotherapy review |

## OSCE Example 1: History in a frail patient with falls

Mr Smith, 88 years old, presents with recent falls.

### Please take a history

- Introduce yourself and clean your hands.
- Explain the purpose of the encounter.
- Make sure that the patient is comfortable and can hear you clearly.
- Ask him to describe his falls:
  - number of falls and where they happen
  - what he is doing before the falls and whether he is aware he is about to fall
  - any injuries, including head injury
  - whether he can get up after falling
  - whether anyone has witnessed his falls
  - his normal mobility and any walking aid.
- Ask focused questions about associated symptoms:
  - loss of consciousness
  - dizziness or vertigo
  - palpitations
  - limb weakness
  - incontinence or tongue biting.
- Ask whether there are any problems with vision, joints or feet.
- Establish whether there is a previous history of diabetes mellitus, heart or stroke disease, or joint disorders.
- Take a drug history, including:
  - new drugs
  - recent changes in drug dosages.
- Assess his social situation, including:
  - Does he live alone?
  - Are there any stairs?
  - Does he have any family or carer support?
- Ask why he thinks he is falling. What is concerning him most?
- Enquire whether there is anything else he can add.
- Thank the patient and clean your hands.

### Summarise your findings

Mr Smith is an 88-year-old man who lives alone in a ground-floor flat, supported by a twice-weekly home help. He is normally able to walk unaided within the house and a quarter of a mile to the local shop with a walking stick. He is generally healthy but takes blood pressure tablets from his doctor. In the past 3 months, he has had two significant falls. On each occasion, he felt drained and dizzy immediately on rising from his chair and collapsed to the floor, sustaining minor bruising. He did not lose consciousness and felt better spontaneously within a couple of minutes. There is no history of incontinence, chest pain, breathlessness, focal weakness or palpitations associated with the falls.

### Suggest a differential diagnosis

Postural hypotension secondary to excessive antihypertensive medication is the likely diagnosis. Paroxysmal arrhythmia, transient ischaemic attacks and episodes of pulmonary embolism are less likely alternatives.

17

## OSCE Example 2: Examination of an acutely confused frail patient

Mrs Collins, 87 years old, has suddenly become confused.

### Please examine the patient

- Introduce yourself and clean your hands.
- Find a quiet place and ask a nurse or family member to be present.
- Ensure that the patient is wearing any glasses and hearing aids.
- Observe the patient's general appearance and behaviour:
  - Is she restless or agitated? Or quiet and withdrawn?
  - Are there any non-verbal signs of pain (see Box 17.6)?
- Look for signs of acute illness:
  - temperature
  - oxygen saturation.
- Check drugs:
  - New drugs?
  - Sudden drug withdrawal?
- Check orientation with simple questions:
  - Where are you?
  - What is today's date?
  - What is your date of birth?
  - What is your age?
- Examine gently, looking for signs of sepsis or sources of pain:
  - chest: crepitations or wheeze
  - abdomen: tenderness or masses; distended bladder
  - skin: rashes, inflammation or sores
  - joints: injuries, pain or inflammation.
- Examine for new neurological features. Observation is helpful if the patient cannot cooperate with formal examination:
  - Is the speech clear?
  - Is the patient moving all limbs equally and purposefully?
  - Can she walk?
- Consider a rectal examination to look for faecal impaction.
- After the examination, help the patient to dress, reassure her and clean your hands.

### Summarise your findings

Mrs Collins is an 87-year-old woman who suddenly became confused this evening. She is disorientated with regard to day, month and place, which is new for her. She appears anxious and did not fully cooperate with the examination but was moving all four limbs purposefully and could speak clearly. Her chart reveals a temperature of 39°C, which is new. She has not been given any drugs that are likely to cause confusion. There are no focal signs in the chest or abdomen.

### Suggest a differential diagnosis

Acute urinary tract infection is the most likely diagnosis, but developing pneumonia is also possible as chest symptoms and signs may take time to appear.

## Integrated clinical examination for the frail patient

- Follow a standard systematic approach, including aspects that are important in frail patients. Remember that examination is tiring for frail patients and may have to be done in stages, and that they benefit from assessment by the full multiprofessional team (see Box 17.1).
- Introduce yourself and clean your hands.
- Ensure that the patient is comfortable and wearing any glasses and hearing aids. Ask if they want someone to be with them.
- Throughout the examination, observe for signs of pain (see Box 17.6) or distress.
- Assess the general appearance: ill-kempt, restless or anxious, withdrawn.
- Test vision and hearing: check with the patient wearing any glasses or hearing aids.
- Assess cognition: screen for cognitive deficit (p. 368), low mood or anxiety.
- Establish nutritional status: body mass index, weight loss or dehydration (see Box 17.5).
- Check skin health: inflammation, ulcers, breaks in pressures areas.
- Look at mobility: decreased balance or gait abnormality.
- Perform a systems examination, noting particularly:
  - Chest: symmetrical air entry, added sounds.
  - Cardiovascular system: cardiac rhythm, heart murmurs, postural blood pressure.
  - Abdomen: distended bladder. Consider rectal examination.
  - Locomotor system: joints – swelling, deformity, pain or inflammation. Feet – overgrown nails, deformities or ulcers.
  - Neurology: abnormal speech, asymmetry of neurology, signs of Parkinson's disease.
- After the examination, help your patient to dress.
- Thank the patient and clean your hands.

17

**Anna R Dover**
**Rosaleen Baruah**

# 18

# The deteriorating patient

Vital signs 394

Early warning scores 394

Initial assessment 395

The ABCDE approach 395

A: Airway 395

B: Breathing 396

C: Circulation 398

D: Disability 398

E: Exposure 399

Point of care ultrasound 399

Sepsis 400

Ongoing management 401

OSCE example: The unwell patient 402

Integrated examination sequence for the deteriorating patient 403

A deteriorating patient is one who becomes acutely unwell in the hospital setting. This can occur at any stage of a patient's illness but is more common if the patient has been admitted as an emergency case, has undergone surgery or has spent time in a high-dependency or intensive care setting. Common causes for deterioration include urinary and chest sepsis, bleeding, myocardial infarction, hypoglycaemia and pulmonary embolism.

Early assessment and intervention are required, as these patients are at a high risk of cardiac arrest. Once this occurs, only 20% of patients survive up to hospital discharge.

## Vital signs

Physiological observations that are routinely monitored in patients who are admitted to hospital include respiratory rate, oxygen saturation, heart rate, blood pressure, temperature and level of consciousness. Additional monitoring may include urine output, pain assessment and blood glucose testing.

## Early warning scores

Vital signs are recorded using track-and-trigger systems in the form of early warning scores designed to assess illness severity. Observations regularly recorded include respiratory rate, the level of oxygen therapy, oxygen saturation, heart rate, blood pressure, temperature and level of consciousness, and scores are assigned for physiological derangement in each domain. The increased frequency of observations is recommended for patients with abnormal signs, and a rising total score triggers a graded response.

In the UK, there is a validated track-and-trigger system, the National Early Warning Score (NEWS2; Fig. 18.1). This system will trigger a graded response due to either an aggregated high score or a single severe physiological derangement, with the urgency and seniority of the team being summoned escalating as the score rises (Box 18.1).

The early warning score is designed to complement clinical judgement. If you or your team are concerned about a patient, do not dismiss this instinct purely because the early warning score is low. A patient may just look unwell or feel cold to the touch and although these features are not captured by the early warning scoring systems, they may signify early deterioration, particularly in young patients with greater physiological reserve.

**Fig. 18.1** An example of a National Early Warning Score (NEWS) chart. The scoring of physiological variables is shown. *BP*, blood pressure; *V/P/U*, responding to voice/pain/unresponsive. Modified from Royal College of Physicians. National Early Warning Score (NEWS) 2. https://www.rcplondon.ac.uk/projects/outputs/national-early-warning-score-news-2.

## 18.1 NEWS thresholds and triggers

| NEWS score | Clinical risk | Response |
| --- | --- | --- |
| Aggregate score 0–4 | Low | Ward-based response |
| A single red score (score of 3 in any individual parameter) | Low-medium | Urgent ward-based response[a] |
| Aggregate score 5–6 | Medium | Key threshold for urgent response [a] |
| Aggregate score 7 or more | High | Urgent or emergency response[b] |

[a]Response by a clinician or team with competence in the assessment and treatment of acutely ill patients, in addition to recognising when the escalation of care to a critical care team is appropriate.
[b]The response team must also include staff with critical care skills, including airway management.
*From Royal College of Physicians. National Early Warning Score (NEWS) 2. https://www.rcplondon.ac.uk/projects/outputs/national-early-warning-score-news-2.*

# Initial assessment

When you review a deteriorating patient, a rapid assessment should replace the usual systematic history taking and physical examination, in order to identify abnormal physiology quickly and to administer immediate life-saving interventions to prevent further deterioration.

This assessment is time-critical. Thus attending to this patient should be prioritised; do not wait to finish other tasks. Make every effort to go and see the patient for yourself, as your immediate first impressions can provide much more information than can be obtained by lengthy discussion by telephone; if patients look sick, they probably are. Have a low threshold for calling for senior help.

## Examination sequence

- Always ensure your own safety and use appropriate personal protective equipment.
- Approach the patient and assess their response by asking 'Are you alright?' Gently shake the patient by the shoulders and shout loudly into both ears if unresponsive. A normal response confirms that the airway is clear and there is perfusion of the brain.
- If the patient is unresponsive, check for a pulse and assess whether the patient is breathing. If in cardiac or respiratory arrest, ask a colleague to summon the cardiac arrest team and begin cardiopulmonary resuscitation in accordance with guidelines.

- Monitor the vital signs; attach a pulse oximeter, non-invasive blood pressure monitor and an electrocardiogram (ECG) monitor as soon as possible.
- Ensure that the patient has a patent intravenous cannula inserted.
- If the patient does not respond or looks unwell, seek senior help immediately.

# The ABCDE approach

The ABCDE approach provides a standardised framework for simultaneously assessing and treating life-threatening problems in critically ill patients. This systematic approach will help you break down complex and stressful clinical situations into more manageable components.

## A: Airway

If a patient is able to speak normally, the airway is patent. If there is no response or if the patient appears to have difficulty in breathing, perform a more detailed assessment. Airway obstruction is a medical emergency; call for expert help immediately.

## Examination sequence

- Look for signs of airway obstruction. There may be use of the accessory muscles of respiration, supraclavicular or subcostal indrawing or paradoxical movements where the abdomen moves out as the chest moves in ('seesaw' breathing).
- Look in the mouth for foreign objects, blood, vomit or secretions. These can be removed by gentle suction with a Yankauer suction catheter, being careful not to cause airway trauma or to push obstructing material further into the airway.
- Listen for abnormal airway noises (Box 18.2).
- Open the airway with a chin-lift or jaw-thrust manoeuvre (Figs 18.2 and 18.3).
- In patients with altered consciousness, it may be necessary to maintain the airway by the insertion of an oropharyngeal (Guedel) or nasopharyngeal airway adjunct (Fig. 18.4). A laryngeal mask airway (LMA; Fig. 18.5) or tracheal intubation may be required, both of which must be performed by an experienced clinician.
- Administer oxygen via a non-rebreather mask at a flow rate of 15 L/minute.

Aim for an oxygen saturation of 94–98% except in patients with severe chronic obstructive pulmonary disease who are at a risk of type 2 (hypercapnic) respiratory failure; in this case, use a lower target of 88–92%.

18

### 18.2 Airway noises

**No noise (the 'silent airway')**

- Implies complete airway obstruction and/or absence of, or minimal, respiratory effort

**Stridor**

- A harsh noise, usually loudest in inspiration, caused by partial obstruction in the trachea or larynx
- In febrile patients, consider supraglottitis
- Other causes are inhaled foreign bodies, laryngeal trauma, burns or tumours

**Snoring/stertor**

- Caused by partial upper airway obstruction from soft tissues of the mouth and oropharynx

**Gurgling**

- Caused by fluids (secretions, blood or vomit) in the oropharynx

**Grunting**

- A grunt during expiration is a sign of respiratory muscle fatigue. It may be present after chest-wall trauma with a flail segment. Grunting improves gas exchange by slowing expiration and preventing alveolar collapse by creating positive end-expiratory pressure

**Wheeze**

- A 'musical' noise, best heard on auscultation
- When loudest in expiration, relates to intrathoracic obstruction of the small bronchi and bronchioles; most often occurs in asthma and chronic obstructive pulmonary disease

**Fig. 18.3 Jaw thrust for opening the airway.** Place your fingers behind the angle of the patient's jaw, and then lift it to open the airway.

**Fig. 18.4 Airway adjuncts.** Guedel airway (top) and nasopharyngeal airway (bottom). Note the 'safety pin', which prevents migration of the proximal end of the airway beyond the nasal orifice.

## B: Breathing

It is vital to identify and treat hypoxia as it can lead rapidly to cardiac arrest and death. Look for life-threatening respiratory compromise due to conditions such as acute severe asthma, pulmonary oedema or tension pneumothorax.

## Examination sequence

- Attach a pulse oximeter to assess peripheral oxygenation. Be alert to circumstances in which this measurement may be unreliable (Box 18.3). In particular, pulse oximetry may fail to detect hypoxaemia in Black patients, and you should have a lower threshold for measuring arterial blood gases in this patient group.
- Look for signs of respiratory distress: sweating, use of accessory muscles or abdominal 'seesaw' breathing. Cyanosis is a late finding and may be absent in severe anaemia or massive blood loss.
- Count the respiratory rate. The normal rate is 12–15 breaths per minute (bpm), but up to 20 bpm is common in anxious

**Fig. 18.2 Chin lift for opening the airway.**

**Fig. 18.5 Laryngeal mask airway (LMA).** From Marten TJ, Elyassnia D. Facelift: Male facelift. In Rubin JP, Neligan PC, editors. Plastic surgery: Volume 2: Aesthetic surgery. 4th edition. Oxford: Elsevier; 2018.

patients. A rising respiratory rate is an early and sensitive sign of deterioration. A respiratory rate of more than 30 bpm is a sign of critical illness and should prompt immediate escalation. Inadequate breathing, which is either a respiratory rate of less than 10 bpm or shallow breathing, requires supported ventilation with a bag-valve mask and should prompt a call to the cardiac arrest team. Look for reversible causes, such as recent exposure to opioids or other sedatives.

• Look for chest wall deformity or injury; observe the depth of inspiration and assess for symmetrical chest-wall expansion.
• Breathing pattern may provide clues to the underlying diagnosis (Box 18.4).
• Palpate the trachea in the suprasternal notch. It should be central; if not, this suggests mediastinal displacement by pneumothorax or lung collapse. Gently palpate any areas of injury to assess for a flail segment, where multiple rib fractures allow a part of the rib cage to move independently. Feel for subcutaneous emphysema indicating pneumothorax or trauma.
• Percuss and auscultate the chest to identify pneumothorax, effusions, consolidation or oedema. A silent chest can occur when airflow is poor, such as in life-threatening asthma.

Consider further evaluation of gas exchange with an arterial blood gas (ABG) measurement; it will give valuable information on arterial oxygen, carbon dioxide and acid–base status, but it

---

### 18.3 Situations in which pulse oximetry may give misleading values

**Inadequate waveform**

• Hypoperfusion – ear-lobe sensor may be better than finger probe in case of poor hand perfusion
• Hypothermia
• Movement artefact
• Rapid irregular pulse – e.g. atrial fibrillation

**Falsely normal or high reading**

• Abnormal haemoglobins:
  ◦ Carboxyhaemoglobin (e.g. carbon monoxide poisoning)
  ◦ Methaemoglobin[a]
  ◦ Sulphaemoglobin[a]
• High levels of $HbA_{1c}$
• Skin pigmentation

**Falsely low reading**

• Severe anaemia
• Abnormal haemoglobin
  ◦ Methaemoglobin
  ◦ Sulphaemoglobin
• Nail varnish, false fingernails
• Excessively dirty fingers

[a]Depending on the levels of methaemoglobin or sulphaemoglobin, pulse oximetry may underestimate or overestimate the true arterial oxygen saturation (usually low).
*$HbA_{1c}$,* haemoglobin $A_{1c}$, glycated haemoglobin.

---

### 18.4 Respiratory patterns: common causes

**Tachypnoea**

| | |
|---|---|
| • Anxiety | • Chest injury |
| • Pain | • Pneumothorax |
| • Asthma | • Pulmonary embolus |
| • Metabolic acidosis | • Brainstem stroke |

**Bradypnoea/apnoea**

| | |
|---|---|
| • Cardiac arrest | • Central neurological causes (stroke, head injury) |
| • Opioids/other sedative overdose | |

**Cheyne–Stokes respiration (waxing and waning tidal volume)**

| | |
|---|---|
| • Left ventricular failure | • Overdose (barbiturates, gamma-hydroxybutyrate, opioids) |
| • Central neurological causes (stroke, head injury) | • Altitude |
| • Can be normal in sleeping elderly | |

**Kussmaul respiration (deep rapid breaths)**

| | |
|---|---|
| • Metabolic acidosis, e.g. diabetic ketoacidosis | • Shock (lactic acidosis) |
| • Uraemia | • Overdose (methanol, ethylene glycol, salicylate) |
| • Hepatic failure | |

**Paradoxical respiration (chest in/abdomen out and vice versa)**

| | |
|---|---|
| • Airway obstruction | • High spinal cord lesions |
| • Respiratory failure | • Guillain–Barré syndrome |
| • Flail segment | |

**18**

requires skill and competence to obtain these parameters. Prolonged attempts at taking an ABG sample should not delay other aspects of resuscitation. It is usually appropriate to obtain a portable chest X-ray in a breathless or hypoxic patient.

## C: Circulation

Consider hypovolaemia as the most probable cause of shock in any acutely unwell patient.

### Examination sequence

- Look at and feel the skin; in hypovolaemic shock, the patient will be cold, and those with lighter skin colours may have pale, white or mottled skin.
- Check capillary refill by pressing on a fingertip (held at the level of the heart) for 5 seconds. This will cause it to blanch. When the pressure is released, the colour should return to the fingertip in less than 2 seconds. This is roughly the same time as it takes you to say 'capillary refill time'. If capillary refill is delayed, this indicates poor peripheral perfusion or shock.
- Assess the pulse rate and rhythm (p. 51). A heart rate of less than 50 beats per minute (bpm) or more than 100 bpm requires further investigation. A heart rate of more than 120 bpm requires immediate attention as this may indicate an abnormal rhythm.
- Palpate peripheral and central pulses, assessing the volume and character (p. 52); poorly felt peripheral pulses may indicate hypovolaemia or poor cardiac output, whereas a bounding pulse may indicate sepsis. As blood pressure falls, peripheral pulses diminish, with loss of the radial, then femoral and finally carotid pulsation. As a rule of thumb, if the radial pulse is present, the systolic blood pressure is likely to be greater than 90 mmHg, but once the femoral pulse becomes impalpable, the systolic blood pressure is likely to be less than 60 mmHg.
- Attach an ECG monitor to the patient to assess their heart rate and rhythm. A 12-lead ECG should also be recorded in patients with suspected acute coronary syndrome or arrhythmia.
- Check the blood pressure (p. 55). Hypotension is a late and serious sign, particularly in young patients who can commonly maintain blood pressure by peripheral vasoconstriction.
- Examine the jugular venous pressure (p. 57). This may be challenging in a tachycardic or tachypnoeic patient.
- Auscultate the heart to identify added sounds or murmurs (p. 81).
- Insert one or more wide-bore (14- or 16-gauge) intravenous cannulae, and take blood for routine haematological, biochemical and coagulation tests and for cross-matching. If the patient is hypotensive, give a bolus of 250–500 mL of warmed crystalloid solution.
- Look for other signs of inadequate organ perfusion such as reduced consciousness (see later) and oliguria (< 0.5 mL/kg/hour). A fluid balance chart should be commenced. Consider urinary catheterisation. Urinary catheters have their own

associated morbidity, in particular catheter-associated urinary tract infection. However, if the patient is obtunded or unable to pass urine, a catheter should be inserted.

## D: Disability

Any change in a patient's conscious level should raise concern. Causes of unconsciousness can include hypoxia, hypercapnia, cerebral hypoperfusion, hypoglycaemia or the use of sedative medications such as opioids.

Conscious level is often recorded using the AVPU scale, which categorises the patient as:

- **a**lert
- responding to **v**oice
- responding to **p**ain
- **u**nresponsive.

This measure is incorporated into many early warning scores and has the advantage of being a fast and easily understood verbal description of the patient's conscious level. It is not designed as a measure to track small changes in a patient's neurological condition.

The Glasgow Coma Scale (GCS) is more sensitive to changes in a patient's conscious level but is more complex. It measures eye opening, vocal and motor responses (Box 18.5). The GCS was initially validated as a measure of conscious level in patients with traumatic brain injury. Its use has been extrapolated to many situations of altered consciousness, and it may not always perform as intended.

| 18.5 Glasgow Coma Scale (GCS) | |
|---|---|
| **Eye opening (E)** | |
| 4 | Spontaneously |
| 3 | To speech |
| 2 | To pain |
| 1 | No response |
| **Best verbal response (V)** | |
| 5 | Orientated |
| 4 | Confused |
| 3 | Inappropriate words |
| 2 | Incomprehensible sounds |
| 1 | No verbal response |
| **Best motor response (M)** | |
| 6 | Obeys commands |
| 5 | Localises painful stimulus |
| 4 | Normal flexion |
| 3 | Abnormal flexion |
| 2 | Extends to painful stimulus |
| 1 | No response |

*Reproduced from Teasdale G, Jennett B. Assessment of coma and impaired consciousness: a practical scale. The Lancet 1974; 304(7872):81–84, with permission from Elsevier Ltd.*

The GCS should always be reported in its component parts – for example, E4 V2 M6 – and it can be useful to describe each component ('E4 eyes open spontaneously; V2 sounds only; M6 obeying commands') when communicating by telephone, to remove ambiguity.

Testing for response to a painful stimulus should be done only if the patient is not responding to speech. The stimulus should be administered centrally by applying firm supraorbital pressure or a trapezius pinch; sternal rub should be avoided, as it can cause distressing bruising to the patient's chest. Peripheral painful stimuli should be avoided, as they can elicit misleading spinal reflexes.

## Examination sequence

- Assess the patient's conscious level using either the AVPU scale or GCS.
- Examine the pupils for size, symmetry and light reflex. Pupil size will vary with ambient lighting, but should be symmetrical and should constrict to light. Symmetrical change in pupil size suggests a drug or metabolic cause.
  *Constricted pupils (miosis):* occur in opioid overdose or organophosphate poisoning
  *Dilated pupils (mydriasis):* seen in toxicity from anticholinergics (e.g. atropine or tricyclic antidepressants) or sympathomimetics (e.g. cocaine).
  *Asymmetrical pupils (anisocoria, xref Ch8):* suggest a structural lesion but can be physiological. A unilateral dilated pupil in a patient with an altered conscious level is a medical emergency and should prompt further investigation with emergency head computerised tomography (CT).
- Check the drug chart for reversible causes of reduced consciousness.
- Check for the capillary blood glucose using a bedside glucose meter. The acronym after ABC of 'DEFG' ('Don't ever forget glucose') is a good reminder. If the blood glucose is less than 4 mmol/L (72 mg/dL) and the patient is unconscious, administer 75–100 mL of 20% glucose intravenously over 15 minutes; thereafter, follow national guidelines for the management of hypoglycaemia.

Delirium is a state of mental confusion that starts suddenly and is caused by a variety of physical conditions including sepsis, alcohol withdrawal and drug toxicity (Chapter 16, OSCE2). It is common, affecting 10–20% of hospital patients, particularly the elderly. Correct identification is important as it may indicate an underlying infection, metabolic derangement, hypoxia or cerebral hypoperfusion.

## E: Exposure

Examine the patient thoroughly while respecting their dignity and minimising heat loss.

## Examination sequence

- Look for evidence of trauma, blood loss and rashes, in particular the non-blanching petechial rash of meningococcal bacteraemia.
- Check the temperature using an infrared tympanic thermometer. Normal mean body temperature is 36.5°C, but it varies diurnally (highest early evening) and according to the site of measurement. A temperature below 35°C indicates hypothermia; this should be confirmed by measuring a core (rectal) temperature and treated by external rewarming using a warming system such as a Bair Hugger. Other forms of active rewarming include warmed intravenous fluids and heated humidified oxygen. A temperature above 37.8°C indicates fever and, if acute, should prompt a search for infection and/or sepsis.

## Point of care ultrasound

Point of care ultrasound (PoCUS), which is the use of portable ultrasound at the bedside by the treating clinician, may provide useful additional information in the assessment of the deteriorating patient. Examples include the rapid assessment of trauma patients, bedside echocardiography and ultrasound assessment of the abdomen, chest and deep venous system. PoCUS is used to answer focused questions; for example, is there a pleural effusion or evidence of consolidation in the chest (Fig. 18.6)? There are many pocket-sized high-quality ultrasound systems now available which allow easy delivery of PoCUS at the bedside (Fig. 18.7). PoCUS does not replace either physical examination or the need for specialist radiological examinations when indicated.

**18**

**Fig. 18.6** [A] point of care ultrasound (PoCUS) image of the right hemithorax of a patient with a new diagnosis of lymphoma and an increasing oxygen requirement. The small particles visible in the large pleural effusion ("plankton sign") are suggestive of an exudative effusion. [B] Cloudy exudate aspirated from the pleural effusion.

**Fig. 18.7** Examples of point of care ultrasound machines. [A] Butterfly Network, Inc, Guilford, CT. [B] Courtesy *Philips, Amsterdam, Netherlands.*

## Sepsis

Sepsis is a condition defined as a life-threatening organ dysfunction due to a dysregulated host response to infection (such as pneumonia, urinary tract infection or intra-abdominal infection). It is the reason for deterioration in approximately 40% of patients who become acutely unwell in medical wards and carries a high mortality risk. Those at greatest risk include elderly or frail patients, those who are immunocompromised or have undergone recent surgery, and those with indwelling lines or catheters. As sepsis progresses, it can lead to septic shock and ultimately multiple organ failure. If it is not identified early, the chance of a good outcome falls rapidly.

Organ dysfunction in suspected sepsis can be measured using the Sequential Organ Failure Assessment (SOFA) score. A bedside modification of this is the quickSOFA ('qSOFA') score which allows rapid evaluation of respiratory, cardiovascular and cerebrovascular dysfunction. The presence of two or more qSOFA points (respiratory rate $\geq 22$ breaths per minute, systolic blood pressure $\leq 100$ mmHg and/or GCS $\leq 15$) in the presence of suspected infection is associated with a greater risk of death than in uncomplicated infection. Septic shock is defined as the presence of sepsis and, despite adequate volume resuscitation, both persistent hypotension requiring vasopressors to maintain a mean arterial pressure $\geq 65$ mmHg and lactate $\geq 2$ mmol/L. The assessment and initial management of sepsis are described by the 'Sepsis Six' screening tool and therapeutic bundle, which aims to deliver three diagnostic and three therapeutic steps within 1 hour of the recognition of sepsis (Boxes 18.6 and 18.7).

---

### 18.6 Identifying sepsis – UK Sepsis Trust sepsis screening tool acute assessment

- Does patient look unwell or NEWS 5 or higher?
- Are there risk factors for sepsis?
  - Age >75
  - Impaired immunity (e.g. diabetes, steroids, chemotherapy)
  - Recent trauma, surgery or invasive procedure
  - Indwelling lines, intravenous drug use, broken skin
- Could this be due to an infection?
  - Likely source: respiratory, urine, joint/skin/wound, indwelling device, brain, surgical
- Any of the following "red flags" present?
  - Objective evidence of new or altered mental state
  - Systolic BP $\leq 90$ mmHg (or drop of >40 from normal)
  - HR $\geq 130$ bpm
  - Respiratory rate $\geq 25$ per minute
  - Needs $O_2$ to keep $S_pO_2$ $\geq 92\%$ (88% in COPD)
  - Non-blanching rash/mottled/ashen/cyanotic
  - Lactate $\geq 2$ mmol/L
  - Recent chemotherapy
  - Not passed urine in 18 hours (<0.5 mL/kg if catheterised)

If yes, start Sepsis Six

- Any of the following "amber flags" present?
  - Relatives concerned about mental state
  - Acute deterioration in functional ability
  - Immunosuppressed
  - Trauma/surgery/procedure in last 8 weeks
  - Respiratory rate 21–24
  - Systolic blood pressure 91–100 mmHg
  - Heart rate 91–130 or new dysrhythmia
  - Temperature <36°C
  - Clinical signs of wound infection

If yes, further review required. Send blood samples, review results and ensure senior review within 1 hour

*Taken from Nutbeam T, Daniels R on behalf of the UK Sepsis Trust. Available at sepsistrust.org/professional-resources/clinical/.*

---

### 18.7 'Sepsis Six' therapeutic bundle

**Complete all actions within 1 hour**

- Ensure that the senior clinician attends
- Oxygen if required: start if $O_2$ saturations less than 92%, aiming for 94–98%. If at risk of hypercapnia, aim for saturations of 88–92%.
- Obtain intravenous access, take blood cultures, blood glucose, lactate, blood count, C reactive protein and clotting
- Give intravenous antibiotics
- Give intravenous fluids: give a fluid bolus of 20 mL/kg or 500 mL balanced crystalloid solution.
- Monitor: Use NEWS2. Measure the urinary output. Repeat lactate at least once per hour, if the initial lactate is elevated or if the clinical condition changes.
- If red flags persist after 1 hour – escalate to consultant now

---

In addition to the routine vital signs, the measurement of urine output and lactate is recommended as a guide to illness severity. Lactate is the product of anaerobic metabolism and is a marker of tissue perfusion. A lactate of >2 mmol/L (18 mg/dL) is abnormal and a level of >4 mmol/L (36 mg/dL) is associated with 30% mortality. A careful search must be undertaken to identify the underlying infection in order to aid diagnosis and guide appropriate choice of antibiotics.

Initial investigations should include the measurement of ABGs, glucose and lactate, blood cultures, full blood count, C-reactive protein, urea and electrolytes and a clotting screen.

Treatment of sepsis with early and appropriate antibiotics, oxygen and intravenous fluids reduces mortality. Patients who fail to respond to initial treatment are very likely to require a higher level of care and must be discussed with a senior clinician.

## Ongoing management

The management of a deteriorating patient must include frequent review of response to therapy. Once you have completed the ABCDE approach, return to the beginning and reassess, if the patient is not improving.

Clear goals of interventions should be communicated to the team (for example, 'The goal of this fluid bolus is to achieve a systolic blood pressure of over 100 mmHg; if this is not achieved, please let me know and we will give a further fluid bolus'). A written management plan should be documented, which should also include the required frequency of observations (such as every 15 minutes until stabilised).

It is particularly important to work as a team when a patient is deteriorating rapidly. A structured approach to communication will help you organise your thoughts and is an effective way to communicate the urgency of the situation to the person you are escalating to. The SBAR tool is particularly useful in this setting (p. 419).

It may be appropriate to move the patient to an area of the hospital able to provide a higher level of care. With increasing

**18**

levels of care, the nurse:patient ratio is higher and increasing numbers of therapeutic interventions can be delivered (Box 18.8).

Finally, consideration should be given to patients with limited reversibility in whom intensive treatment may not be appropriate. It is important to acknowledge and communicate the uncertainty of outcomes in these cases (p. 407) and to ensure early discussion of resuscitation status and agreed goals of care.

---

### 18.8 Levels of clinical care

| | |
|---|---|
| Level 0 | Suitable for patients whose needs can be met through normal ward care in an acute hospital. |
| Level 1 | Suitable for patients at risk of their condition deteriorating or those recently relocated from higher levels of care, whose needs can be met on an acute ward with additional advice and support from the critical care team. |
| Level 2 | Suitable for patients requiring more detailed observations or interventions, including support for a single failing organ system, or recently relocated from a higher level of care. Also known as 'high dependency units' (HDUs). |
| Level 3 | Suitable for patients requiring advanced respiratory support alone or basic respiratory support together with support of at least two organ systems. This level includes all complex patients requiring support for multi-organ failure. Also known as 'intensive care units' (ICUs) or 'intensive treatment/therapy units' (ITUs). |

*Data from NHS Data Model and Dictionary. https://www.datadictionary.nhs.uk/attributes/critical_care_level.html. Contains information from NHS Digital, licensed under the current version of the Open Government Licence.*

---

### OSCE example: The unwell patient

Mr Green, 50 years old, had a laparotomy and small-bowel resection 5 days ago. He has an elevated temperature of 38.6°C and is tachycardic with a heart rate of 98 beats per minute.

#### Please assess this unwell patient

- Prioritise seeing this patient.
- Introduce yourself and clean your hands.
- Is the patient responsive? If unconscious, are they in cardiac arrest?
- Assess the airway. Is the patient speaking to you? Look for airway obstruction, supraclavicular or subcostal indrawing, or paradoxical movements of the chest and abdomen.
- Assess breathing for rate and depth. Attach pulse oximeter. Look for chest asymmetry. Palpate the trachea in the suprasternal notch. Percuss and auscultate, looking for pneumothorax, consolidation or effusion.
- Assess the circulation. Examine for skin pallor, clamminess and capillary refill time. Assess the pulse for tachycardia. Measure the blood pressure with a manual sphygmomanometer.
- Assess the conscious level. Is the patient confused?
- Measure blood glucose.
- Comment on the presence of red flags and signs of systemic infection.
- Examine the abdomen for signs of infection or bleeding.
- Call for senior help and document the management plan.

#### Summarise your findings

Mr Green is a 50-year-old man who had a small-bowel resection 5 days ago and has now become drowsy and febrile. He is hypotensive at 95/60 mmHg, with a tachycardia of 98 beats per minute and an elevated respiratory rate of 28 breaths per minute. He is rousable and responds appropriately to questions, but looks unwell. Abdominal examination reveals a recent laparotomy scar and generalised tenderness with rebound.

#### Suggest a differential diagnosis

The likely problem is sepsis from an intra-abdominal infection. This is an emergency situation requiring urgent resuscitation.

#### Suggested investigations

Lactate, full blood count, blood cultures.

#### Advanced level comments

Immediate resuscitation is appropriate as per the 'Sepsis Six' bundle: oxygen, fluids and antibiotics, with early senior review. Review the effects of resuscitation on blood pressure and urine output, and repeat the measurement of lactate concentration. Escalation to critical care should be considered, and exploratory surgery may be required for source infection control.

## Integrated examination sequence for the deteriorating patient

- General appearance:
  - If the patient is unconscious, are they in cardiac arrest?
  - If they look unwell, call for help.
- Airway:
  - Is the airway clear?
  - Is patient able to speak?
  - Look for signs of airway obstruction: supraclavicular, subcostal indrawing or paradoxical movements or 'seesaw' breathing.
  - Listen for abnormal airway noises.
  - Open the airway with airway manoeuvres if required.
  - Administer high-flow oxygen via a facemask.
- Breathing:
  - Measure the respiratory rate and assess peripheral oxygenation using pulse oximetry.
  - Look for signs of respiratory distress: use of accessory muscles, abdominal 'seesaw' breathing, chest deformity or trauma, asymmetrical movement.
  - Palpate the trachea in the suprasternal notch and palpate any areas of injury.
  - Percuss and auscultate the chest.
- Circulation:
  - Examine the skin: is it cold, pale or mottled? Check capillary refill time.
  - Assess the rate and volume of the pulse; palpate peripheral pulses.
  - Check the blood pressure.
  - Examine the jugular venous pressure and auscultate the heart.
  - Measure the urine output and assess cerebral perfusion.
  - Obtain intravenous access and perform a 12-lead electrocardiogram.
- Disability:
  - Assess conscious level using the AVPU or Glasgow Coma Scale scores.
  - Examine pupils for symmetry, size and reaction to light.
  - Measure capillary blood glucose.
  - Check the drug chart for reversible causes of reduced consciousness.
- Exposure:
  - Check the temperature.
  - Look for trauma, bleeding and rashes.

**18**

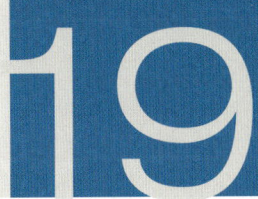

Kirsty Boyd
Nazir Lone

# The dying patient

**Assessing a dying patient 406**
Physiology 406
The history 406
The physical examination 406
Care in the last days of life 407
Communication with patients and families 407

**Verifying and certifying death 408**
The history 408
The physical examination 408

Communication with families 409
Medical certification of death 409

**Looking after yourself and others 409**
**OSCE example 1: Informing relatives that a patient is nearing death 410**
**OSCE example 2: Verification of death 411**
**Integrated examination sequence for a patient in the last days of life 412**
**Integrated examination sequence for verifying death 412**

Around 1% of the population in high-income countries die each year. Although some deaths are unexpected, the majority are the result of one or more advanced, progressive conditions and occur in hospital, at the patient's home or care home, or in a hospice. It is important to identify whether an acute deterioration or a new complication from an underlying health problem is reversible. This change may represent an anticipated decline and indicate that the person is approaching the end of their life. Recognising where a person is on their current illness trajectory and identifying their priorities, goals and preferences allows shared decisions to be made with the patient and their relatives about what further investigations and treatments are appropriate, and about their preferred place of care or death.

# Assessing a dying patient

## Physiology

There are three broad illness trajectories (Fig. 19.1):

- progression of a life-limiting condition with a clear terminal phase: for example, advanced cancer where oncology treatment is no longer of benefit or is given for symptom management.
- fluctuating decline with intermittent, potentially life-threatening, acute exacerbations or complications that may result in death: for example, advanced respiratory, heart, kidney or liver disease.
- prolonged, gradual decline with acute episodes that may be the final illness such as a chest infection: for example, dementia, general frailty in older age or advanced neurological conditions.

Many physiological and functional changes occur in the final weeks or months of life. General indicators of deteriorating health include:

- performance status that is poor or worsening, with the person in bed or in a chair for more than half the day.

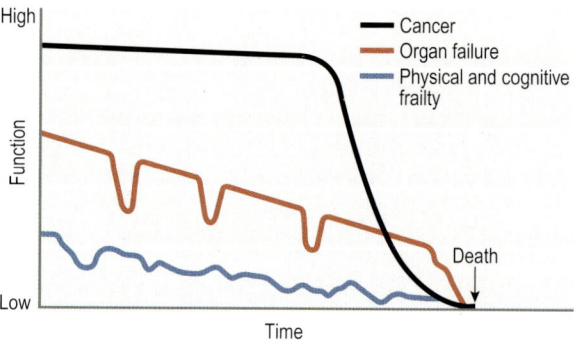

**Fig. 19.1 Illness trajectories towards the end of life.** Adapted from Lynn J, Adamson DM. Living well at the end of life. In: Adapting Health Care to Serious Chronic Illness in Old Age. Washington: Rand Health; 2003. With permission from RAND Corporation, Santa Monica, California, USA. *https://www.rand.org/pubs/white_papers/WP137.html.*

- increasing number of unplanned hospital attendances or admissions.
- persistent symptoms despite optimal treatment of underlying conditions.
- progressive weight loss with low muscle mass (cachexia), or difficulty maintaining normal weight.
- increasing dependency on others for care and support due to physical and/or mental health problems.

Having considered these clinical indicators of deteriorating health, it can be helpful to ask yourself: 'Would I be surprised if this person died in the next few months, weeks or days?' Patients may be close to death when they first present or may fail to improve with treatment, so it becomes clear that they will die soon. It is crucial that we recognise when a person is so unwell that they could die.

In the last days of life, people eat and drink less, sleep more and have physiological changes in breathing patterns, circulation, and in the level of consciousness.

## The history

The clinician may already know the patient well, for example, if they are the general practitioner. If not, it is important to gather information about the patient's underlying conditions, presenting illness, current and previous treatment, family and social/cultural context.

### Background information

Use all available sources to determine the patient's previous health status in addition to their presenting problems. Review referral letters, primary care and hospital records, and previous discharge summaries. Check for advance/anticipatory care plans, emergency treatment plans or any advance directive/decision. Find out if the person has a legally appointed, proxy decision-maker or a registered Power of Attorney. Look for any record of previous discussions or decisions about cardiopulmonary resuscitation (CPR). Find out if the person has a pacemaker or any other device that will need to be deactivated now or removed after death; record this clearly.

### Establishing the broader context

Build up a picture of the patient's overall health status and any recent changes, not only the presenting symptoms. A family member or friend can provide valuable additional information and support the patient. If the patient or family cannot provide information, contact someone who knows the person, such as the general practitioner, another member of the primary care team, their hospital specialist or any senior nurse involved in their care.

## The physical examination

People may retain some awareness, even when close to death. Speak to the person by name and to others in the room as you would when your patient is awake. Always introduce yourself and

Some patients will benefit from carefully selected investigations to confirm whether their condition is reversible, to guide specific palliative treatments or to clarify the prognosis.

## Care in the last days of life

If the patient is likely to die soon, their care needs to be planned. Anticipate and address potential problems with symptom management and emotional distress. This includes making sure suitable medications are prescribed and available, regularly and as needed. Treatments for underlying conditions need careful review to avoid burdening people with medications that are no longer of benefit while continuing to manage symptoms effectively. It is important to review a patient who is dying at least daily, and more often if they are unsettled or have complex clinical problems. If a patient deteriorates rapidly or their symptoms change, urgent assessment is required. Find out if the other people who are caring for the dying patient have any concerns, especially family members who are caring for the person at home, and work with them to maintain the patient's comfort and dignity. Involve and support family members and close friends. A clear explanation of the dying process, good communication and effective palliative care from the multidisciplinary team helps families prepare for the person's death and improves outcomes for the bereaved.

Cultural, religious and spiritual care are very important when a person is dying, around the time of death and afterwards. Always ask the person and those close to them about how they would like to be cared for and what you and other staff members can do to help support them. This may include making plans for visiting by family members and/or a spiritual care provider, specific wishes about how the person is touched or cared for after death, and funeral arrangements.

## Communication with patients and families

If you believe a patient could be approaching the end of their life, it is important to share this information with them and their family in a timely way so that they have opportunities to address personal priorities and concerns. The 6-step REDMAP framework is recommended to guide conversations about treatment and care at the end of life (Box 19.2). It includes helpful words and phrases that can be adapted to the person, their family and the context of the conversation. Begin by finding out what people know and expect before sharing information in small chunks, with pauses. Next, explore what matters to this person and their family, then discuss treatment and care that takes account of available options and the person's priorities, and agree on an individualised care plan.

Many countries now have policies and processes for decision making about treatments at the end of life, and specifically for cardiopulmonary resuscitation (CPR). Decisions are based on a clinical assessment of treatment benefits, burdens and outcomes but also involve shared decision-making discussions with patients and/or legally appointed proxies. It is important to talk about treatments in context and based on a mutual understanding of the patient's current health situation and priorities. If

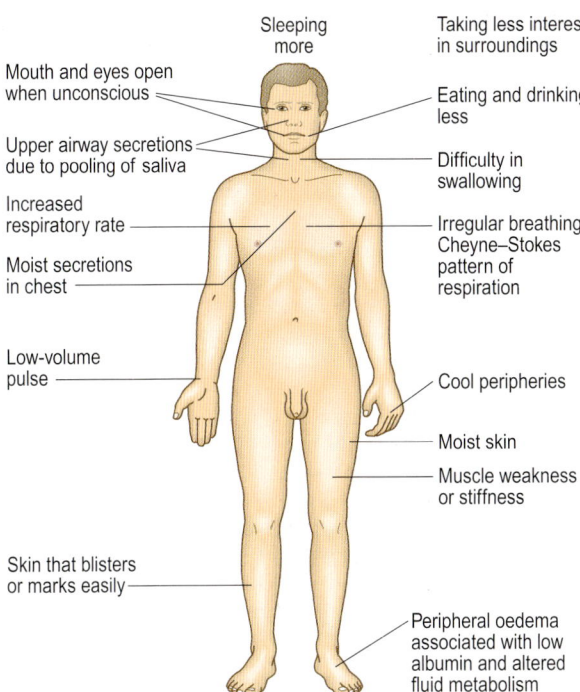

Sleeping more

Taking less interest in surroundings

Mouth and eyes open when unconscious

Eating and drinking less

Upper airway secretions due to pooling of saliva

Difficulty in swallowing

Increased respiratory rate

Irregular breathing/ Cheyne–Stokes pattern of respiration

Moist secretions in chest

Low-volume pulse

Cool peripheries

Moist skin

Muscle weakness or stiffness

Skin that blisters or marks easily

Peripheral oedema associated with low albumin and altered fluid metabolism

**Fig. 19.2** Signs that suggest a patient will die soon.

| 19.1 Common potentially reversible causes of deterioration in advanced illness |
|---|
| • Dehydration |
| • Infection |
| • Opioid toxicity or other drug toxicity or poisoning; recreational drugs |
| • Glucocorticoid withdrawal or a new diagnosis of adrenal insufficiency |
| • Acute kidney injury |
| • Delirium |
| • Hypercalcaemia |
| • Hypoglycaemia or hyperglycaemia |
| • Hyponatraemia |
| • Hypothermia |

explain your role in the team. Your assessment begins with observing whether the patient looks comfortable and confirming this with other staff and the family. Non-verbal ways of showing concern for the person (tone, gentle touch, gestures of kindness) have a significant impact on the patient and the patient's family.

While it can be difficult to decide when a person has entered the last days of life, there are clinical signs that suggest a patient will die soon (Fig. 19.2). Even in this situation, a focused examination looking for reversible causes of deterioration is always indicated (see the integrated examination sequence at the end of the chapter). Common, potentially reversible causes of deterioration in people with advanced conditions are shown in Box 19.1.

**19**

| 19.2 REDMAP: Talking about care planning in the last days of life | |
|---|---|
| **R**eady | Can we talk about your health and care? <br> Who should be involved in this conversation? |
| **E**xpect | How have you been recently? What has changed? <br> What do you **know** about your health problems? <br> What do you think **might happen**? <br> Do you want to **tell/ask** me about anything? |
| **D**iagnosis | We **know** you are less well because… <br> We **hope** you will improve, but I **am worried** that…. <br> It **is possible** you will not get better…. <br> I'm sorry but you **could die soon** with this illness <br> Do you have questions or worries we can talk about? |
| **M**atters | What is **important** to you and your family? <br> How **would you like** to be cared for? <br> Is there anything you **would not want**? <br> What would (*patient's name*) **say** about this situation if we could ask them? |
| **A**ctions | What we **can do** is… Options that **can help** are…. <br> This **will not help** because…. That **does not work** when… <br> I **wish** that was possible, let's talk about **what we can do**. |
| **P**lan | Let's make a **plan** for you and your family. <br> This is how we care for someone who is dying. <br> We are not sure how quickly things will change…. |
| Used with permission from the author, Dr. Kirsty Boyd. | |

the patient already has a recorded decision that CPR will not be given, this should be documented clearly and shared within the healthcare team. If a patient has advanced illness and is dying, CPR will not have a medically successful outcome. Ask what the patient and family know about CPR. Explain that CPR is a treatment to restart the heart and/or breathing after they have stopped, which does not work when a person is dying. It is better to focus on planning good care. Be clear that any other treatments that can help the person will still be offered. Do not ask people if they 'want' to be resuscitated when it is not a realistic treatment option for them. Occasionally, a patient with one or more advanced conditions deteriorates more rapidly than expected or a decision that CPR will not be given has not been made in advance. In those situations, professionals present must decide if CPR should not start or be stopped.

Explain what happens when a person is dying. Talk about changes that may be seen and what they mean. Explain why the focus of treatment, monitoring and care is changing to making sure the person is comfortable. Plan visiting arrangements suited to this person and their family and find out who to contact if the patient deteriorates or dies. Explain what to expect when

someone dies and what to do if the person is at home. Most people stop breathing gradually but may take a final breath after a long pause. A brief muscle spasm may be observed at that time, so warn relatives about this.

# Verifying and certifying death

The verification and medical certification of death are important to allow the legal requirements and cultural and religious traditions that happen after a person has died to be completed in a timely way. Some people will have decided to be organ or tissue donors in advance or be eligible under 'opt-out' legislation in some countries. It is important to contact the organ donation service as soon as the possibility of donation is identified, and to inform and involve family members.

In the UK, death is defined as 'the irreversible loss of the essential characteristics necessary to the existence of a living person – to be able to sense and interact with the environment and to maintain the fundamental bodily functions of respiration and circulation'. Consciousness and respiratory and circulatory function are controlled within the brainstem. Irreversible damage to the brainstem, either after cardiorespiratory arrest or due to direct damage to the brainstem itself, always results in death.

## The history

If you are not familiar with the patient and their recent medical history, always read the patient record before going to see them or speaking to their family. Being aware of whether the death was sudden or expected and how the person has been during their final illness helps you to prepare. Check with clinical colleagues whether there is anything you should know about this patient and family.

## The physical examination

After the person has died, it is important for the clinical team to continue to care for them as they would any other patient. This includes speaking about the person by name to family members who are present at the time of death or while you are carrying out the examination to verify death. As some relatives choose to remain in the room, you need to explain each part of the examination in simple terms and conduct it in a respectful and professional manner.

To verify death, clinical examination and observation should take place over a minimum of 5 minutes to establish that irreversible cardiorespiratory arrest has occurred. This provides an opportunity for you to spend time supporting and listening to any family members who are present. After death, the body cools gradually and stiffens; bowel sounds may persist for a time until the sphincters relax and the bowels and bladder empty.

## Diagnosing death using neurological criteria

The diagnosis of death using neurological criteria must be made by at least two doctors who have been fully registered for at least 5 years. They should have experience in the assessment of brainstem function. One of the doctors must be a consultant or equivalent senior physician. The tests are performed on two occasions. The first set of tests is to diagnose brainstem death. The second set is to confirm the diagnosis. There is no minimum time required between tests; they can occur concurrently. If the tests demonstrate that brain death has occurred, then the time of death is recorded as the time when the first set of tests was completed.

## Communication with families

Communicating with family members to tell them that someone has died should be done as soon as possible. If in hospital, speak to relatives in a quiet, private room and try to avoid interruptions. If the death is sudden and unexpected, this will be breaking bad news so needs clear and sensitive communication. When contacting a family member by telephone to inform them of a patient's death, it is important to decide if it is safe to do so or whether it would be better to contact someone such as the police and ask them to go and inform the family member in person. Explain what has happened and what will happen next. Offer the family time with the person who has died if they wish. Respect and support cultural or religious requirements after death and ensure you are aware of any plans already made with the patient and family. Rapid provision of the medical certificate of death is important for some faith groups.

## Medical certification of death

Document the place, time and date of death in the patient's medical record. In some countries, the time of death is when the person was observed to have died by those present or the person was found to have died. In other countries, the time of death is when death is verified by a doctor or another suitably trained health professional, so make sure you know which time to record. Include details of who was present when the person died and what the primary and secondary causes of death were. In hospital, the cause of death must be discussed and confirmed with a senior colleague, usually a consultant. Some medical certificates of death require additional information, such as the duration of the final illness, so make sure you are familiar with these requirements. You should also know or seek advice about when a medical certificate of death should not be issued because the death has to be reported for further investigation (Box 19.3).

## Looking after yourself and others

Although caring for a patient who is dying and their family is extremely rewarding, it can also be stressful and emotionally demanding. It is important to recognise this and look for help and personal support when you need it. You may need advice on how to manage a patient's symptoms, decide on a care plan or communicate sensitively and effectively with people who are experiencing loss and bereavement. Talk to your medical colleagues and other members of the healthcare team and support them too. If a death has been particularly challenging, a senior clinician may invite the team members involved to take part in a debriefing session soon after the death or later. This is an opportunity for everyone to share how they are feeling and talk about what the team and service can learn from the situation.

**19**

---

### 19.3 Deaths that may require further investigation

- The cause of death is unknown.
- Death was violent or unnatural.
- Death was sudden and unexplained.
- The person who died was not visited by a medical practitioner during their final illness.
- A medical certificate is not available.
- Death occurred during an operation or before the person came round from the anaesthetic.
- The medical certificate suggests that the death may have been caused by an industrial disease or industrial poisoning.
- Death occurred in legal custody.
- A complaint has been received over the medical treatment or standards of care received by the deceased.
- Death was due to a notifiable disease.

## OSCE example 1: Informing relatives that a patient is nearing death

Mr. David Jenkins, 80 years old, has severe chronic obstructive pulmonary disease. He is on home oxygen therapy and was admitted to the ward 3 days ago with severe pneumonia. Despite initially responding to treatment, his condition has now deteriorated, and he is becoming breathless, confused and distressed. He has been assessed by the intensive care consultant, who recommended that Mr. Jenkins should stay on the ward with a focus on good symptom management and care appropriate for the last days of life. The nurses ask you to speak with Mr. Jenkins' son about what is happening and the care plan for his dad. You should explore his understanding and what he thinks his dad would say about the situation. Explain why ward-based care has been recommended as the best option for a comfortable and dignified death, and why cardiopulmonary resuscitation will not work or help when his dad dies.

- To prepare for this conversation:
  - Find a private room.
  - Ask if you can leave your bleep/mobile phone with nursing staff.
  - Introduce yourself by name and role to the son and clarify his relationship to the patient.
  - Outline the reason for the meeting, and check if anyone else should be contacted.
    - "Hello, my name is Dr. Jenny Smith and I am the ward doctor on duty today. Are you David Jenkins' son, Kiron Jenkins? Thank you for coming in to see me. I'm sorry but your dad has become much more unwell today. I'd like to talk with you about what is happening with his treatment and care. Is there anyone else you'd like us to contact at this time?"
- Find out what Kiron knows and expects:
  - "Can I start by asking what you know about your dad's illness and what's happened so far"'
- Explain the diagnosis using clear language free of jargon:
  - "As you know, he's been unwell for a while with his lung disease and has not been out of the house for several months. He's been in hospital three times over the last year with chest infections and never really seemed to get back to where he was before. This time he has a severe chest infection sometimes called pneumonia."
- Explain that, because Mr. Jenkins has advanced lung disease and is not responding to treatment, he is likely to deteriorate further.
  - "We were hoping that your dad would improve with the antibiotics and oxygen on the ward, but we are worried about how he is doing. It is possible he will not get better this time. He has been seen by his own consultant and a senior doctor from the intensive care unit who agree that his underlying lung condition and the pneumonia are the reason for this."
  - Pause.
  - Explain that this means Mr. Jenkins is likely to die.
    - "I'm sorry, but he could die soon with this illness."
- Pause to give Kiron time to respond. Address any concerns or questions Kiron may have. Explore what would be important for Mr. Jenkins and his family.
  - "Your dad is not able to tell us what would be important for him and his family. Can you tell me what you think he would say in this situation?"
- Sensitively cover the following aspects of care for a dying patient:
  - Say that you are not sure how soon he will die, but it could be in the next few days or even sooner.
  - Explain that some people can improve for a short while and then become less well again, and that occasionally unexpected improvement occurs but this is now very unlikely.
  - State that the most important thing now is to make sure Mr. Jenkins has the right care and medicines to keep him as comfortable and free of symptoms as possible.
  - Outline treatments he might receive now and explain that subcutaneous administration of drugs is often used in palliative care (for example, a syringe pump). Explain about stopping treatments that will no longer be beneficial and having 'as needed' medications available.
  - Ask if Kiron knows about cardiopulmonary resuscitation or CPR. Explain that when a person dies, their heart and breathing stop. Giving treatment to restart the heart does not work in this situation and is, therefore, not the best way to care for them. A decision about CPR is made in advance and recorded so that everyone knows about it.
  - Ask about any religious, spiritual or cultural practices.
  - Ask if Kiron would like you to talk to anyone else, and about who is supporting him.
  - Ask if there are any other questions or things you can help with.
  - Explain how to contact you or a colleague later if he has further questions or worries.

## OSCE example 2: Verification of death

The nurse-in-charge calls you to tell you that Mrs. Williams, a 70-year-old inpatient, has died.

### Please describe the process for verifying death, and how you would communicate with staff and family

- Introduce yourself to the nursing team on the ward.
- Ask if the death was expected and when Mrs. Williams died, as well as if anyone was present when she died.
- Confirm that a 'Not for cardiopulmonary resuscitation' decision had been made in advance and recorded.
- Ask if the team knows why Mrs. Williams was in hospital and what the likely cause of death might be. Find out if any family members would like to be present when you see her.
- Read the patient's medical record and check that you have the correct name, hospital number and date of birth. Check if any specific infection control measures are needed.
- On entering the patient's bed space:
  - Clean your hands and introduce yourself to any relatives or staff present.
  - Express your condolences and explain why you need to examine the patient:
    - "I'm sorry to intrude at a sad time. I'm here to examine Mrs. Williams to confirm that she has died. You are welcome to stay with her if you would like to. I'll explain what I am doing but if you have any questions about what is happening, please ask me."
  - Check the patient's identity on their wristband.
  - Clinical observations and examination should take place over a minimum period of 5 minutes.
  - From the end of the bed, respectfully inspect the patient. If necessary, make sure the patient looks dignified before continuing with your examination: for example, position their head, clean any obvious secretions, and move their limbs into appropriate and peaceful positions.
  - Gently stimulate the patient and say their name:
    - "Mrs. Williams, Mrs. Williams, can you hear me?"
  - Look for any respiratory effort, carotid pulsation or limb movement.
  - Note the colour and temperature of the skin.
  - Palpate for carotid pulsation for 1 minute.
  - Listen for heart sounds for 1 minute.
  - Listen for breath sounds for 1 minute.
  - Say:
    - "I'm just going to look into your eyes."
  - Respectfully retract the eyelids and inspect the eyes. The pupils should be dilated and unresponsive.
  - Shine a torch into each eye, looking for both a direct response and a consensual response.
  - Test for corneal reflexes by stimulating the cornea with cotton wool and look for a motor response. To ensure that the cornea is stimulated, the cotton wool must touch the area over the iris. Close the eyelids gently after examination.
  - Apply supraorbital pressure and check for a response.
  - Respectfully expose the upper anterior chest wall and palpate for a pacemaker on both sides. This is felt as a firm, subcutaneous object with a clear geometrical shape and an associated linear operation scar.
  - Cover the patient in a dignified manner, leaving the face visible.
  - Check if any relatives present have questions or would like help with anything.
  - Clean your hands.
- Document the examination and verification of death in the notes:
  - Date and time of death:
    - Mrs. Williams died at 01:00h on 4th January 2022.
    - People present when the patient died, or none.
    - No response to stimulation.
    - Pupils unreactive to light and dilated.
    - No corneal reflex.
    - No central pulse palpated for 1 minute.
    - No heart sounds auscultated for 1 minute.
    - No breath sounds auscultated for 1 minute.
  - Write your full name, qualifications, contact number and formal signature.
  - If appropriate, write the cause of death in the notes, indicating that this will need to be discussed with a senior member of the team before a medical certificate of death can be issued.
- If appropriate, make arrangements for the patient's relatives to be informed.
- Thank the nursing staff on the ward.

**19**

## Integrated examination sequence for a patient in the last days of life

- Look at how the patient is breathing. Does their chest sound moist? You do not need to auscultate the chest to identify chest secretions.
- Is the respiratory rate raised (sepsis, metabolic disorders, persistent hypoxia or brain injuries)?
- Is the breathing pattern changing? Irregular breathing, with phases of rapid or deeper breathing followed by periods of apnoea, is called Cheyne–Stokes breathing.
- If secretions are present and clinically assisted hydration or nutrition is being given, consider stopping these to avoid worsening symptoms due to fluid overload and reduced excretion.
- Review monitoring charts and decide when pulse, temperature and blood pressure monitoring can stop. For many people with diabetes, blood glucose monitoring can be stopped along with medications. A once-daily capillary blood glucose test in insulin-dependent patients may be needed, along with a small dose of maintenance, long-acting insulin.
- Skin care: patients are moved for comfort and a special mattress may be used.
- Bladder care: you may need to check for signs of urinary retention (lower abdominal discomfort and bladder dullness on suprapubic percussion).
- Bowel care: the bowels may still open even after a person stops eating, so consider a gentle rectal examination and a suppository if this could be causing discomfort or restlessness.
- Mouth care: check the lips and mouth are clean and being moistened regularly with water and oral gel.
- Check for reduced blinking and drying of the eyes and prescribe a lubricant.
- Ensure that medication for symptom management is prescribed and review it in line with 'as-needed' use and whether the patient appears comfortable.
- If the patient has a subcutaneous infusion of medication for symptom management, check that this is running correctly. If the site is red or swollen, the infusion may need to be re-sited.

## Integrated examination sequence for verifying death

- Review the clinical notes and check that there is a 'Do not attempt cardiopulmonary resuscitation' (DNACPR) form or appropriate documentation.
- Confirm the patient's name on their wristband.
- Clinical observations and examination should take place over a minimum period of 5 minutes.
- Look for any obvious signs of life: spontaneous movement, respiratory effort.
- Look for any obvious signs of death: rigor mortis, pallor mortis – dependent pooling of blood causing distinct paleness, decomposition.
- Approach the person and say their name.
- Gently stimulate the person, such as by gently shaking their shoulder and repeating their name.
- Listen for heart sounds for 1 minute.
- Feel for a central pulse (carotid or femoral) for 1 minute.
- Listen for breath sounds for 1 minute.
- Press firmly over the supraorbital ridge and look for a motor response to stimulation.
- Gently retract the eyelid and shine a bright light into each eye, looking for both direct (constriction of the pupil that the light is being shone into) and indirect pupillary responses (constriction of the opposite pupil to that which the light is being shone into).
- Test for corneal reflexes by stimulating the cornea with cotton wool and look for a motor response. To ensure that the cornea is stimulated, the cotton wool must touch the area over the iris.
- Make sure the person is lying in a dignified position with a cover over their body.
- Document the verification of death in the notes: the person's name, the date and time of death, people present when the patient died (or none) and, if appropriate, primary and secondary causes of death.

# Section 4

## Putting history and examination skills to use

20. Reaching and communicating a diagnosis  415

21. Adapting skills for practice  423

22. Preparing for assessment  427

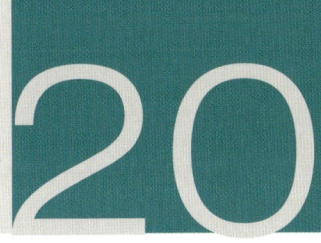

Karen Fairhurst
Anna R Dover
J Alastair Innes

20

# Reaching and communicating a diagnosis

Reaching a diagnosis 416
Pretest probability 416
Rare diseases 416
Multimorbidity 417
Diagnostic error 417

Biopsychosocial model 417

Approach to the patient with medically unexplained symptoms 417

Communicating a diagnosis 418

Shared decision-making 418

Diagnostic and therapeutic uncertainty 419

Documenting your findings 419

Communicating with colleagues 419
Verbal communication 419
Written communication 422

History taking, examination and investigation are the methods by which clinicians gather information to allow them to understand patients' problems. Clinical reasoning is the analytical process by which this information is translated into diagnoses, therapeutic possibilities and prognoses. This chapter addresses how the clinical skills described in this book enable clinicians to reach diagnoses and other clinical decisions and communicate these to patients and colleagues in everyday practice.

# Reaching a diagnosis

Doctors recognise patterns of symptoms and signs, then apply clinical reasoning to interpret them and formulate diagnostic possibilities or probabilities. Sometimes, doctors instantly recognise a condition based on previous experience ('spot diagnoses', p. 38). Visual patterns are particularly likely to lead to such recognition: for example, a typical rash. More commonly, elements of the history and examination together trigger pattern recognition. This process relies on comparing a patient's presentation to cases encountered before and remembered as illness scripts. With increasing experience, less typical presentations are encountered and recalled, and doctors are increasingly able to recognise more exceptional cases.

## Pretest probability

When doctors are unable to recognise patterns in presentations quickly, various refinement strategies are used to arrange the possible diagnoses in order of probability. The pretest probability of a disease is the proportion of people in a population at risk who have the disease. For an individual with a new symptom, the pretest probability of disease depends on the context in which the symptom has appeared because the prevalence of disease varies between populations. In general practice populations, the incidence of serious disease, for example, colorectal cancer, is much lower than in hospital populations, although serious conditions still usually need to be excluded. In practice, the pretest probability of a disease is the clinician's judgment of the likelihood of a particular disease based on the information gathered to date and their understanding of the context in which they work. Clinicians need a mental map of how likely different diseases are and how those probabilities shift as they gather and synthesise information. This may involve identification of 'red flag' or 'alarm' symptoms and signs of serious disease, for example, or the use of clinical prediction rules, such as the Wells score for deep vein thrombosis. Positive 'alarm' features or above-threshold prediction scores increase the probability of a disease in individuals and generally trigger further investigation. Clinicians also rely on understanding the sensitivity, specificity and predictive value of symptoms for the diagnosis of a particular condition in the population with which they work. For example, chest pain is a highly sensitive symptom in the diagnosis of acute coronary syndromes (ACS) as a high proportion of people who have an eventual diagnosis of ACS experience chest pain. However, it is not a specific symptom as many people who do not have an eventual diagnosis of ACS will also have chest pain.

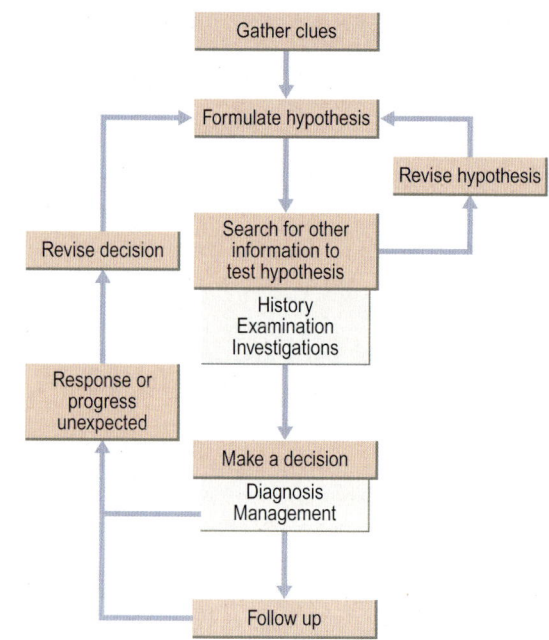

**Fig. 20.1** The hypothetico-deductive method of decision-making.

If the presence of chest pain alone were used to diagnose, ACS would therefore be overdiagnosed. The predictive value of symptoms is more useful in clinical practice than either sensitivity or specificity as it predicts the likelihood that a person with a particular symptom has the associated condition. Like pretest probability, it is affected by the prevalence of the disease in the population. For example, the positive predictive value of rectal bleeding in the diagnosis of colorectal cancer is higher in older populations than in younger ones.

Additional factors affecting the pretest probability of disease in patients with the same presenting symptoms include age, gender, past medical history, family history and lifestyle. Few doctors use formal probabilistic reasoning in making diagnoses, but most know the relationship between these factors and the likelihood of a specific disease and use this understanding intuitively to select likely diagnoses to subject to hypothetico-deductive reasoning (Fig. 20.1). Initial history, examination and investigation results are used to develop a list of possible diagnoses – the hypotheses. Further history, examination and investigation are used to support or refute each of these putative diagnoses until a final diagnosis is determined. Returning to clarify the history or re-examine matters when signs are ambiguous allows an iterative approach and more accurate diagnosis.

## Rare diseases

While diagnosis by probability works in most cases, rare diseases also occur, and to the affected patients and their families, they are not rare. Avoid the trap of thinking that all patients have common conditions, and symptoms that do not fit with common diagnoses are less important. Indeed, occasional patients with a credible and consistent history of unusual symptoms may actually merit more, not less, investigation. The art is to listen carefully, keep an open mind and pick up the uncommon situation when the usual patterns of presentation really do not fit the facts of a case.

## Multimorbidity

The application of clinical skills in diagnosis is complicated when patients have multiple morbidity. New symptoms arise in the context of existing physical and psychological illness and may represent new manifestations or complications of a known condition, of more than one known condition, or of a new disease altogether. Typically, patients with multiple morbidities do not experience their diseases discretely and therefore may report symptoms in an indistinct or incoherent way. Furthermore, their symptoms might interact with each other, and present differently compared to a single disease. Faced with this atypical pattern of symptoms, it is not easy for clinicians to reach distinct diagnoses.

## Diagnostic error

Diagnosis is not easy, and all clinicians, irrespective of expertise, make diagnostic errors. Errors are more common when presentations are atypical or nonspecific, when patients have comorbidities, or when the underlying condition is rare. Most errors occur because of defects in diagnostic thinking, of which the most common error is heuristic-based thinking. Heuristics are cognitive shortcuts used to solve problems; they are quick and reflexive and used to generate an approximate answer to a reasoning question. They are used, for example, in spot diagnosis, pattern recognition and hypothetico-deductive approaches but are prone to produce error by disproportionately diagnosing conditions that are at the forefront of the clinician's mind. This could be due to:

- seeing several recent cases
- missing a diagnosis
- settling on a hypothetical diagnosis without gathering enough information to confirm or refute it
- interpreting new information in a way that supports rather than refutes a hypothetical diagnosis, or
- using stereotyping or profiling in clinical reasoning, for example, deciding that a drug-using patient presenting with back pain is seeking drugs rather than investigating the cause of their pain.

Many strategies have been proposed to debias diagnostic thinking. Metacognition is one such strategy. It promotes awareness and understanding of your own thinking as a way of recognising and minimising unconscious bias or errors. It encourages you to check for conflicting evidence and consider alternatives to the decision you have arrived at. For example, in reaching a diagnosis, it may be helpful to stop and ask yourself:

- 'What else could this be?'
- 'How much is my decision being influenced by the fact I am running late?'

- 'How much is my decision being influenced by the patient I misdiagnosed last week?'

As a reflective process, metacognition can be learnt and practised.

## Biopsychosocial model

Much of this book deals with the association between a patient's history and examination findings and the presence of underlying disease that can be viewed independently from the person who is suffering from it. However, patients often experience symptoms that either cannot be explained wholly by disease or occur in the absence of underlying pathology altogether. Symptoms are, consequently, not synonymous with disease but subjective experiences with many possible sources: pathological, physiological, psychological, cultural, behavioural and external. Therefore, understanding what has caused a patient to be ill often requires the clinician to consider their symptoms within a wider biopsychosocial framework rather than a limited biomedical one.

## Approach to the patient with medically unexplained symptoms

Symptoms that impair function but do not fit characteristic patterns of disease and persist despite normal examination and investigations are often called 'functional', 'medically unexplained symptoms' (MUS, Fig. 20.2) or, more recently, 'persistent physical symptoms'. In this chapter 'medically unexplained symptoms' will be used. Over 30% of patients attending their

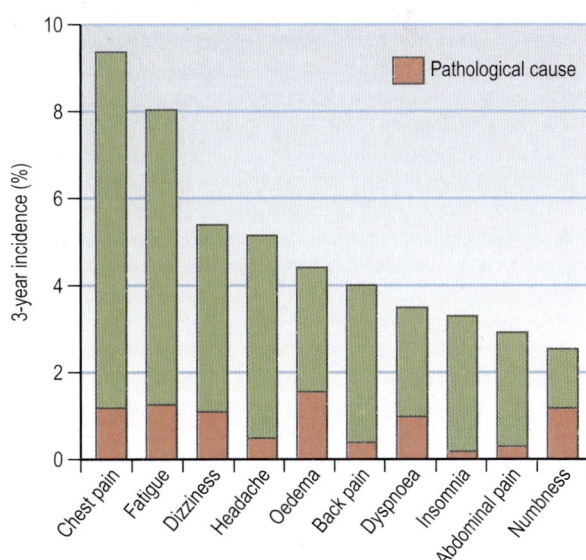

**Fig. 20.2** Percentage of symptoms presenting in primary care with an underlying pathological cause.

20

**20.1 Aetiological factors for medically unexplained symptoms**

- Precipitating: stress, depression, anxiety and sometimes disease and injury, especially if associated with fears of or belief in disease
- Predisposing: fear of disease from previous experience
- Perpetuating: inappropriate attempts to alleviate symptoms (e.g. excessive rest) failure to address patient's concerns

general practitioner have MUS, and they are also common in secondary care, although disease prevalence is much higher there. Some symptoms are more likely to be medically unexplained than others: for example, persistent fatigue, abdominal pain and back pain. The causes of MUS are poorly understood, but various predisposing and precipitating factors (Box 20.1) may contribute. Most functional symptoms are transient, but some become persistent, causing similar disability to those resulting from disease and also significant emotional distress. If MUS are not recognised and managed appropriately, attempts to alleviate them can result in harm from fruitless investigations, inappropriate interventions or drugs, and increased fear of disease.

Patients with MUS commonly feel that clinicians do not think their symptoms are real, leading to a breakdown in trust between patient and clinician and frustration for both. Crucially, clinicians must use an empathic and non-judgemental approach, so the patient feels believed. Keep an open mind and accept all the patient's symptoms at face value. Remember that patients with MUS may also have or develop disease. Even if a functional diagnosis is suspected, a comprehensive history and examination remain imperative. This helps patients to feel that they are being taken seriously; in addition, organic disease, however unlikely, is less likely to be missed.

Patients' illness beliefs matter hugely and should be explicitly acknowledged. What do they think is wrong? Why have they come to you now, and what do they hope you can do for them? Inconsistencies in the history should be explored with the patient; for example, a patient with severe chest pain and normal coronary angiography may still firmly believe they have angina. Normal investigations need to be explained clearly to help demonstrate that the evidence does not support their belief.

Patients may complain about previous clinicians or treatments. Allowing a patient to express dissatisfaction shows interest and helps to avoid suggesting treatments they are likely to reject. Always remain professional and avoid being drawn into criticism of other healthcare providers.

Patients can be acutely sensitive to questions that suggest a clinician thinks there is a psychological basis for their symptoms ('all in the mind'). Frame questions carefully in terms of their symptoms: for example, 'Do your symptoms ever make you feel down or frustrated?' rather than 'Do you ever feel depressed?' Abuse is one possible precipitant of MUS but seek this history judiciously. Follow local guidelines for any abuse you discover.

The physical assessment includes observing the patient throughout the consultation. Watch for inconsistent signs, although this does not indicate whether they are consciously or subconsciously produced. Usually, there are no physical signs, but some non-pathological signs are associated with MUS; for instance, in irritable bowel syndrome, you may find evidence of bloating and some tenderness, but otherwise, gastrointestinal examination will be normal. The history often suggests MUS, so focus on excluding any unexpected physical findings, as well as demonstrating to patients that you are taking them seriously. Any signs you do find may vary between examinations, but overall, the examination is commonly normal with MUS.

Investigations are used in MUS mainly to reassure both clinician and patient. Exhaustive investigations to exclude all physical illness are costly and unhelpful, risk side effects, and do not reassure patients in the longer term. Before requesting investigations, discuss with the patient the likelihood and significance of a normal result. Patients are more likely to be satisfied when your explanation makes sense to them, removes blame and helps to generate ideas about how they can manage their symptoms.

## Communicating a diagnosis

Clinicians routinely inform patients about new diagnoses, and, even if not life threatening, many will be unwelcome to patients. Inappropriate communication, such as an abrupt or harsh disclosure, can be psychologically devastating to the patient. Effectively communicating a diagnosis to a patient requires an understanding of the key medical and informational needs of the patient, and an appreciation of the patient's prior knowledge and beliefs about their health. Ask, 'What do you already know about your illness?', or 'Would you like me to tell you the details of the diagnosis?'' For disclosure of bad news, it is usual to give a 'warning shot' (e.g. 'I'm afraid I have bad news for you'). Information should be given in small chunks and aligned with what the patient knows or believes already. Misconceptions should be corrected. The language used should be free from medical jargon. Patients should be given time to absorb the information given, and clinicians should check their understanding often, clarify any misunderstandings and reinforce important information. Responding empathetically to the patient's emotions at this stage allows the patient to feel heard and provides support if the news is bad.

## Shared decision-making

To share decision-making with the patient about treatment, the clinician requires an understanding of the patient's needs, values, goals and preferences regarding care, including their desired degree of involvement in decision-making. Available options for treatment can then be explored with the patient. Again, information should be given in "chunks" and the patient's understanding of information checked. Choices should be discussed openly with the patient, and the clinician should be clear about the potential harms and benefits of different treatment options. Risk information should be presented numerically whenever possible, using consistent denominators (e.g. 'Of 100 children with otitis media, 84 would be free from pain at 2 to 3 days even without antibiotics, 11 will not be pain-free even with antibiotics, and only 5 will have their pain relieved by receiving antibiotics, so antibiotics only help in about 1 in 20 cases.') For complex information such as this, visual decision aids may present information in a way that the patient can better understand; examples of these can be found at Dr. Chris Cates' EBM website, nntonline.net. Information should be provided in absolute as well as relative terms and attention should be paid to the way information is framed. Equivalent information can be more or less attractive depending on what features are highlighted, and the framing of health information can lead to different decisions and health behaviours. Positive framing (e.g. chance of survival) is more effective than negative framing (e.g. chance of death) in persuading people to take risky treatment options, such as surgery, whereas 'loss' framing (e.g. the potential losses from not having a mammogram) influences screening uptake more than 'gain' framing.

Patients should be encouraged to consider 'what matters most to them', and to determine their preferences for treatment. It is often helpful for patients to consider what would happen if they chose not to take up any of the treatment options. Clinicians should accept that patients may not share their views about the balance of risks, benefits, and side effects of treatments. Many studies demonstrate a correlation between effective clinician-patient communication and improved health outcomes. If patients feel they have been listened to, and understand the problem and proposed treatment plan, they are more likely to follow the plan and less likely to reattend.

## Diagnostic and therapeutic uncertainty

In practice, not all diagnoses are reached with certainty despite diligent application of clinical methods and reasoning to patients' problems. Patient frailty may, for example, make definitive tests too risky. Similarly, treatment choices are not always straightforward even when the diagnosis is clear. For some diseases, there is no clear-cut evidence that one treatment option is superior to others. Sharing uncertainty about diagnosis and treatment with patients is a key component of patient-centred care and goes beyond simple exchange of information. With careful explanation, most patients understand and accept unavoidable uncertainty, but in this situation it is especially important to agree with the patient on the appropriate course of action after full discussion.

## Documenting your findings

Documenting clinical findings in a clear and concise medical record is a crucial aspect of medical practice. It should include a structured account of the history and examination – both positive and important negative findings. Some circumstances demand additional detail: for example, forensic documentation of the length and position of wounds.

The appropriate level of detail varies with the context, but you should adopt and use a consistent format. This format quickly becomes a habit, reduces your need to think about what to record next, and lessens the likelihood of forgetting something important. A consistent format also allows others to locate specific information quickly in your documentation. An example of clear and concise clinical documentation of a case is shown in Fig. 20.3.

## Communicating with colleagues

An essential part of a clinician's work is the accurate and timely sharing of information about patients with colleagues. Communication failures are strong predictors of healthcare-related harm.

Typical situations include:

- referral of a patient from the community to a hospital (Box 20.2)
- request for advice or immediate help
- discharge of a patient back to the community from a hospital (Box 20.3)
- outpatient clinic letter to the general practitioner or referring consultant
- referral of a patient to another consultant
- referral of a patient to other hospital or community services (such as a social work referral or referral to a specialist service, such as palliative care).

### Verbal communication

Verbal communication about a patient needs to be structured and concise to be effective. Be clear about your expectations of the person you are communicating with, especially if you are requesting that they do something, such as coming to review the patient.

SBAR (situation, background, assessment, recommendation) is a simple tool to help standardise communication. It is recommended by the World Health Organization for use as a tool to increase patient safety. It allows staff to share similar expectations about what is to be communicated and how the communication is structured. SBAR can be used face to face, over the telephone or even in some written communication.

#### Using situation, background, assessment, recommendation

First, collect the information you need to pass on, and think through what you want to achieve by the communication, for example, informing a colleague, asking for immediate help or requesting advice. Consider some brief notes under the SBAR headings.

Attract the attention of the person you are communicating with. Introduce yourself. If face to face, make eye contact. If possible, use the person's name: 'Hello, Dr Jones. My name is Dr Smith. I'm one of the junior doctors in the emergency department.'

- **Situation:** give a one- or two-sentence description covering why you are calling, what is happening and what the acute change is.

Date: 02.Oct.21   Time: 17.00

Emergency admission to CCU
Consultant: Dr J G Macgregor

Mary Brown
32 Tartan Crescent
Edinburgh EHx xPX
CHI 1209431111

**History**
**PC:** Chest pain, Breathlessness

**HPC:**
Pain: Severe, band-like, onset while watching TV, has lasted 2 hours despite GTN and aspirin.
Radiates to jaw and inner aspect of L arm. Previous similar pain in past 6/12 only with exertion.
Increased episodes recently, after 200m on flat. GP diagnosed angina 2/12 ago, treated with daily
aspirin and GTN as required

Breathlessness: Began gradually during first hour of pain. Now present at rest, worse if reclining.

**PH:**
Tonsillectomy 1958, Perf. peptic ulcer 1983, COPD diagnosed by GP 2008.  °MI, °DM, °↑BP, °stroke

| **DH:** | Dose | Frequency | Duration |
|---|---|---|---|
| Salbutamol inhaler | 2 puffs | as required | 13 years |
| GTN spray | 1 puff | as required | 2 months |
| Aspirin | 75mg | once daily | 2 months |
| °Known allergies | | | |

**FH:**
Aunt died age 57 of MI, no other significant h/o premature heart disease or other familial diseases.
Nil else of note. NOK: daughter (lives nearby, visits regularly).

**SH:**
Retired cleaner, widowed 3 years, lives alone in ground floor sheltered housing. Smokes 20/day since
age 19. No alcohol. HH once a week for cleaning and shopping.

**SE:**
CVS: see above
RS: Chronic morning cough with white sputum. Chronic mild exertional breathlessness on hills and
stairs
GI: Good appetite, weight steady, bowels regular, °blood in stools
CNS/GUS: Nil of note

1

**Fig. 20.3** Example of initial clerking documentation for an acute admission: *CHI*, Community Health Index (Health Service patient identifier); *HH*, home help; *NOK*, next of kin; *ESM*, ejection systolic murmur; *LLSE*, lower left sternal edge; *PN*, percussion note; *LKKS*, palpable liver, kidneys, spleen; *VR*, vocal resonance.

**O/E:**
Looks pale, anxious, sweaty, with tachypnoea
<u>CVS</u>: P90 regular, BP 150/100, JVP +3cm
HS I+II + 2/6 ESM at LLSE °radiation, no leg oedema
<u>RS</u>: Tachypnoea 22/minute, mild hyperinflation. No palpable LN. Expansion reduced but symmetrical.
PN normal. Scanty fine inspiratory crackles at both bases. VR normal
<u>AS</u>: Old epigastric surgical scar. Abdo soft and non-tender. °LKKS, °masses. PR not done

Scar

<u>CNS</u>: Alert and orientated.
Cranial nerves: Normal except fundoscopy shows mild hypertensive retinopathy (AV nipping)
Limbs – Power, tone sensation normal and symmetrical. Reflexes present and symmetrical.

**Summary:**
Recent onset of pain at rest typical of cardiac ischemia in a patient with a clinical diagnosis of
angina and a background of mild COPD.
Risk factors: 1. Smoking 2. BP and fundoscopy suggest possible underlying hypertension. 3. ESM
suggests possible aortic valve disease – will need echocardiogram to assess
Breathlessness, tachypnoea and basal crackles suggest early pulmonary oedema

**Provisional diagnosis:**
Acute coronary syndrome, possible MI, possible early pulmonary oedema

**Immediate plan:**
Oxygen to maintain saturation >94%
Establish IV access and ECG monitoring
Give pain relief – morphine and metoclopramide
Give oral aspirin 300mg
12 lead ECG: shows diagnostic ST elevation so refer to cardiology for reperfusion therapy
Blood for FBC, U&E and Troponin
Transfer to specialist cardiology unit for further care

Signed: *Dr A P Smith*          Designation: <u>FY1 doctor, Acute Medicine</u>

Print name: <u>Dr. A. P. Smith</u>          Date: <u>2/10/21</u>

2

20

**Fig. 20.3** Con't

## 20.2 Contents of a referral letter

- Demographic details about the patient and the referring doctor practice
- Consultant/receiving practitioner and/or clinic, ward, or specialty
- The urgency of the referral

### Clinical information:

- History of presenting symptoms/examination findings/results of any investigation
- Reason for referral and expected outcome
- Past medical history
- Current and recent medication (including any complementary therapies and self-medication known to the referring doctor)
- Clinical warnings (e.g. allergies, blood-borne viruses)
- Smoking status/alcohol history
- Additional relevant information, e.g.:
  Relevant social or personal circumstances
  Patient/family's understanding of the condition and their expectations
  Information about any advanced directives or resuscitation orders
- Name and contact information of referring clinician.

Similar information will be required when a patient is referred internally to another hospital consultant.

## 20.3 Contents of a patient discharge letter following a hospital admission

Demographic information about the patient, the consultant and the preferred GP (the GP who has been most involved, if known)

- Ward
- Date of discharge/transfer or date of death
- Reason for admission/transfer
- Mode of admission: elective, emergency, or transfer
- Source of admission
- Diagnosis/problem list
- Significant operations/procedures (dates)
- Relevant investigations
- Complications/adverse reactions
- Medication (including start and stop dates, recommendations for altering dose or stopping medication after discharge, use of aids such as a dosette box)

### Discharge plans:

- Further information about destination
- Care package
- Primary care support needed
- Information given to patient/carers
- Results awaited
- Hospital review plan/referral to other hospital services
- Other relevant clinical or personal information
- Contact name and telephone number of author

'I'm concerned about a 53-year-old man who came into the emergency department this morning complaining of severe headache. His headache's getting worse, and he's begun to vomit.'

- **Background:** the information needed to make an assessment.
- **Relevant history:** What were the key events leading up to the present situation?
- **Vital signs:**
  - 'Mr Jackson had a sudden onset of severe headache after waking at about seven this morning. The pain hasn't improved despite painkillers, and he appears to be getting worse. He's hypertensive at 210/110 and vomiting.'
- **Assessment:** what is your assessment of the problem?
  - 'I'm concerned that Mr Jackson may be having an intracranial bleed.'
- **Recommendation/request:** what do you think should be done? What assistance are you asking for? Be clear about what you need and when you need it.
  - 'I'd like you to come and review the patient urgently, please.'

If you are feeling out of your depth and need support from a senior colleague, be clear about that. It is better to endure the brief discomfort of having to admit that you need help than put a patient's well-being in jeopardy.

SBAR can be applied as a standard framework to transfer important information in many situations. By using this method,

you are proactively giving the listener the information that they need to assess the problem. You save time by assimilating and presenting information in a structured way.

## Written communication

Conventionally, information was transferred between doctors by post, but nowadays, much communication is conducted electronically. Whatever the medium, the quality of written communication is crucial. Handwritten forms must be clear and legible. Clinicians should write clear, well-structured referral, discharge or transfer letters (see Boxes 20.2 and 20.3). More and more, these letters are copied to or read by patients as well as other clinicians, so they must always contain appropriate language.

Clinical information is confidential and sensitive. It should never be transmitted by insecure electronic means. Nor should it be stored on or copied to equipment that could be stolen or lost, breaching confidentiality. Encryption should be used wherever possible to protect electronic records, and all clinical information should always be managed in accordance with local information governance regulations.

J Alastair Innes
Karen Fairhurst
Anna R Dover

# Adapting skills for practice

**Adapting to different presentations 424**
Presentation in emergency 424
Presentation with localised illness 424
Presentation with non-specific symptoms 424

**Adapting to different working environments 425**
Assessing patients in the community 425
Remote consultation 425

**Adapting clinical skills over a career 426**

The previous chapters have covered the idealised process of taking a history and examining each system in depth. This chapter considers how this 'toolbox' of skills can be used selectively and adaptively to address the patient's needs in specific circumstances.

# Adapting to different presentations

## Presentation in emergency

Patients presenting with collapse or multiple injury may clearly be unable to engage in the normal systematic process of history taking and examination. The approach to the acutely ill or deteriorating patient is covered in depth in Chapter 18, but this clinical context demands a different approach:

- Triage of airway, breathing and circulation for immediate stabilisation
- Identifying the key elements of the history from a third party (witness, family) – including the patient's normal level of functioning, the time course of the illness, major prior illnesses and any key precipitating events (e.g. medication taken, injury sustained).
- Interleaving further selected elements of examination with critical investigations (e.g. chest x-ray, ultrasound) and resuscitation treatments such as establishing intravenous access and administering fluids and/or emergency drug treatment.

Seamlessly merging these elements of assessment, triage and treatment is a skill which becomes highly developed in Emergency Department clinicians but should be practiced by all, as the sudden need to assist a collapsed or injured patient is something with which any clinician may be faced unexpectedly (see below).

## Presentation with localised illness

Some patients present with a well-defined clinical problem in a specific system, for example, an infected insect bite or a localised bony injury. In this situation, the temptation may be to confine history and examination to the affected incident and area. However, despite the resulting saving of time, this may not serve the patient well. Although a comprehensive history and examination may not be appropriate or even possible in this situation, nevertheless, some broader questioning is nearly always required. For example, an infection may indirectly reveal previously undiagnosed diabetes, so a brief enquiry about recent weight loss, polyuria and polydipsia may be helpful. Similarly, the injured patient should always be asked about the context of the injury in case there are underlying episodes of syncope or seizure, or a background of alcohol excess, which also need to be addressed. Consider also the impact of the illness in the context of the patient's life. For example, a hand injury may directly threaten the livelihood of a manual labourer, sports professional or musician, and may compromise the ability of frail or isolated patients to maintain their self-care.

## Presentation with non-specific symptoms

While many patients volunteer distinctive symptoms suggesting particular disease processes, others offer less specific or more unusual clues and require a more broad-ranging approach. There are a number of possible reasons for this:

- The patient finds it hard to express what they are feeling in terms understandable to the clinician.
- They are actually suffering from more than one ailment at a time (multimorbidity); this is increasingly common in elderly or frail patients.
- Their disease is rare and the symptoms are genuine but unfamiliar to the doctor.
- Their disease process has begun to affect their health insidiously and generally (e.g. chronic poisoning, deficiency states, haematological malignancies or insidious autoimmune diseases such as Addison's disease or pernicious anaemia).

In a further group of patients, a wide range of seemingly unrelated symptoms are reported but no abnormality is found on examination or investigation. These patients are not uncommon, particularly in primary care, and this presentation is covered on page 417 (see Chapter 20).

These are the situations where a structured approach to the integrated general examination (Box 21.1) can be most useful. Students taught in a system-based approach may initially find this difficult, however with practice an integrated examination becomes a quick and efficient tool for excluding serious

| 21.1 One system for performing an integrated physical examination | |
|---|---|
| Greeting and introduction | Clearly identify yourself and establish a rapport |
| Observation of whole patient | Demeanour, gait, ease of movement, speech, eye contact, obesity/cachexia, plethora/pallor, 'spot diagnosis' signs |
| Hands | Pallor, cyanosis, clubbing, wasting, palmar erythema, joint deformity, radial pulse |
| Face | Symmetry, complexion, spot diagnoses (e.g. myotonic dystrophy) |
| Mouth | Central cyanosis, tongue fasciculation or wasting, oropharynx |
| Neck | Lymphadenopathy, goitre, trachea |
| Thorax | Scars, respiratory rate/movements, heart, lungs, breasts, axillae |
| Abdomen | Tenderness/guarding, liver, spleen, kidneys, masses, aorta, hernial orifices, (+ if needed, with consent, genitalia/PR) |
| Lower limbs | Oedema, circulation, mobility, joints, neurology |
| Upper limbs | Mobility, joints, neurology, blood pressure |
| Cranial nerves | Including eye movements, visual fields and fundoscopy |
| Bedside testing | Temperature, pulse, blood pressure, height, weight, urinalysis |

underlying problems or revealing the unexpected (e.g. a painless abdominal mass).

# Adapting to different working environments

Clinicians who have developed their examination and history-taking skills at the bedside may need to adapt how these skills are applied to other situations.

## Assessing patients in the community

Those delivering non-urgent care in the community frequently need to assess patients in their home environment, where constraints of mobility, space, time and privacy can compromise many aspects of conventional examination. It is important here to recognise the limitations of what is possible and to focus on what the patient needs – if they cannot be assessed adequately at home, day hospital attendance or outpatient investigations can be arranged to ensure that the correct diagnosis is reached for the patient.

In remote and rural settings, a local primary care or community healthcare setting may be available, which offers better space, privacy and access to examination equipment and near-patient testing. However, complex illness is equally common in remote settings and it is important for the local clinician to be able to recognise when travel to a hospital for investigations such as imaging or endoscopy is required, despite the inconvenience involved.

The constraints on usual practice are particularly acute for clinicians who find themselves attending to unexpected emergencies outside of their workplace in the community ('Good Samaritan' work), yet important and life-saving assessment and care can still be performed pending the arrival of emergency services. In this situation, the ethical obligation to treat the patient in need is foremost. However clinicians should, where possible, obtain patient consent, keep a written record of events and recognise the limits of their competence while doing their best for the patient until emergency help arrives.

Situations vary widely; common scenarios include accidental injury, cardio-pulmonary resuscitation following cardiac or respiratory arrest, seizures and syncope. Early intervention from a bystander can be crucial. Even the simple act of placing an unconscious patient in the recovery position (having first considered an unstable neck injury) may prevent a devastating aspiration pneumonia. Maintenance of the airway, control of bleeding by pressure and assessment and recording of conscious level (GCS p. 398) are other examples of vital immediate intervention. Collecting basic information about the circumstances and initial clinical observations can be invaluable later to the emergency team. In some societies, the fear of litigation can discourage those offering emergency help, but the needs of the patient should always come first, as courts will generally strive to support the well-intentioned efforts of a trained individual offering first aid in an emergency. Many medical indemnity organisations offer cover for such 'Good Samaritan' work. In some countries, the law specifically protects clinicians who assist patients in emergencies (e.g. the Social Action, Responsibility and Heroism Act (2015) in England).

## Remote consultation

The Covid-19 pandemic has highlighted both the value and the limitations of remote consultation by telephone or video link. Whilst it offers the patient significant benefit in terms of reduced travel time, remote consultation is not appropriate for all situations. Advance consideration of a number of factors should be used to select whether remote consultation is appropriate in particular circumstances (Box 21.2).

### Telephone consultation

Clinical consultations by telephone are particularly challenging for both patients and clinicians because they remove the rich source of information normally available to both from non-verbal cues. This loss is very difficult to mitigate, and the limitations of telephone consultation should be recognised explicitly. First check that the patient is happy to communicate by phone, that the timing is convenient and, if necessary, allow them time to find a private space where they are unlikely to be overheard. Clinicians, on the telephone, should always allow the patient extra time to volunteer concerns, taking care not to dominate the interaction

| 21.2 Factors that determine whether remote consultation may be appropriate | | |
|---|---|---|
| Factor | Favours remote | Favours face to face |
| Patient | Willing/eager for remote contact<br>Mobility problems | Unwilling to engage with remote contact<br>Hearing or speech impairment<br>Language barrier<br>Learning or cognitive difficulty<br>Unable to consent |
| Clinician | Already knows patient<br>Medical records available | New to patient<br>No medical records available |
| Clinical problem | Follow-up of known condition | New problem for diagnosis |
| Patient environment | Private space available<br>Lives far from hospital | No privacy possible |
| Equipment | Telephone, computer or tablet + software available<br>Technically skilled | Lacks computer or mobile device<br>Lacks digital skills |
| Specialty | Relies more on history or results of investigations (e.g. nephrology, gastroenterology) | Relies more on physical examination (e.g. otolaryngology, dermatology, orthopaedics) |

21

with their directed questions. Reflection is also vital, repeating to the patient what you understand to be their symptoms and concerns and seeking confirmation or correction if you have misinterpreted. The telephone should not be used routinely to communicate bad news or sensitive results, as there is limited opportunity to gauge non-verbal reaction or to offer additional support.

## Video consultation

Video consultation adds back some, but not all, of the non-verbal communication at the cost of requiring the patient to have and engage with adequate technology for a successful call. This may limit the applicability of video consultation to vulnerable patients with physical or mental frailty or deprived circumstances, potentially exaggerating health inequalities. Again, it is vital to give the patient time to express their concerns adequately and to cross-check that you have understood these concerns correctly during the video consultation.

## Examination and investigation

Even video consultation clearly removes the capacity to undertake physical examination apart from the purely observational aspects (joint deformity, skin lesions etc.). Simple tests such as observing the patient touching their toes or getting up from a chair and crossing the room ('get up and go test' (p. 387)) may be possible to perform with patience and a cooperative patient but are at the limit of what is reasonably possible for most patients. One possible hybrid solution is for the patient to be accompanied on the remote call by a local clinician who can perform simple tests and examination on behalf of the specialist. However, this approach has not yet been widely validated.

Emailed photographs are used increasingly for dermatological consultations but require an adequate camera and lighting as well as skill and motivation on the part of the patient to provide images of sufficient quality from several angles, including standard objects to reveal scale. To prevent health inequality, it is important to recognise when such efforts fall short and to arrange for conventional face-to-face interaction to ensure good quality care.

Portable devices which allow patients to make remote observations (which, if automatically transmitted to a receiving unit, is referred to as telemetry), can allow useful information to be gathered remotely in specific situations. In particular, home monitoring of blood pressure, blood glucose, oxygen saturation and spirometry is now used widely in specific patient groups. There is emerging evidence that some conditions such as diabetes and chronic heart failure can be monitored remotely with regular home recording of clinical measurements such as weight, blood pressure and blood glucose. However, this practice is relatively new and the risk of missing important findings such as new onset atrial fibrillation or retinopathy remains to be assessed.

## Communicating with patients by message

Asynchronous communication with patients using email or web-based applications has been adopted by some clinicians. These interactions are most commonly administrative but may also include online consultation and online triage of problems for onward referral. However, this is not yet widely seen as a viable alternative to face-to-face consultation or synchronous remote consultation, and concerns remain about the security of confidential information transmitted in this way.

While the convenience of remote consultation is popular with some groups of patients, it remains very important to meet patients directly at regular intervals because even the best quality remote assessments are rarely a complete substitute for conventional face-to-face clinical assessment.

# Adapting clinical skills over a career

The skills described in this book are best regarded as a 'toolbox' which different clinicians will draw on differently as their careers diverge. With increasing clinical expertise, this solid foundation can be adapted for use in many different clinical and community settings. The progressive emergence of remote consultation is one example of how the environment in which medicine is practiced evolves over time and influences the selective use of skills. However, the clinician with a well-stocked and well-maintained toolbox will always be well placed to serve their patients in whatever clinical environment they find themselves.

Anna R Dover
J Alastair Innes
Karen Fairhurst

# 22

# Preparing for assessment

General principles 428

Methods of assessment 428
Clinical simulation 428
OSCEs 428

Marking structures 430

Approach to preparation 430

Approach to assessment 432
Professionalism 432
Managing time 432
Communication during assessment 432
Managing unexpected difficulties 433

Putting it all together 433

# General principles

Clinical assessments are integral to undergraduate and post-graduate medical education and training, and are designed to verify that those involved in the care of patients meet safe clinical standards. Assessments can be formative and/or summative. Formative assessments (such as workplace-based assessments and progress tests) allow you to receive feedback on and monitor your own performance. Assessments such as these can be highly effective adjuncts to learning if they promote reflection on your own performance and recognition of areas for improvement and further development. Summative assessments, on the other hand, are used to evaluate whether you have achieved a required competence or standard of proficiency in terms of knowledge, skills or performance, which may be set by licensing bodies such as the General Medical Council in the UK or postgraduate colleges. Assessments can also be used to provide evidence of safe practice: for example, simulation assessments for doctors in difficulty, or for recruitment and selection into specialty training.

This chapter provides an overview of the spectrum of clinical assessment methods, with a particular emphasis on objective structured clinical examinations (OSCEs) and clinical simulation scenarios. Guidance is offered on how to prepare for formal assessment, including the role of deliberate rehearsal, along with suggestions for optimising your performance in clinical and communication skills assessment.

# Methods of assessment

The most widely used clinical assessment methods include OSCEs, short cases, long cases and clinical simulation scenarios (Box 22.1), during which you may be observed performing an integrated sequence of clinical, practical and/or communication skills.

Different assessment formats test different aspects of your professional competence or expertise. Short cases, for example, will usually focus on testing either your clinical examination skills or your ability to take a history from a patient. Modern assessment methods, such as OSCEs and clinical simulation, allow assessment of knowledge, skills and professional behaviours in an integrated manner and can permit candidates to demonstrate a higher level of performance through 'showing how' and 'doing' (Fig 22.1). Increasingly, assessment of communication skills is being undertaken remotely. In this situation, the focus of the assessment is likely to be on taking a history, or giving explanation and/or advice to a patient or surrogate in a community setting. Make sure that your remote environment is suitable for the assessment, with adequate technology and lighting, and be aware that you may lose some of the non-verbal cues that you might ordinarily rely on during an in-person consultation (see p. 4 for guidance on remote consultations).

Assessments are linked to the learning outcomes of a course or curriculum, and 'blueprinting' is used to ensure that there is appropriate coverage of the required knowledge, skills and behaviours across the examination. To perform well in clinical assessments, it is therefore crucial that you familiarise yourself with both the curriculum and the domains or skills on which you are being assessed. Not all skills will be assessed at each examination (Box 22.2).

Once you have achieved a standard of competence in a clinical skill or domain, you may be considered 'entrustable' in this professional activity. For example, a final-year medical student may be 'entrusted' to perform peripheral cannulation on a patient if they have demonstrated competence in the specified domains (such as obtaining consent from a patient for the procedure and technical competence in the procedure itself).

# Clinical simulation

Clinical simulation, using either high-fidelity patient mannequins or simulated patients, is increasingly employed for teaching and learning in healthcare, as it supports deliberate rehearsal of clinical skills in a realistic setting without compromising patient safety. Experiential learning such as this ('learning by doing') also supports the transition from theory to practice. Clinical simulation is commonly included in both undergraduate and postgraduate assessments to evaluate a candidate's ability to integrate a number of complex skills or domains, which may include clinical examination, practical skills and drug or fluid prescribing. Often the scenario will involve an acutely unwell patient who is experiencing a medical emergency such as life-threatening asthma, where the use of a real patient is not feasible (Box 22.3). The patient mannequin is set up in a realistic clinical environment (such as a simulated ward), with real props and equipment (such as a nebuliser mask), and there is often an additional member of staff in the room (playing the role of the nurse, for example) who can perform tasks and provide results of investigations if requested by the candidate. Sometimes a facilitator may also be the 'voice' of the patient, giving important prompts ('I can't breathe' or simulating an audible wheeze). The candidate instructions will clarify what is expected of you, but it is likely that you will be assessed on your competence in physical assessment, communication skills and the initial management of the patient.

# OSCEs

These are widely used in undergraduate and postgraduate assessments and are commonly designed to assess communication/consultation skills, practical skills, examination skills or an integrated combination of all of these. OSCEs consist of multiple clinical encounters or 'stations' (generally between 6 and 12). Candidates rotate through each station, which will be assigned a fixed duration (usually 8 to 12 minutes).

OSCEs may use a combination of real patients with good clinical signs, simulated patients who often participate in the communication skills stations, simulation mannequins (who may be put in the role of an acutely unwell patient when using a real patient is not feasible or safe) and/or part-task trainers (lifelike models of body parts) for assessment of procedural skills such as venepuncture (Box 22.4).

## 22.1 Clinical assessment formats

| Assessment format | Patient/mannequin | Marking structure | Example |
|---|---|---|---|
| Objective structured clinical examination | Either, in multiple stations testing different domains | Checklist or global judgement | 8-minute OSCE station where the candidate is required to obtain consent from a simulated patient for venepuncture and then perform this procedure on a part-task trainer (often 6–12 stations per OSCE) |
| Short case | Patient | Domain-based marking and/or global judgement | 22-minute station where the candidate is required to examine three patients with evident physical signs (systolic murmur, abdominal mass and abnormal gait) and present the findings |
| Long case | Patient | Domain-based marking and/or global judgement | 60-minute station where the candidate is required to take a full history and examine a patient with chronic liver disease. The candidate is expected to formulate a differential diagnosis and plans for investigation and management (not normally during the case but the candidate presents to the examiner afterwards) |
| Clinical simulation scenario | Mannequin | Often domain-based marking, e.g. behavioural marker system with areas such as communication, leadership, situation awareness, task management | 22-minute station in which the candidate is required to assess and treat a simulated mannequin patient who is having an anaphylactic reaction |

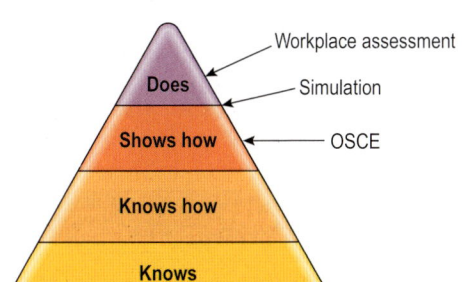

Fig. 22.1 Miller's pyramid of clinical competence and assessment methods. *OSCE,* Objective structured clinical examination. (Adapted from Miller G. The assessment of clinical skills/competence/performance. *Acad Med.* 1990;65[suppl]:S63–S67.)

**22**

## 22.2 Example OSCE blueprint

| OSCE station | Gastroenterology curriculum | Respiratory curriculum | Cardiology curriculum | Procedural skills | Resuscitation skills | Communication skills |
|---|---|---|---|---|---|---|
| 1. Venepuncture | | | | ✔ | | ✔ |
| 2. Cardiovascular examination | | | ✔ | | | |
| 3. History taking | | ✔ | | | | ✔ |
| 4. Abdominal examination | ✔ | | | | | |
| 5. Advanced life support | | ✔ | | | ✔ | |
| 6. Explanation and advice | | ✔ | | | | ✔ |

## 22.3 Clinical simulation station

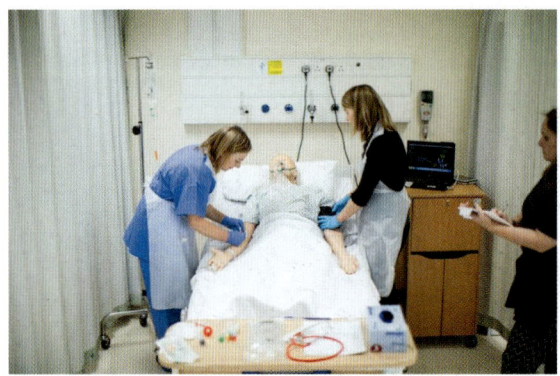

Life-threatening asthma.

You are a junior doctor on the admissions unit. The nurses ask you to see a 25-year-old male patient (the mannequin) with breathlessness whom they are concerned about. There is also a nurse present who can help you with appropriate tasks.

*Typical domain-based mark sheet: life-threatening asthma simulation station*

| | Fail | Borderline | Good | Excellent |
|---|---|---|---|---|
| Structured initial assessment | | | ✓ | |
| Recognition of severity of illness | | | ✓ | |
| Initial management and resuscitation | ✓ | | | |
| Interpretation of results | | ✓ | | |
| Safe and appropriate prescribing | | ✓ | | |
| Escalation of care | | ✓ | | |
| Formulation of an ongoing management plan | | ✓ | | |

### Comments

Good initial A–E assessment + recognition of life-threatening asthma. Did not prescribe oxygen or nebulisers. Failed to ask for a blood gas. Called for help but quite late on. Recognised that patient needs critical care.

## Marking structures

Examiners award marks for your performance in assessments using a standardised marking structure. While this varies from one type of examination to another, some common marking approaches are used, and you should be familiar with these.

Many assessments will employ a 'checklist' format that allows the examiners to award your score objectively. These checklists are commonly used in OSCE stations, where the assessment is broken down into its individual components (e.g. 'Introduces self to patient'), each component is allocated a range of marks, and your score is calculated as the sum of the component marks (see Box 22.4). Often a significant number of marks will be allocated to generic aspects of the encounter (such as hand washing, obtaining consent to proceed, and demonstrating kindness and respect). There may also be some elements of the OSCE that are mandatory to achieve a pass (such as administering oxygen to a simulated patient with acute asthma or addressing the patient's concerns in a communications station). By familiarising yourself with the marking structure for the examination, you can ensure that you tailor your preparation to maximise your chance of success.

Another common examination marking approach is the use of domain-based marking. Marks are awarded as a rating of performance or competence in particular domains or distinct observed behaviours (such as 'Identifying clinical signs' or 'Maintaining patient welfare', see Box 22.3). Where domain-based marking is used, make sure you know what domains are being assessed. Examiners will usually also be asked to make a global judgement of the candidate's performance overall on the station. This is used to determine the pass score for each station. If the assessment has included a simulated or real patient, they may also be asked for their global judgement of your performance.

In the majority of clinical examinations, the purpose of assessment is to distinguish candidates who are competent, and those who are not yet competent for their stage of training. Examiners undergo detailed and specific training before participating in assessments, and they participate in calibration of examination scenarios to establish what performance would be deemed 'not yet competent' in each of the domains.

## Approach to preparation

Make sure that you start to prepare well in advance and familiarise yourself with the format of the assessment: know how many stations there are, how long you have for each station and what domains or skills are being assessed. Most institutions will readily help you understand what standard is expected from a candidate to pass each station, and there may be useful information available online. For example, to achieve a pass in a physical examination OSCE you may be required to perform a systematic examination, correctly identify the physical signs, create a sensible differential diagnosis and suggest an appropriate initial management plan. Remember that assessments are 'blueprinted' (that is, they will be mapped to the learning outcomes from your curriculum; Box 22.2) and you should therefore use the curriculum to guide your learning.

To some extent, the cases you are likely to be presented with in an examination can be predicted. Institutions will typically have a cohort of volunteer patients with common chronic stable diseases (such as pulmonary fibrosis or a renal transplant) or pathognomonic signs (retinitis pigmentosa or acromegaly) who have volunteered to participate. These patients may have helped in examinations before and will be well prepared to cooperate

## 22.4 Venepuncture OSCE station

Assessment of venepuncture using a part-task trainer.

You are a junior doctor on the medical unit and have been asked to check Mrs. Jones's full blood count. Please carry out the procedure on the mannequin while interacting with the actual patient.

**Typical checklist mark sheet**

| Observed skill or behaviour | Potential score | Actual score |
|---|---|---|
| Cleans hands | 0,1 | 1 |
| Introduces self to patient | 0,1,2 | 0 |
| Checks patient details | 0,1,2 | 1 |
| Explains procedure | 0,1,2,3 | 2 |
| Allows patient to ask questions | 0,1 | 1 |
| Gains consent | 0,1,2 | 1 |
| Applies tourniquet to arm and chooses vein | 0,1,2 | 2 |
| Releases tourniquet | 0,1 | 1 |
| Gathers equipment and checks expiry date | 0,1,2,3 | 2 |
| Cleans hands and puts on appropriate PPE | 0,1,2 | 0 |
| Cleans skin and allows to dry | 0,1 | 0 |
| Reapplies tourniquet | 0,1 | 1 |
| Inserts needle at 15 degrees | 0,1 | 1 |
| Attaches blood tubes while holding needle steady | 0,1,2,3,4 | 3 |
| Releases tourniquet and removes blood tube | 0,1,2 | 1 |
| Removes needle and presses on wound with cotton swab | 0,1,2 | 2 |
| Immediately disposes of needle in sharps bin | 0,1 | 1 |
| Labels and packages bloods | 0,1,2,3 | 3 |
| Appropriately disposes of waste and cleans hands | 0,1,2 | 0 |
| Documents in patient notes | 0,1 | 1 |
| Simulated patient global assessment | 0,1,2,3 | 2 |
| **TOTAL MARK (MAXIMUM 40)** | 40 | 26 |

*PPE*, Personal protective equipment.

22

with your physical assessment. Occasionally it is necessary to use a surrogate patient with normal clinical findings; in this situation, you must remember that the purpose of the assessment is to allow you to demonstrate that you can perform a systematic examination. It is unusual to be asked to examine a patient who is acutely unwell, and therefore conditions such as severe asthma or pulmonary oedema will usually be tested only in simulated scenarios. Remember that there are certain rare conditions, many of which are covered in earlier sections of this book that may be over-represented in certain examinations. Where possible, speak to other candidates who have taken the examination in the past, or refer to past papers or revision aids where they are available.

Take every opportunity you can to practise what will be expected of you on the day, informally with peers or more formally in preparatory courses if these are available to you. Many institutions run revision courses or mock examinations, and these can be excellent ways to experience what the examination itself will be like. Daily clinical encounters are always opportunities for practice, as are more formal encounters with senior colleagues such as workplace-based assessments and bedside or simulation-based teaching events. Make sure that you also ask colleagues for honest and critical feedback after clinical encounters so that you can reflect on which areas you can improve.

You may be offered technical and non-technical (such as team working and leadership) skills training in your local clinical skills centre, and these occasions will also allow you to repeatedly practise the techniques that you will be asked to demonstrate during assessments. Deliberate practice, repeating the skills and sequences of examination that you will be expected to execute on the day, helps to make these behaviours automatic and reduces the chances of you forgetting an aspect of history taking or physical examination under pressure.

# Approach to assessment

## Professionalism

Make sure that you are smartly dressed, look professional and adhere to any local infection control and uniform policies. Most institutions would expect you to be bare from the elbows down and to have long hair tied back. Ensure that you have the appropriate clinical equipment with you (such as stethoscope, pen torch and so on) and are familiar with their use. If you are going to have physical contact with a patient during the assessment, always clean your hands with alcohol-based gel or soap and water (Fig. 3.1) and observe basic safety principles, including the use of personal protective equipment and safe sharps disposal.

## Managing time

Managing your time, both in advance of and during the assessment, can have a major impact on your performance. Make sure that you know where the examination is to be held,

rehearse your journey to the venue and give yourself plenty of time to get there. If the examination is remote, make sure that you have the necessary internet browser and version, and where possible, that others are not using your Wi-Fi connection at the same time as your exam.

Pay particular attention to the timings within the examination and ensure that you have practised completing your assessment within the allocated time. Some assessments will be broken into different stages, and it is worth finding out as much as you can about the format; you may think you have 10 minutes to complete the OSCE station but in reality you may be allowed to spend only part of the time with the patient, with the remaining time reserved for questioning from the examiners. Marks will be awarded for your answers to these questions. If you take too long assessing the patient, you may not be able to take advantage of these marks. Assessments will often have short breaks between stations to allow candidates to read the instructions for the next station; once again, it is helpful to familiarise yourself with these aspects of the examination in advance to reduce any uncertainty. However, be reassured that the staff at the assessment will be monitoring the timings of the examination and will lead you smoothly through the stations.

## Communication during assessment

It is vital in any assessment that you communicate with the examiners and patients in a polite and professional manner, as you would in real clinical practice. Always obtain consent from the patient to be examined, be sure not to cause any physical discomfort and thank them at the end of the station. Examiners will be assessing your communication skills and bedside manner, as well as your clinical examination technique.

Listen carefully to the instructions from the examiners, as these are often very specific ('Examine this patient's precordium'). You may also be told whether you should present your findings as you go along or at the end of your examination. Pause for a moment once you have finished your physical examination to consider whether your findings make sense, and ready yourself to present them in an organised and logical manner. When presenting your clinical findings, try to sound confident about them, avoid using language that indicates uncertainty in your own abilities and never report findings that you have not actually elicited. Use a succinct and structured format when presenting, highlighting important positive findings and describing only the relevant negative findings (Box 22.5); listing all negatives wastes valuable time. If there is an obvious abnormality (such as a patient who is jaundiced), it is sensible to mention this early in your case presentation so that examiners see that you have noted the important finding. Do not expect any feedback from your examiners at the end of each station, as they are generally asked to avoid giving you an indication of how you have performed.

In communication stations involving simulated patients, you may be asked to take a focused history, to discuss a specific issue such as consent or to break some difficult news. The simulated patients will have been given a standardised scenario or brief that often includes information that they will volunteer to

## 22.5 Presenting your findings: examination of the cardiovascular system

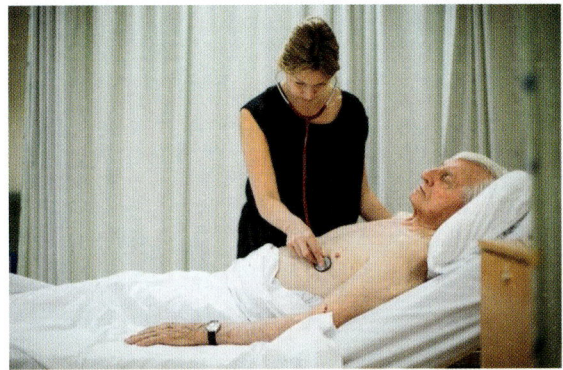

'Mr. Scott is a 65-year-old male. On general inspection, the patient looks comfortable at rest and has a normal respiratory rate. Examination of the hands does not show any abnormality such as splinter haemorrhages. The pulse is regular and is slow rising in character with a rate of 80 beats/min; there is no evidence of a collapsing pulse. The JVP is not elevated; I did not detect any central cyanosis. Examination of the precordium revealed no evidence of scars; the apex beat is palpable in the fifth intercostal space and there are no thrills or heaves. On auscultation, the heart sounds are normal and there is a grade 3/6 ejection systolic murmur, loudest over the aortic area and radiating to the carotids. To conclude my examination, I would like to measure the blood pressure, listen to the lung bases, check for peripheral oedema and assess peripheral pulses. The most likely diagnosis in this patient is that of aortic stenosis'.

you from the outset, and further information that they will divulge only if asked. It is therefore important to ensure that you take a structured approach to your questioning, making sure that you start with open questions and listen carefully to the information the patient is sharing. You should then focus on pertinent

aspects of the history using more direct questioning. It is important to enquire about the patient's own concerns. It can be helpful to summarise the information back to the patient towards the end of the consultation, as this allows you to distill the key points in your own mind and gives the patient an opportunity to add any information that you may have missed.

## Managing unexpected difficulties

Even with thorough preparation, things may not go to plan, because of examination pressure or nerves, or by misunderstanding the format of a station or the question you are asked. Remember that examiners generally want you to succeed and will have experienced similar assessments themselves. They will understand that you may be very nervous and will try to support you if you are finding the experience difficult. If you feel you have performed poorly in a station, try to put it behind you and focus your attention on the next one, where you may be able to recover your position. Remember that in most assessments your final mark will be a composite of all of the components of the assessment, and it is often possible to fail a station or two and still pass overall.

## Putting it all together

Preparing for assessment starts long before the examination itself. Deliberate repeated practice of clinical and communication skills is key to performing well on the day. This should include timed practice within the format itself, as well as practice in presenting your findings to a surrogate examiner. A detailed understanding of the examination format and timing, as well as the marking structure, will help to ensure that you are well prepared.

Take time to review the information provided in the relevant system-based chapters, as well as the more general guidance in Section 1, and watch the clinical videos for examples of comprehensive systematic examination techniques.

Good luck!

**22**

# Index

Page numbers followed by "*f*" indicate figures, and "*b*" indicate boxes.

## A

Abbreviated Mental Test (AMT), 374, 374b
ABCDE approach, 395–399
  airway, 395, 395b, 396f–397f
  breathing, 396–398, 397b
  circulation, 398
  disability, 398–399, 398b
  exposure, 399
Abdomen
  acute. *See* Acute abdomen
  palpation, enlarged organs, 119
Abdominal aortic aneurysm (AAA), 73, 73f
Abdominal distension, 112, 112f
  and bloating, 248
Abdominal examination
  for peripheral arterial disease, 75b–76b
  in babies, 348–349, 348b
  in children, 362–364
Abdominal hernia, 125
Abdominal pain, 73, 108–110, 131b
  associated symptoms, 109–110
  characteristic of, 109
  diagnosing, 109b
  exacerbating and relieving factors in, 110
  in later pregnancy, 258
  non-alimentary causes of, 110b
  onset of, 108
  radiation in, 109
  severity of, 110, 110b
  site of, 108, 108f–109f
  timing of, 110
Abdominal reflexes, 156b–157b
Abdominal scars, in gastrointestinal disorders, 119, 119f
Abdominal swelling, in gastrointestinal disorders, 119
Abducens (VI) nerve, 144
Abnormal beliefs, 370, 370b
Abnormalities, 327
Abscesses, 329b
  Bartholin's, 251f
  peritonsillar, 210f
Abuse, of children, 364, 364b
Accessory (XI) nerve, 148–149, 148f, 149b
Accessory breast tissue, 240f
Accommodation, 182, 182b

Achalasia, 111
Achondroplasia, 40, 40f
Acne neonatorum, 343
Acrocyanosis, in babies, 342
Acromegaly, 227
  physical examination for, 227, 227b, 228f
Active listening, 5
Activities of daily living (ADL), 387
Acute abdomen, 110, 111b
  specific signs in, 120b. *See also specific conditions*
Acute appendicitis, 111b
  abdominal pain and, 110
Acute coronary syndromes (ACS), 419
Acute diarrhoea, 113
Acute kidney injury (AKI), 275–276
  causes of, 275, 275b
  definition of, 275, 275b
  intrinsic, 276
  postrenal, 276
  prerenal, 275
Acute limb ischaemia, 72, 72b
Acute mesenteric ischaemia, 111b
Acute otitis media, 199f
Acute pancreatitis, 111b, 121f
Acute tonsillitis, 210f
Acute vertebral collapse, in abdominal pain, 110b
Adapting skills, for practice, 423–426
  in career, 426
  presentations, 424–425
    in emergency, 424
    with localised illness, 424
    with non-specific symptoms, 424–425, 424b
  working environments, 425–426
    patient assessment in community, 425
    remote consultation, 425–426, 425b
Addison disease, 228–229
  physical examination for, 228–229, 229f
Adherence, 14
Adie's pupil, 182–183
Adrenal gland disorders, 228
  anatomy and physiology in, 228
  common presenting symptoms in, 228–231, 229b
  past history in, 231

Adrenal gland disorders (*Continued*)
  physical examination for, 231
Adrenocorticotrophic hormone (ACTH), 28
Adult breast, 240, 240f
Adult-onset Still disease, 291
Agitation, 369
  clinical vignette for, 375b
Airway, 395, 395b, 396f–397f
  adjuncts, 396f
  inflammation, 87b
  noises, 396b
Albinism, 28
Alcohol, 16
  consumption, in gastrointestinal disorders, 116
Allergy, in respiratory disease, 90, 90b
Allodynia, 134
Altered bowel habit, 112–113
Altered vision, 172f, 173, 174b–175b
Amaurosis fugax, 174b
Amniotic fluid, 256b
Anaemia, 28
Analgesia, 134
Angina pectoris, 45
  functional classification of, 45b
  medication and, 49b
  unstable, 45
Angioedema, 34, 35f, 329b
Angiotensin-converting enzyme inhibitors, side effects of, 293b
Angle-closure glaucoma, 177b
Angor animi, 45
Angular stomatitis, 29, 30f, 213f
Anisocoria, 181, 181b
Ankle, 316–319
  anatomy of, 316–317, 316f–317f
  clonus, 153b–154b
  history of, 317, 317f
  physical examination of, 317–318
    achilles tendon, 318–319, 318f
    feel, 317b–318b
    look, 317b, 318f, 318b
    Morton neuroma, mulder sign for, 319
    move, 317b–318b
    Thomson, 319
Ankyloglossia, 345–346
Annular, 329b
Anorexia
  abdominal pain and, 109–110

Anorexia (*Continued*)
  in gastrointestinal disorders, 106–107
Anorexia nervosa, 112
Anosmia, 142b–144b
Antiepileptics, side effects of, 293b
Aorta, coarctation of, 54, 54f, 347
Aortic dissection, 45, 54
Aortic regurgitation, 66f
Aortic stenosis, 60, 65f
Apex beat, 59–60
Apgar score, 343
Aphthous stomatitis, 214f
Apnoea, 397b
Appearance, of patient, 369
Apraxia, 159, 159b
Arcuate, 329b
Argyll Robertson pupil, 183
Arms, 295b–296b. *See also* Upper limb
Arrhythmias
  extrasystoles, 47–48, 48b
  supraventricular tachycardia, 48, 48b
  syncope and, 49
  ventricular tachycardia, 48, 48b. *See also* Arterial pulses
Arterial pulses, 52–55, 52b
  rate and rhythm, 52–54, 53b
  waveforms, 54f. *See also* Arrhythmias; *individual arteries*
Arthralgia
  cause of, 288, 288b
  clinical vignette of, 289b. *See also* Joint pain
Arthritis
  polyarthritis, 290, 290f
  psoriatic, 292b
  reactive, 292b
  rheumatoid. *See* Rheumatoid arthritis
  septic, 292b
Ascites, 123–124, 123b–124b
  causes of, 125b
Aspirin, drug history, 14b
Assessment, 427–433
  approach to preparation, 430–432
  communication, 432–433, 433b
  general principles, 428
  managing unexpected difficulties, 433
  marking structures, 430, 431b
  methods of, 428, 429f, 429b
    clinical simulation, 428

Assessment (*Continued*)
objective structured clinical examinations, 428, 429b–430b
professionalism, 432
time management, 432
Asterixis, 118
Asthma, 85, 87b
Astrocytes, 134
Asymmetric tonic neck reflex, 350b–351b
Asymptomatic ischaemia, 70–71
Atenolol, drug history, 14b
Athetosis, 153
Atrial fibrillation, 48b, 53f, 53b
JVP and, 57b–58b
Atrial septal defect, 63f
Atrophy, 329b
Attention, impaired, 372–373
Attitude, of doctor, 7
Auditory canal abnormalities, 199f
Auscultation, 60–66, 61f, 61b
in babies, 347f
in gastrointestinal disorders, 124–125, 124b–125b
of kidney, 280b–281b
in respiratory disease, 98–99, 98b
*See also* Heart sounds
Austin Flint murmur, 64–66
Axial spondyloarthritis, 292b
Axillary nodes, 37f, 37b–38b
Axillary vein thrombosis, 80f

**B**
Babies, 341–366
classification of, 342b
developmental attainment of, 353b
examination sequence for, 343b
integrated, 366b
head circumference of, 352f
head shapes in, 344b
history in, 342–343
birth, 342
infant's progress and, 342
maternal, 342
physical examination of, 343–352
general, 343–346
timing and efficacy of, 343
presenting problems and definitions in, 342–343
weighing and measuring of, 352, 352b. *See also* Children; *specific disorders*
Babinski sign, 156b–157b
Bad breath, 106
Balance, in frail elderly, 384
Ballism, 153
Barlow manoeuvre, 351b, 352f
Bartholin's abscess, 251f
Basal cell carcinoma, 334f
Basal ganglia, 151f
lesions of, 150–151
Beau's lines, 27f
Beckwith-Wiedemann syndrome, 345–346
Behaviour
of doctor, 7
of patients, 369b
Beighton scoring system, 296b
Bell palsy, 147
Bell phenomenon, 147
Benign prostatic hyperplasia, 127–128
Bilateral testicular atrophy, 268
Bilirubin, 115. *See also* Jaundice
Bimanual examination, of female reproductive system, 252–253, 252f, 252b, 253f, 253b
Biopsy
endometrial, 253, 255f
skin, 336

Bivalve speculum, 251f
Bleeding, gastrointestinal, 113–115
haematemesis, 113–114
melaena, 114
rectal, 114–115
Rockall and Blatchford score, 114, 114b
Blind spot, 183–184
Blister, 329b
Blood pressure, 55–57
ambulatory monitoring of, 67
in frail elderly, 384b
in renal disease, 279
Korotkoff sounds, 56–57, 56f
measuring, 55, 56f. *See also* Hypertension; Hypotension
Bloody diarrhoea, 113
Blue toes, 73–74
Blunting, 369b
Bone pain, 288
Borborygmi, 112
Bouchard nodes, 294, 295f
Bovine cough, 87
Bowel habit, altered, 112–113. *See also* Constipation; Diarrhoea
Brachial plexus injuries, 350
Brachial pressure index, 76–77, 77b
Brachial pulse, 52b, 53f
Brachycephaly, 344b
Bradycardia, 52–53
Bradypnoea, 397b
Brain, 134. *See also individual regions*
Brainstem, 134
death, 408–409
lesions of, 161–162
Breast disorders
cancer, 242f, 244
cysts, 245f
gynaecomastia, 242, 242b
investigations in, 244, 245f
lump, 241
nipple changes, 241–242, 242f
pain (mastalgia), 241
skin changes, 241, 242f
Breast examination, 240, 242b, 243f, 268b
anatomy and physiology in, 240, 240f
common presenting symptoms in, 241–242
Breath sounds, in auscultation, 98
Breathing, 396–398, 397b
Breathlessness. *See* Dyspnoea (breathlessness)
Bristol stool form scale, 113, 113f
Broca's area, 140
Brown-Séquard syndrome, 161
Brudzinski sign, 139b
Bruising, in frail elderly, 385
Buerger's test, 76, 76b
Bulbar palsy, 140b
Bulimia, 112
Bulla, 329b
Burning retrosternal pain, 89
Burrow, 329b

**C**
CAGE questionnaire, 374b
Callus (callosity), 329b
Cannon waves, 58, 59b
Cardiac catheterisation, 70
Cardiac output, mechanical obstruction, 49
Cardiac tamponade, 55f
Cardiomegaly, 347
Cardiovascular disease
common symptoms of, 44–49, 44b
history for, 44–50
drug, 49
family, 49–50

Cardiovascular disease (*Continued*)
past medical, 49, 50b
social, 50
other symptoms of, 49, 50f
physical examination for, 50–66.
*See also specific disorders*
Cardiovascular examination
in babies, 346–347, 346b
in children, 362
in frail elderly, 386
Cardiovascular system, 43–82, 82b
Carotene, 28
Carotid artery, pressure, 57b
Carotid pulse, 52b, 53f
Carpal tunnel syndrome, features of, 162
Cataract, 174b–175b, 176f
Catastrophic reaction, 369b
Cauda equina syndrome, 300
Cellulitis, orbital, 177b–178b
Central abdominal pain, 109
Central ataxia, 151b
Central cyanosis, of tongue, 95, 95f
Central retinal arterial occlusion, 174b, 175f
Central retinal vein occlusion, 174b, 175f
Cephalhaematoma, 344
Cerebellum, 134
Cerebral infarct, vision and, 174b
Cerebrospinal fluid (CSF), 134
Cervical nodes, 37f, 37b–38b
Cervical smear, 251–252, 252f, 252b
Cervical spine disorders, 297–298
anatomy and physiology in, 297–298
history of, 298
physical examination for, 298, 298f, 298b
feel, 298b
look, 298b–299b
move, 298f, 298b. *See also* Neck
Cervix, 245–246
Chest deformity, in respiratory disease, 92–93, 93f
Chest pain, 45–46, 88–89
acute, 45–46
angina pectoris causing, 45
cardiovascular causes of, 46b
intermittent, 45
Chest wall deformity, in deteriorating patient, 396b–397b
Chest wall pain, 89
Chest X-ray, 67, 69f
Cheyne-Stokes respiration, 93, 397b
Chilaiditi's sign, 122
Children, 341–366
abdominal examination in, 362–364
cardiovascular examination in, 362
developmental attainment of, 353b
growth and development in, 357–359, 358f
neurological, 357–359
history in, 353–357
birth, 356
common presenting symptoms in, 353–356, 354b–355b, 356f
compared with adults, 353
developmental, 356
drug, 356
family and social, 356–357
past medical, 356
systematic enquiry in, 357
vaccination, 356
neglect or abuse of, 364b
neurological examination in, 364
pain in, 353–356, 354b–355b, 356f
physical examination of, 357–364
acutely unwell child, 360, 361b
ears, nose, and throat in, 361–362, 362f

Children (*Continued*)
general, 360, 361f
height in, 360, 361f
lymphadenopathy in, 361–362, 362b
similarities with adults, 359
techniques in, 359–360
preschool, 361–362
protection of, 364
puberty. *See* Puberty
respiratory examination in, 362
school-age, 357
sick, identification of, 363f, 364, 364b
vital signs in, 360, 361b. *See also specific disorders*
Cholestatic jaundice, 115
Cholesteatoma, 199f
Chordee, 349, 350f
Chorea, 153
Chromosomal abnormalities, 39–40.
*See also specific abnormalities*
Chronic cough, 365b–366b
Chronic kidney disease (CKD), 276–277
definition of, 276, 276b
Chronic obstructive pulmonary disease (COPD), 85, 87b
Chronic pain syndrome. *See* Fibromyalgia
Chronic skin excoriation, in children, 356
Chronic venous ulceration, 78–80
Circinate, 329b
Circle of Willis, 137f
Circulation, 398
Circumstantiality, 370b
Clang associations, 369b
Cleft palate, 346
Clinical reasoning, 416
Clinical vignettes, 375b
for confusion, agitation, and hostility, 375b
for fatigue, 376b
for overdose, 375b
for paranoid thoughts, 376b
Clitoris, 245
Clonus, 153b–154b
Coarctation of the aorta, 54, 54f
Coarse crackles, 98–99
Co-codamol, drug history, 14b
Cog wheeling, 154
Cognition, 372–373
in frail elderly, 381–382
Cognitive difficulties, 19
Cognitive impairment, 380
Colicky pain, 109
Collapsing pulse, 52b
Collateral history, 374
Coloboma, 345, 345f
Colour, of hands, 25, 26f
Coma
Glasgow Coma Scale (GCS), 398b, 401. *See also* Consciousness
Comedo, 329b
Common peroneal nerve, 164, 164b
Communication, 418
with colleagues, 419–422
verbal, 419–422, 422b
written, 422, 422b
during assessment, 432–433
in frail elderly, 381–382, 381b
terminally ill patient and, 408–409, 410b–411b
Comorbidities, 381, 383b
Compartment syndrome, 72–73
Compassion, 7
Compulsion, 369b
Computed tomography (CT), 70
Concentration, impaired, 372–373
Concordance, 14
Concrete thinking, 370b

Confabulation, 372
Confidentiality, clinical encounters and, 7
Confusion, 382, 387b–388b
clinical vignette for, 375b
Conjunctiva, 170
Conjunctival pallor, 29, 30f
Conjunctivitis, 177b
allergic, 177b–178b
bacterial, 177b–178b
viral, 177b–178b
Consciousness
assessment of, 139
clouding of, 372
level of, 372
transient loss of, 136
Consent, clinical encounters and, 7
Constipation, 113, 113f
Constructional apraxia, 159
Continuous murmurs, 66
Conventional smear, cervical, 252b
Coordination, motor system and, 158–159, 158b–159b
Cord compression, in abdominal pain, 110b
Cornea
infection of, 177b
reflex of, 144b, 145f, 145b
ulcer/abrasion in, 177b–178b
Corneal arcus, 52, 52f, 386
Corneal disease, 174b
Cortical function, 140–142, 141f
Costochondritis, 89
Cough, 86–87
causes of, 86, 87b
Courvoisier's sign, 123
COVID-19, ophthalmic examination and, 189–192
Crackles, 98–99, 386
Cranial nerves, 142–149, 143f, 143b. See also individual nerves
Cremasteric reflex, 156b–157b
Crust (scab), 329b
CSF. See Cerebrospinal fluid
CT. See Computed tomography
Cultural factors, in managing clinical encounters with patient, 4
Cushing syndrome, 28, 229–231, 230f
physical examination for, 231
Cyanosis, 30–31
in babies, 342
central, 31, 31f
peripheral, 31
Cyst, 329b
Cystocoele, 249

D
Deafness, 381b. See also Hearing loss
Death, 408–409, 411b
brainstem, 408–409
care for others after, 409–412
communication with families, 409, 410b–411b
definition of, 408
history of, 408
medical certification of, 409, 409b
physical examination and, 408–409
Decision-making
capacity, 373
shared, 418–419
Deep vein thrombosis, 80b
Dehydration, in frail elderly, 385b
Delirium, 381b
assessment of, 376b–377b
Delusional beliefs, 371
Delusional perception, 370b
Demeanour, of patients, 5, 25
Dementia, 19, 381b
Dental caries, 214f
Dentition, 209f

Depersonalisation, 371b
Depression, 381, 381b
Derealisation, 371b
Dermatitis herpetiformis, 328
Dermatoscopy, 336, 336f
Dermatoses, 327
Dermis, 326
Dermopathy, 222–224
Deteriorating patient, 393–403
ABCDE approach to, 395–399
airway, 395, 395b, 396f–397f
breathing, 396–398, 397b
circulation, 398
disability, 398–399, 398b
exposure, 398b, 399
early warning scores of, 394
initial assessment of, 395
ongoing management of, 401–403, 402b
sepsis in, 400–401, 401b
point of care ultrasound, 399, 400f
vital signs of, 394
Deterioration, 407, 407f, 407b
Developmental attainment, 353b
Diabetes mellitus, retinal abnormalities in, 186, 188f
Diabetes, 232
anatomy and physiology in, 232, 233b
common presenting symptoms in, 233–234
investigations in, 236b
past medical, drug, family and social history, 234, 234b
physical examination for, 234–238
assessment of newly diagnosed diabetic patient, 234–235, 234b, 235f, 235b
diabetic foot, 235–238, 236b, 237f
hypoglycaemia, 233–234
routine review of diabetic patient, 235, 235b
Diabetic foot, 235–238, 236b, 237f
example of, 238b
risk assessment, 237b
Diabetic ketoacidosis, in abdominal pain, 110b
Diabetic maculopathy, gradual loss of vision and, 174b–175b
Diagnosis, 415–422
approaching patient with medically unexplained symptoms, 417–418, 417f, 418b
biopsychosocial model, 417
communication, 418
with colleagues, 419–422
decision-making, 418–419
documentation, 419, 420f–421f
reaching, 416–417
error, 417
multimorbidity, 417
pretest probability, 416
rare diseases, 416–417
uncertainty, diagnostic and therapeutic, 419
Dialogue, 5, 7
Diarrhoea, 131b, 365b
Diascopy, 336
Diastolic murmurs, 64–66
Digital ischaemia, 73–74
Digital mammography, 245f
Diplopia, 173–176. See also Double vision
Direct inguinal hernia, 125–126
Disability, 398–399, 398b
Discharge, from eye, 176, 179b
Discoid, 329b
Discolouration, 29–31, 30f
Disinhibition, 369b

Dissecting aortic aneurysm, in abdominal pain, 110b
Disturbance of smell, 204
Dix–Hallpike positional test, 201–202, 201f
Dizziness, 48, 138
Doctors, duties of, 6, 7b
Documentation, 419
Dolichocephaly, 344b
Doll's-eye reflex, 184, 184b, 185f
Domestic activities of daily living, 387
Dorsal root, peripheral nerves and, 161, 163f
Dorsalis pedis pulse, 75b, 76f, 76b
Double vision, 173–176, 177b, 179f, 191b
Down syndrome, 39, 40f, 256b
glossoptosis, 345–346
Dressing apraxia, 159
Driving, 384
Drug-induced gastrointestinal conditions, 116b
Drugs
adverse musculoskeletal effects caused by, 293b
allergies, 14–15
history, 14–15, 14b
in respiratory disease, 90, 90b
Dry eyes, 177b–178b
Dry mouth, 106
Dupuytren contracture, 25, 25f
of palmar fascia, 118
Dysaesthesia, 134
Dysarthria, 19, 139–140, 381b
Dysdiadochokinesis, 159
Dysmorphism, in babies, 343
Dysmotility-like dyspepsia, 108
Dyspareunia, 248
Dyspepsia, 108
Dysphagia, 110–111, 211
Dysphasia, 19, 140, 140b, 381b
expressive (motor), 140
global, 140
receptive (sensory), 140
Dysphonia, 140, 211, 211b, 381b
Dyspnoea (breathlessness), 46–47, 85, 85b
causes of, 85, 86f
in later pregnancy, 258
medication and, 49b
paroxysmal nocturnal, 47, 47f
Dystonia, 153
Dysuria, 272–273

E
Ear discharge, 195
Ear disorders
common presenting symptoms in, 195–196
ear discharge, 195
hearing loss, 195–196, 196b
nystagmus, 196, 197b
pain and itching, 195, 195b
tinnitus, 196
vertigo, 196, 197b
drug history and, 196
family history and, 196
investigations in, 202f, 202b, 203
past medical history in, 196
physical examination for, 197–203, 217b
in babies, 346, 346b
in children, 361, 361b
inspection in, 197–198
otoscopy in, 197–198, 198f
palpation in, 197–198
testing hearing, 198–201
testing vestibular function, 201–203
social history, 196

Ear, 193–217
anatomy and physiology of, 194
external ear, 194, 194f
inner ear, 194
middle ear, 194, 194f
Earache, 195b
Easy bruising, 29
Ecchymosis (bruise), 329b
ECG. See Electrocardiography
Echocardiography, 67
Echolalia, 369b
Ectopic beats (extrasystoles), 47–48
Eczema, 328
EEG. See Electroencephalography
Elbow, 306–307
anatomy and physiology of, 306
golfer elbow, 307
physical examination of, 306
feel, 306b
look, 306b
move, 306b
tennis elbow, 307
Elderly, frail. See Frail elderly
Electrocardiography (ECG), 67, 68f
ambulatory, 67
exercise, 67
Electroencephalography (EEG), 165
Electromyography (EMG), 166
Emmetropia, 171, 171f
Empathy, 11
Endocrine disease
adrenals, 228
anatomy and physiology in, 228
common presenting symptoms in, 228–231
past history in, 231
physical examination for, 231
clinical features of, 220b
diabetes, 232
anatomy and physiology in, 232, 233b
common presenting symptoms in, 233–234
investigations in, 236b
past medical, drug, family and social history, 234, 234b
physical examination for, 234–238
gonads, 231
parathyroids, 225
anatomy and physiology in, 225
common presenting symptoms in, 225–226
past medical, drug, family and social history in, 226
physical examination for, 226, 226b
pituitary, 226
thyroid, 220–222
anatomy and physiology in, 220–222, 221f, 222b
common presenting symptoms in, 222
past medical, drug, family and social history of, 222
physical examination for, 222–225
Endocrine system, 219–238
Endometrial biopsy, 253, 255f
End-stage renal disease, 277
Enlarged organs, in gastrointestinal disorders, 121
Enterocoele, 249
Epidermis, 326
Epididymal cyst, 267
Epididymitis, 267
Epilepsy. See Seizure
Episcleritis, 177b–178b
Epistaxis, 204
Epitrochlear nodes, 37f, 37b–38b

Epstein's pearls, 345
Epworth Sleepiness Scale, 90
Erb palsy, 350, 350f
Erectile dysfunction, 264–265
Erosion, 329b
Error, diagnostic, 417
Erythema ab igne, 29, 29f
Erythema multiforme, in children, 354
Erythema toxicum, 343
Erythema, 329b
    tint of, 331
Erythroderma, 329b
Essential tremor, 153
Estimated date of delivery (EDD), 256b
Exanthem, 329b
Excoriation, 329b, 332
Exertional dyspnoea, 46–47
Exomphalos, 348, 348f
Exposure, of deteriorating patient, 398b,
    399
External abdominal hernia, 125
External auditory meatus, exostosis of,
    199f
Extraocular muscles, 170–171, 171f
Extrasystoles, 47–48, 48b
Eye, 170, 170f
    movements of, 170–171, 171f, 184,
        184b
    refractive elements of, 171, 171f
Eye disorders
    coloboma as, 345, 345f
    discharge, 176, 179b
    examination, in babies, 344–345,
        345f
    musculoskeletal conditions and,
        294
Eyelid, 170
    ptosis, 180b–181b

F
Face, examination of
    for heart diseases, 51–52, 51b
    for respiratory disease, 95, 95f, 95b
Facial (VII) nerve, 145–148, 146f–147f,
    147b
Facial expression, 25, 25b
Facial flushing, 30f, 31b
Facial nerve palsy, 350
Facial pain, 204–205
Facial weakness, types of, 147f
Faecal incontinence, 387b
Faecal masses, 127
Fallopian tubes, 246
Falls, 381–382, 387b–388b
Family history, 15, 15f
Fasciculation, 153
Fast alcohol screening test (FAST)
    questionnaire, 375b
Fat intolerance, in dyspepsia, 108
Fatigue, 289b
    clinical vignette for, 376b
Female reproductive system disorders,
    245–246
    anatomy and physiology in, 245–246,
        246f
    common presenting symptoms in,
        247–249
        abnormal vaginal bleeding, 247
        abdominal distension and
            bloating, 248
        lower abdominal pain, 247–248
        prolapse, 248–249, 249f
        urinary incontinence, 248
        vaginal discharge, 248
    drug history in, 249
    family and social history in, 249
    investigations in, 253, 254b, 255f
    physical examination for, 249–253,
        250b
    sexual history in, 249, 249b

Females
    puberty in, 359f
        stages of, 360f
    urinary tract, 273f
Femoral hernia, 126
Femoral nerve stretch test, 301, 302f
Femoral pulses
    examination of, for peripheral arterial
        disease, 75b, 76f, 76b
    in babies, 346f, 347
Femoral triangle, 75f
Fetor hepaticus, 118
Fever, 89
Fibromyalgia, 289, 289b
Fine crackles, 98–99
Finger clubbing, 26–28, 26b, 27f, 51,
    94, 118
Finger jerk, 156b–157b
Fingers
    deformities of, 304f
        rotational, 304f
    flexors and extensors of, testing,
        305f
Finger-to-nose test, 158f, 158b–159b
Fissure, 329b
Fistula test, 202–203
Fitzpatrick scale of skin types, 328b
FLACC scale, 354b
Flashes, 173
Flattening, 369b
Flatulence, 112
Flights of ideas, 370b
Floaters, 173
Fluid thrill, in ascites, 123b–124b, 125f
Focal seizure, 136–137
Foetal movements, reduced, in later
    pregnancy, 258
Fontaine classification, of lower limb
    ischaemia, 70b
Food intolerances, in gastrointestinal
    disorders, 116
Foot drop, 151b
Foot ulcer, 388b
Foreign body, corneal, 177b
Fornices, 245–246
Fracture, 319–320
    pain, 288–290
    history of, 319, 319f
    physical examination of, 319–320
        feel, 317b–318b
        look, 319f, 319b–320b
        move, 317b–318b, 321f
Frail elderly, 379–391, 391b
    assessment of, 380–382
    cognition and mood of, 381–382
    communication difficulties in,
        381–382, 381b
    functional decompensation in, 381f
    history of, 382–384
        drug, 382–383, 383b
        factors influencing, 381–382
        family, 383
        past medical, 382
        presenting symptoms in, 382
        social and functional, 383–384
        systematic enquiry in, 384
    interpretation of findings in, 388–391
    multiprofessional team in, 381b
    physical examination of, 384–388,
        384b
        cardiovascular, 386
        functional assessment in,
            387–388
        gastrointestinal, 386
        general, 385
        musculoskeletal, 386
        neurological, 386
        respiratory, 386
        sequence of, 387b–388b
        systemic, 385–386

Frail elderly (Continued)
    presentation of
        factors influencing, 381–382
        with decreased mobility, 382,
            387b–388b
Freckle, 329b
Frontal lobe, 142
Functional assessment, in frail elderly,
    387–388
Functional gait, 151b
Fundus, 185f
Furuncle, 329b

G
Gait, 25, 296
    increased tone of, 296
    pain, 296
    structural change of, 296
    weakness, 296
Gait abnormalities, 151, 151b, 152f
    antalgic gait, 296
    in frail elderly, 386
Gait apraxia, 151b
Galactorrhoea, 242
Gallbladder, 107b
GALS screen, 296
    initial questions in, 294–296, 295f
Gastrointestinal disorders
    history of
        drug, 116, 116b
        family, 116
        past medical, 116
        social, 116
    investigations in, 128–132, 129b,
        130f–131f
    symptoms of, 106–116
    mouth, 106. See also specific
        disorders
Gastrointestinal examination, 116–128
    abdominal, 118–125
    auscultation in, 124–125
    general, 117–118
    in frail elderly, 386
    inspection in, 118–119
    palpation in, 119–121
    percussion in, 122–124
    proctoscopy in, 128
    rectal, 126–128, 126b
    sequence of, 117f, 117b–119b,
        121b–127b
Gastrointestinal system, 105–132
    anatomy and physiology of, 106,
        106f–107f, 107b
    integrated examination sequence for,
        132b
Gastro-oesophageal reflux disease,
    107
Gastroschisis, 348
General examination. See Physical
    examination
Genital examination. See Reproductive
    system
    Gestation, 256b. See also Pregnancy
Giant cell arteritis, 174b
Gibbus, 297, 297f
Gilbert's syndrome, 115
Glabellar tap, 158b
Glandular fever. See Infectious
    mononucleosis
Glasgow Coma Scale (GCS), 398b, 401
Glaucoma, 174b–175b
    angle-closure, 177b–178b
    haloes and, 173
Glossopharyngeal (IX) nerve, 148, 148f,
    148b
Glossoptosis, 345–346
Glucocorticoids, side effects of, 293b
Goitre, 222
Gonads, 231
'Good Samaritan', 425

GORD. See Gastro-oesophageal reflux
    disease
Gout, 288, 288f, 292b
Gouty tophi, 294, 295f
    in frail elderly, 386
Graphaesthesia, 160b–161b
Grasp reflex, 158b
Grasp response, 350b–351b
Graves disease, 220
Graves hyperthyroidism, 221f, 222b
Groin swellings, 115–116
Grommet in situ, 199f
Growth, in children, 357–359, 358f
Grunting, 396b
Gurgling, 396b
Gynaecological malignancy, 127
Gynaecomastia, 118, 242, 242b
Gyrate, 329b

H
Haemarthrosis, 291f
Haematemesis, 113–114
Haematoma, 198f, 329b
    cephalhaematoma, 344
Haematuria, 274
    non-visible, 274
    principal sources of, 274, 274f
    visible, 274
Haemochromatosis, 28, 29f
Haemodialysis, 277
    fistula, 278, 279f
Haemoptysis, 87–88
Haemorrhoids, 127
Haemosiderin, 29
Hair, 325–337
    anatomy of, 327
    asynchronous cycles of, 327
    signs, 335, 335f–336f
Hair loss, in children, 356
Half-and-half (Lindsay's) nails, 278, 278f
Halitosis, 106
Hallucination, 371b
Haloes, 173
Hand hygiene, 23f
Hand, 302–306
    extra-articular signs of, 303b–306b
    finger clubbing, 51
    history of, 303, 303b
    physical examination of, 303–306,
        304f–305f
        active movement, 303b–306b
        feel, 303b–306b
        for heart diseases, 51, 51b
        look, 303b–306b
        move, 303b–306b
        for respiratory disease, 94, 94f,
            94b, 95f
        swelling, 303b–306b
        T1 root lesion and, 305f
Head impulse test, 202
Head thrust test, 202
Head tremor, isolated, 153
Head
    examination of, in babies, 344, 344b
    shapes of, neonatal, 344b
Headache, 134–136, 136b
    history of, example of, 167b
Hearing loss, 195–196, 196b, 385
Hearing, testing of, 198–201, 203f
Heart block, 59b
Heart failure
    causes of, 46b
    JVP and, 59b
    New York Heart Association
        classification of, 47b
Heart murmurs, 64–66, 64b
    continuous, 66
    diastolic, 64–66
    systolic, 64, 64b
Heart rate, in babies, 346–347, 346b

Heart sounds, 62–64, 62f, 62b, 64b
Heart valves, 44f
  mechanical, 64
Heart, 44
  anatomy and physiology of, 44, 44f
  auscultation of, 60–66, 61f, 61b
  normal resting pressure (mmHg), 44f
  palpation of, 59–60, 60f, 60b
  surface anatomy of, 59f
Heartburn, 107
Heberden's nodes, 294, 295f
Heel-to-shin test, 158b, 159f, 159b
Hemiparesis, 34
Hemiplegic gait, 152
Hepatic encephalopathy, grading of, 123b
Hepatic jaundice, 115
Hepatomegaly, 121, 121f
  causes of, 122b
  palpation for, 346b
Hernias, 116, 125–126, 125f, 125b–126b
  anatomical structure of, 126f
Herpes simplex virus keratitis, 175f
Herpes zoster infection
  in abdominal pain, 110b
  in chest pain, 89
  trigeminal nerve and, 145, 146f
High-volume diarrhoea, 113
Hip, developmental dysplasia of, 351b, 352f
Hirsutism, 231, 335
History taking, 9–19
  in babies, 342–343
  beginning the history, 10–11
  in children, 353–357
  concordance and adherence in, 14
  consultation and, 10–11
  in difficult situation, 17–19
  drug history for, 14–15, 14b
  empathy during, 11
  family history in, 15, 15f
  gathering information during, 10–17
  history of the presenting symptoms, 11–13, 11b–13b
  importance of a clear history in, 10
  of mental illness/learning disability, 368
    general approach to, 368
    sensitive topics in, 368
    uncooperative patient in, 368
  past medical history for, 14
  preparation for, 10
  social history and lifestyle in, 15–17
  systematic enquiry in, 17. See also
    Physical examination
Hoarseness, 215b. See also
  Dysphonia
Hoffmann reflex, 156b–157b
Holmes-Adie syndrome, 182–183
Home environment, 383
Hoover sign, 155, 156f
Horn, 329b
Horner's syndrome, 182
Hostility, clinical vignette for, 375b
Hydration, 33–34
  in frail elderly, 385, 385f, 385b
Hydrocephaly, 344b
Hydrocoele, 266, 349
Hyperaesthesia, 134
Hyperalgesia, 134
Hyperandrogenism, 231
Hypercarotenaemia, 29, 29f
Hyperkeratosis, 329b
Hyperlipidaemia, 52f
Hypermetropia, 171, 171f
Hypermobility, 296
  Beighton scoring system, 296b
Hyperreflexia, 157
Hypertension, 55–56

Hypertension (Continued)
  secondary, 55–56
  white coat, 55
Hypertensive retinopathy, 56, 186–187, 189f
Hypertonia, 154
Hypertrichosis, 335
Hypoaesthesia, 134
Hypochondriasis, 370b
Hypoglossal (XII) nerve, 149, 149f, 149b
Hypoglycaemia, 233–234
Hypogonadism, 231
Hyponatraemia, 388b
Hypopituitarism, 28, 227
  physical examination for, 227, 227b
Hyposmia, 142b–144b
Hypospadias, 349, 350f
Hypotension
  abdominal pain and, 110
  postural, 48
Hypothetico-deductive reasoning, 416, 416f
Hypothyroidism, 220–222
Hypotonia, 154
  in babies, 343
Hysterosalpingogram, 255f

I
Ichthyosis, 329b
Idiopathic cough, 87b
Iliac fossa pain, 248
Illness trajectories, 406, 406f
Illusion, 371b
Immunosuppressants, side effects of, 293b
Incongruity, 369b
Incontinence, in frail elderly, 387b–388b
Indirect inguinal hernia, 126
Infants. See Babies
Infectious mononucleosis, 210, 210f
Infective diarrhoea, 113
Infective endocarditis, 49
Inguinal hernia, 126, 126f, 348
Inguinal nodes, 37, 37b–38b
Insight, 373
Intelligence, 373
Intention tremor, 153
Intermittent claudication, 71, 71b
Interstitial lung diseases, 87b
Intestinal obstruction, 111b
Intracranial lesions, 161–162
Itching
  in ear, 195. See also Pruritus

J
Janeway lesions, 51, 51f
Jaundice, 29, 115, 115f, 115b, 131b–132b
  in babies, 343
  hepatic, 115
  posthepatic/cholestatic, 115
  prehepatic, 115
  urine and stool analysis of, 115b
Jaw jerk, 144b, 145f, 145b
Jendrassik manoeuvre, 156b–157b
Jitteriness, in babies, 343
Joint pain, 288b, 289
  exacerbating factors of, 290
  investigations, 320–323, 320b–321b
  progressive, 289
  radicular, 289b
  referred, 289b
  severity of, 290
Joints
  erythema, 291
  extra-articular symptoms of, 291–292, 292b
  GALS screen, 295–296
  involvement, patterns of, 290
  locking and triggering, 291

Joints (Continued)
  physical examination of, 281, 293–296
  position sense, 160b–161b
  stiffness, 290
  structure of, 288f, 290
  swelling, 290–291, 291f
  warmth, 291
  weakness, 291. See also
    Musculoskeletal disorders.
  See also individual joints
Jugular venous pressure (JVP), 57–58, 57b, 58f, 58b, 95–96, 280
  abnormalities of, 59b
  carotid artery pressure versus, 57b
JVP. See Jugular venous pressure

K
Keratosis, 329b
Kernig sign, 139f, 139b
Kidney, 107b
  anatomy of, 272, 272f
  auscultation of, 280b–281b
  inspection of, 280f, 280b–281b
  nephron, 272f
  palpation of, 280b, 281f, 281b
  percussion of, 280b–281b. See also
    entries under renal
Klinefelter syndrome (47XXY), 40, 231
Klumpke palsy, 350
Knee, 312–316
  anatomy of, 312–313, 314f
  history of, 313
  physical examination of, 314–315
    anterior cruciate ligament, 315–316
    collateral ligament, 315–316, 315f
    feel, 314f, 314b–315b
    look, 314b–315b
    meniscal provocation test, 316
    meniscal tears, tests for, 316
    move, 314b–315b
    patella, 316
Koebner (isomorphic) phenomenon, 329–330, 331f
Koilonychia, 27f
Korotkoff sounds, 56–57, 56f, 57b
Kussmaul respiration, 397b
Kussmaul's sign, 58
Kyphosis, 297, 297f

L
Labia majora, 245
Labia minora, 245
Lability, 369b
Laryngomalacia, 347
Last menstrual period (LMP), 256b
Lateral cutaneous nerve, of thigh, 164, 164b
Left ventricular hypertrophy, 60
Leg pain, 70–73
  Legs, 295b–296b. See also Lower
    limb
Lentigo, 329b
Leuconychia, 27f, 118
Leukoplakia, 214f
Lichen planus, 329–330, 333f
Lichenification, 329b
Lifestyle, 15–17
Light reflex, direct and consensual, 182, 182b
Light touch, 160b–161b
Light swelling, 78
Limbs
  examination of, in babies, 351–352, 351b
  lower. See Lower limb
  upper. See Upper limb

Linea nigra, 256b
Liquid-based cytology, cervical smear
  and, 252f, 252b
Liquor, 256b
Live birth, 256b
Liver, 107b
Liver disease, 117f, 118
  risk factors for, 116
Localised oedema, 34
Locking, 291
Loin pain, renal disease causing, 273–274
Long-standing dysphagia, 111
Loosening of associations, 370b
Lordosis, 297, 297f
Low back pain, 299, 299b
Lower abdominal pain, 108
  female reproductive system and, 247–248
Lower limb, 309–319
  hip, 309–312
    anatomy of, 309, 310f, 311b
    peripheral arterial disease and, 75b–76b
    physical examination of, 311–312
      feel, 307b–309b, 311b–312b
      look, 307b–309b, 311b–312b
      move, 311f, 311b, 312f, 312b
      shortening, 312, 312b, 313f
      trendelenburg sign, 312, 313f. See
        also individual parts
Lower motor neuron, lesions of, 150, 150b
Lower urinary tract, functional
  assessment of, 282b
Low-volume diarrhoea, 113
Lumbar puncture, 165
Lumbar spine, 299–301
  anatomy and physiology of, 299
  physical examination of, 300, 301f
    feel, 300b
    look, 300b
    move, 300b, 301f
    special tests for, 301
Lumbar spine disorders, history of, 299–301
Lumps
  breast, 241
  groin, 34–36, 35f, 36b, 115–116
  neck, 211, 212b, 213f, 216b. See
    also Swelling
Lung cancer, 87b
  in pleuritic pain, 89
Lungs. See Respiratory disease
Lymph nodes, 34–38, 36f, 37b–38b
Lymphadenopathy, in children, 361–362, 362b
Lymphoedema, 34, 34f
  of breast, 241

M
Macroglossia, 345–346
Macular degeneration
  dry age-related, 174b–175b, 176f
  wet age-related, 174b, 175f
Macular purpura, 331
Macule, 329b
Magical thinking, 370b
Magnetic resonance imaging (MRI), 70
Male reproductive system disorders, 262–263
  anatomy and physiology in, 262–263, 262f
  common presenting symptoms in, 263–265
    erectile dysfunction, 264–265
    penile discharge or dysuria, 263
    penile skin lesions, 264, 265f
    scrotal swelling or pain, 244b, 263–264, 264f

Male reproductive system disorders (*Continued*)
  urinary symptoms, 263
  drug history in, 265
  investigations in, 268–269
  past medical history in, 265
  physical examination for, 265–268
    penis, 266, 266b
    prostate, 268, 268b
    skin, 265–266, 265b
    scrotum, 266–268, 266b, 267f
  social history in, 265
Males
  puberty in, 359f
    stages of, 360f
  urinary tract, 273f
Mallory-Weiss syndrome, 113–114
Malnutrition Universal Screening Tool (MUST) score, 385f
Marfan syndrome, 33, 33f
'Mechanical' dysphagia, 111
Mechanical heart valves, 64
Meconium, 348b
Median nerve, 162, 162b
Medical Research Council (MRC) breathlessness scale, 85, 85b
Medically unexplained symptoms, 417f
  approach to patient with, 417–418
  aetiological factors for, 418b
Medication
  angina pectoris and, 49b
  dyspnoea and, 49b
  oedema and, 49b
  palpitation and, 49b
Megalencephaly, 344b
Melaena, 114
Melanin, 28
Melanocytic naevi, 334, 344
Memory, 372
Men. *See* Males
Meningeal irritation, 139, 139f, 139b
Meninges, 134
Meningism, 139
Mental disorder, 369, 372
Mental illness/learning disability, patients with, 367–377
  clinical vignettes for, 374–377, 375b–377b
  collateral history in, 374
  history of, 368
    general approach to, 368
    sensitive topics in, 368
    uncooperative patient in, 368
  integrated examination sequence for, 377b
  physical examination for, 373–374
Mental state examination (MSE), 368–373
  appearance in, 369
  behaviour in, 369b
  capacity in, 373
  cognition in, 372–373
  insight in, 373
  mood in, 369–370, 369b
  perceptions in, 371–372, 371b
  personal, 368b
  psychiatric, 368b
  risk assessment in, 373
  speech in, 369
  thought content in, 370–371, 370b
  thought form in, 370, 370b
Mesenteric ischaemia, 73
Metacognition, 417
Microcephaly, 344b
Microglial cells, 134
Micrognathia, 346
Microtia, 198f
Migraine, vision and, 174b
Milia, 329b, 343

Miller's pyramid, 429f
Mini-Mental State Examination (MMSE), 374
Miscarriage, 256b
Mitral regurgitation, 64, 65f
Mitral stenosis, 62, 64–66, 66f
Mobility, 382, 387, 387b–388b
Mongolian blue spot, 344, 344f
Mood
  in frail elderly, 381–382
  of patient, 369–370, 369b
Morbid thinking, 370b
Moro reflex, 350b–351b
Motor retardation, 369b
  Motor system, 150–159, 150f. *See also* Muscles; Tendon reflexes
Mouth disorders, 208–209
  anatomy and physiology in, 208–209, 208f
  common presenting symptoms in, 209–211
    sore mouth, 209–210, 210b
  drug history in, 212
  investigations in, 214–217, 215b
  past medical history in, 211
  physical examination for, 213–214, 213f–214f
    in babies, 345–346, 345b
  signs, 335, 335f–336f
  social history in, 212. *See also specific disorders*
MRI. *See* Magnetic resonance imaging
Muehrcke's lines, 278, 278f
Multimorbidity, 380, 417, 424
Murmurs, of heart, 346b
Murphy's sign, 123
Muscle bulk, 152–153
Muscle pain, 288, 289b
Muscles
  fasciculation and, 153
  inspection and palpation of, 152–153, 152b
  myoclonic jerks and, 153
  power, 154–155, 154b, 156f
  tendon reflexes
    deep, 155–158, 156f, 156b, 157f, 157b
    primitive, 158, 158b
  tone, 153–154, 153b–154b
  tremor. *See* Tremor
Musculoskeletal chest pain, 89
Musculoskeletal disorders
  extra-articular symptoms of, 291–292, 292b
  general examination of, 293–296
  history of, 288–293
    drug, 292, 293b
    family, 292
    past medical, 292
    social, 293
  look-feel-move in, 293
  physical examination for, 293–296
  presenting symptoms of, 288–292. *See also specific disorders*
Musculoskeletal system, 287–323
  detailed examination of, 296–319
  of frail elderly, 387b–388b
Mutism, 369b
Myalgia. *See* Muscle pain
Mycology, 336
Myocardial infarction, 45, 46b
  in abdominal pain, 110b
Myoclonic jerks, 153
Myopathic gait, 151b
Myopia, 171, 171f
Myotonia, 154

**N**

Naevus, 329b
Nail disorders

Nail disorders (*Continued*)
  history in, 327
  common presenting symptoms in, 327–328
  family and social history in, 328
  past medical and drug history, 328. *See also specific disorders*
Nail-fold infarcts, 294f, 303b–306b
Nails, 26–28, 26b, 27f, 325–337
  investigations in, 336
  physical examination of, 303–306, 328–336
  signs in, 335, 335f–336f
  splinter haemorrhages, 51, 51f
  structure of, 327f
Nasal abnormalities, 205f
Nasal deformity, 205, 205f
Nasal discharge, 204
Nasal obstruction, 204
Nasal pain, 204–205
Nasal polyps, 205f
Nasal septum perforation post-surgery, 205f
National Early Warning Score (NEWS), 394
Nausea and vomiting, 111–112
Neck lump, 211, 212b, 213f, 216b
Neck, 208–209
  anatomy and physiology of, 209, 209f
  common presenting symptoms in, 209–211
    neck lump, 211, 212b, 213f, 216b
  drug history in, 212
  investigations in, 214–217, 215b
  past medical history in, 211
  physical examination in, 214, 214b, 215f
    for peripheral arterial disease, 75b–76b
    for respiratory disease, 95–96, 96f, 96b
    in babies, 346, 346b
  social history in, 212
  stiffness of, 139b
    in children, 364
  swelling of, 346b
Neck swelling, 238b
Necrobiosis lipoidica diabeticorum, 330f
Neglect, of children, 364, 364b
Nelson syndrome, 28
Neologism, 369b
Neonates. *See* Babies
Nephron, 272f
Nephrotic syndrome, 274–275
Nerve conduction studies, 165
Nervous system disorders, 133–168
  anatomy and physiology in, 134, 135f
  cranial nerves, 142–149, 143f, 143b
  examination of, 139–142, 281
  history of, 134–139
    common presenting symptoms, 134–138
    drug history, 138
    family history, 138
    occupational history, 139
    past medical history, 138
    social history, 138–139
  integrated examination sequence for, 168b
  interpretation of findings in, 164–165
  investigations in, 165–168
    initial, 165, 165f–166f
    lumbar puncture, 165
    neurophysiological tests, 166–168
  motor system, 150–159, 150f

Nervous system disorders (*Continued*)
  peripheral nerves, 162–164
  sensory system, 159–162, 163f.
    *See also specific disorders*
Neurocardiogenic syncope, 48–49
Neurofibromatosis, 31, 32f
Neurological dysphagia, 111
Neurological examination
  in babies, 349–351
  in children, 364
  in frail elderly, 386
Neurological symptoms, functional, 138
Neuromuscular dysphagia, 111
Neuron, 134
Neurophysiological tests, 166–168
Newborn child, integrated examination sequence for, 366b
Night pain, 72
Night sweats, 89
Nipple, 240
  changes in, 241–242, 242f
  discharge, 242
  inversion, 242
  Paget's disease of, 242
Nocturia, 274
Nodules, 294, 294f–295f, 329b
Non-pieuritic chest pain, 89
Nonverbal communication, 5
Nose and sinuses, disorders of
  anatomy and physiology in, 203–204, 205f
  common presenting symptoms in, 204–205
    epistaxis, 204
    nasal discharge, 204
    nasal obstruction, 204
    disturbance of smell, 204
    nasal and facial pain, 204–205
    sneezing, 204
    nasal deformity, 205, 205f
  drug history in, 206
  family history in, 206
  investigations in, 207, 207f, 207b
  past medical history in, 205–206
  physical examination for, 206–207, 206f, 217b
    in babies, 345, 345b
    in children, 361–362
  social history in, 206. *See also specific disorders*
Nummular, 329b
Nutrition, in frail elderly, 385
Nystagmus, 184, 196, 197b
  testing for, 201

**O**

Obesity, 32
Objective structured clinical examinations (OSCEs), 428, 429b–430b
Obsessions, 370b
Obstetric history and examination, of reproductive system, 254
  checklist for, 255b
  drug, alcohol and smoking history in, 254
  family history in, 254, 256b
  information of previous pregnancies, 255b
  investigations in, 256, 257b
  occupational history in, 256, 256b
  past medical history in, 254
  social history in, 255–256
Obstructive jaundice, 115
Obstructive sleep apnoea (OSA), 89
Obstructive sleep apnoea/sleep hypopnoea (OSASH), 89
Occipital lobe, 142
Occupational disorder, 16, 17b

Occupational exposure, in respiratory disease, 91
Occupational history, 16
Ocular alignment, 184
Ocular pain, 173, 177b
Oculocephalic reflex, 184, 184b, 185f
Oculomotor (III) nerve, 144
Odours, 32
Odynophagia, 108
Oedema
  cardiac, 49
  medication and, 49b
  peripheral, 280
Oesophageal
  dysmotility, 111
  pain, 45, 46b
  reflux, 87b
Olecranon bursitis, 291f
Olfaction, 204
Olfactory (I) nerve, 142–144, 142b–144b
Oligodactyly, 352
Oligodendrocytes, 134
Oligohydramnios, 256b
Oliguria, 274
Omphalocoele, 348
Onycholysis, 27f, 329b
Ophthalmology, integrated examination sequence for, 192b
Ophthalmoscopy, 181f, 184–186, 185b
  in babies, 345
Optic (II) nerve, 144
Optic disc pallor, differential diagnosis of, 187b
Optic disc swelling, causes of, 186, 186b
Optic neuritis, 174b, 175f, 177b
Optic neuropathy
  anterior ischaemic, 174b
  compressive, 174b–175b, 176f
Oral thrush, 214f
Orbit, 170
  examination of, 180–181, 180b, 181f, 181b
Orientation, 372
Orthopnoea, 47
Osler's nodes, 51, 51f
Osteoarthritic changes, in frail elderly, 386
Osteoarthritis, 294, 295f
Osteogenesis imperfecta, 38–39
Otitis externa, 199f
Otitis media, 199f
  fluid level, 199f
  with effusion, 199f
Ovaries, 246
  pain in, 247–248
  torsion of, 110b
Overdose, clinical vignette for, 375b
Overvalued ideas, 370b, 371

P
Paget's disease, of nipple, 242
Pain
  abdominal. See Abdominal pain
  chest. See Chest pain
  in breast (mastalgia), 241
  in children, 353–356
  in ear, 195, 195b
  in frail elderly, 385, 386b
  in gastrointestinal disorders, 107–110
  loin, renal disease causing, 273–274
  mouth, 107, 107f
  musculoskeletal, 288
    associated symptoms of, 289
    character of, 290
    exacerbating factors of, 290
    onset of, 288
    radiation in, 289

Pain (Continued)
    severity of, 290
    site of, 288
    timing of, 289–290, 289b
  ocular, 173, 177b
Painful hands, 322b
Pallor, 29–30
  conjunctival, 29, 30f
  in babies, 342
Palmar erythema, 118
Palmomental reflex, 158b
Palpable mass, in gastrointestinal disorders, 120–121, 121f
Palpable purpura, 331
Palpation, 59–60, 60f, 60b
  in gastrointestinal disorders
    enlarged organs, 121
    hepatomegaly, 121
    palpable mass, 120–121
    spleen, 122f
  in gastrointestinal disorders, 119–121
    spleen, 123
    tenderness, 119–120
  in respiratory disease, 96–97, 96b, 97f
  of kidney, 280b, 281f, 281b
Palpitation, 47–48
  medication and, 49b
Pancreas, 107b, 232
Pansystolic murmurs, 64
Papilloma, 329b
Papule, 329b
Paradoxical respiration, 397b
Paraesthesia, 134
Paranasal sinuses, 207f
Paranoid thoughts, clinical vignettes for, 376b
Paraphimosis, 265f
Parathyroid disease, 225, 226f
  anatomy and physiology in, 225
  common presenting symptoms in, 225–226
  past medical, drug, family and social history in, 226
  physical examination for, 226, 226b
Parietal lobe, 142
Parity, 256b
Parkinson disease, tremor and, 153
Parkinsonian gait, 151b, 152f
Parosmia, 142b–144b
Parotid duct, 208
  pus in, 213f
Parotid gland, 208
Paroxysmal nocturnal dyspnoea, 47, 47f
Past medical history, 14
Patch testing, 336–337, 337f
Patch, 329b
Patent ductus arteriosus, 347
Patients
  appearance of, 369
  behaviour of, 369b
  clinical encounters with, 3–8
    addressing the problem during, 6
    clinical environment and, 4–5, 4f
    concerns during, 5–6
    concluding, 6
    cultural sensitivity and, 6
    dialogue with, 7
    empathy in, 6
    gathering information during, 5
    opening, 5
    personal responsibilities in, 7–8
    professional responsibilities in, 6–7, 7b
    reasons for, 4, 4b
    sensitive information and third parties in, 5
  uncooperative, 368
  with cognitive difficulties, 19

Patients (Continued)
    with communication difficulties, 17–19
    emotional or angry, 19
    interpreted consultation, 17–19
    with mental illness/learning disability, 367–377
Peau d'orange, of breast, 241, 242f
Pedigree chart, 15f
Pedunculated, 329b
Pelvic inflammatory disease, 110b–111b
Pelvic masses, 248
Pelvic response to back stimulation, 350b–351b
Pelvis, 245, 246f
  pain in, 248b
  ultrasound of, 255f
Penile discharge or dysuria, 263
Penile skin, 262
  lesions, 264, 265f
Penis, 262, 262f
  physical examination of, 266, 266b
Perceptions, 371–372, 371b
Percussion
  in gastrointestinal disorders, 122–124, 122f, 122b–123b
    ascites, 123–124
    splenomegaly, 123
  in respiratory disease, 97–98, 97f, 97b
  of kidney, 280b–281b
Perforated peptic ulcer, with acute peritonitis, 111b
Pericardial constriction, 59b
Pericardial effusion, 59b
Pericardial pain, 45, 46b
Pericardial rub, 64
Perineum, 245
  in babies, 348–349, 348b–349b
Peripheral arterial system, 70
  anatomy and physiology, 70, 70f
  history for
    drug, 74
    family, 74
    past medical, 74
    social, 74
  history for, 70–74
  investigations for, 77, 77b
  physical examination of, 74–77, 75b–76b
Peripheral nerve map, 163f
Peripheral nerves, 134, 162–164
Peripheral oedema, 280
Peripheral venous system, 77, 78f–79f, 79b
  investigations for, 81–82
  past history for, 81b–82b
  physical examination of, 80–81, 80b–81b
Peritoneal dialysis, 277
Peritonsillar abscess, 210, 210f
Perseveration, 370b
Personal responsibilities, of doctor, 7–8
Personality disorder, 374b
Petechiae, 38, 38f, 51, 51f, 329b
Phaeochromocytoma, 56b
Phenothiazine-induced pigmentation, 30f
Phobia, 370b
Physical examination, 21–40
  equipment for, 22b
  initial observations in, 24–25, 24f
  of babies, 343–352
  of children, 357–364
  of frail elderly, 384–388, 384b
  of mental illness/learning disability, 373–374
  preparing for, 22, 22b
  sequence for, 23–24

Physical examination (Continued)
    spot diagnoses, 38–40, 38b, 39f.
    See also specific body systems
Physiological symptoms, in later pregnancy, 258
Physiological tremor, 153
Pierre Robin syndrome, 346
Pigmentation, 329b
Pigmented lesion, 337b
Pinna, 198, 198f
Pipelle, for endometrial biopsy, 255f
Pituitary gland, 226
Pituitary macroadenoma, 227f
Pituitary tumours, 226–227
Pityriasis rosea, 328–329
Place-and-step reflexes, 350b–351b
Plantar response, 156b, 157f, 157b
Plaque, 329b
Pleural rub, 99
Pleurisy, in abdominal pain, 110b
Pleuritic pain, 89
Pneumaturia, 274
Pneumonia, in pleuritic pain, 89
Pneumothorax, in pleuritic pain, 89
Poikiloderma, 329b
Polyarthritis, 290, 290f
Polycythaemia, 30
Polydactyly, 352
Polyhydramnios, 256b
Polypharmacy, 382–383
Polyuria, 274
Pons, lesions of, 147f
Popliteal pulse, examination of, for peripheral arterial disease, 75b, 76f, 76b
Posterior tibial pulse, examination of, for peripheral arterial disease, 75b, 76f, 76b
Posthepatic jaundice, 115
Postural hypotension, 48
  in frail elderly, 384b
Posture, 25
Posturing, 369b
Precordium, 58–66, 60f
Pre-eclampsia, in later pregnancy, 258
Pregnancy, routine antenatal check in, 257
  common presenting symptoms in, 258
    abdominal pain, 258
    breathlessness, 258
    foetal movements, reduced, 258
    physiological symptoms, 258
    pre-eclampsia, 258
    pruritus, 258
    vaginal bleeding, 258
  history in, 257
  investigations in, 257b, 260–261
  physical examination in, 258–260, 258b–260b
Prehepatic jaundice, 115
Preoccupations, 370b
Preschool child, 361–362
  examination of throat in, 361–362, 361b, 362f
Pressure of speech, 369b
Pressure of thought, 369b
Presyncope, 48–49
Primary dysmenorrhoea, 248
Primitive reflexes, 158, 158b, 350–351, 350b, 351f, 351b
Proctoscopy, 128, 128b
Professionalism, 432
Prolactinoma, 227
Prolapse
  assessment of, 250b–251b, 252f
  female reproductive system, 248–249, 249f

Prostate, 262–263
  physical examination of, 268, 268b, 281
Prostatitis, 272–273
Proteinuria, 274–275
  quantification of, 277b
Pruritus, 337b
  in later pregnancy, 258
Pseudobulbar palsy, 144b–145b
Pseudohallucination, 371b
Psoriatic arthritis, 292b
Psychiatric assessment, integrated examination sequence for, 377b
Psychiatric interview, 368
Psychiatric rating scales, 374
Puberty, 359
  stages of, 360f
  timing of, 359f
Puerperium, 256b
Pull test, 152
Pulmonary embolism, JVP and, 59b
Pulmonary embolus, in chest pain, 89
Pulmonary infarcts, in pleuritic pain, 89
Pulmonary regurgitation, 66
Pulse pressure, in renal disease, 279
Pulse rate, in frail elderly, 384b
Pulse. See Arterial pulses
Pulse volume, 54–55
Pulsus alternans, 54
Pulsus bisferiens, 54
Pulsus paradoxus, 54–55
Pupillary pathways, 172, 172f
Pupils, 181–183
  defects of
    Adie's pupil, 182–183
    Argyll Robertson pupil, 183
  examination of, 181–183
Purpura, 329b, 332f
Pustule, 329b
Pyrexia. See Fever

**Q**

Quinolones, side effects of, 293b
Quinsy, 210

**R**

Radial nerve, 164, 164b
Radial pulse, 52b, 53f
Radionuclide studies, 67
Ramsay Hunt syndrome, 147
Ranula, 346
Rare diseases, 416–417
Rash
  distribution of, 328–329, 330f
  morphology of, 329–330, 331f
  pattern of, 329–330
Raynaud phenomenon, 74, 74f, 292
Reactive arthritis, 292b
'Rebound tenderness', 120
Rectal bleeding, 114–115
Rectal examination, 126–128, 127f, 127b
  abnormal stool appearance in, 128b
  indications for, 126b
  position in, 127f
Rectocoele, 249
Red eye, 173, 177b–178b
Reducible hernia, 126
Reflexes. See Tendon reflexes
Reflux-like dyspepsia, 108
Refractive error, gradual loss of vision and, 174b–175b
Relative afferent pupillary defect (RAPD), 182, 182b
Remote consultation, 425–426, 425b
  communication by message, 426
  examination, 426
  investigation, 426
  telephone consultation, 425–426

Remote consultation (*Continued*)
  video consultation, 426
Renal disease
  abdominal examination in, 280–281, 280b–281b
    auscultation, 280b–281b
    inspection, 280f, 280b–281b
    palpation, 280b, 281f, 281b
    percussion, 280b–281b
  anatomy and physiology in, 272
  end-stage, 277
  fluid balance assessment, 279–280
    charts, 280
    chest examination, 280
    general appearance, 279
    weight, 280
  history of, 272–278
    drug, 277
    family, 277–278
    past medical, 277
    social, 278
  integrated examination sequence for, 286b
  interpretation of findings in, 281
  investigations in, 281–286
    blood and urine, 283b
    imaging for, 283b
  OSCE example on, 284b–285b
  physical examination for, 278–281
    dialysis access, 278, 279f
    face, 278
    general appearance, 278–279
    hands, 278, 278f
    skin, 278–279, 279f
  presenting symptoms of, 277
  storage symptoms of, 274
  voiding symptoms of, 274. See also specific disorders
Renal system, 271–286
Renal transplant, 277
Reproductive system disorders, 239–269
  breast, 240
    anatomy and physiology in, 240, 240f
    common presenting symptoms in, 241–242
    investigations in, 244, 245f
    physical examination for, 242–244, 242b, 243f, 268b
  female, 245–246
    anatomy and physiology in, 245–246, 246f
    common presenting symptoms in, 247–249
    drug history in, 249
    family and social history in, 249
    investigations in, 253, 254b, 255f
    physical examination for, 249–253, 250b
    sexual history in, 249, 249b
  male, 262–263
    anatomy and physiology in, 262–263, 262f
    common presenting symptoms in, 263–265
    drug history in, 265
    investigations in, 268–269
    past medical history in, 265
    physical examination for, 265–268
    social history in, 265
  obstetric history and examination, 254
    routine antenatal check in later pregnancy, 257
    common presenting symptoms in, 258
    history in, 257
    investigations in, 257b

Reproductive system disorders (*Continued*)
    physical examination in, 258–260
    investigations in, 260–261
Respiration, haemodynamic effects of, 54b
Respiratory disease
  findings of, interpretation of, 99, 99b
  history, 84–92, 84b, 101b
    drug and allergy, 90, 90b
    family, 90
    occupational, 91, 91b
    past medical, 90, 90b
    social, 91–92
  home circumstances in, 91
  investigations in, 99–103, 100b
  physical examination for, 92–99, 102b
    auscultation in, 98–99, 98b
    inspection in, 92–96, 92f–93f
    sequence of, 93b, 94f, 94b, 95f, 95b, 96f, 96b, 97f, 97b–98b, 103b
  symptoms of, 85–90
  systematic enquiry in, 92. See also specific disorders
Respiratory distress, in babies, 342
Respiratory examination
  in babies, 347, 347b
  in children, 362
  in frail elderly, 386
Respiratory rate
  in babies, 347b
  of deteriorating patient, 396b–397b
Respiratory system, 83–103, 84f
Rest pain, 72
Reticulate, 329b
Retinal detachment, 174b, 175f
Retinitis pigmentosa, 174b–175b, 176f
Retinopathies, 186–188
  hypertensive, 186–187, 189f
Retraction pocket, of pars tensa, 199f
Retrobulbar neuritis, 174b
Rheumatoid arthritis, 292b
Rheumatoid nodules, 294, 294f
Rhinitis, with postnasal drip, 87b
Rhinophyma, 206f
Right acoustic neuroma, 202f
Right shoulder pain, 322b
Rigidity, 154
Rigors, 89
Rinne's test, 200–201, 200f, 200b
Risk assessment, 373
Rockall and Blatchford score, 114, 114b
Romberg's test, 151b
Root compression tests, 301
Root-and-suck responses, 350b–351b
Roth's spot, 51, 51f
Rumination, 370, 370b
Ruptured aortic aneurysm, 111b
Ruptured ectopic pregnancy, 111b

**S**

Sacroiliac joints, 301–302
Sacrum, examination of, in babies, 349, 349b
Salbutamol, 14b
Saliva, 208
Salivary glands, 208, 208f
SBAR (situation, background, assessment, recommendation) tool, 419–422
Scabies, 332, 333f
Scale, 329b
Schober test, 301, 301f
School-age child, 357
Sciatic nerve
  flip test, 301, 302f
  stretch test, 301, 302f

Scleritis, 177b–178b
Scoliosis, 297, 297f
Scratch marks, 332
Scrotum, 262, 262f
  physical examination of, 266–268, 266b, 267f
  swelling or pain, 263–264, 264f, 264b, 269b
  in babies, 349b
Scurvy, 31f
Seborrhoeic dermatitis, 328–329
Seizure, 136–137, 137b
  focal, 136–137
  tonic-clonic, 136–137
Seminal vesicles, 262–263
Sensitive situations, 19
Sensory ataxia, 151b, 152f
Sensory impairment, in frail elderly, 384, 386b
Sensory inattention, 160b–161b
Sensory system, 159–162, 160b–161b
  anatomy of, 159–160, 163f
  peripheral nerve map, 163f
  sensory modalities, 161–162
Sepsis, in deteriorating patient, 400–401, 401b
Septic arthritis, 292b
Serpiginous, 329b
Sexual history, 17
  in female reproductive system, 249, 249b
Shifting dullness, in ascites, 123b, 124f, 124b
'Shooting' pain, 289
Short stature, 33
Shoulder, 307–309
  anatomy and physiology of, 307
  history of, 307, 307b, 308f
  physical examination of, 307–309
    feel, 307b, 308f
    look, 307b, 308f
    move, 307b–308b, 309f, 309b, 310f
Silent airway, 396b
Simmond's test. See Thomson's test
Single testis, 268
Sinus tachycardia, 48b
Sinuses. See Nose and sinuses
'Sister Mary Joseph's nodule', 121
Sjögren's syndrome, 292b
Skin changes, 78–80
  in breast, 241, 242f
Skin dimpling, in breast, 241
Skin disorders
  history in, 327–328
    common presenting symptoms in, 327–328
    family and social history in, 328
    past medical and drug history, 328
  investigations in, 336
  physical examination for, 28–31, 293–296, 328–336
    in cardiovascular disease, 51
    in frail elderly, 385
    in gastrointestinal disorders, 118
Skin turgor, in frail elderly, 384b
Skin, 325–337
  anatomy and physiology of, 326–327
  biopsy of, 336
  Fitzpatrick scale of, 328
  functions of, 327b
  integrated examination sequence for, 337b
  lesions of, morphology of, 332–335, 334f
  structure of, 326f
  supplementary examination techniques for, 336
Skull, fetal, 345f

Sleepiness, 89–90
Sleepiness scores, 90
Sleep-related breathing disorder, 89
Slow-rising pulse, 54
Smell, disturbance of, 204
Smoking, 16, 16b, 91
  cough and, 87
  gastrointestinal disorders and, 116
Sneezing, 204
Snellen chart, 180
Snoring/stertor, 396b
Snout reflex, 158b
Social history, 15–17
  alcohol and, 16
  lifestyle and, 15–17
  occupational history and, 16
  sexual history and, 17
  smoking and, 16, 16b
  travel history and, 16
Social media, clinical encounters and, 7
Soft tissues, physical examination in,
    293–294
Somatic pain, 108
Somatotopic homunculus, 141f
Sore mouth, 209–210, 210b
Sore throat, 210, 210f
Spastic gait, 151b
Spastic hemiparesis, 152f
Spasticity, 154
Speculum, in female reproductive
    system, 249–251, 250b, 251f,
    251b
Speech, abnormalities, 25
Speech
  nervous system and, 139–140, 140b
  of patient, 369
  definitions of, 369b
Spider naevi, 118
Spina bifida occulta, 349
Spinal cord, 134
  lesions of, 161
Spine, 295b–297b, 297–302
  cervical, 297–298
  definitions of, 297–302
  examination of, in babies, 349, 349b
  lumbar, 299
  thoracic, 298–299
Spleen, 107b
Splenomegaly, 122f, 123, 124b
  causes of, 124b
  palpation for, 348b
Splinter haemorrhages, 51, 51f
Spot diagnoses, 38–40, 38b, 39f
Sputum, 87
  colour of, 87, 88f
  consistency of, 87, 88f
  volume of, 87
Squamous cancer, of ear, 198f
Squint, detection of, 184, 184b
Stance, motor system and, 151–152,
    151b
Statins, side effects of, 293b
Stature, 33
Steatorrhoea, 113
Steppage gait, 152f
Stereognosis, 160b–161b
Stethoscope, in auscultation, 98–99
Stiffness, joint, 290
Still birth, 256b
Stomas, in gastrointestinal disorders,
    119, 119f
Stork's beak marks, 343, 344f
Stress, in gastrointestinal disorders, 116
Stria(e), 329b
Striae gravidarum, 256b
Stridor, 88, 210–211, 347, 396b
Stroke, 74, 137–138, 137b
Sturge-Weber syndrome, 344
Subconjunctival haemorrhage,
    177b–178b

Subcutaneous metastases, from lung
    tumours, 94, 94f
Subcutis, 327
Submandibular gland, 208
Suicidal risk, assessment of, 376b
Sun exposure, skin damage from, 328
Superficial pain, sensory system and,
    160b–161b
Superficial venous thrombophlebitis, 80
Superior vena cava obstruction, 95, 95f
  JVP and, 59b
Supraventricular tachycardia, 48, 48b
Swelling
  joint, 290–291, 291f
  neck, 346b
  optic disc, 186, 186b
  scrotal, 348b, 349f, 349b
  wrist, 302–306. See also Lumps
Swollen eyes, 176
Symptoms, medically unexplained. See
    Medically unexplained
    symptoms
Syncope, 48–49, 136
Syndactyly, 352
Systemic inflammatory response
    syndrome (SIRS) criteria,
    402b
Systemic lupus erythematosus, 292b
Systemic sclerosis, 292b, 293, 294f
Systolic murmurs, 64, 64b

**T**

Tachycardia, abdominal pain and,
    110
Tachypnoea, 397b
Talipes calcaneovalgus, 352
Talipes equinovarus, 352
Tall stature, 33
Tamoxifen, in female reproductive
    system, 249
Targetoid, 329b
Teeth
  anatomy and physiology of, 204–205,
    209f
  drug history in, 212
  eruption of, 346
  investigations in, 214–217
  past medical history in, 211
  physical examination of, 214f
  social history in, 212
Telangiectasia, 329b
Telephone consultation, 425–426
Temperature
  in frail elderly, 384f
  sensory system and, 160b–161b
Temporal lobe, 142
Tenderness, in gastrointestinal
    disorders, 119–120, 120f,
    120b, 121f
Tendon reflexes, 349b
  deep, 155–158, 156b–157b
    testing, 157f
  primitive, 158, 158b
Tendon xanthomata, 51, 52f
Terminal hair, 327
Terminally ill patient, 412b
  assessment of, 406–408
  broader context in, 406
  care for, 407
  communication with patients and
    families of, 407–408
  death of, 408–409, 411b
    brainstem, 408–409
    care for others after, 409–412
    communication with families,
      409
    definition of, 408
    history of, 408
    physical examination and,
      408–409

Terminally ill patient (Continued)
    history of, 406
    physiology of, 406, 407f
Testes, 262
  torsion of, 110b
Testicular tumour, 267
Thoracic spine, 298–299
  anatomy and physiology of, 298
  cause of, 298b
  history of, 299
  physical examination of, 299
    feel, 299b
    look, 299b
    move, 299b
Thorax
  anatomy of, 84, 84f
  examination of, in respiratory
    disease, 96
Thought broadcasting, 370b
Thought content, 370–371, 370b
Thought form, of patient, 370, 370b
Thought insertion, 370b
Thought withdrawal, 370b
Throat disorders, 208–209
  anatomy and physiology in, 208
  common presenting symptoms in,
    209–211
    dysphagia, 211
    dysphonia, 211, 211b
    sore throat, 210, 210f
    stridor, 210–211
  drug history in, 212
  investigations in, 214–217, 215b
  past medical history in, 211
  physical examination for, 213–214,
    217b
    in children, 361, 362f
  social history in, 212
Thrombosis, oedema and, 34, 34f
Thyroglossal cyst, 215f
Thyroid acropachy, 221f
Thyroid disorders, 220–222
  anatomy and physiology in, 220–222,
    221f, 222b
  common presenting symptoms in,
    222
    hyperthyroidism, 222
    hypothyroidism, 222
    neck pain, 222
    neck swelling, 222, 238b
  past medical, drug, family and social
    history of, 222
  physical examination for, 222–225
    eyes, 225, 225b
    general, 224f, 224b
    general, 222–224
    thyroid gland, 224–225, 224b–225b.
      See also specific disorders
Thyroid enlargement, 223f
Thyroid eye disease, 177b–178b
Thyrotoxicosis, 220
Tics, 153
Tietze's syndrome, 89
Time management, 432
Timed Get Up and Go test, 387f
Tinnitus, 196
Tissue loss, 72
Tone, motor system and, 153–154,
    153b–154b
Tongue, 31
  ankyloglossia, 345–346
  glossoptosis, 345–346
  macroglossia, 345–346
Tonic-clonic seizure, 136–137
Torsion, of testis/ovary, in abdominal
    pain, 110b
Torus palatinus, 213f
Transient ischaemic attack, 137–138
Transient murmurs, 347
Trauma, red eye and, 177b–178b

Travel history, 16
Tremor, 153
  example of, 167b
Tricuspid regurgitation, JVP and, 59b
Tricuspid stenosis, JVP and, 59b
Trigeminal (V) nerve, 144–145, 144f,
    144b–145b
Triggering, 303b–306b
Trimester, 256b
Trisomy 21. See Down's syndrome
Trochlear (IV) nerve, 144
Trousseau sign, 226f
Tubal pregnancy, in abdominal pain,
    110b
Tuning fork tests, 200–201, 201b
Turbinate hypertrophy, 205f
Turner syndrome (45XO), 39, 40f
Tympanic membrane abnormalities,
    199f
Tympanosclerosis, 198

**U**

Ulcer, 329b
Ulcer-like dyspepsia, 108
Ulnar nerve, 164, 164b
Umbilical hernia, 348
Umbilication, 329b
Uncertainty, diagnostic and therapeutic,
    419
Uncooperative patient, 368
Undernutrition, 385
Unterberger's test, 202
Upper limb, 302–309
  peripheral arterial disease and,
    75b–76b
  respiratory disease and, 94, 94f, 94b.
    See also specific parts
Upper motor neuron, lesions of, 150,
    150b
Uraemia, 277
Uraemic fetor, 32
Urinalysis, 281–282, 282b
Urinary incontinence, 248, 250b, 387b
Urinary symptoms, of male reproductive
    system, 263
Urinary tract
  lower, functional assessment of,
    282b
  male, 273f
  female, 273f. See also individual parts
Urine dipstick test, 282, 282b
Urine
  blood. See Haematuria
  investigations, 283b
  jaundice and, 115b
  protein. See Proteinuria
  test. See Urinalysis
Urological disease, investigations of
  blood and urine, 283b
  imaging for, 283b
Urticaria pigmentosa, 332
Urticaria, 328
Uterine examination, in later pregnancy,
    258b, 259f–260f, 260b, 261f
Uterus, 246
  external prolapse of, 249f
Uveitis, 177b
  acute anterior, 177b–178b

**V**

Vagina, 245–246
  bleeding
    abnormal, 247, 250b
    in later pregnancy, 258
  discharge in, 248, 250b
  Vaginal wall prolapse, 249f
Vagus (X) nerve, 148, 148f, 148b
Varicocoele, 266
Vasculitic rash, 278–279, 279f
Vasculitis, 331, 332f

Veins, examination, in gastrointestinal disorders, 118
Vellus hair, 327
Ventral suspension, 350b–351b
Ventricular tachycardia, 48, 48b
Verbal communication, 419–422, 422b
  SBAR (situation, background, assessment, recommendation) tool, 419–422
Verrucous, 329b
Vertigo, 138, 196, 197b
Vesicle, 329b
Vestibular function, testing of, 201–203
Vestibulocochlear (VIII) nerve, 148
Vibration, sensory system and, 160b–161b
Video consultation, 426
Visceral abdominal pain, 108
Vision, examination of, in frail elderly, 385
Visual acuity, 180, 180b
  in frail elderly, 385
Visual fields, 183–184, 183f, 183b–184b
  defects, 172f
Visual loss, example of, 191b
Visual pathway, 172, 172f
Visual system, 169192
  anatomy and physiology of, 170–172, 170f

Visual system (Continued)
    extraocular muscles, 170–171, 171f
    eye, 170, 170f
    pupillary pathways, 172, 172f
    refractive elements of eye, 171, 171f
    visual pathway, 172, 172f
  history, 173–179
    common presenting symptoms, 173–176
    drug and allergy history, 178
    family history, 178–179
    past medical history, 178
    past ocular history, 178
    social history, 179
  investigations for, 188, 190b
  COVID-19 and, 189–192
  physical examination of, 179–188
    general examination, 179
    ocular alignment and eye movements, 184
    ophthalmoscopy, 184–186
    orbit and periorbital examination, 180–181, 180b, 181f, 181b
    pupils, 181–183
    retinopathies, 186–188, 188f–189f
    visual acuity, 180

Visual system (Continued)
    visual fields, 183–184, 183f. See also Eye disorders. See also specific parts
Vital signs
  in children, 360, 361b
  of deteriorating patient, 394
Vitiligo, 28, 28f
Vitreous haemorrhage, 174b
Vocal resonance, 99
Vomiting. See Nausea and vomiting
Vulva, 245
  inspection of, 251f

W
Weakness
  facial, 147f
  gait, 296
  joint, 296
Weber's test, 200, 200f, 200b
Weight gain. See Obesity
Weight loss, 32
  in gastrointestinal disorders, 106–107
  in respiratory diseases, 89
Weight, 32, 32b
Wells score, for deep vein thrombosis, 416
Wernicke area, 140

Wheal, 329b
Wheeze, 85–86, 98, 396b
  polyphonic, in children, 362
Whispered voice test, 198
'Whispering pectoriloquy', 99
'Whistling' sounds, in wheeze, 85
'White coat hypertension', 55
Whispered voice test, 198
Wind, 112
Women. See Females
Wood's lamp, 336
Word salad, 370b
Wrist, 302–306
  assessing, 295f
  extra-articular signs of, 303b–306b
  history of, 303, 303b
  physical examination of, 303–306
    active movement, 303b–306b
    feel, 303b–306b
    look, 303b–306b
    move, 303b–306b
Written communication, 422, 422b

X
Xanthelasma, 52, 52f
Xerosis, 329b

Y
Yellow nail syndrome, 94
Young person, 353